Caring in Nursing Classics

Marlaine C. Smith, PhD, RN, AHN-BC, FAAN, is dean and Helen K. Persson Eminent Scholar in the Christine Lynn College of Nursing at Florida Atlantic University (FAU). From 1988 to 2006 she was on the faculty of the University of Colorado Health Sciences Center, School of Nursing, serving as associate dean for Academic Affairs and the director of the Center for Integrative Caring Practice for 6 years. She has been a nurse educator since 1976 with other faculty appointments at Duquesne University, the Pennsylvania State University, and LaRoche College in Pittsburgh. Dr. Smith's research has focused on outcomes of touch therapies as an expression of caring. She has written a variety of theoretical, philosophical, research, practice, and review articles related to caring. Her most recent work has been the development of a middle range theory of unitary caring. With Marilyn Parker she co-edited the third edition of *Nursing Theories and Nursing Practice*. Dr. Smith completed her BS in nursing at Duquesne University, her MPH and MNEd in oncology nursing and nursing education at the University of Pittsburgh's Graduate School of Public Health and School of Nursing, and her PhD in Nursing at New York University.

Marian C. Turkel, PhD, RN, NEA-BC, FAAN, is the director of Professional Nursing Practice and Research at Einstein Health care Network (EHN) and faculty associate of the Watson Caring Science Institute (WCSI). In her role at EHN she is responsible for advancing Watson's Theory of Human Caring, integrating research and evidence-based practice initiatives, and creating a professional practice environment. Under her leadership and guidance, EHN received designation in 2010 as a WCSI affiliate. As part of the faculty of WCSI, Dr. Turkel works with various hospitals on the practical application of the theory and does presentations on caring science with an emphasis on education, leadership, practice, and research. Her commitment to advancing caring science and valuing caring being the essence of nursing practice and a substantive area of study within the discipline started in 1989 when she returned to school for a master's in Nursing Administration at Florida Atlantic University (FAU). After graduation, Dr. Turkel enrolled in the University of Miami's PhD program and in 1997 she returned to FAU as an assistant professor and taught undergraduate and graduate theory, research, and leadership courses. In 2002, she relocated to Chicago and began consulting with various hospitals on developing practice innovations related to Magnet, creating research initiatives, implementing Watson's Theory of Human Caring into the practice setting, and working with leaders to understand the core value of caring in nursing practice. Over the course of her career she has worked in collaboration with Dr. Marilyn Ray and was the co-principal investigator on almost $1 million in federal research funding to study the relationship among caring, economics, and patient outcomes. Dr. Turkel authored a textbook on strategies for obtaining Magnet Program Recognition®, published in peer-reviewed journals, contributed chapters in nursing textbooks, and presented at numerous national and international conferences. She has been actively involved with the International Association for Human Caring for approximately 20 years and assumed the role of president in June 2012. *Nursing Caring and Complexity Science for Human Environment Well Being* that she co-edited with the late Dr. Alice Davidson and Dr. Marilyn Ray received the *American Journal of Nursing* Book of the Year Award (2011).

Zane Robinson Wolf, PhD, RN, FAAN, is dean emerita and professor, School of Nursing and Health Sciences at La Salle University. She returned to full-time teaching in the fall of 2012. She practiced as a critical care and medical surgical nurse and has worked in nursing education, teaching in diploma, associate, baccalaureate, master's, and doctoral nursing programs. She teaches courses on patient safety, nursing research, evidence-based practice, and caring and continues to conduct qualitative and quantitative research on medication errors, nurse caring, nursing education concerns, and other topics. Dr. Wolf is a board member of the Institute for Safe Medication Practices and she is a member of the Patient Safety Committee of St. Christopher's Hospital for Children. She reviews manuscripts for various nursing and health care journals. Dr. Wolf has been an editor of the *International Journal for Human Caring* since 1999. She is a former board member and past president of the International Association for Human Caring and has hosted three International Caring Conferences in Philadelphia. The Christine E. Lynn College of Nursing at Florida Atlantic University honored her by designating her as caring scholar.

Caring in Nursing Classics
An Essential Resource

MARLAINE C. SMITH, PhD, RN, AHN-BC, FAAN

MARIAN C. TURKEL, PhD, RN, NEA-BC, FAAN

ZANE ROBINSON WOLF, PhD, RN, FAAN

Editors

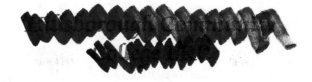

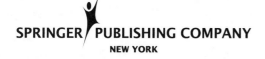
SPRINGER PUBLISHING COMPANY
NEW YORK

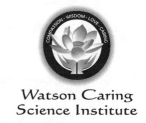
Watson Caring
Science Institute

Springer Publishing Company, LLC
11 West 42nd Street
New York, NY 10036
www.springerpub.com

Acquisitions Editor: Allan Graubard
Composition: diacriTech

ISBN: 978-0-8261-7111-5
E-book ISBN: 978-0-8261-7112-2

PowerPoint presentation ISBN: 978-0-8261-7108-5
Essential Resource Guide ISBN: 978-0-8261-7109-2

Qualified Instructors may request these supplements by emailing textbook@springerpub.com

13 14 15/ 5 4 3 2

The author and the publisher of this Work have made every effort to use sources believed to be reliable to provide information that is accurate and compatible with the standards generally accepted at the time of publication. Because medical science is continually advancing, our knowledge base continues to expand. Therefore, as new information becomes available, changes in procedures become necessary. We recommend that the reader always consult current research and specific institutional policies before performing any clinical procedure. The author and publisher shall not be liable for any special, consequential, or exemplary damages resulting, in whole or in part, from the readers' use of, or reliance on, the information contained in this book. The publisher has no responsibility for the persistence or accuracy of URLs for external or third-party Internet websites referred to in this publication and does not guarantee that any content on such websites is, or will remain, accurate or appropriate.

Library of Congress Cataloging-in-Publication Data

Caring in nursing classics: an essential resource / Marlaine C. Smith, RN, PhD, AHN-BC, FAAN, Marian C. Turkel, RN, PhD, NEA-BC, Zane Robinson Wolf, PhD, RN, FAAN, editors.
    pages; cm
    Includes index.
    ISBN 978-0-8261-7111-5
    1. Nursing. 2. Nursing—Standards. I. Smith, Marlaine C. (Marlaine Cappelli)
II. Turkel, Marian C. III. Wolf, Zane Robinson.
    RT85.5.C37 2013
    610.73—dc23
                                                                                    2012041557

Special discounts on bulk quantities of our books are available to corporations, professional associations, pharmaceutical companies, health care organizations, and other qualifying groups. If you are interested in a custom book, including chapters from more than one of our titles, we can provide that service as well.

For details, please contact:
Special Sales Department, Springer Publishing Company, LLC
11 West 42nd Street, 15th Floor, New York, NY 10036-8002s
Phone: 877-687-7476 or 212-431-4370; Fax: 212-941-7842
Email: sales@springerpub.com

Printed in the United States of America by Bang Printing.

I dedicate this book to:

- The pioneering caring scholars who had the vision and courage to create the path we walk today. Madeleine, Jean, Sister Simone, Anne, Savina, Dee, Dolores, Kathleen.... You stood in the center of your truth and formed the foundation for the caring science, art, pedagogy, and practice that is humanizing nursing and health care today. Without you we wouldn't need this book. You are my heroes and I thank you.
- The past and present faculty, staff, alumni, students, and friends of the Christine Lynn College of Nursing at Florida Atlantic University. I was drawn here because of our shared conviction that nursing is a professional discipline grounded in caring and because Dr. Anne Boykin, the iconic founding dean, presided over the growth of a college that bears witness to this conviction. I look forward to continuing to build upon this legacy.
- The past and present scholars who have contributed and will continue to contribute to the body of caring knowledge. Some of your work appears in this book; some does not. Please know that we value all your work and wish we could transcend the page limits.
- My former students. Thank you for inspiring me, teaching me, and helping me to grow.
- My dad, Deno Cappelli, whom I lost in April 2010 as we were working on this book. Through your example I learned about love, courage, and living caring. You planted in my heart a passion for education and the moral imperative to care for others. I miss you every day.

—*Marlaine C. Smith*

As I reflected on my dedication, I remembered starting graduate school at Christine Lynn College of Nursing at Florida Atlantic University in 1989 with a curriculum grounded in caring. I always thought of myself as a "caring" nurse but soon learned that there was an ontology and epistemology of caring, that caring was informed by multiple ways of knowing, and that nursing was being and becoming through caring. I wish I had this book when I took my first course with Dr. Anne Boykin in 1989 when we had to find five articles on caring per week over the course of 12 weeks, and analyze them in the multiple ways of knowing—not easy before the Internet and electronic search engines. This book is dedicated to my mentors and guides on my journey to understanding the scholarship of caring science. Dr. Anne Boykin, Dr. Carolyn Brown, Dr. Marilyn Parker, Dr. Marilyn Ray, Dr. Savina Schoenhofer, and Dr. Jean Watson provided ongoing love, nurturance, and inspiration as I came to understand the meaning of caring as a substantive area of study within the discipline.

To the faculty and board of directors of the Watson Caring Science Institute (WCSI) whom I am privileged to work with for being there and holding the energetic field for me the past few months.

To my colleagues at Einstein Health care Network for valuing my commitment to caring and being on the journey with me to transform practice.

To registered nurses in the practice setting who are creating caring moments every day, and to the Caritas Coaches that I have had the honor to serve and guide. Remember the journey never ends; you only continue to grow.

Most important is the special dedication to my husband, Brooks Turkel. He truly understands my love for caring science, is supportive of my work with WCSI and the International Association for Human Caring, and encourages the dissemination of caring in terms of writing and publishing. Thank you for giving up so many weekends to do the household tasks and errands while I was writing. This is a formal recognition for Husband of the Year for 2011.

—*Marian C. Turkel*

I dedicate this book to the many scholars whose work we selected for this publication and for the many caring experts who authored excellent publications on nurse caring over the past decades. I also dedicate this work to past, present, and future nursing students.

I am in awe of our colleagues' commitment and excellence when investigating and seeking to understand what nurse caring really means for patients, families, communities, students, nurses, researchers, and administrators. I enjoy their writing when I discover it while searching the literature and as editor of the *International Journal for Human Caring*.

I also dedicate this book to my husband, Charles J. Wolf, MD, for his constant support and love.

—*Zane Robinson Wolf*

Contents

Foreword Jean Watson, PhD, RN, AHN-BC, FAAN *xi*
Preface *xiii*

PART I CARING AND THE DISCIPLINE OF NURSING
Marlaine C. Smith

>   *Questions for Reflection* *8*

PART II ANALYZING THE CONCEPT OF CARING
Zane Robinson Wolf

1. Concepts of Caring and Caring as a Concept *19*
    Janice M. Morse, Shirley M. Solberg, Wendy L. Neander, Joan L. Bottorff, and Joy L. Johnson
    Questions for Reflection *31*

2. Caring in Nursing: Analysis of Extant Theory *33*
    Anne Boykin and Savina Schoenhofer
    Questions for Reflection *42*

3. Caring and the Science of Unitary Human Beings *43*
    Marlaine C. Smith
    Questions for Reflection *57*

4. What Is Known About Caring in Nursing Science: A Literary Meta-Analysis *59*
    Kristen M. Swanson
    Questions for Reflection *102*

5. Metasynthesis of Caring in Nursing *103*
    Deborah Finfgeld-Connett
    Questions for Reflection *115*

PART III THEORETICAL PERSPECTIVES ON CARING
Marlaine C. Smith

6. Caring—An Essential Human Need: Proceedings of Three National Caring
    Conferences *127*
    Madeleine M. Leininger
    Questions for Reflection *141*

7.   Nursing: The Philosophy and Science of Caring   143
     Jean Watson
     Questions for Reflection   153

8.   Foundations of Humanistic Nursing   155
     Josephine G. Paterson and Loretta T. Zderad
     Questions for Reflection   163

9.   Caring: The Human Mode of Being   165
     M. Simone Roach
     Questions for Reflection   180

10. New Dimensions of Human Caring Theory   181
     Jean Watson
     Questions for Reflection   191

11. Caring Science in a New Key   193
     Katie Eriksson
     Questions for Reflection   200

12. Five Basic Modes of Being With Another   201
     Sigridur Halldorsdottir
     Questions for Reflection   210

13. Empirical Development of a Middle Range Theory of Caring   211
     Kristen M. Swanson
     Questions for Reflection   221

14. Nursing as Caring: A Model for Transforming Practice (Chapters 1 and 2)   223
     Anne Boykin and Savina O. Schoenhofer
     Questions for Reflection   236

15. The Theory of Human Caring: Retrospective and Prospective   237
     Jean Watson
     Questions for Reflection   241

16. Nursing: The Philosophy and Science of Caring (Revised Edition)   243
     Jean Watson
     Questions for Reflection   264

PART IV SEMINAL RESEARCH RELATED TO CARING
Zane Robinson Wolf

17. Development of a Theoretically Adequate Description of Caring   271
     Delores A. Gaut
     Questions for Reflection   281

18. Important Nurse Caring Behaviors Perceived by Patients With Cancer   283
     Patricia J. Larson
     Questions for Reflection   291

19. Noncaring and Caring in the Clinical Setting: Patients' Descriptions   293
     Doris Johnston Riemen
     Questions for Reflection   298

20. Oncology Nurses' Versus Cancer Patients' Perceptions of Nurse Caring Behaviors: A Replication Study   *299*
    Deborah K. Mayer

    Questions for Reflection   307

21. The Theory of Bureaucratic Caring for Nursing Practice in the Organizational Culture   *309*
    Marilyn A. Ray

    Questions for Reflection   320

22. Caring About–Caring For: Moral Obligations and Work Responsibilities in Intensive Care Nursing   *321*
    Agneta Cronqvist, Töres Theorell, Tom Burns, and Kim Lützén

    Questions for Reflection   332

PART V RESEARCH DESIGNS AND METHODS FOR STUDYING CARING
Zane Robinson Wolf

23. Caring Inquiry: The Esthetic Process in the Way of Compassion   *339*
    Marilyn A. Ray

    Questions for Reflection   345

24. Dimensions of Nurse Caring   *347*
    Zane Robinson Wolf, Eileen Riviello Giardino, Patricia A. Osborne, and Marguerite Stahley Ambrose

    Questions for Reflection   356

25. Metasynthesis of Qualitative Analyses of Caring: Defining a Therapeutic Model of Nursing   *357*
    Gwen D. Sherwood

    Questions for Reflection   370

26. A Standard of Care for Caring: A Delphi Study   *371*
    Zane Robinson Wolf, Margaret Miller, Dawn Freshwater, Rebecca A. Patronis Jones, and Gwen D. Sherwood

    Questions for Reflection   384

PART VI CARING-BASED NURSING PRACTICE MODELS
Marian C. Turkel

27. The Quality-Caring Model©: Blending Dual Paradigms   *395*
    Joanne R. Duffy and Lois M. Hoskins

    Questions for Reflection   406

28. Creating a Caring Practice Environment Through Self-Renewal   *407*
    Marian C. Turkel and Marilyn A. Ray

    Questions for Reflection   413

29. The Attending Nurse Caring Model®: Integrating Theory, Evidence, and Advanced Caring–Healing Therapeutics for Transforming Professional Practice   *415*
    Jean Watson and Roxie Foster

    Questions for Reflection   422

PART VII CARING, HEALTH POLICY, AND THE COMMUNITY
Marian C. Turkel

30. Watson's Philosophy, Science, and Theory of Human Caring as a Conceptual Framework for Guiding Community Health Nursing Practice   *431*
    Adeline R. Falk Rafael

    Questions for Reflection   444

31. Earth Caring   *445*
    Eleanor A. Schuster

    Questions for Reflection   450

32. Caring on the Ragged Edge: Nursing Persons Who Are Disenfranchised   *451*
    Joyce V. Zerwekh

    Questions for Reflection   464

PART VIII CARING LEADERSHIP AND ADMINISTRATION
Marian C. Turkel

33. The Effects of Care and Economics on Nursing Practice   *473*
    Jan Nyberg

    Questions for Reflection   480

34. Struggling to Find a Balance: The Paradox Between Caring and Economics   *481*
    Marian C. Turkel

    Questions for Reflection   495

35. Exploration of the Relationship Between Caring and Cost   *497*
    Kathleen L. Valentine

    Questions for Reflection   506

36. Leading Via Caring–Healing: The Fourfold Way Toward Transformative Leadership   *507*
    Jean Watson

    Questions for Reflection   512

37. Love and Caring: Ethics of Face and Hand—An Invitation to Return to the Heart and Soul of Nursing and Our Deep Humanity   *513*
    Jean Watson

    Questions for Reflection   519

PART IX SYNTHESIS AND EPILOGUE
Marlaine C. Smith, Marian C. Turkel, and Zane Robinson Wolf

Index   525

Foreword

This collected work by noteworthy scholars Smith, Turkel, and Wolf stands as a classic indeed. It offers nursing and related fields a repository and living history of the evolution of nursing within a caring science paradigm over a 40-year span from foundational ideas and developments, to current work in education, research, and institutional/community practices of caring. It lays the foundation for understanding core concepts, theoretical views, and seminal forms of caring inquiry, study designs, and methods.

The book is organized clearly, as it carries us through the intellectual foundation of caring as a serious epistemic endeavor, not just a "nice" way of being. From there, this classic includes caring in relation to health policy, eco-caring, as well as caring within a communitarian framework.

Lastly, caring leadership, administrative practices, and system approaches are represented, concluding with the latest thinking on the state of Caring Science. This overview highlights and summarizes the historic classic cross-sections of writing from the literature. The closing Epilogue offers mature implications for continual evolution of Caring Science, including reflective future directions.

Because of the span of this collection, it will quickly become essential reading for all nursing faculty, graduate students, and current scholars in related fields while also educating a new generation of students, scholars, and educators/practitioners into Caring Science and its distinct disciplinary foundation of nursing. It is through such work, as contained in *Caring in Nursing Classics*, that we can find our way home again to sustain and advance the philosophical-ethical-theoretical guide to the nursing discipline, which is being threatened. Indeed there are new generations of nurses who have not studied the core disciplinary foundation of the profession. This work offers informed caring scholarship that, in turn, provides a broader foundation upon which to guide the development of the profession, from the inside out.

This timeless, historical nursing caring scholarship occurred in some ways parallel to, and outside of, the mainstream thinking in nursing at the time it was written. Now, however, this history promises to be reclaimed and rediscovered from within and without as nursing undergoes its next major transition as a mature health and healing profession.

This work requires attention like never before, or nursing may become even more detoured from its disciplinary essence, and in turn lose its meta-story. The meta-story of caring scholarship in this book helps to carry forward the heritage, history, values, goals, theories, ethics, knowledge, and philosophical views of humanity that guide the future professional and profession.

Without such works as *Caring in Nursing Classics,* nursing is in danger of losing a core story of its scholarly evolution, and caring, as a specific disciplinary endeavor, necessary for nursing to continue to mature within a unified paradigm that sustains and advances knowledge of human caring to serve humanity.

Jean Watson
Founder, Watson Caring Science Institute

Preface

Descriptions of what caring in nursing really means range from the essence of nursing to an often repeated phrase spoken by nurses who provide direct patient care every day. Many nurse scholars and clinicians have offered their perspectives on caring, realizing its importance to professional nursing practice. But the significant work of caring scholars began to emerge during the 1970s, laying the foundation for current conceptualizations in the discipline. This book honors the scholars who, early on, called our attention to nurse caring and the other colleagues who persisted and produced an abundance of work in the ensuing years.

Caring in Nursing Classics includes selected, foundational, scholarly work for nursing students, faculty, researchers, administrators, and those who care for patients to examine and enjoy. We have provided a reflection on each set of manuscripts and have posed questions for reflection for baccalaureate, master's, and doctoral students.

Part I sets the stage for the book, with in-depth analysis of the evolution of caring scholarship. Review of the narratives in Part II, "Analyzing the Concept of Caring," includes systematic reviews on the concept of caring. Part III, "Theoretical Perspectives on Caring," reveals conceptual orientations, middle-range theories, and grand theories on nurse caring. Part IV, "Seminal Research Related to Caring," contains qualitative and quantitative examples of research beginning with Delores Gaut's (1983) work on the meaning of the word caring and essential conditions for actions to be considered caring. In this section, noncaring nursing is described by Doris Johnston Riemen (1986). Furthermore, instruments to measure caring are introduced. In Part V, "Research Designs and Methods for Studying Caring," research designs, with both quantitative and qualitative examples, are reviewed and are elaborated.

Part VI, "Caring-Based Nursing Practice Models," references professional practice models and theoretical frameworks for the integration of caring within the contemporary hospital-based practice environment. The focus of Part VII, "Caring, Health Policy, and the Community," is on caring theory guiding the practice of nursing with the context of community as practice environment. Part VIII, "Caring Leadership and Administration," highlights research related to caring and economics, and includes exemplars related to caring science guiding the practice of nursing leaders. Part IX forecasts the future of caring science contextualized by the works that have preceded it.

As a collection of important work, we think *Caring in Nursing Classics* is a unique contribution to professional nursing. We also hope that all nurses and other colleagues continue to create and share scholarly and clinical publications on nurse caring and find this book and the authors represented in it stimulating and inspiring.

Caring in Nursing Classics: An Essential Resource is supplemented by the *Teachers' and Students' Resource Guide*. The guide includes three syllabi for a course on caring in nursing at three educational levels: baccalaureate, master's, and doctoral. Nine sections reflect each part of the *Caring in Nursing Classics* book. Parts I through VIII incorporate multiple-choice test questions, a matching test, and a nursing situation with reflective questions for discussion. PowerPoint slides are also included for Parts I through VII. Part IX has a matching test and a critique examination for both a quantitative and a qualitative caring research study. **These are available from Springer Publishing Company for qualified instructors by emailing textbook@springerpub.com.**

ACKNOWLEDGMENTS

We are indebted to colleagues from the International Association for Human Caring and the Watson Caring Science Institute for their belief in this caring work. Their financial support enabled us to obtain copyright clearances for many of the caring classics contained within. Our colleagues in caring likewise supported the idea of this book by helping us to identify the market interest in such a publication.

We also would like to thank Lisa Willie, administrative assistant, Dean's Office, School of Nursing and Health Sciences of La Salle University for her support throughout this book project and Suzanne Riley and Christine Seixeiro, undergraduate students, for their steadfast assistance.

We are grateful to Allan Graubard, former Executive Editor, Springer Publishing Company, for his guidance and support during the process and to Christina Ferraro, former assistant editor, nursing, for her attention to the details of the process.

Marlaine C. Smith
Marian C. Turkel
Zane Robinson Wolf

I

Caring and the Discipline of Nursing

MARLAINE C. SMITH

The inclusion of caring as a central concept in the discipline of nursing has been the topic of passionate debate. Despite the disagreement, over the past 40 years, an emerging science of caring has been developed with substantive theories, research, and practice models. The art of caring in nursing has been expressed in the practice of individual nurses and captured through a variety of art forms. There have been about 60 books and thousands of journal articles published on the phenomenon. The International Association for Human Caring (IAHC) is nearly 25 years old, and the 35th annual conference will be held in 2013. The *International Journal of Human Caring* was established in 1997, and has been a vehicle to advance the work of caring scientists, artists, and practitioners. Yes, caring in the discipline of nursing has come of age. The purpose of this chapter is to describe the importance of caring within the discipline of nursing, to review the historical debate around caring in the discipline, and to provide a brief overview of two philosophies that have informed nursing theories and conceptualizations of caring.

Caring has been at the heart of nursing's identity before its recognition as a profession or discipline. The root of the word "nursing" means nurturance or care. Nursing, as a set of nurturing activities focused on caring for the sick, was assigned or ascribed as a role in all societies to healers, members of religious orders, or women in their homes before the role became formalized. In these myriad variations, the role of the one performing these activities has been imbued with qualities of protection, nurturance, and altruism.

Florence Nightingale (1860) professionalized western nursing when she asserted that specific knowledge and training were needed to practice well. According to Nightingale, this knowledge focused on the activities associated with putting a person in the best condition for nature to act. For Nightingale, nature was the inherent healer, and the nurse's activities focused on creating the environment that facilitated this natural process of healing. One cannot read Nightingale's writings without finding caring within them. Her references to the importance of sensitivity to the person's experience, tender attendance to the needs of the suffering person, and to nursing as a spiritual practice affirm the primal connection between nursing and caring.

As modern nursing evolved under the shadow of medicine, its relationship to caring became less explicit, and as the quest for scientific legitimacy consumed this early modern consciousness, some considered the "feminine" or "soft" side of nursing as a threat. However, the terms "care" and "caring" were always a part of the traditional nursing lexicon, with common references to "patient care" or "nursing care" (Smith, 1999). In the early 1970s, there was an urgent call to distinguish nursing as a discipline in its own right, separate from medicine. A discipline is characterized by "a unique perspective, a distinct way of viewing all phenomena, which ultimately defines the limits and nature of its inquiry" (Donaldson & Crowley, 1978, p. 113). A discipline has a substantive body of knowledge that students learn, faculties teach, practitioners apply, and scientists expand through research.

Several scholars attempted to identify the unique perspective or the substantive focus of the discipline of nursing. Donaldson and Crowley (1978) identified the unique perspective of nursing as:

> (1) concern with principles and laws that govern the life processes, well-being and optimum functioning of human beings—sick or well; (2) concern with the patterning of human behavior in interaction with the environment in critical life situations; and (3) concern with the processes by which positive changes in health are affected. (p. 113)

Jacqueline Fawcett (1984) coined the nursing metaparadigm as person, environment, health, and nursing in an effort to name the uniqueness of the discipline of nursing. To Fawcett, nursing is the study of person–environment relationships that facilitate health. The inclusion of the word "nursing" in the metaparadigm seemed tautological to many. Although Fawcett's intent in using "nursing" is to reflect the processes or activities that affected health (also identified by Donaldson and Crowley), it is awkward to define the discipline nursing by using "nursing" as one of the defining concepts.

In the 1970s, Madeleine Leininger (1978) identified care as the essence of nursing, and this idea captured the imaginations of some scholars. She stated, "Caring is the dominant intellectual, theoretical, heuristic and practice focus of nursing, and no other profession is so totally concerned with caring behaviors, caring processes, and caring relationships than nursing" (p. 33). Following Leininger,

Watson (1979, 1985) proposed that nursing is the art and science of human caring. At a major conference in 1989, leaders of the American Academy of Nursing and Sigma Theta Tau concurred that "caring" should replace "nursing" in the metaparadigm (Stevenson & Tripp-Reimer, 1990). In this way, the focus of the discipline might be stated as the study of person–environment relationships that facilitate health through caring. In 1991, Newman, Sime, and Corcoran-Perry published a landmark article focussing the discipline of nursing. They submit that "nursing is the study of caring in the human health experience" (Newman, Sime, & Corcoran-Perry, 1991, p. 3). The authors cite the theoretical linkages between caring, health, healing, and well-being that appeared in the literature. (Benner & Wrubel, 1989; Leininger, 1989; Watson, 1979, 1985). In a similar way, M. C. Smith (1994) linked these concepts by asserting that nursing is the study of human health and healing through caring.

In 2008, Newman and another group of colleagues (Newman, Smith, Dexheimer-Pharris, & Jones, 2008) published a paper that revisited the focus of the discipline. In this chapter, the authors suggested that theoretical perspectives are shifting to a unitary-transformative paradigm,

> from looking at the whole as sum of parts to looking at the whole as primary, from seeking to solve a problem to seeking to know the pattern, and from embracing an action-reaction causal approach, to realizing the mutuality of the unfolding, rhythmic process through which insight arises. (p. E16)

These authors reflected that relationship was emerging as the central focus of the discipline.

> It is the nature of the nurse–patient relationship that unites the practice of nursing as it occurs in myriad settings throughout the world at every moment of every day. Whether it be a neonatal nurse applying

knowledge of highly technical treatments aimed at preserving the life of the baby of the parents before her, a nurse sitting on the cot of a person dying of a chronic illness in a remote village, or a nurse working with community members faced with an epidemic, nursing actions occur within the context of a unified commitment. That commitment is to a caring relationship focusing on understanding the meaning of the current situation for the people involved and appreciating the pattern of evolving forces shaping health, so that appropriate actions can be taken. (p. E-17)

In the published summary of a symposium held at the IAHC conference, Cowling, Smith, and Watson (2008) offered their reflections on the unifying concepts of wholeness, consciousness, and caring as emergent themes in the disciplinary discourse within nursing.

> We are essentially whole beings, but our human perceptions get in the way of experiencing and realizing this. Blake said, "If the doors of perception were cleansed, everything would appear . . . as it is, Infinite." Caring cleanses the doors of perception so that we can see ourselves and others as they are—whole." As we become more aware of and awake to this universal oneness, we grow in caring and love for ourselves, others and our environment. When we see ourselves as separate from others, we focus on our differences and it is easier to judge, label, objectify, fix, advise, intervene, and order. We may more easily be called to intolerance, conflict, apathy, and disrespect. When we see others as whole we can marvel, appreciate, journey with, partner with, accompany, support and facilitate. Seeing others as whole is a different ontology and a different ethical starting point. . . . When we see self as integral with all that is, we are more likely to live life with reverence, harmony and peace. (pp. E-45–E-46)

Through caring, we apprehend the whole, and through caring for others, we come to apprehend their own wholeness, their integral nature, or who they truly are. Caring deepens with expanding consciousness. The caring consciousness is

qualitatively different in that it is focused in the transcendent present and connected to the universal consciousness. This is what Watson refers to as the caring occasion (p. E-46).

THE CRITIQUE OF CARING AS CENTRAL TO THE DISCIPLINE OF NURSING

Although we, the editors, obviously agree that caring is a central and identifying concept in the discipline of nursing, there are those who have questioned this. It is important to represent these views to readers as part of the historical scholarly debate on the topic within nursing.

Martha Rogers (1992) was one of the most vocal opponents for defining nursing with the concept of caring. She was adamant that "there is something to know in nursing," that anti-intellectualism is pervasive in nursing and has eroded the progress of the discipline, and that identifying nursing with caring would undermine the progress of building nursing science through identifying it with an affect instead of substantive knowledge.

Similarly, Mary Jane Smith (1990) wrote a short but powerful article raising the question: Is caring ubiquitous or unique? In this chapter, she argues that disciplines have unique perspectives and that caring does not provide this unique perspective; therefore, it should not be a defining element for the discipline of nursing. She states that caring is present in many professions. For example, pastoral care providers, physicians, psychologists, teachers, and counselors care within their professional practices. So defining nursing by caring does not provide the uniqueness that is needed for nursing to distinguish its area of inquiry.

Morse, Solberg, Neander, Bottorff, and Johnson (1990) published an article raising issues about the conceptual clarity related to the use of caring in the nursing literature. They stated that reviewing the literature on caring produces confusion, and if caring is to be advanced as a distinguishing concept in nursing, it must be clarified.

John Paley (2001) provided a challenging critique on the body of developing literature on caring. He takes issue with nursing's persistent interest in caring as an object of study. Paley uses Foucault's archaeology of knowledge to critique the current knowledge of caring, saying that it is limited to "knowledge of things said" that is presented in associations, attributes, and aggregations (p. 190). Paley argues that theoretical and research literature related to caring becomes circular, endless, and useless, prescientific, irrelevant, and irretrievable, and he compares it to what can be found in a thesaurus. He concludes that caring is ". . . an elusive concept, which is destined to remain elusive" (p. 196).

RESPONSE TO THIS CRITIQUE

Caring scholars have responded thoughtfully to these critiques. M. C. Smith (1999) acknowledged the lack of clarity in the use of the term *caring*. She suggests that the concept of caring is different depending on the theoretical perspective in which it is situated. So, to clarify the concept, it is essential to be clear about the assumptions and worldview within which caring is being conceptualized. As far as the argument about the ubiquitous nature of caring, it is true that caring as a dimension of human relating is important for all professions and arguably in all human relations. But nursing is the only discipline developing knowledge about "how this quality of relationship facilitates health, healing and the quality of life" (Smith, 1999, p. 19). In addition, caring is the art of nursing, and any discipline seeks to understand the art of its practice. "There is substantive knowledge related to nursing's art and this is a legitimate area of scholarship" (p. 19). For those concerned

about defining nursing exclusively with caring, it is the interrelationship of caring with health and healing that distinguishes the focus of the discipline: "Is nursing caring? No. But neither can nursing exist without caring" (p. 18).

Watson and Smith (2002) respond to Paley's critique of caring knowledge. They state that he ignored the discussion in the literature related to how different worldviews shape the meaning of caring. "Caring looks differently depending upon the ontological and ethical perspective in which the approaches and categories are located. Without specifying the ontology one cannot understand caring within it" (p. 454). In addition, Paley, in his critique, engages in the same approach to analyzing caring knowledge that he criticizes. He "accumulates words and total lists, categories and approaches to the study of caring . . . derived from a detached analysis of text, without an engagement with the ideas of caring or context espoused by the authors" (p. 454). Watson and Smith note that there is a call to examine nursing knowledge within the context of deliberation and moral action. Without addressing ontological foundations and the moral-ethical context, what results is a superficial analysis of the knowledge of caring. "Understanding caring is not a spectator sport; the scholar must invest in the deep understanding of the moral, ethical foundations where caring is understood as a value-laden relation of infinite responsibility to self and others" (p. 455). Perhaps caring is ineffable and unknowable in its totality. When engaging in caring science, we are entering a mystery.

> Indeed knowledge of caring is, like most of the important ideas in history of humankind that seek to define and sustain our humanity, ineffable, difficult to describe and incomprehensible. However, just because concepts such as caring, suffering, love, beauty and God are elusive we struggle to capture their essence because of

their importance. We always fall short, and will continue to fall short. Nevertheless, we strive to know them through many different methods and approaches; we seek descriptions, qualities, attributes as well as experience. (p. 455)

PHILOSOPHICAL FOUNDATIONS OF CARING

Milton Mayeroff

American philosopher Milton Mayeroff (1925–1979) offered his philosophy of caring in a primer that informed the work of many caring scholars in nursing. In *On Caring* (Mayeroff, 1971), he provided the definition and ingredients of caring that elaborate his perspective on the meaning of the concept. According to Mayeroff, caring is helping the other to grow. The "other" can be a person, an animal, idea, or object. He states, "I experience what I care for . . . as an extension of myself and at the same time separate from myself" (p. 7). As an extension of self, one who cares recognizes himself in the experience of the other; there is a recognition of a shared humanity. But Mayeroff differentiates caring from a parasitic relationship in that instead of trying "to dominate or possess the other" the one caring wishes the other to grow into his or her own right and not in the preferred image of the one caring. (p. 8). Caring is being needed by the other, but the response to this need does not reflect a "power over" the other; instead, there is acknowledgment of the other's agency and personhood. Mayeroff asserts,

> In helping the other to grow I do not impose my own direction; rather, I allow the direction of the other's growth to guide what I do, to help determine how I am to respond and what is relevant to such response. (p. 9)

Devotion is an essence of the caring relationship, and it involves a commitment to self and others (Mayeroff, 1971, p. 5). Devotion is "being there for the other" in a way that is the opposite of being equivocal about entering into this relationship. (p. 11). The well-being of the one caring is "bound up" in the well-being of the other: "I respond affirmatively and with devotion to the other's need, guided by the direction of its growth" (p. 12). Helping the other to grow means helping him or her care for self and to discover areas of life in which his or her care is invested. When Mayeroff describes caring as helping the other to grow, he refers to helping the person become more self-determining, making decisions based on his or her own values. (p. 13). Human growth is becoming who the person truly wants to be.

The major ingredients of caring are: (1) knowing, (2) alternating rhythms, (3) patience, (4) honesty, (5) trust, (6) humility, (7) hope, and (8) courage. Mayeroff states that caring involves knowing about many things. "I must know who the person is, what his strengths and limitations are, what his needs are, and what is conducive to growth; I must know how to respond to his needs, and what my own powers and limitations are . . ." (p. 19). So caring involves knowing self and others. Caring involves implicit and explicit, direct and indirect knowledge, and knowing that and knowing how. Alternating rhythms refer to "moving back and forth between a narrower and a wider point of view" to understand fully (p. 22). Patience is "enabling the other to grow in its [sic] own time and in its [sic] own way" (p. 23). "Patience is not waiting passively for something to happen, but is a kind of participation with the other in which we give fully of ourselves" (p. 24). The one caring believes in the potential for the other's growth and must be patient with his or her own growth in caring (p. 24). Honesty refers to being true to self and open with others, seeing truly. Honesty is the foundation for authentic presence.

> I must be genuine in caring for the other. I must "ring true." There must not be a

significant gap between how I act and what I really feel, between what I say and what I feel. To be present for the other, so that the other can be present for me, I must be open to the other. Pretending to be what I am not interferes with being able to relate to the other as an individual in its [sic] own right: I cannot be fully present for the other if I am more concerned about how I appear to other people than I am with seeing and responding to its needs. (p. 26)

Mayeroff (1971) asserts that caring is trusting that the person will grow in his or her own time and way (p. 27). This involves letting go of control of the other and trying to impose one's own will on the other. From this perspective, the nurse who labels someone as "noncompliant" or "nonadherent," falls short in the ingredient of trust in caring. Humility is understanding that there is always more to know about the other, that the one caring is always learning. The one caring does not have all the answers: "Through caring I come to a truer appreciation of my limitations as well as my powers" (p. 31). Hope is the seventh caring ingredient. For Mayeroff (1971), hope is the belief in the plentitude of the present, "a present alive with a sense of the possible" (p. 32). Finally, courage is living caring through the ability to journey into the unknown with the other.

Mayeroff's philosophy of caring informed the philosophies and theories of nurse scholars such as Paterson and Zderad, Boykin and Schoenhofer, and Watson. According to Mayeroff, caring is helping the other to grow through coming to know self and others, moving with alternating rhythms, learning more about self and others with humility, trusting that the other knows what is best for self, being honest with self and others in living authentic presence, being patient in the unfolding process of becoming, focusing on possibilities in the moment, and having the courage to journey with the other in the process of becoming.

Emmanuel Levinas

Emmanuael Levinas (1906–1995) was a Lithuanian Jewish philosopher who has influenced the thinking of Jean Watson, Katie Eriksson, and others. He studied under Martin Heidegger, and introduced Husserlian and Heideggarian phenomenology to France; however, later in his life, he renounced Heidegger for his connections to the Nazis.

Levinas (1969) is known for his assertion of ethics as first philosophy. Although the conventional philosophy of the time placed ontology, the study of being or existence, as the primary question, Levinas argued that belonging or being for another was most essential. While Heidegger's emphasis was *dasein* or being in the world or being with the other, Levinas' philosophy is belonging for the other, which includes the responsibility to care, and to act to alleviate suffering. In this way, his writing holds profound meaning for the caring theorists.

Levinas (1969) argues that the human condition implies responsibility and commitment to the other. Caring for another implies being face-to-face in a human encounter. This human encounter, gazing into the eyes of the other, breaks through the mask of objectivity. Levinas (1969) stated that "the eyes break through the mask—the language of the eyes, impossible to dissemble" (p. 66). In his ethic of face, he reminds us that looking on the face of the other connects one to the humanity of the other. "The face of the Other at each moment destroys and overflows the plastic image it leaves me [. . .]. The face is a living presence; it is expression" (Lavoie, De Koninck, & Blondeau, 2006, p. 225). This face-to-face encounter illuminates both connection and separation. The subjectivity of the self is known through apprehending the subjectivity of the other through this face-to-face encounter. By knowing self as subject and other as subject, there is an experience of shared humanity. At the same time, by knowing self as subject, there is a recognition of the other as separate from the self. In the face-to-face encounter, we touch Infinity (Levinas, 1969).

Levinas' (1969) work is an ethic in that it lays a foundation for the moral imperative of caring. The ethic of face compels care. "The human face obliges each and every one of us, leaving no possibility "to remain deaf to its appeal" or to "cease being responsible" (Lavoie et al., 2006, p. 228). Indeed the human being is a responsible being (p. 228). This responsibility gives life meaning. There is the responsibility to be *available* for the other, not only being with the other. Levinas emphasizes goodness and compassion at the very heart of care (Lavoie et al., 2006, p. 230). Compassion is expressed in action; it is not sufficient to feel with the other, and this is a strong foundation for caring in nursing.

In this introductory chapter to our anthology, we present an overview of the central place of caring in the discipline of nursing. We offered an overview of the dialogue surrounding this. Finally, we summarized Mayeroff's and Levinas' philosophies that serve as the foundation to classic nursing texts on caring. The readers are invited to go deeper into these philosophies to more fully comprehend their meaning. This chapter is an invitation to enter into an exploration of the classic works on caring within nursing.

REFERENCES

Benner, P., & Wrubel, J. (1989). *The primacy of caring: Stress and coping in health and illness.* Menlo Park, CA: Addison-Wesley.

Cowling, W. R., Smith, M. C., & Watson, J. (2008). The power of wholeness, consciousness and caring: A dialogue on nursing science, art and healing. *Advances in Nursing Science, 31*(1), E41–E51.

Donaldson, S., & Crowley, D. (1978). The discipline of nursing. *Nursing Outlook, 26*(2), 113–120.

Fawcett, J. (1984). The metaparadigm of nursing: Current status and future refinements. *Image Journal of Nursing Scholarship, 16,* 84–87.

Lavoie, M., De Koninck, T., & Blondeau, D. (2006). The nature of care in light of Emmanuel Levinas. *Nursing Philosophy, 7,* 225–234.

Leininger, M. (1978). Transcultural nursing theories and research approaches. In M. Leininger (Ed.), *Transcultural nursing: Concepts, theories and practices.* Thorofare, NJ: Slack.

Leininger, M. (1989). Historic and epistemologic dimensions of care and caring with future directions. In: Stevenson JS, Tripp-Reimer T, eds. Knowledge About care and Caring. Proceedings of a Wingspread Conference, February 1-3, 1989. Kansas City, Mo: American Academy of Nursing.

Levinas, E. (1969). *Totality and infinity: An essay on exteriority.* Pittsburgh, PA: Duquesne University Press.

Mayeroff, M. (1971). *On caring.* New York, NY: Harper and Row.

Morse, J. M., Solberg, S. M., Neander, W. L., Bottorff, J. L., & Johnson, J. L. (1990). Concepts of caring and caring as a concept. *Advances in Nursing Science, 13*(1), 1–14.

Newman, M. A., Smith, M. C., Dexheimer-Pharris, M., & Jones, D. (2008). The focus of the discipline revisited. *Advances in Nursing Science, 31*(1), E16–E27.

Newman, M.A., Sime, A.M., Corcoran-Perry, S.A. (1991) The focus of the discipline of nursing. Advances in Nursing Science, 14(1), 1-6.

Nightingale, F. (1860). *Notes on nursing: What it is and what it is not.* London, England: Harrison.

Paley, J. (2001). An archaeology of caring knowledge. *Journal of Advanced Nursing 36*(2), 188–198.

Rogers, M. E. (1992). Nursing science and the space age. *Nursing Science Quarterly, 5,* 27–34.

Smith, M. C. (1994). Arriving at a philosophy of nursing: Discovery, constructing, evolving. In Kikuchi & Simmons (Eds.), *Philosophy in the nurse's world.* Thousand Oaks, CA: Aspen.

Smith, M. C. (1999). Caring and the science of unitary human beings. *Advances in Nursing Science, 21*(4), 14–28.

Smith, M. J. (1990). Caring: ubiquitous or unique? *Nursing Science Quarterly, 3,* 54.

Stevenson, J. S., & Tripp-Reimer, T. (1990) (Eds.). *Knowledge about care and caring. Proceedings of a cingspread conference.* February 1–3, 1989. Kansas City, MO: American Academy of Nursing.

Watson, J. (1979). *Nursing: The philosophy and science of caring.* Boulder, CO: University of Colorado Press.

Watson, J. (1985) *Nursing: Human science and human care: A theory of nursing.* New York, NY: National League for Nursing.

Watson, J., & Smith, M. C. (2002). Caring science and the science of unitary human beings. *Journal of Advanced Nursing, 37*(5), 452–461.

QUESTIONS FOR REFLECTION

Baccalaureate

- How did Newman, Sime, and Corcoran-Perry define the focus of the discipline of nursing?
- Identify, describe, and provide an example of two of Mayeroff's caring ingredients.
- What is your definition of the focus of the discipline of nursing? Is caring a part of that definition? Why or why not?

Master's

- What is the difference between a discipline and a profession? How do Donaldson and Crowley characterize a discipline?
- What was Martha Rogers' concern about the emphasis on caring in nursing? How would you respond to her concern?
- Provide an example of how humility is an important ingredient of living caring in nursing.

Doctoral

- Should caring be a defining element in the nursing metaparadigm? Support your answer.
- Respond to Paley's analysis that caring knowledge is no better than consulting a thesaurus on the term "caring."
- Provide a brief synopsis of Levinas' ethic of face and relate it to one nursing theory related to care or caring.

II

Analyzing the Concept of Caring

ZANE ROBINSON WOLF

The words care and caring have appeared in nursing literature and everyday talk for more than 150 years. Various authors have questioned whether caring has been adequately defined as a concept or construct or even if caring could be defined at all. This ongoing conversation has stimulated interesting and sometimes contentious debate and resulted in an abundance of literature. Furthermore, scholars have pointed out that a great deal of emotion surrounds, frames, and sometimes obscures the analysis of the concept of caring for the nursing profession. The implication is that logic or systematic study has been insufficient. Caring as a concept or construct has not readily generated direct measurement as some concrete physical and physiological concepts have height, weight, serum potassium, and glycosylated hemoglobin. Because of this fact, scholars have pursued other analytical approaches, among them concept analysis strategies.

Concept analysis approaches are used when theoretical literature exists as a body of work, and investigators review it to determine the consistencies and inconsistencies in its use. Definitions are examined starting with a preliminary definition reflecting the occurrence of the concept in nursing situations. Nursing literature is carefully analyzed just as the literature of other disciplines is carefully questioned (Brink & Wood, 1998, p. 242).

Many theorists have defined the concept of caring using inductive or deductive approaches. The available research on caring has been chiefly qualitative. This is not surprising, considering one argument that asserts that human phenomena, such as caring and caring moments, are not like objects, but are about ". . . modes of existing and the meaning of being" (Watson, 2012, p. 95). However, few have systematically conducted an in-depth analysis of the concept; some of these important works are presented in this section.

Morse, Solberg, Neander, Bottorff, and Johnson (1990) acknowledged the importance of considering caring as the core or essence of nursing and simultaneously confronted an intellectual challenge. Moreover, they used concept analysis to explore the definitions of caring and its main characteristics, illustrated in a figure and specifying the authors who framed the definitions in theoretical perspectives. Initially, examining the difficulty of understanding the differences among the terms caring, care, and nursing care, they discussed the conceptualizations of caring, the adequacies and inadequacies of these conceptualizations, and assessed the concept's application to nursing practice. They also identified trends and gaps in caring research (Morse et al., 1990, p. 2). They first identified 35 authors who defined caring and representations of its main characteristics. They next organized 25 authors' work from the viewpoint of the basis of their perspectives. In doing so, Morse et al. (1990) revealed the complexity of the literature reviewed but did not suggest causal relationships.

The following five categories of caring were identified and included: *caring as a human trait, caring as a moral imperative or ideal, caring as an affect, caring as an interpersonal relationship, and caring as a therapeutic intervention*. The authors uncovered two outcomes of caring, implying that caring was an intervention: caring as a subjective experience of the patient and as a physical response.

Caring as a human trait incorporates the notion that humans have the potential to care, yet this position is modified by the need for nurses to become professionalized by acquiring knowledge and skill. Furthermore, the human trait of caring might motivate nursing actions, yet its meanings are culturally derived. Caring as a moral imperative or ideal is grounded in nursing's value of preserving the dignity and integrity of the patients. Caring needs to be supported by a workplace that values nurses' work by providing working conditions that help caring to flourish (Morse et al., 1990). Caring as an affect corresponds with the emotional or empathetic feeling for the patient experience. The affect is experienced by the nurse with the patient and is considered intimate during interaction. Both the nurse and the patient are vulnerable throughout this involvement. Caring is further inhibited by warnings that nurses remain objective, not too involved with the patients. Nurse caring is distracted by technology and deterred by unresponsive patients. Morse and colleagues emphasized that the workplace of nurses devalued caring.

Caring as the nurse–patient interpersonal relationship is the medium through which caring is expressed, according to Morse et al. (1990). The nurse–patient relationship is equated with the essence of nursing and the interaction between the nurse and the patient and as such expresses and

defines caring. Next, caring as therapeutic intervention connects actions that enable or assist the patients. In this conception, knowledge and skill are emphasized and nursing actions are associated with the patients' needs. Furthermore, the patients' perceptions of caring are valued in the literature selected by Morse and colleagues. They contrast perceptual differences between instrumental behaviors (patients') and expressive aspects (nurses') of caring actions. Finally, the outcomes of care and caring are described using physiological and psychological organizers. Mortality, morbidity, length of hospital stay, number of incident reports, pressure ulcers, and subjective responses are the outcomes reflecting nurses' concerns with quality assurance.

Morse et al. (1990) also reviewed Orem's Self-Care Deficit Theory of Nursing, Watson's Theory of Human Care, and Leininger's Theory of Transcultural Care Diversity and Universality. Watson's theory is evaluated very carefully, with Morse and colleagues (1990) questioning its connection to nursing situations, for example, those in which length of hospitalization is short or the patients are unconscious, thus unable to interact with the nurses. The contribution of Leininger's theory is valued through its focus on the need to consider cultural values and practices that influence patterns and meanings of care.

According to the investigators, caring as a process required additional study, as did caring as a uniform state. The latter perspective suggested that the authors who see caring as a human trait might assume that nurses should be more caring than nonnurses or manifest caring differently than lay or natural caregivers. Morse et al. (1990) called for more research on nurse caring behaviors, assuming that they are adjusted in response to suffering or depressed patients. Finally, they affirmed that caring should alter patient responses. They considered nursing's treatment of caring to be in its adolescence and provided questions raised through their analysis of the works cited about whether patients can be cured without caring or whether nurses could practice safety without caring. While they praised the divergent theoretical approaches provided by different caring theories, they also focused future debates on caring as intervention versus caring as interaction. They reiterated their concerns about the workplaces of nurses, declaring that care was restricted due to the expectations of health care agencies.

Boykin and Schoenhofer (1990) also recognized the scholarly work of nurses describing caring in nursing. They used five categories of questions proposed by Roach (1987) to analyze the concept. They discussed related literature framed by five questions as follows: (1) *ontological* ("being" of caring), (2) *anthropological* (what it means to be a caring person), (3) *ontical* (function and ethic), (4) *epistemological* (the ways caring is known [personal knowing, empirical knowing, ethical knowing, and esthetic knowing]), and (5) *pedagogical (teaching and learning)*.

The authors systematically considered the five questions. First, the ontological questions addressed the being of caring examined by nurses as well as the scholars of other disciplines. As a human mode of being, the ability to care is inseparable from that of being human. Person-to-person caring involves seeing the value of each person as important in itself. Persons are affected in caring and respond to caring affectively. They are both whole and holy. In this way and consistent with Roach (1987), body–mind–spirit are joined.

Boykin and Schoenhofer (1990) cited Watson (1985) who proposed that caring is an intersubjective human process in which interpersonal human care transactions occur. Individuals are authentically present and unique, together in caring. The call and the response involves the risk of being with another, connecting in moments of joy

(Parse, 1981). Mayeroff (1971) saw caring as a process, an end in itself and not a product.

Several scholars' views correspond with Boykin and Schoenhofer's (1990) analysis. Common elements consist of the importance of the authentic presence and connectedness of the persons in the caring situation. Caring is conceptualized as a mutual human process in which the nurse responds with authentic presence to a call from another. Caring is the center and integral to nursing.

Examining what it means to be a caring person from an anthropological perspective, Boykin and Schoenhofer (1990) reviewed Roach's (1987), Watson's (1985), and Mayeroff's (1971) work. Although the capacity to care may lie dormant, someone or something that matters helps individuals actualize the capacity to care and perform specific behavior, in this instance, caring behavior. The intersubjective process of caring preserves a common sense of humanity. Transpersonal caring includes a moral commitment to an end and affirms the subjective significance of the person. The caring nurse is a co-participant in the human care process. In offering authentic presence as the human mode of being, the nurse chooses to offer presence. Being a caring person involves being entrusted with the care of another at the same time living the meaning of a person's own life. Caring is an actualizing experience for the nurses and the patients. According to Boykin and Schoenhofer (1990), Leininger (1988) provided another view such as care being essential for human survival, growth, and development and is determined through the person's meanings, symbols, patterns, and expression of cultural care and nursing from a holistic perspective (Leininger, 1988, p. 153).

The ontical questions focus on function and ethic, which is what nurses do when they are caring for others. The literature of Roach, Watson, and Leininger were again analyzed by Boykin and Schoenhofer

(1990), considering what nurses do when they are caring and what their obligations are as they care. For example, what nurses do as they care varies from culture to culture. Caring nurses deliberate about how caring can best be accomplished; they are compassionate and professional. Competent caring includes knowledge, skill, and judgment as well as other skills so that nurses respond appropriately and compassionately to care recipients. Caring nurses are committed to serving humanity through caring.

Next, the epistemological questions about caring focus on the ways in which caring is known. The authors framed their analysis with Carper's (1978) patterns of knowing: personal, empirical, ethical, and esthetic. Nursing situations require knowing self objectively and subjectively, knowing self professionally, and knowing the patient. Awareness of self and others is essential and the nurses and the patients take on risk when engaging in knowing self and other.

Empirical knowing incorporates facts, principles, theories, and explanations based on observations and experiments. Caring theories can be used to frame research and generate findings. Next, ethical knowing is based on philosophical systems, judgment, and normative action. Caring involves nurses' commitment to the persons cared for and respects their right to self-determination. Caring protects human dignity and preserves humanity. Conscience directs behavior and caring nurses live their values and beliefs. (Noddings, 1984; Roach, 1984; Watson, 1985). Finally, esthetic knowing helps nurses to understand human experience through art forms, including music, poetry, literature, and so on. Artistic nurses create unique approaches to caring as they respond to the dreams and goals of patients.

The authors proposed that the pedagogical questions on caring address teaching and learning efforts. Teaching and learning activities need to be based on the values of caring and reflect the previous categories of questions used in Boykin and Schoenhofer's (1990) analysis. They also maintained that students need to perform exercises to assist them to know themselves and suggested that curriculums might follow Carper's (1978) patterns of knowing to organize teaching. Boykin and Schoenhofer (1990) affirmed that caring should be lived in the classroom. They argued that caring might unify nursing practice, education, administration, and research.

Marlaine Smith (1999) added to the debate on the concept of caring, asserting that it was a central unifying concept for nursing and did not need to be buried as others suggested. She studied caring within Rogers' framework of the Science of Unitary Human Beings (SUHB). She labeled her analytic approach as concept clarification, which was comprised of the following: background and analysis of the dialogue regarding caring in nursing, explication of the process developed to clarify the concept within the unitary perspective, and the presentation and discussion of the findings of the clarification. Dr. Smith also noted that Rogers was a serious opponent to the position that caring was a defining attribute of nursing.

Smith (1999) cited the then 20-year history of the discourse on caring in the nursing discipline, explaining that the terms care and caring for patients described the patient provider covenant in health care and the activities performed to fulfill the covenant (Smith, 1999, p. 15). She provided some historical details on Leininger's, Watson's, Ray's, Roach's, Gadow's, and Boykin and Schoenhofer's works to make her case, revealing the continuing resistance of scholars in the SUHB tradition. Caring was considered trite and intimate care was mocked. Nonetheless, Smith pointed out the need to study caring in nursing frameworks; not to do so would result in caring being poorly understood, sentimental, and task oriented. Caring was positioned in the nursing paradigm and linked to the quality of the relationship that helps the nurses and the patients connect.

Caring began to gain stature in the discourse of the discipline as a concept worthy of study, but disagreements continued. Its ubiquitous nature was restated; it was seen as a *scrap basket* or synonym for nursing practice associated with women and not necessarily men (Smith, 1999). It was not viewed as a dominating concept of the discipline at this time, however, during these conversations, caring and health were connected.

Smith (1999) outlined the concerns gleaned from her historical review of the literature about caring as a defining focus of nursing care as follows: ambiguity (lack of clarity), limiting and perspectival (too narrow and not common to all conceptualizations of nursing), ubiquitous (present in all human service areas, not unique to nursing), nonsubstantive (as affect or activities, not substantive body of knowledge), nongeneralizable (different across cultures and national boundaries), and feminine (associated with women's sensibilities) (Smith, 1999, p. 17). She called for a clear conceptualization, preferably framed by assumptions and the worldview of a conceptual model or grand theory. She next proposed that although nursing does not equal caring, nursing cannot exist without caring; caring transcends specific theories and is central to the art or practice of nursing. While caring is present in professional relationships of nursing and other disciplines, nursing may generate in-depth knowledge on how caring in relationships facilitate health, healing, and quality of life. Dr. Smith argued that both the science and art of caring need to be studied.

Smith (1999) contended that in addition to the concept of caring, other defining concepts of the discipline will not survive the challenge of cultural transcendence, but rather different meanings and acts will be seen as caring in different cultures. As far as caring being feminine, Smith stressed its association with nursing, not gender.

Finally, Dr. Smith (1999) questioned what is caring within "the theoretical niches" of SUHB. She assumed that caring is a way of participating knowingly in human-environmental field patterning and is the manifestation of human-field patterning in this process of participation. She identified the process of concept clarification to identify the essential meanings of the concept of caring from the unitary (SUHB) perspective. Findings revealed constitutive meanings supported through semantic expressions of caring as follows: manifesting intentions, appreciating pattern, attending to dynamic flow, experiencing the infinite, and inviting creative emergence. Each expression included a selection of phrases from relevant literature.

The author provided an instantiation (tangible or concrete example) of the concept of caring. She did this through narratives reflecting the constitutive meanings of caring. Stories illustrated caring in the context of SUHB. She left readers with a compelling argument to consider the concept carefully and intellectually and to frame the conversation in the theories of nursing.

Kristen Swanson (1999) performed a substantive analysis of caring in nursing science through a literary meta-analysis. She reviewed the literature and analyzed citations in the four selections in this section of the book. Similar to other authors, she described the importance of the Wingspread Caring Conference, sponsored by the Robert Wood Johnson Foundation and the American Academy of Nursing. Caring became more visible to scholars after this event, according to Swanson. However, Dr. Swanson's position was that not all of nursing care (practice) equates with nurse caring (way of caring) (Swanson, 1999, p. 32). She analyzed approximately 130 works, published between 1980 and 1996, and included data-based investigations on the concept of caring, both interpretive and empiric analytic. She focused on the findings as a framework for analyzing the studies.

Swanson derived the levels of inquiry and arranged them hierarchically based on assumptions. Level I inquiry showed findings identified what were the characteristics of persons with the capacity for caring, examining whether such traits and characteristics were inherent (nature) or environmentally enhanced or diminished (nurture). Level II included concerns and commitments, looking at beliefs or values framing caring actions. Level III described conditions or patients, nurses, or organization-related circumstances enhancing or diminishing the likelihood that caring transactions take place. Level IV specified caring actions, behaviors, or therapeutic interventions. Level IV used Swanson's five caring categories and provided a conceptual framework for caring actions and empirical support to her middle range caring theory Level V, the positive and negative consequences of caring, including intentional and unintentional outcomes of caring (Swanson, 1999, p. 33).

Swanson contrasted substantive to formal theory and made the case that her literary meta-analysis unearthed the concept of caring in nursing science and thus generated a formal theory. Level I, the capacity for caring category. Here, the findings of 21 studies were examined under capacity for caring and yielded results indicating how a caring person is. Caring is compassionate, empathic, knowledgeable, confident, and reflective. Level II, concerns/commitments category, analyzed studies on the beliefs or values underlying nurse caring. Values supporting nursing practices were composed of professional identity, seeing persons as unique beings, being compassionate and empathetic, and

believing that relationships should be therapeutic (p. 36). Level III, conditions, focused on questions about what affects or enhances caring or inhibits the occurrence of caring. Nurse and patient experiences, backgrounds and/or personalities, society, organizations, health status, and disease complications influenced whether or not caring occurred (p. 37). Dr. Swanson suggested that biases, legal constraints, and cultural influences might affect nurse caring. Furthermore, nurse-related (personal and professional resources constraints and demands) conditions, such as family history and personality and education and experience, affected caring (p. 39). Patient- (communication, personality, health problems, care needs, nurse–patient relationship, and other) and organization-related (personnel or role-related, technology, administration, and work or practice) conditions also positively or negatively affected caring.

Level IV category, caring actions, was developed from a review of quantitative and qualitative studies on caring actions. Larson's (1984) CARE-Q, subsequent articles on the CARE-Q, and Cronin and Harrison's (1988), Wolf's (1986), and Gardner and Wheeler's (1981, 1987) instruments along with others were compared to Larson's original CARE-Q items. Nurses, nursing students, faculty, and patients responded to the instruments. Both nurses' and patients' most highly ranked nurse caring behaviors were reported, with Swanson pointing out the differences between nurses and patients. She also classified caring actions from 67 investigations. She identified 20 groupings of actions and compared the actions using inductively derived categories from Swanson's middle-range theory, identifying themes and references.

Level V, the caring consequences category, addressed caring transactions that improved the situation of the health care provider and care receiver. Swanson located a few quantitative studies connecting caring-based therapeutic interactions with outcomes. For example, Duffy (1992) linked nurse caring with patient satisfaction, health status, length of stay, and health care costs. Another study (Duffy, 1993) evaluated nurse administrators' caring with staff nurse job satisfaction and turnover rates. Qualitative studies reviewed specified enhanced patients' well-being, classified as emotional–spiritual (enhanced self-esteem, etc.), physical (physical healing, etc.), and social (meaningful reciprocal relationship, etc.) as a result of caring. The consequences of caring for nurses were categorized as professional (e.g., enhanced intuition, empathy, and clinical judgment) and emotional–spiritual (e.g., feeling important, accomplished, and purposeful) outcomes. Social outcomes for nurses were feeling connected to their patients and colleagues (p. 53). Swanson briefly discussed the consequences of noncaring.

Dr. Swanson completed her in-depth, high-level analysis by acknowledging the plethora of interpretive studies on caring. She asserted that the five levels of discussion (capacity for caring, concerns and commitments underlying caring, conditions inhibiting or enhancing caring, caring actions, and caring consequences) that she induced should be used in scholarly discourses on caring. This substantive work will continue to serve nursing scholars interested in examining the concept of caring.

Deborah Finfgeld-Connett (2008) met her own scholarly challenge by describing some of the underpinnings of the concept of caring. She understood that the concept was imprecise as acknowledged by different scholars. At the same time, she valued the importance of caring as a professional nursing concept worthy of investigation. She noted that only one metasynthesis was available in the literature and decided to examine the concept through an inductive metasynthesis approach using qualitative studies as sources. She found that the number of qualitative studies on the concept had predominated over several decades.

Dr. Finfgeld-Connett (2008) located citations from the nursing literature exclusively. She searched the Cumulative Index of Nursing and Allied Health Literature from 1988 to 2006 using caring in combination with concept analysis, qualitative studies, phenomenology, grounded theory, and ethnography. Excluded were the terms care and caring presence. She carefully detailed inclusion and exclusion criteria. This metasynthesis examined 49 qualitative sources of investigations and 6 concept analyses on caring. An important point made was about being flexible when reviewing earlier studies applying her approach. She noted that the standards of methodological rigor changed over time.

Using process as a theoretical framework for her study of caring, Deborah Finfgeld-Connett (2008) applied the methods of grounded theory and constant comparative analysis initially to analyze data. The process orientation of Strauss and Corbin (1998), including causal conditions, context, action/interactional strategies, and consequences, was followed during the data analysis phase. Codes and categories resulted. Next, Walker and Avant's (2005) process categories helped Dr. Finfgeld-Connett create a new conceptualization of caring.

Dr. Finfgeld-Connett represented caring as ". . . an interpersonal process, characterized by expert nursing, interpersonal sensitivity, and intimate relationships" (Finfgeld-Connett, 2008, p. 198). The process of caring was depicted in a figure that detailed its antecedents, attributes, and outcomes. Antecedents encompass the care recipient (need for caring and openness to caring) and the nurse (professional maturity and moral foundations) in the context of a conducive work environment. The attributes of the caring process include expert nursing, interpersonal sensitivity, and intimate relationships. Outcomes for the patient are physical and mental well-being and for the nurse, mental well-being.

Of interest is Dr. Finfgeld-Connett's statement that the findings allow for cultural or situational circumstances. Her findings also fit with the results of factor analytic studies on caring behaviors (e.g., Wolf, Giardino, Osborne, & Ambrose, 1994; Wu, Larrabee, & Putman, 2006). In addition, she connected this study to a previous metasynthesis she conducted on the construct of caring presence and emphasized the need to compare related nursing terminology through systematic approaches. She made the point that advanced concept analysis techniques need to be used to help with the development of concepts for theoretical frameworks used in research.

Ultimately, the complexity of describing the process of caring is revealed in Finfgeld-Connett's study. Her concern about how difficult it is to overcome the patients' reticence to caring emphasizes the need to investigate the patients' openness to caring. She asserted that her findings refuted Paley's (2002) position that caring represents a slave mentality.

The publications in this section reveal the ongoing interest of scholars in clarifying the concept of caring for nursing. In general, their approaches can be termed concept analyses, yet they take different approaches. They leave us with some clarity but also the realization that more work is needed.

REFERENCES

Boykin, A., & Schoenhofer, S. (1990). Caring in nursing: Analysis of extant theory. *Nursing Science Quarterly, 3*, 149–155.

Brink, P. J., & Wood, M. J. (1998). *Advanced design in nursing research* (2nd ed.). Thousand Oaks, CA: Sage.

Carper, B. (1978). Fundamental patterns of knowing in nursing. *Advances in Nursing Science, 1*, 13–23.

Cronin, S. N., & Harrison, B. (1988). Importance of nurse caring behaviors as perceived by patients after myocardial infarctions. *Heart and Lung, 17*, 374–380.

Duffy, J. R. (1992). Impact of nurse caring on patient outcomes. In D. A. Gaut (Ed.), *The presence of caring in nursing* (pp. 113–136). New York, NY: National League for Nursing.

Duffy, J. R. (1993). Caring behaviors of nurse managers: Relationships to staff nurse satisfaction and retention. In D. Gaut (Ed.), *A global agenda for caring* (pp. 365–377). New York, NY: National League for Nursing.

Finfgeld-Connett, D. (2008). Metasynthesis of caring in nursing. *Journal of Clinical Nursing, 17*, 196–204.

Gardner, K. G., & Wheeler, E. (1981). Patients' and staff nurses' perceptions of supportive nursing behaviors: A preliminary analysis. In M. M. Leininger (Ed.), *Caring: An essential human need* (pp. 109–113). Thorofare, NJ: Slack.

Gardner, K. G., & Wheeler, E. (1987). Patients' perceptions of support. *Western Journal of Nursing Research, 5*, 313–324.

Larson, P. J. (1984). Important nurse caring behaviors perceived by patients with cancer. *Oncology Nursing Forum, 11*(6), 46–50

Leininger, M. (1988). Leininger's theory of nursing: Cultural care diversity and universality. *Nursing Science Quarterly, 1*, 152–160.

Mayeroff, M. (1971). *On caring*. New York, NY: Harper Collins.

Morse, J. M., Solberg, S., Neander, W. L., Bottorff, J. L., & Johnson, J. L. (1990). Concepts of caring and caring as a concept. *Advances in Nursing Science, 13*(1), 1–14.

Noddings, N. (1984). *Caring: A feminine approach to ethics and moral education*. Berkeley, CA: University of California Press.

Paley, J. (2002). Caring as slave morality: Nietzshean themes in nursing ethics. *Journal of Advanced Nursing, 40*, 25–35.

Parse, R. R. (1981). Caring from a human science perspective. In M. Leininger (Ed.), *Caring: An essential human need*. Thorofare, NJ: Slack.

Roach, S. (1984). *Caring: The human mode of being, implications for nursing*. Toronto, Canada: Faculty of Nursing, University of Toronto.

Roach, S. (1987). *The human act of caring*. Ottawa, Canada: Canadian Hospital Association.

Sherwood, G. D. (1997). Metasynthesis of qualitative analysis of caring. *Advanced Practice Nursing Quarterly, 3*, 32–42.

Smith, M. C. (1999). Caring and the science of unitary human beings. *Advances in Nursing Science, 21*(4), 14–28.

Strauss, A., & Corbin, J. (1998). *Basics of qualitative research: Techniques and procedures for developing grounded theory*. Thousand Oaks, CA: Sage.

Swanson, K. M. (1999). What's known about caring in nursing: A literary meta-analysis. In A. S. Hinshaw, J. Shaver, & S. Feetham (Eds.), *Handbook of clinical nursing research* (pp. 31–60). Thousand Oaks, CA: Sage.

Walker, L. O., & Avant, K. C. (2005). *Strategies for theory construction in nursing*. Upper Saddle River, NJ: Pearson/Prentice Hall.

Watson, J. (1985). *Nursing: Human science and human care, a theory of nursing*. Norwalk, CT: Appleton-Century-Crofts.

Watson, J. (2012). *Human caring science: A theory of nursing* (2nd ed.). Sudbury, MA: Jones and Bartlett Learning.

Wolf, Z. R., Giardino, E. R., Osborne, P. A., & Ambrose, M. S. (1994). Dimensions of nurse caring. *Image: Journal of Nursing Scholarship, 26*(2), 107–111.

Wolf, Z. R. (1986). The caring concept and nurse identified caring behaviors. *Topics in Clinical Nursing, 8*(2), 84–93.

Wu, Y., Larrabee, J. H., & Putman, H. P. (2006). Caring behaviors inventory: A reduction of the 42-item instrument. *Nursing Research, 55,* 18–25.

1

Concepts of Caring and Caring as a Concept

Janice M. Morse, Shirley M. Solberg, Wendy L. Neander,
Joan L. Bottorff, and Joy L. Johnson

*I*f caring is to be retained as the "essence" of nursing, and if research in this area is to advance, then the various perspectives of caring must be clarified, the strengths and the limitations of these conceptualizations examined, and the applicability of caring as a concept and theory to the practice of nursing identified. Examination of the concept of caring resulted in the identification of the following five epistemological perspectives: caring as a human state, caring as a moral imperative or ideal, caring as an affect, caring as an interpersonal relationship, and caring as a nursing intervention. The following two outcomes of caring were identified: caring as the subjective experience and as the physiologic responses in patients. The authors concluded that knowledge development related to caring in nursing is limited by the lack of refinement of caring theory, the lack of definitions of caring attributes, the neglect to examine caring from the dialectic perspective, and the focus of theorists and researchers on the nurse to the exclusion of the patient.

In the past decade, nurse theorists have identified caring as a paradigm unique to nursing. Caring has been described as the "core"[1] or the "essence" of nursing.[2–5] There is no doubt that as a concept, caring

has had a profound influence on nursing philosophy, education, and research. Literature expounding on the nature of caring and its implication for practice is rapidly increasing. Recognizing the complexity and significance of the concepts of care and caring, groups of scholars, such as those at the Center for Human Caring at the University of Colorado Health Science Center, have concentrated research efforts on exploring the nature of caring and its relationship to and ramifications for the profession. Moreover, annual conferences and think tanks, such as the one sponsored by the American Academy of Nursing and Sigma Theta Tau in 1989, have focused on this topic.

Despite these efforts, caring as a concept remains elusive. At this time, instead of enlightening the reader, examination of the literature only increases confusion. There is no consensus regarding the definitions of caring, the components of care, or the process of caring. Articles frequently appear repetitive without contributing further information, and different perspectives appear contradictory. Furthermore, in nursing, authors have not debated, commented on, or analyzed these different meanings and perspectives associated with

This research was supported by the National Center for Nursing Research (NIH), No. R01 NR02130-01, and by a Medical Research Council/National Health Research Development Program Award (Canada) to Dr J. Morse.

From Morse, J. M., Solberg, S., Neander, W. L., Bottorff, J. L., & Johnson, J. L. (1990). Concepts of caring and caring as a concept. *Advances in Nursing Science, 13*(1), 1–14. Permission to reprint granted by Wolters Kluwer.

the term *caring*. From the literature, it is difficult to discern the differences between the terms *caring*, *care*, and *nursing care*. Some of the diversity in these perspectives comes from the use of care as a noun or caring as a verb. Care or caring may specify the actions performed, as in *to take care of*, or the concern exhibited, as in *caring about*, the former having a more specific sense and the latter a more general one.[6] It is also possible that in a given situation, the word "care" may encompass both meanings, as was the case in some of the conceptualizations reviewed in this chapter. To make this review as comprehensive as possible, all of these usages were included. Clearly, it is imperative that if *caring* is to be retained as the essence of nursing and if research in this area is to advance, then these various perspectives of caring must be clarified and the strengths and the limitations of the conceptualizations must be identified. Therefore, the purpose of this chapter is to discuss the various conceptualizations of caring, to explore the adequacies and inadequacies of these conceptualizations, to evaluate the applicability of caring as a concept to the practice of nursing, and to identify trends and gaps in caring research. It is hoped that examining the literature will raise questions that will facilitate and stimulate debate among nurse scholars pertaining to these conceptualizations of care and caring.

PERSPECTIVES OF CARING

Confining the review to the nursing literature, the researchers identified 35 authors' definitions of caring and the main characteristics of their perspectives. Content analysis of these 35 authors who either explicitly or implicitly defined caring revealed five perspectives on the nature of caring. Of these definitions, the conceptualizations of 25 authors are organized, not according to the major focus of their theory but rather according to the basis from which their perspective was derived.

When caring was not explicitly defined, theoretic perspectives were identified and classified from the examination of research approaches and their underlying assumptions. For example, Stevenson[7] reviewed the quantitative literature and sampled all nursing articles that used *care* in the title, thus implying that care is inherent in all nursing procedures. On the other hand, Aamodt[8,9] explored care from the patient's perspective, implying that care is a concept that is reflected in nursing behaviors and is recognizable by the patient. When the conceptualization of caring was described as a process, the explicit or implied linkages are shown with arrows (Figure 1.1). Some theorists did not view the concept as a process. For example, Forrest[10] and Fanslow[11] view caring as an affect, do not consider outcomes, and therefore remain within that category. The categories are not intended as rigid or inflexible cells, nor is any value judgment intended as to the appropriateness or inappropriateness of the derivations of the conceptualizations. They are merely identified to clarify aspects inherent in the complexity of the literature rather than to imply causal relationships.

The five categories of caring identified were caring as a human trait, caring as a moral imperative or ideal, caring as an affect, caring as an interpersonal relationship, and caring as a therapeutic intervention. In addition to these, two outcomes that were identified were caring as the subjective experience of the patient and caring as a physical response (Figure 1.1). In each case, the decision to classify a definition was based on the theorist's epistemological perspective. If the theorist viewed caring as a process and described the means and outcomes of caring or the changing nature of the caring relationship, then these pathways linking categories were shown (Figure 1.1). For example, Leininger[3–5,12–17] reiterates that humans are caring beings and that caring is a universal trait vital to human survival; therefore, this definition was categorized with those

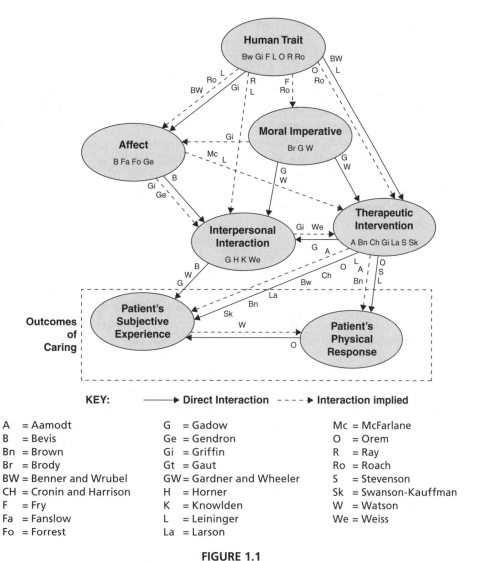

FIGURE 1.1

The interrelationship of five perspectives of caring.

who purported that caring is a human trait. The examples of care constructs identified by Leininger are behavioral attributes representative of caring; consequently, her definition of caring extends from the human-trait category to "the direct (or indirect) nurturant and skillful activities related to assisting people"[4](p. 4) or the therapeutic intervention category.

Caring as a Human Trait

From this perspective, caring is an innate human trait, the "human mode of being,"[18](p. 2) a part of human nature, and essential to human existence.[5,16] Although all humans have the potential to care, this ability is not uniform. Roach[18] suggests that one's own experience in being cared for and expressing caring influences one's ability to care. The nurse's educational experience professionalizes this caring through the acquisition of knowledge and skills. Despite this assertion that one's ability to care is influenced by life experiences in being cared for and in expressing caring, research that verifies this by examining the early experiences of nurses has yet to test this relationship. Alternatively, Leininger states that diverse expressions, meanings, patterns, and modalities of caring are culturally derived.[5] Attributes of professional caring, such as Roach's[18] dimensions of compassion, competence, confidence, conscience, and commitment, or Leininger's 55 carative constructs, are derived from or have their locus in caring. According to these definitions, the human trait of caring is the motivator of nursing actions.

Benner and Wrubel[19] concur that caring is the "basic way of being in the world"[19(p. 398)] from which all nursing practice evolves. They agree that one's ability to care is enhanced by learning and that differences in nursing practice reflect different levels of expertise in understanding the meaning of the patients' experiences of health and illness. Similarly, Griffin[20] views caring (and Orem[6] considers self-care) as a human trait underlying nursing practice. However, Orem[6] believes that caring consists of actions by others, which become necessary when self-care requirements cannot be met.

The universal concept of care is extended by Ray,[21–24] who examines the human aspects of caring in the context of bureaucratic hospital organizations. Because all cultures have developed social organizations to some degree, this description of caring is universally apropos. Ray's description of care encompasses a synthesis among political, economical, legal, and technological aspects as well as humanistic dimensions of caring. As such, this theory of "bureaucratic caring" has implications that extend beyond the nursing profession.

Caring as a Moral Imperative or Ideal

Authors in this category describe caring as a "fundamental value" or moral ideal in nursing.[1,25–29] For example, Gadow[28] and Watson[1,29] suggest that the substantive base of nursing is preserving the dignity of patients. From this perspective, caring is not manifest as "a set of identifiable behaviors,"[26(p. 48)] images, or traits evident in the caring nurse (e.g., sympathy, tenderness, or support[28]) nor does it encompass all that nurses *do*. Rather, caring is the adherence to the commitment of maintaining the individual's dignity or integrity. In contrast to Gadow's[28] realistic and attainable view for praxis, Watson suggests that caring actions revealed in the nurse–patient encounter are merely "approximations of caring" and not a "pure form of caring."[29(p. 34)] According to Watson, caring remains an unattainable ideal.

Nevertheless, in agreement with the theorists who adhere to the human-trait perspective, theorists who describe caring as a moral imperative concur that caring provides the basis for all nursing actions. Thus, the environment in which nurses work must facilitate and support caring. Paradoxically, nurses are caught in a dilemma created by a mandate to care in a society that does not value caring.[30] Nurses are expected to care for others as a duty (i.e., to be altruistic), yet they are unable to exercise their right to control their own practice (i.e., without professional autonomy). Fry[26] notes that if, as a profession, nursing holds caring as a moral ideal and present working conditions increasingly limit the opportunity to care (e.g., unsafe staffing conditions persist), then the survival of the nursing profession remains in question.

Caring as an Affect

The authors who define caring as an affect emphasize that the nature of caring extends from emotional involvement with or an empathetic feeling for the patient experience.[10,11,31–34] For example, McFarlane[34(p. 189)] states that caring "signifies a feeling of concern, of interest, of oversight with a view to protection." Bevis[32] considers caring to be a feeling of dedication, a feeling that motivates nursing actions. It is a response that is primarily focused on increasing intimacy between the nurse and the patient, which in turn enhances mutual self-actualization and consists of the following four developmental stages: attachment, assiduity, intimacy, and confirmation, each with its own tasks to be accomplished. Without successful progression through each stage, caring does not take place; instead, it becomes "warped, non-functional or stagnant" and it becomes distorted, changed, and "no longer caring."[32(p. 51)] From the perspective of caring as an affect (reflecting nursing as a female profession with historical roots in religion[35]), the nurse is moved to act selflessly without immediate gratification or expectation of material reward.[32] The personal vulnerability of the nurse who becomes involved with a patient or patient's family as a result of an empathetic identification with the patient's experience can be potentially damaging to the nurse, but support and recognition from colleagues may alleviate personal frustrations and maintain the nurse's ability to care.[10,19]

Unfortunately, the affectual nature of caring may be jeopardized or devalued in some situations. For example, constraints on nursing time (e.g., the increased demand for technical skills), technological demands (e.g., the distraction of monitors),[11] and unattractive patient characteristics (e.g., rejecting or unresponsive behaviors)[36] may inhibit the development of a caring feeling toward the patient. Furthermore, institutional incentive for the nurse to care is lacking, and professional socialization to remain objective, such as warnings not to get "too involved" with patients, continues to contribute to the devaluation of the importance of caring as an affect in nursing.

Caring as the Nurse–Patient Interpersonal Relationship

In contrast to those who view the caring relationship between the nurse and the patient as the foundation of human caring or the medium through which it is expressed, authors who believe caring is an interpersonal relationship suggested that the nurse–patient relationship *is* the essence of caring.[37–40] Those with this perspective believe the interaction between the nurse and the patient both expresses and defines caring. Caring encompasses both the feeling and the behaviors occurring within the relationship.[39] For example, the relationship (i.e., feeling) and content (i.e., behavior) of caring include aspects such as "showing concern" and "health teaching."[37] Alternatively, these may be manifested in the supportive relationships that nurses have with their patients.[38]

Caring as a Therapeutic Intervention

By defining specific nursing interventions or therapeutics as caring[7,41–48] or by describing conditions as necessary for caring actions,[43] these theorists have linked caring more directly than others to the work of nurses. Caring actions may be specific, such as attentive listening, patient teaching, patient advocacy, touch, "being there," and technical competence,[41,44,46–48] or caring may include all nursing actions (i.e., all nursing procedures or interventions[7]) that enable or assist patients.[45] Emphasis is placed on the necessity for adequate knowledge and skill as a basis for these caring actions as well as on the congruence between nursing actions and the patient's perception of need.

Several researchers obtained patients' perceptions of the importance of preselected nursing behaviors and interventions in relation to being cared for,[42,44,45] implying that these nursing behaviors and interventions are caring. Two investigations[41,42] included an open-ended question asking patients to describe situations in which they felt cared for. These data were used to verify the "caringness" of interventions included in the questionnaire rather than to define caring per se.

On the other hand, several authors have focused on the patient as the authority who determines what caring interventions are. It is the patient who defines caring and the components of caring, thus enabling the researcher to delineate the concept of care.[8,9,49–54] This type of research permits patients to identify indicators of nurses' caring behaviors, to recognize qualities of caring, and to report their caring needs, thus providing another way of eliciting appropriate nursing interventions that signify caring. For instance, researchers have noted that patients repeatedly report that they feel cared for when they are treated as individuals, when they receive help in dealing with their illness experiences, when nurses anticipate their needs, when they believe that nurses are available, and when nurses appear relaxed and confident.[41,42,50,51,54] Despite this, comparisons of the patients' and the nurses' perceptions of care reveal discrepancies between the two perspectives and identify different, significant caring behaviors, with patients focusing on instrumental behaviors of nursing practice and the nurses focusing on involvement and the affectual or expressive aspects of caring actions. Recognizing the incongruity between these perspectives adds credence to the significance of considering patient satisfaction and goals in the preparation of care plans.[44,45] But at the same time, these discrepancies may be expected, as patients may not be aware of all of the nurses' intentions underlying nursing actions.

OUTCOMES OF CARE AND CARING

Rather than studying the concept of care and caring, some researchers have examined the concept of care by exploring patient physiologic or psychologic outcomes. This perspective is primarily used by those researchers who focus on quality assurance and use physiologic outcomes as indicators of care (e.g., injuries from patient falls). For example, these outcomes may be the level of care, determined using selected statistical indices, such as morbidity and mortality statistics, length of stay (hospitalization), or the number of patient-incident reports, thus removing the indicators of care to the group level. Alternatively, researchers and auditors may use a physical examination to observe for the absence of indicators of poor care, such as skin conditions (decubitus and abrasions), poor muscle tone, or even the patient's state of hygiene to ensure that an individual patient has been cared for. Attempts are now being made to include patients' subjective responses to care as part of quality assurance programs.

THEORIES OF CARE AND CARING FOR NURSING

Thus far, three major theories of caring have been developed for nursing. The first is Orem's[6,55] Self-Care Deficit Theory of Nursing. It includes three interrelated theories of self-care deficit, self-care, and nursing systems. Assuming that human beings need "continuous self-maintenance and self-regulation"[6(p. 39)] through actions referred to as "self-care"[6(p. 39)] and that their ability to meet this need can vary, caregivers may be required to perform specific actions to assist patients in meeting their self-care requisites when they are unable to do so themselves. The main caring functions identified by Orem are part of a "helping system"[6(p. 149)] and include doing for or acting for another, guiding another, supporting another (physically and psychologically), providing environmental conditions that support personal development, and teaching.[6] However, the values inherent in this self-care theory reflect those of western society and may not be appropriate in other societies, including multicultural ones.[56,57]

The second caring theory, the Theory of Human Caring, developed by

Watson[1,29,58] explicates the kind of relationships and transactions that are necessary between the caregiver and care receiver to promote and to protect the patient's humanity, thereby influencing the patient's healing potential. In describing the processes involved in caring as well as the outcomes of care, Watson[1,29] emphasizes the psychological, emotional, and spiritual dimensions of care—almost to the exclusion of other characteristics of everyday tasks inherent in nursing care, such as bathing or procedures involving technical expertise. Combinations of interventions related to the process of human care are presented as carative factors (e.g., a "humanistic altruistic system of values"[1(p. 9)] and "installation of faith-hope"[1(p. 75)]) that are enacted in the context of the caring relationship.

Several questions arise regarding Watson's[1,29,58] theory. First, there is a broad gap between the nurse caring process and the clinical reality, and some authors have suggested that this gap reduces clinical relevance.[59] Second, the depth of the nurse–patient relationship required in Watson's theory may be impossible to attain in many nursing situations in which the length of hospitalization is short, the nurse–patient contact is brief (as with minor surgical admissions), or the patients are unable to interact with the nurses (as in the case of unconscious or cognitively impaired patients). Third, if this theory accurately describes caring in nursing, and one of nursing's major responsibilities is to care, then one may question whether nurses are really nursing in situations when the caring relationship has not developed. Finally, it is difficult to discern a unique caring role for nurses on the basis of this theory. As Ryan points out, "not all human caring is nursing."[60(p. 243)] Thus, the theory may also be useful to other professionals involved in caring, such as psychologists, theologians, and social workers.

The third theory, Leininger's[3,12,13] Theory of Transcultural Care Diversity and Universality, has matured from a static taxonomy of caring constructs to a theory that predicts culturally specific "nursing care actions"[5(p. 212)] that are beneficial to and congruent with the client's expectations and beliefs.[61] Although some of the care "patterns, processes and acts"[5(p. 210)] may be universal, cultural diversity, human variation, and ecologic variation result in some "care diversities."[5(p. 210)] Three nursing care actions—maintenance, negotiation, and restructuring—assist the client to change health, life patterns, or "life ways."[5(p. 209)] Leininger's[5,61] Sunrise Model is intended as a "wholistic conceptualization to help the researcher systematically study the theory's diverse components."[61(p. 157)] As yet, the theory is described in general abstract terms (e.g., "cultural care preservation/maintenance" or "assistive, supportive or enabling professional actions and decisions"[61(p. 156)]) that encompass a broad range of undelineated nursing activities.[61] Leininger[61] calls for further research to identify these nursing actions and decisions and to explore their conditions and consequences. Nevertheless, Leininger's Theory of Transcultural Care Diversity and Universality has alerted nurses to the need to consider cultural values and practices that influence patterns and meanings of care, and this contribution is significant.

PROCESS OF CARING

Although the authors have been classified, into the above categories on the basis of the primary emphasis they have given to caring, many have also drawn links to other categories. Other authors have described caring as a process that moves from one of the categories in Figure 1.1 to another and not as a process that changes within an identified category. For example, Leininger, who views caring as a human trait that motivates caring actions, links her ideas concerning caring to the categories of therapeutic interventions and the patient's subjective experience. On the other hand, on the basis of an ethical foundation, Gadow[28] draws implications for caring in nurse–patient interactions using the nursing actions of truth telling and touch and links the moral imperative to therapeutic intervention. In other words, the subjective (rather than the objective) interaction between the nurse and the patient results in a change in the patient's subjective experience. Watson's[29] theory fits into the moral imperative category, and as she sees the nurse–patient relationship and how this affects health and healing, her theory is also linked to the interpersonal relationship category. Again this extends to the patient's subjective experience, "restoring inner harmony and potential healing"[29(p. 58)] of the patient.

Many of these linkages are ill-defined or implicit rather than clearly described. These implied linkages are shown in Figure 1.1 as broken-line arrows. Using these inferences, the outcome of caring in nursing is a change in the patient's physical and psychological experience through nursing actions and work. However, these linkages are often tenuous and need further development.

CARING AS A UNIFORM STATE

Is caring a constant and uniform characteristic, or may caring be present in various degrees within individuals? To date, some authors have described caring as an ideal and an affect that makes nursing tasks humanistic. It is an emotion that motivates nurses to act and is an essential component of a good nurse. Although the authors who claim that caring is a human trait note that caring is present in all humans, they imply that nurses should be more caring than non-nurses. Alternatively, nurses may manifest their caring in different ways from non-nurses, and this assumption is reflected by authors who attempt to differentiate professional nurse caring from lay or "natural" caring.[18,33,62,63]

Researchers who view caring as an interpersonal interaction consider that a caring mode of interacting may be learned through instruction in counseling techniques, by modeling, or by trial and error in the clinical setting.[37,62] Consequently, if caring is conceived to be learnable, then caring skills can be acquired, practiced, perfected, demonstrated, and taught. When applied to caring, this implies that caring will be evident in various skill levels, and nurses will exhibit varying abilities or levels of caring.

On the other hand, when considering caring as a moral imperative, caring becomes a constant, an obligation to care for the patient according to patient needs, regardless of the nurses' experience or abilities or the patient characteristics or patient receptivity. The implication is that patients with similar needs are cared for equally, that nurses do not lavish more care on one patient than another; each is cared for in turn.

Still there is little evidence that caring is a uniform state. We know from the reports of burnout theory that without sabbaticals, caring as an emotional state may dissipate.[64] Is this because the caring affect may be depleted? Or is it because the nurse's personal needs for emotional protection take precedence over the human trait of caring for others? If caring is viewed as a therapeutic intervention, then physical exhaustion may reduce the nurse's ability to continue to provide care. Yet the relationship between caring theory and the concept of burnout continues to be queried,[19] and rather than approaching it from a dialectic perspective by examining uncaring or careless encounters, researchers continue, with few exceptions,[50,52] to examine caring in caring situations.

From their clinical practice, the authors know that nurses do not use the same caring behaviors with all patients;

instead, they use different styles of interactions with different patients. The process of assessment and of styles of care is poorly understood outside the context of counseling. Nurses have the ability to adjust their approach and their style of interaction as they move from patient to patient, altering not only the nature of dialogue and the tone of voice to meet each patient's needs, but also adjusting their affective response. For example, to the patient who is perceived to be suffering, the nurse's tone may be quiet and empathetic; to the confused patient, directive or persuasive; to the patient experiencing chronic pain, encouraging; and so forth. Moreover, to the depressed patient who is beginning to respond, the nurse may be teasing, or to the young orthopedic patient, the nurse may be authoritarian. Delineation of these behaviors would be a significant contribution, yet to date these styles of care have not been explored.

THE FOCUS OF CARE

It is the authors' opinion, albeit often implicit, that the ultimate outcome of caring is to alter patient responses. Those theorists who have explicitly extended this caring to the patient largely focus on the patient's subjective experience and, with the exception of Orem[6] and Stevenson,[7] do not include the patient's physical responses (Figure 1.1). Others who consider outcomes have used global indices, such as health[61] and well-being.[29] Yet, if the goal is changing patient outcomes, then why is the theoretic link from nurse caring to the patient outcome inexplicit and often tenuous? In particular, among those theorists who perceive caring to be an affect, little attention is given to the patient; research efforts focus on the nurse. For example, research may be conducted from this perspective to develop scales to measure nurses' propensity to care or to predetermine nurse caring behaviors.[41,42,44–46] Such approaches may have only limited usefulness in

nursing, especially given the evidence for the patient's low valuing of the nurses' affect.[44,45] It is apparent that the concept of caring has not yet matured beyond the stage of adolescence; it is imperative that researchers mature and move forward to focus on the patient.

Many questions are yet to be answered about the therapeutic nature of caring. Can caring be nontherapeutic? Can a nurse care too much? There is evidence that a nurse may become overinvolved with a patient so that the nurse's commitment to the patient as a person takes precedence over the nurse's commitment to the patient's treatment goals.[65] Consequently, the nurse may serve to assist the patient to bend or to break institutional rules or to avoid therapy, which, from a curative perspective, is not in the patient's best interests. Alternatively, the nurse may relish a caring relationship and foster patient dependency to meet his or her own needs for caring, thus interfering with treatment goals that work toward patient autonomy and health. These unseemly aspects of the caring relationship have yet to be addressed by contemporary nurse theorists.

THE CONSEQUENCES OF CARING

It is unquestionable that caring has limited utility for meeting all patients' needs. Gadow writes, "it is not that caring will achieve a cure . . . it will not arrest pathology"[28(p. 31)]; and Leininger[5] notes that caring is a necessary but insufficient condition for cure. Yet, conversely, can a cure be realized without caring? Reflections on the efficacy of caring, on the health outcomes of caring actions, and, to take this one step further, on quantifying caring and communicating caring epidemiologically with morbidity and mortality, have not been attempted.

A related question is whether a nurse can provide safe practice without caring. Gadow[66,67] notes that sometimes it may be necessary to practice without care. It is paradoxical that for a nurse to care, he or she must be embodied and totally immersed in the patient's experience. Yet to inflict pain—an often necessary part of any procedure—the nurse must be disembodied from the pain experience. Paradoxically, while the nurse is in this state of disembodiment, the suffering patient is immersed in the experience, in a state of total embodiment. This introduces an important question as follows: If nurses must become detached from caring to perform pain-inducing nursing procedures, in other words, to nurse, how can caring retain its seminal, theoretic position as the essence of nursing?

Analysis of the concept of caring and the identification of the five conceptualizations of care are important. The breadth of these conceptualizations, whether caring is "only" an affect or whether caring may also encompass technical tasks (as in nursing care), is significant for the critics who have difficulty seeing the clinical relevance of caring as a concept[59] and who for that reason have rejected the concept of caring. Clearly, further conceptual development and refinement of caring are important. The first desperately needed step is to develop a clear conceptualization of caring that encompasses all aspects of nursing. Until this is accomplished, progress will be restricted.

The beginning move away from the exclusive development of nurse-focused theories of care to include patient-centered theory is significant. Until this move is developed—until patient outcomes of caring are considered—caring will remain an inadequate and only partially useful concept for nursing. Although caring has been called the glue that holds nursing together, at this time it does not appear to have the pragmatic implications necessary for the practice of nursing per se. In addition, none of the authors

suggested or developed a model that includes caring as a minor component. It was always suggested that other constructs (e.g., Leininger's[16] care constructs and Watson's[1,58] carative factors) might be a part of caring, not the reverse. Caring as a component of a more encompassing construct, such as comfort, may be a perspective worthy of consideration.

In a closely related step, the focus of theory and research must shift to incorporate a focus on the patient, asking, "What difference does caring make to the patient?" If caring changes the course of illness for the patient, then the concept may be useful enough to retain its lofty position as the "essence of nursing." If the question cannot be answered or if a negative answer is forthcoming (i.e., a careless nurse can still provide satisfactory care—even in some conditions), then the concept of care is inappropriate or inadequate to stand alone as the central or encompassing theory for nursing.

As distressing as removing caring as the central paradigm may seem, caring may not be totally discarded. Even if caring is the main ingredient that makes nursing humanistic, what else is essential to nursing? Clues are emerging as qualitative research increases and as patients' "stories" or case studies, such as those now published in the *American Journal of Nursing*,[68] become increasingly available. Thus far, this material has not contributed to the theory development beyond Benner's[69] concept of the expert nurse, and inductive theory development from these case histories is sorely needed. This approach can complement the ongoing philosophic inquiry.

Of special concern, discrepancies remain among the various conceptualizations of care, especially between those who view caring as an interaction process and those who view care as an intervention. The bedside nurses must contend with the crosscurrents of these two divergent concepts of care competing for their allegiance. Thus, the administrator's goal is to achieve the tasks of nursing as efficiently (i.e., quickly) and as economically (i.e., with minimal staff) as possible. It is clear that tension may develop between these administrators and nurses who value caring as an interpersonal interaction. Administrators seek to control nursing actions, to limit caring time, and to require concrete, measurable outcomes to justify their actions, while nurses beg for time for caring tasks (e.g., listening to the patient's concerns) that do not have solid, quantifiable outcomes other than patient satisfaction. Even in their own arena, the bedside nurses do not have professional control of their own practice[11,26]; consequently, they may be forced to resort to deviant and defiant behaviors to maintain minimum staffing levels and a safe and caring practice.

Finally, although the divergent perspectives of care and caring as described by the nurse theorists provide eclectic and diverse conceptualizations that strengthen the concept, further development is needed. Meanwhile, it is imperative that conceptualizations and theories of care and caring must be debated, queried, and clarified so that the concept, when developed, will be applicable to the art and science of nursing.

REFERENCES

1. Watson, J. (1988). *Nursing: Human science and human care a theory of nursing.* New York, NY: NLN.
2. Leininger, M. M. (1978). Transcultural nursing: A new and scientific subfield of study in nursing. In M. M. Leininger (Ed.), *Transcultural nursing: Concepts, theories and practices.* Thorofare, NJ: Slack.
3. Leininger, M. M. (1978). Transcultural nursing theories and research approaches. In M. M. Leininger (Ed.), *Transcultural nursing: Concepts, theories and practices.* Thorofare, NJ: Slack.
4. Leininger, M. M. (1984). Care: The essence of nursing and health. In M. M. Leininger (Ed.), *Care: The essence of nursing and health.* Thorofare, NJ: Slack.
5. Leininger, M. M. (1985). Transcultural care diversity and universality: A theory of nursing. *Nursing Health Care, 6*(4), 209–212.
6. Orem, D. E. (1985). *Nursing: Concepts of practice* (3rd ed.). Chevy Chase, MD: McGraw-Hill.
7. Stevenson, J. (1990). A review of the quantitative literature on care. In J. Stevenson & T. Tripp-Reimer (Eds.), *Knowledge about care and caring: State of the art and future development.* Kansas City, MO: American Academy of Nursing.
8. Aamodt, A. M. (1984). Themes and issues in conceptualizing care. In M. M. Leininger (Ed.), *Care: The essence of nursing and health.* Thorofare, NJ: Slack.
9. Aamodt, A. M. (1989). Ethnography and epistemology: Generating nursing knowledge. In J. M. Morse (Ed.), *Qualitative nursing research: A contemporary dialogue.* Rockville, MD: Aspen Publishers.
10. Forrest, D. (1989). The experience of caring. *Journal of Advanced Nursing, 14,* 815–823.
11. Fanslow, J. (1987). Compassionate nursing care: Is it a lost art? *The Journal of Practical Nursing, 37*(2), 40–43.
12. Leininger, M. M. (1981). The phenomenon of caring: Importance, research questions and theoretical considerations. In M. M. Leininger (Ed.), *Caring. An essential human need. Proceedings of three national caring conferences.* Thorofare, NJ: Slack.
13. Leininger, M. M. (1981). Cross-cultural hypothetical functions of caring and nursing care. In M. M. Leininger (Ed.), *Caring. An essential human need. Proceedings of three national caring conferences.* Thorofare, NJ: Slack.
14. Leininger, M. M. (1984). Caring: A central focus on nursing and health care services. In M. M. Leininger (Ed.), *Care: The essence of nursing and health.* Thorofare, NJ: Slack.
15. Leininger, M. M. (1984). Caring is nursing: Understanding the meaning, importance, and issues. In M. M. Leininger (Ed.), *Care: The essence of nursing and health.* Thorofare, NJ: Slack.
16. Leininger, M. M. (1988). History, issues, and trends in the discovery and uses of care in nursing. In M. M. Leininger (Ed.), *Care. discovery and uses in clinical and community nursing.* Thorofare, NJ: Slack.
17. Leininger, M. M. (1981). Some philosophical, historical, and taxonomic aspects of nursing and caring in American Culture. In M. M. Leininger (Ed.), *Caring. An essential human need. Proceedings of three national caring conferences.* Thorofare, NJ: Slack.
18. Roach, M. S. (1987). *The human act of caring: A blueprint for health professions.* Toronto, Ontario: Canadian Hospital Association.

19. Benner, P., & Wrubel, J. (1989). *The primacy of caring: Stress and coping in health and illness.* Menlo Park, CA: Addison Wesley.

20. Griffin, A. P. (1983). A philosophical analysis of caring in nursing. *Journal of Advanced Nursing, 8,* 289–295.

21. Ray, M. A. (1984). The development of a classification system of institutional caring. In M. M. Leininger (Ed.), *Caring. The essence of nursing and health.* Thorofare, NJ: Slack.

22. Ray, M. A. (1987). Health care economics and human caring in nursing: Why the moral conflict must be resolved. *Family and Community Health, 10*(1), 35–43.

23. Ray, M. A. (1987). Technological caring: A new model in critical care. *Dimensions of Critical Care Nursing, 6*(3), 166–173.

24. Ray, M. A. (1989). The theory of bureaucratic caring for nursing practice in the organizational culture. *Nursing Administration Quarterly, 13*(2), 31–42.

25. Brody, J. K. (1988). Virtue ethics, caring, and nursing. *Scholarly Inquiry for Nursing Practice, 2*(2), 87–101.

26. Fry, S. T. (1988). The ethic of caring: Can it survive in nursing? *Nursing Outlook, 36*(1), 48.

27. Fry, S. T. (1989). Toward a theory of nursing ethics. *ANS, 11*(4), 9–22.

28. Gadow, S. A. (1985). Nurse and patient: The caring relationship. In A. H. Bishop & J. R. Scudder (Eds.), *Caring, curing, coping.* Birmingham: University of Alabama Press.

29. Watson, J. (1985). *Nursing: Human science and human care, A theory of nursing.* Norwalk, CT: Appleton-Century-Crofts.

30. Reverby, S. A. (1987). Caring dilemma: Womanhood and nursing in historical perspective. *Nursing Research, 36*(1), 5–11.

31. Bevis, E. O. (1978). *Curriculum building in nursing: A Process* (2nd ed.). St Louis, MO: Mosby.

32. Bevis, E. O. (1981). Caring: A life force. In M. M. Leininger (Ed.), *Caring: An essential human need. Proceedings of three national caring conferences.* Thorofare, NJ: Slack.

33. Gendron, D. (1988). *The expressive form of caring.* Toronto, Ontario, Canada: University of Toronto.

34. McFarlane, J. (1976). A charter for caring. *Journal of Advanced Nursing, 1,* 187–196.

35. Kalisch, P. A., & Kalisch, B. J. (1986). *The advance of American nursing* (2nd ed.). Boston, MA: Little, Brown.

36. Kahn, D. L., & Steeves, R. H. (1988). Caring and practice: Construction of the nurse's world. *Scholarly Inquiry for Nursing Practice, 2*(3), 201–216.

37. Knowlden, V. (1988). Nurse caring as constructed knowledge. In *Caring and nursing explorations in the feminist perspectives.* Denver, CO: School of Nursing, University of Colorado Health Sciences Center.

38. Gardner, K. G., & Wheeler, E. C. (1981). The meaning of caring in the context of nursing. In M. M. Leininger, (Ed.), *Caring: An essential human need. Proceedings of three national caring conferences.* Thorofare, NJ: Slack.

39. Horner, S. (1988). Intersubjective co-presence in a caring model. In *Caring and nursing explorations in the feminist perspectives.* Denver, CO: School of Nursing, University of Colorado Health Sciences Center.

40. Weiss, C. J. (1988). Model to discover, validate, and use care in nursing. In M. M. Leininger, (Ed.), *Care. Discovery and uses in clinical and community nursing.* Detroit, MI: Wayne State University Press.

41. Brown, L. (1986). The experience of care: Patient perspectives. *Topics in Clinical Nursing, 8*(2), 56–62.

42. Cronin, S. N., & Harrison, B. (1988). Importance of nurse caring behaviors as perceived by patients after myocardial infarction. *Heart and Lung, 17*(4), 374–380.

43. Gaut, D. A. (1983). Development of a theoretically adequate description of caring. *Western Journal of Nursing Research, 5*(4), 13–324.

44. Larson, P. (1987). Comparison of cancer patients' and professional nurses' perceptions of important caring behaviors. *Heart and Lung, 16*(2), 187–193.

45. Mayer, D. K. (1986). Cancer patients' and families' perceptions of nurse caring behaviors. *Topics in Clinical Nursing, 8*(2), 63–69.

46. Peterson, B. H. (1985). A qualitative clinical account and analysis of a care situation. In M. M. Leininger, (Ed.), *Qualitative research methods in nursing.* New York, NY: Grune & Stratton.

47. Poulin, M. A. (1987). Leadership and the caring role. *IMPRINT, 34*(6), 51–56.

48. Wolf, Z. R. (1986). The caring concept and nurse identified caring behaviors. *Topics in Clinical Nursing, 8*(2), 84–93.

49. Clayton, G. M. (1989). Research testing Watson's theory. In J. Riehl-Sisca (Ed.), *Conceptual models for nursing practice* (3rd ed.). Norwalk, CT: Appleton & Lange.

50. Drew, N. (1986). Exclusion and confirmation: A phenomenology of patients' experiences with caregivers. *Image, 18*(2), 39–43.

51. Paternoster, J. (1988). How patients know that nurses care about them. *The Journal of the New York State Nurses Association, 19*(4), 17–21.

52. Riemen, D. J. (1986). Noncaring and caring in the clinical setting: Patients' descriptions. *Topics in Clinical Nursing, 8*(2), 0–36.

53. Swanson-Kauffman, K. M. (1986). Caring in the instance of unexpected early pregnancy loss. *Topics in Clinical Nursing, 8*(2), 37–46.

54. Swanson-Kauffman, K. M. (1988). Caring needs of women who miscarried. In M. M. Leininger (Ed.), *Care: Discovery and uses in clinical and community nursing.* Detroit, MI: Wayne State University Press.

55. Orem, D. E. (1971). *Nursing: Concepts of practice.* New York, NY: McGraw-Hill.

56. Fawcett, J. (1989). Orem's self-care framework. In J. Fawcett (Ed.), *Analysis and evaluation of conceptual models of nursing.* Philadelphia, PA: FA Davis.

57. Meleis, A. J. (1985). *Theoretical nursing: Development and progress.* Philadelphia, PA: JB Lippincott.

58. Watson, J. (1979). *Nursing: The philosophy and science of caring.* Boston, MA: Little, Brown.

59. Dunlop, M. J. (1986). Is a science of caring possible? *Journal of Advanced Nursing, 11,* 661–670.

60. Ryan, L. G. (1989). A critique of nursing: Human science and human care. In J. Riehl-Sisca (Ed.), *Conceptual models for nursing practice.* Norwalk, CT: Appleton & Lange.

61. Leininger, M. M. (1988). Leininger's theory of nursing: Cultural care diversity and universality. *Nursing Science Quarterly, 1,* 152–160.

62. Kitson, A. L. (1987). A comparative analysis of lay-caring and professional (nursing) caring relationships. *International Journal of Nursing Studies, 24*(2), 155–165.

63. Hernandez, C. G. (1988). A phenomenologic investigation of the concept of the lived experience of caring in professional nurses. In *Caring and nursing explorations in the feminist perspectives.* Denver, CO: School of Nursing, University of Colorado Health Sciences Center.

64. Maslach, C. (1982). *Burnout: The cost of caring.* Englewood Cliffs, NJ: Prentice Hall.

65. Morse, J. M. Involvement and commitment in the nurse–patient relationship. In review.

66. Gadow, S. A. (1988). Covenant without cure: Letting go and holding on in chronic illness. In J. Watson & M. A. Ray (Eds.), *The ethics of care and the ethics of cure: Synthesis in chronicity.* New York, NY: NLN.

67. Gadow, S. A. (1989). Clinical subjectivity. Advocacy with silent patients. *The Nursing Clinics of North America, 24,* 535–541.

68. Dyck, B. (1989). The paper crane. *The American Journal of Nursing, 89,* 824–825.

69. Benner, P. (1984). *From novice to expert: Excellence and power in clinical nursing practice.* Menlo Park, CA: Addison Wesley.

QUESTIONS FOR REFLECTION

Baccalaureate

1. What did Morse and colleagues confront as a difficulty as they searched the literature on caring in an effort to examine different conceptualizations of caring?

2. How many perspectives of caring did Morse et al. (1990) describe? List them.

3. What did you observe about caring as a core concept of nursing as you read Morse et al.'s (1990) chapter?

Master's

1. How is caring as a human trait explained by Morse et al. (1990)?

2. What is the meaning of caring as a moral imperative or ideal?

3. What was the importance of Morse et al.'s (1990) discussion of the outcomes of caring?

Doctoral

1. What were the critical points Morse et al. made about the caring theories they reviewed?

2. How might you answer the question posed by Morse et al. (1990) about whether caring can be therapeutic?

3. What does the analysis of concepts of caring and caring as a concept reveal in that the investigators (Morse et al., 1990) specified five conceptualizations of care?

2

Caring in Nursing: Analysis of Extant Theory

ANNE BOYKIN AND SAVINA SCHOENHOFER

Caring in nursing as a substantive area of nursing science has been the focus of considerable scholarly effort. Based on the assumption that caring is the central concept in nursing and is uniquely known and expressed in nursing, this chapter focuses on an analysis of major theoretical works related to the concept. Five categories of questions provide a framework for the analysis: ontological, anthropological, ontical, epistemological, and pedagogical.

Caring is a concept that is increasingly recognized as having central importance to nursing (Leininger, 1981; McBride, 1989; Roach, 1987; Watson, 1985). Considerable scholarly work to explicate the substantive contribution of the concept is being undertaken by nursing scholars (Gaut, 1984; Leininger, 1988; Parse, 1981; Ray, 1981; Roach, 1984, 1987; Watson, 1985). Illuminating caring in nursing, a complex phenomenon reflecting the richness of persons-in-relationship requires a multidimensional approach.

The purpose of this chapter is to analyze the theory about caring in nursing using the following categories of questions posed by Roach (1987); ontological, anthropological, ontical, epistemological, and pedagogical. Each of these categories comprises a section of the chapter. The first three categories, ontological, anthropological, and ontical, contribute to the analysis and integration of extant theory. The fourth and fifth categories, epistemological and pedagogical, guide the organization of substantive knowledge for purposes of teaching and learning.

ONTOLOGICAL

The ontological questions focusing on the "being" of caring are addressed by scholars in nursing and other disciplines. Caring may be understood as the human expression of respect for and response to wholeness, an active engagement in the person-to-person process of being and becoming.

Caring as an intrinsically human expression is powerfully conveyed in Roach's (1987) statement that "caring is the human mode or manifestation of being" (p. 45) and as such "entail(s) the capacity or power to care, a capacity linked with and inseparable from our nature as human beings" (p. 47). Roach's primary thesis is that caring is person-to-person recognition of intrinsic value and response to that value. She focuses on the recognition and response to the value of person as "important-in-itself," being both affected and responding affectively. The intrinsic value that persons reflect and to which they respond is the sanctity of persons, an ultimate metaphysical value that suggests a correspondence between the terms "wholeness" and

From Boykin, A., & Schoenhofer, S. (1990). Caring in nursing: Analysis of extant theory. *Nursing Science Quarterly, 3,* 149–155. Permission to reprint granted by Sage Publications, Inc.

"holiness." Both terms convey a sense of understanding of the body–mind–spirit and address the transcendent nature of being human.

Watson (1985) described caring as the "moral ideal of nursing" (p. 29), a moral commitment toward protection, enhancement, and preservation of human dignity. Watson's theory of human care addresses values associated with respect for the mystery of being-in-the-world and acknowledges the three spheres of being as mind–body–soul. The dimension of soul acknowledges the spiritual or inner self aspects, which are not bound by time and space.

Explicit in Watson's work is the idea that caring is an intersubjective human process. The ideal of intersubjectivity is based on a belief that "persons learn from one another how to be human by identifying ourselves with others or finding their dilemmas in ourselves" (Watson, 1985, p. 59). Through interpersonal human care transactions, there is a reciprocity between persons that allows for a unique and authentic quality of presence in the world of the other. The togetherness in the caring I–Thou encounter described by Buber (1970) facilitates spiritual growth, creates meaning for the experience, and potentiates transcendence.

Parse (1981) defines the ontology of caring as "risking being with someone toward a moment of joy" (p. 130). In this definition, the ideas of choice, authentic presence, and realization of meaning are brought together in relation to the human science theme of call and response. According to Parse (1981), the beingness is risking, which includes having the courage to be authentic in a situation. Through being with another, connectedness occurs and moments of joy are experienced by both the one caring and the one being cared for.

Although Paterson and Zderad (1988) did not elaborate directly on the topic of caring, their conceptualization of humanistic nursing conveys values and understanding similar to those of Roach, Watson, and Parse as they contribute to an ontology of caring. They acknowledge that nursing is not only concerned with well being but also with more being, becoming "more as humanly possible" in the particular life situation (Paterson and Zderad, 1988, p. 12). The authentic and active being within a nursing situation communicates connectedness and development of the "between" (Buber, 1970; Paterson and Zderad, 1988) in which nurturance occurs.

Mayeroff (1971) offers a substantial link between generic caring and caring as it is uniquely expressed in nursing. His description of caring as helping the other grow complements Watson's concept of intersubjective ideal. The essential concept here is the importance of viewing others as an extension of self and yet as independent, and needing to grow in special and unique ways. Mayeroff (1971) discussed the primacy of caring as process in contrast to caring as product, viewing caring as an end in itself and not merely a means to some future end. Certain "ingredients" of caring were described by Mayeroff (1971): knowing, alternating rhythm, patience, honesty, trust, humility, hope, and courage.

The being of caring as described by Roach (1984), Watson (1985), and Parse (1981), as well as by Paterson and Zderad (1988) and Mayeroff (1971), have common elements. Each stresses the importance of authentic presence and connectedness with the other. Caring in nursing is viewed as a mutual human process in which the nurse responds with authentic presence to a call from another.

Nursing is described by Roach as the professionalization of caring, and she states that "the affirmation of caring as the human mode of being is a presupposition for all the activities that are designed to develop the capacity to care professionally" (1987, p. 49). Roach (1984) stresses that an understanding of caring is integral to nursing and that ". . . without a focus on caring, reflections about nursing and their application to education, service, administration, and research would be analogous to spokes of a wheel deprived of both hub and rim—removed from focus, center, and identifiable boundaries" (p. 4).

Examination of extant theory leads to reflections on the ontological dimensions of caring in nursing. Understanding centers on valuing and celebrating human wholeness, the human person as being and becoming, and active personal engagement with others.

ANTHROPOLOGICAL

The anthropological category addresses the issue of what it means to be a caring person (Roach, 1987). In this context, being a caring person means engaging in the struggle to grow, being truly human, and creating meaning and order in life.

The meaning of being a caring person is reflected in the ongoing struggle of human experience. Although the capacity to care is innately human (Roach, 1987), this capacity may lie dormant. Roach (1987) postulates certain entailments of caring as the human mode of being: having the capacity or power to care, the calling forth of this capacity, responsivity to being called by someone/something who matters, actualization of the capacity to care, and performance of the ability through specific behavior (p. 55). Therefore, in actualizing the capacity to care through self-transcendence and self-donation, Roach (1987) says, "I live the meaning of my own life" (p. 56).

Watson (1985) made the point that the intersubjective process of caring preserves a common sense of humanity and even "teaches us how to be human by identifying ourselves with others" (p. 33), such that the humanity of one is reflected in the other. She notes that the most abstract response of a caring person is the ability to respond to a person as unique, or as Roach states as important-in-itself (1987, p. 55). The meaning of transpersonal caring includes moral commitment to a particular end, the intent and will to affirm the subjective significance

of the person, the ability to realize and assess another's being in the world, and to feel a union with another (p. 63). This is congruent with Roach's description of the entailment of being a caring person.

Watson (1985) discusses what it means to be a caring nurse, one who as coparticipant in the human care process, engages fully as an experiencing person in the process. Paterson and Zderad (1988) affirm that in offering authentic presence as the human mode of being, the nurse must choose to offer and that such choosing requires a belief in the value of presence.

Mayeroff (1971), relating how caring provides meaning and order, writes:

> In the context of a man's life, caring has a way of ordering his other values and activities around it. When this ordering is comprehensive, because of the inclusiveness of his caring, there is a basic stability in his life; he is "in place" in the world instead of being out of place, or merely drifting or endlessly seeking his place. Through caring for certain others, by serving them through caring a man lives the meaning of his own life. In the sense in which a man can ever be said to be at home in the world, he is at home not through dominating, or explaining, or appreciating, but through caring and being cared for. (p. 2)

Mayeroff (1971) expresses ideas about the meaning of being a caring person when he refers to the caring relationship being experienced as a trust, "being entrusted with the care of another" (p. 4). He speaks of both "being with" the other and "being for" (p. 31) the other, experiencing the other as an extension of self and at the same time "something separate from me that I respect in its own right" (p. 3). To be a caring person means "living the meaning of my own life" (p. 45), having a sense of stability and basic certainty which enables an openness and accessibility, experiencing belonging, living congruence between beliefs and behavior, and expressing a clarity of values which enables living a simplified rather than a cluttered life. Other aspects of personal meaning of caring include the sense that the process of life is enough, being at home in the world, and appreciating the unfathomable mystery of existence, having a sense of autonomy—being both free and responsible, and experiencing confidence in and gratitude for life (Mayeroff, 1971).

Leininger (1988), a forerunner in the care movement in nursing, speaks of care as the "essence of nursing and the central, dominant, and unifying feature of nursing" (p. 152). She focuses on cultural care differences and similarities as a theoretical basis for nursing practice. Care from Leininger's theory is determined through the emic views of the "meanings, symbols, patterns, and expressions of cultural care and nursing from a holistic perspective" (p. 153). Her anthropological finding that care is essential for human survival, growth, and development supports Roach's thesis of caring as the human mode of being.

With the exception of Leininger, there seems to be congruence among the various authors as to what it means to be a caring person. Leininger's works have provided significant insight into various cultural care practices. From her perspective, a caring person would implement actions "directed toward assisting, supporting, or enabling another individual (or group) with evident or anticipated needs to ameliorate or improve a human condition or lifeway" (1988, p. 156).

Watson (1985), Roach (1987), Paterson and Zderad (1988), and Mayeroff (1971) offer a more existential answer to the question posed. Living the meaning of one's life actualizes the capacity to be a caring person. As a person more fully experiences being-in-the-world, the ability to express caring behaviors with self and others is enhanced. Therefore, caring in nursing is an actualizing experience for the nurse as well as the client.

ONTICAL

The ontical category focuses on questions that address function and ethic, including normative statements or statements of obligation and facts in science and everyday life. Roach (1987) provides examples of ontical questions in relation to caring in nursing, such as "what is a nurse doing when she or he is caring" and "what obligations are entailed in caring" (p. 45). It now becomes increasingly apparent that these categories of questions are overlapping and assist in the holistic rather than reductionistic understanding of caring.

Roach finds that caring is the locus for rules, principles, and norms governing professional conduct. She points out that nurses do not deliberate whether to care, for care is the end of nursing, but rather how caring can best be accomplished (Roach, 1987). Attributes of caring include the following: compassion, competence, confidence, conscience, and commitment (Roach, 1987, p. 58).

Compassion is operationalized as participation in the experience of another while being fully immersed in the condition of being human (Roach, 1987). Watson (1985) describes the truly caring nurse as one who forms union with others that transcends the physical, preserving the subjectivity and physicality of persons without reducing them to objects (p. 68). The nurse, according to Watson, attends to the dignity of person as an important end, demonstrating respect for human life, and expressing nonpaternalistic values related to human autonomy and freedom of choice. These views complement Roach's description of compassion. Through compassion, an individual is freed up to fully experience his humaneness and interconnectedness.

Competence is expressed as having the knowledge, skill, energy, motivation, judgment, and experience necessary to respond appropriately to one's professional responsibilities (Roach, 1987). These competencies are humanized by compassion. Care and caring can be understood as action patterns that are helping and enabling (Gaut, 1984; Leininger, 1981).

Leininger (1981) stated that the relationship between the caregiver and recipient appears to be the heart of the therapeutic help. Based on her theory of transcultural nursing, Leininger (1988) asserts that what nurses do to provide care differs from culture to culture.

Caring enacted as confidence fosters a trusting relationship "without dependence, communicates truth without violence, and respect without paternalism, fear, or powerlessness" (Roach, 1987, p. 64). Confidence is an integrated action form of Mayeroff's caring ingredients of trust, hope, and courage. A nurse must have the confidence and competence as described by Roach to enter nursing situations in a meaningful way.

Conscience is recognized as directing one's behavior toward the "moral fitness of things" (Roach, 1987, p. 64). Conscience grows out of the experience of valuing. It is closely related to Mayeroff's caring ingredient of humility.

Commitment is a convergence between preference and choice that shows itself as devoted, conscious, willing, and positive action (Roach, 1987). Commitment is the embodiment of function and ethic. The caring nurse is living the personal commitment of service to humankind, sending forth through caring an affirmation of personhood within the rubric of the nursing relationship.

The works of Roach (1984, 1987), Watson (1985, 1987), and Leininger (1981, 1988) provide insight as to what a nurse is doing when he or she is caring. Roach and Watson find caring expressed through commitment, compassion, confidence, conscience, and competence. Leininger describes caring within nursing as actions which are helping or enabling, more directly addressing the specific obligation to be competent in transcultural knowledge.

EPISTEMOLOGICAL

Epistemological questions are concerned with the ways in which caring in nursing is known. Carper (1978) described patterns of knowing fundamental to nursing similar to Phenix's (1964) realms of meaning. Carper's patterns of knowing: personal, empirical, ethical, and esthetic, provide an organizing framework for asking the epistemological questions of caring in nursing. To experience in knowing the "whole" of a nursing situation with caring at the center, each of these patterns comes into play. Personal knowing focuses on knowing and encountering self and other, empirical knowing addresses the science of caring in nursing, ethical knowing focuses on what "ought to be" in nursing situations, and esthetic knowing is the integration and synthesis of all the patterns of knowing in relation to a particular situation. Through the richness of the knowledge gleened, the nurse as artist creates the caring moment.

In this section of the chapter, the epistemology of caring in nursing will be addressed within each of the four patterns of knowing.

Personal Knowing

The initial focus of understanding in any nursing situation would be on the personal and professional self of the nurse and personal knowing of the client. Paterson and Zderad (1988) state that for nursing practice to be humanistic, and therefore caring, awareness of self and others is essential. The importance of knowing self is integral to knowing others and to the "therapeutic use of self." Knowing self-caringly requires being able to objectively and subjectively experience self, feeling at one with self rather than estranged (Mayeroff, 1971).

Personal knowing requires that the one caring demonstrate humility, courage, and trust. Humility implies openness between people that makes the exchange of information unencumbered. One who cares is genuinely humble in being ready and willing to know more about self and others. Humility involves the realization that learning is continuous and the recognition that each experience is new and unique. The essence of humility is captured in the verse:

> If only
>
> I could throw away
>
> The urge
>
> To trace my patterns
>
> In your heart
>
> I could really see you. (Brandon, 1976, p. 47)

To know self and other requires authenticity or genuineness. Roach (1984) says that being for others is authentic if it results in freedom of others, and inauthentic if it is permeated by dominance and depersonalization. This freeing of self and others requires trust and courage. Mayeroff (1971) says that caring involves "trusting the other to grow in its own time and in its own way" (p. 20). The establishment of trust is essential to a therapeutic relationship and requires risk taking and courage. Trusting self implies confidence in judgments made and courage to learn from mistakes. Trusting others activates the person cared for to trust in his own growing and to justify the trust of the other (Mayeroff, 1971). Carper's description of personal knowing is congruent with Mayeroff's direct knowing. It is only through entering the interpersonal space of others that authentic knowing can occur. Buber (1970) speaks of this as the "between" that is common to both. The unfolding of this sphere is the dialogical. Meaning extracted from the dialogue is found neither in the one caring nor in the one cared for, not in both together, but in their interchange. This intense awareness rescues personal knowing lest the experience be cold and impersonal.

In a similar vein, Parse (1981) states that the "essence of a subject-to-subject experience originates in coexistence with others and is man's genuine presence with the interrelational" (p. 32). To elicit true meaning from nursing situations, the nurse and client must incur the risks required to know self and other. Personal knowing of both joy and risk contributes essential understanding of caring in nursing situations. Compassion is born out of "awareness of one's relationship to all living creatures; engendering a response of participation in the experience of another" (Roach, 1987, p. 20).

The use of personal knowing as an organizing structure to study nursing situations assists the learner to appreciate and respect the uniqueness of each person. Focusing on the meaning inherent in the particular situation fosters the compassion essential to I–Thou relationships and enhances the capacity to care in the one caring.

Empirical Knowing

Empirics, according to Phenix (1964), includes the sciences that study living things, the physical world, and man. The knowledge gleaned from these areas provides factual descriptions, principles, theoretical formulations, and explanations that are "based on observations and experiments in the world of matter, life, mind, and society" (Phenix, 1964, p. 6).

Empirical knowledge from nursing and related disciplines provides a theoretical basis for understanding the phenomenon of caring. The empirical knowledge base of caring in nursing is a rapidly developing area of nursing scholarship. For example, Leininger's (1988) theory of cultural care offers a framework for understanding the one being cared for. This theory can be used to understand cultural differences, cultural conflicts, and care in different cultures. It is also useful in generating research findings and structuring a component of the empirical knowledge base. Empirical knowing of caring in nursing is further enhanced by the research of scholars such as Ray on technological and bureaucratic caring (1987, 1988), Rieman on the structure of a caring interaction (1986), and Larson on nurse-caring behaviors and attributes (1987).

Mayeroff's (1971) caring ingredient of alternating rhythms offers a perspective for viewing the application of empirical knowing. Rhythm is involved as situations are studied from narrowing and then widening viewpoints. Through authentic presence, the nurse experiences the one being cared for from his world. With this personal knowing in place, the nurse detaches from the situation and reflects on the relevant empirical knowledge to enhance understanding of caring in the particular nursing situation. Competence on the part of the one caring is essential in order to extract relevant meaning from empirical generalizations. Bruner (1962) described detachment as caring based, expressed through a "deep need to understand something, . . . to render a meaning" (p. 24).

What can be known of caring in nursing through the methods of science is essential knowledge for practice. Empirical analysis takes on new meaning when alternated with the unique perspective of particular situations.

Ethical Knowing

Ethical knowing involves examination of philosophical systems, judgment, and normative action in general and particular situations. Roach (1984) says, "caring is the locus of nursing ethics in the universe, the foundation for, the center of nursing ethics . . . caring is living in the context of relational responsibilities—responsibilities to self and to the other" (p. 27). Ethical knowing provides then another lens through which caring in nursing situations should be studied.

Noddings (1984) posits the concept of ethics as arising from the consciousness of self as one-caring, with ethical behavior being founded in "natural caring." Commitment to act on behalf of the cared-for and a continual interest in the reality of the cared-for are the essential ethical elements in caring situations (Noddings, 1984).

The nurse is obligated to consider the nature of the cared-for and to respect his right to self determination. In a caring or relational ethic, Noddings (1988) states the primary concern is "in the relation itself—not only what happens physically to others involved in the relation and in connected relations but what they may feel and how they may respond to the act under consideration" (p. 219).

The protection of human dignity and preservation of humanity as described by Watson (1985) presupposes ethical knowing and valuing the process of becoming through caring. As Roach (1987) points out, conscience is a state of moral awareness that directs behavior according to the moral fitness of things. Nurses continuously face difficult ethical dilemmas in which they are asked to clarify and verify their values and philosophical positions.

Implicit in this clarification process is honesty, which implies genuineness or realness. Caring involves truly seeing self and others as they are (Mayeroff, 1971). The nurse brings to each nursing situation values and beliefs to which he or she must be committed. Nurses must acknowledge and respect the differences in values between the one caring and the one cared for. Caring requires that those caring have the courage and honesty necessary to live their values and beliefs. To substitute institutional goals and policies for what the one caring and the one cared for believe to be right is a breach of ethics. Basic to the ethical dimension is respect for person as person and, therefore, respect for the individual's right to self-determination. Ethical knowing highlights the issue of autonomy and represents Roach's (1987) "important-in-itself" value. What is known of caring in nursing through the pattern of ethical knowing contributes to the framework of an active value system as normative background for decision-making and caring action.

Esthetic Knowing

It is through the esthetic dimension that the art of nursing is illuminated. Esthetic knowing is described by Carper (1978) as experience involving the "creation and/ or appreciation of a singular, particular, subjective expression of imagined possibilities or equivalent realities which resist projection into the discursive form of language" (p. 16). The capacity for esthetic knowing in nursing is enhanced by engaging in esthetic encounters with human experience through art forms such as music, poetry, literature, painting, and the like. Drawing on personal, empirical, and ethical knowing in esthetic knowing, the nurse transcends the moment to envision and create possibilities within the specific nursing situation.

The artistry of esthetic knowing calls for the caring ingredients of patience and hope. According to Mayeroff (1971), "patience is not waiting passively for something to happen, but it is a kind of participation with the other in which we give fully of ourselves" (p. 17). The nurse allows the one cared for enough time and space to unfold and demonstrates hope that becoming will facilitate the achievement of dreams and goals. It is through experiencing the other that the moment becomes alive with possibilities, that the nurse as artist creates unique approaches to care based on the dreams and goals of the one cared for. In the realm of the esthetic, the nurse is free to know and express the beauty of the caring moment. It is in this full engagement within the nursing situation that the nurse truly knows caring in nursing.

The epistemology of caring in nursing is thus guided by an understanding of the patterns of knowing described by Carper (1978). What can be known about caring in nursing is significantly enhanced by going beyond empirics, into realms of personal, ethical, and esthetic knowing.

PEDAGOGICAL

The pedagogical category examines questions related to teaching and learning. Sound educational practice requires that methodology is appropriate to the subject matter. Therefore, teaching–learning activities must be congruent with the values of caring. Each of the prior categories

of questions, ontological, anthropological, ontical, and epistemological, offers meaning to the pedagogical process. The pedagogy of caring in nursing begins with knowing self as caring and cared for and progresses to knowing others as caring and worthy of care, knowing nursing as a uniquely lived form of caring, and creating personal and social environments to sustain caring nursing situations.

Students of nursing must be presented the opportunity to know themselves ontologically as caring persons and professionals and to understand how caring orders their lives. Through this experience, students develop self-insight that enhances the capacity for knowing others. Activities that teach students how to focus on and know the inner self-assist with this process.

A beginning way for students to learn the anthropological perspective is through studying and appreciating the college culture of which they are an integral part. Through studying their immediate surroundings, students can learn to truly know persons from different cultural backgrounds, their values and beliefs, and the meaning of health in various cultures. Students can be challenged to create a caring environment in the educational milieu. Additional understanding can be gained through empirical knowing, videotapes, role playing, and nursing practice opportunities to "be with" and "experience" diverse cultural groups.

Understanding the values and beliefs of various cultures and individuals is fundamental to care and caring in nursing. Teaching strategies that assist in this learning process should be integral to the curriculum and should arise from the value of caring in nursing. Students are continuously confronted with ontical issues in nursing situations: issues of health policy and health care economics, for example. Guided discussion in both practice and classroom settings can assist the student to develop analytic and decision-making patterns that retain caring as the core value of nursing, relevant to the most emergent or wide-ranging issues.

Carper's (1978) patterns of knowing can be used as an infrastructure to organize lessons, courses, and entire programs of nursing education with caring as the unifying concept. The authors have been involved in design and implementation of graduate and undergraduate curricula based on this structure. Content is presented for study in the form of nursing situations, defined as "a lived experience in which the caring between nurse and client promote the process of being and becoming."

Within this context, there is a strong focus on personal knowing for the student of nursing. Exercises that offer the student the experience of knowing self and that encourage expression of this discovery enhance personal knowing. Expert faculty play a vital role in modeling for students in the practice arena how to enter the world of another as the ground of meaning on which nursing practice is based. Students generally gain empirical knowledge from textbooks, journals, records, and similar sources. Certain moral obligations emanate from caring as the core of nursing practice. Noddings (1988) says that moral education involves modeling, dialogue, practice, and confirmation. According to this perspective, teachers are committed to encouraging self-affirmation in students, to open, nonjudgmental dialogue, to living the caring ideal in the classroom, and to developing the person's ethical ideal. Issues of relational ethics, including the response to person as person and person as important-in-itself, are addressed. The esthetic dimensions are illuminated by removing constraints in the teaching–learning situation and encouraging students to take risks to discover and express self. Rather than dictate to students the best method for integration of learning, the teacher allows choices for the expression of learning. Opportunities to engage in knowing human experience through dance, art, music, poetry, and other media of expression are made available. The uniqueness and artistry of the student is born in nursing when the teachers nurture its emergence through caring.

CONCLUSION

This chapter has focused on the contributions of scholars whose works have added valuable insights for understanding the substantive concept of caring in nursing. Five categories of questions provided an organizing framework for examining caring in nursing: ontological, anthropological, ontical, epistemological, and pedagogical. Systematic analysis of extant theory about caring in nursing promoted discovery of common themes and unique nuances that offer a basis for future study. Organization of substantive nursing knowledge of caring requires patterns of knowing and instructional design that reflects the richness and creative potential inherent in the phenomenon. As the concept of caring, unique to nursing, is further explicated, caring will emerge as a new model with the power to unify nursing practice, education, administration, and research.

REFERENCES

Brandon, D. (1976). *Zen in the art of helping*. New York, NY: Dell.

Bruner, J. (1962). *On knowing*. Cambridge, MA: Belknap Press.

Buber, M. (1970). *I and thou*. W. Kaufman (Trans.), New York, NY: Scribner.

Carper, B. (1978). Fundamental patterns of knowing in nursing. *Advances in Nursing Science, 1*, 33–24.

Gaut, D. (1984). A theoretic description of caring as action. In M. Leininger (Ed.), *Caring: The essence of nursing and health* (pp. 17–24). Thorofare, NJ: Slack.

Larson, P. (1987). Comparison of cancer patients' and professional nurses' perceptions of important nurse caring behaviors. *Heart and Lung, 16*, 187–193.

Leininger, M. (1981). *Caring: An essential human need*. Thorofare, NJ: Slack.

Leininger, M. (1988). Leininger's theory of nursing: Cultural care diversity and universality. *Nursing Science Quarterly, 1*, 152–160.

Mayeroff, M. (1971). *On caring.* New York, NY: Harper & Row.

McBride, A. (1989). Knowledge about care and caring: State of the art and future development. *Reflections, 15,* 5–7.

Noddings, N. (1984). *Caring: A feminine approach to ethics and moral education.* Los Angeles, CA: University of California Press.

Noddings, N. (1988). An ethic of caring and its implications for instructional arrangement. *American Journal of Education, 97,* 215–230.

Parse. R. R. (1981) Caring from a human science perspective. In M. Leininger (Ed.), *Caring: An essential human need* (pp. 129–132). Thorofare, NJ: Slack.

Paterson. J., & Zderad, L. (1988). *Humanistic nursing.* New York, NY: National League for Nursing, Pub. No. 41–2218.

Phenix, P. (1964). *Realms of meaning.* New York, NY: McGraw-Hill.

Ray, M. (1981). Philosophical analysis of caring. In M. Leininger (Ed.), *Caring: An essential human need* (pp. 25–36). Thorofare, NJ: Slack.

Ray, M. (1987). Technological caring: A new model in critical care. *Dimensions in Critical Care Nursing, 6,* 166–173.

Ray, M. (1988). The theory of bureaucratic caring for nursing practice in the organizational culture. *Nursing Administration Quarterly, 13,* 31–42.

Rieman, D. (1986). The essential structure of a caring interaction: Doing phenomenology. In P. Munhall & C. Oiler (Eds.), *Nursing research: A qualitative perspective.* Norwalk, CT: Appleton-Century-Crofts.

Roach, S. (1984). *Caring: The human mode of being, implications for nursing.* Toronto, ON: Faculty of Nursing, University of Toronto (Perspectives in Caring Monograph 1).

Roach, S. (1987). *The human act of caring.* Ottawa, Canada: Canadian Hospital Association.

Watson J. (1985). *Nursing: Human science and human care, a theory of nursing.* Norwalk, CT: Appleton-Century-Crofts.

Watson J. (1987). Nursing on the caring edge: Metaphorical vignettes. *Advances in Nursing Science, 10,* 10–18.

QUESTIONS FOR REFLECTION

Baccalaureate

1. What did you learn about theories of nurse caring when you read Boykin and Schoenhofer's (1990) chapter?
2. What does the phrase caring involves ". . . a moral commitment toward protection, enhancement, and preservation of human dignity" mean to you?
3. What did you learn about empirical knowledge from nursing? What does it mean?

Master's

1. What did you observe about the steps Boykin and Schoenhofer (1990) followed to describe caring in nursing?
2. Think of an example from your practice in which *ethical knowing* might be illustrated when you stood your ground and had the courage and honesty to act according to your values and beliefs. How did you feel in this situation?
3. How do nurses know caring through esthetic expressions?

Doctoral

1. How has Leininger's theory influenced the analysis of caring in nursing as described by Boykin and Schoenhofer (1990)?
2. How is the anthropological category explained by Boykin and Schoenhofer (1990) in relation to what it means to be a caring person?
3. How does Mayeroff (1971), as cited by Boykin and Schoenhofer (1990), contrast generic caring and nurse caring?

3

Caring and the Science of Unitary Human Beings

Marlaine C. Smith

The purpose of this chapter is to clarify the ambiguity surrounding the concept of caring through situating it within one conceptual system, the Science of Unitary Human Beings. An analysis of the dialogue on caring in nursing is presented. A process of concept clarification was developed to examine points of congruence between existing literature on caring and theoretical niches expressing similar meanings in the Science of Unitary Human Beings. The process resulted in the synthesis of five constitutive meanings of caring in the Science of Unitary Human Beings: manifesting intentions, appreciating pattern, attuning to dynamic flow, experiencing the infinite, and inviting creative emergence. Narratives were developed to ground the abstract meanings in concrete human experience.

The inclusion of caring as a central and defining concept within the discipline of nursing has generated contentious debate. Although some nursing scholars assert that caring is central to nursing science and art, others argue that caring is ubiquitous among all professions and does not reflect the uniqueness of the knowledge and practice of nursing.[1] Rogers was one of the most vocal advocates of the latter position. She stated, "It's time that we bury the whole idea of caring

as the essence of nursing and begin to look at some substance."[1(p. 39)]

If caring has been buried in the Science of Unitary Human Beings (SUHB), it may be time to exhume it for the purpose of examining some of the legitimate concerns about its inclusion as a central and significant concept within nursing, and then to resurrect it within the context of the SUHB. This will be approached through a process of concept clarification developed in response to Paley's[2] critique of existing methods of concept analysis. The thesis of this chapter is that caring is a central and significant concept within the discipline of nursing and that caring can be conceptualized congruently within the SUHB.

This chapter is organized in three sections: a background and analysis of the dialogue regarding caring in nursing, an explication of the process developed to clarify the concept of caring within the unitary perspective, and the presentation and discussion of findings of the concept clarification.

THE DISCIPLINARY DIALOGUE ON CARING

Historical Background

It is important to review the history and content of the debate surrounding the inclusion of caring as a central and defining

From Smith, M. C. (1999). Caring and the science of unitary human beings: A trans-theoretical discourse for nursing knowledge development. *Advances in Nursing Science, 21*(4), 14–28. Permission to reprint granted by Wolters Kluwer.

concept within the discipline. The use of the terms "care" and "caring for patients" have been part of the common professional language of nursing. These terms refer to both the patient–provider covenant in health care and the activities carried out in the fulfillment of that covenant. For example, it is common to refer to providing "patient care" or "nursing care." Madeleine Leininger[3] was the first to describe caring as the central focus of nursing. She stated: "Caring is the dominant intellectual theoretical, heuristic, and practice focus of nursing, and no other profession is so totally concerned with caring behaviors, caring processes, and caring relationships than nursing."[4(p. 33)] Leininger supported this position stating that the term "nursing" actually is derived from the word "nurturance," which by definition means caring, growth, and support.[4] Watson's two books, published in 1979[5] and 1985,[6] as well as her numerous journal publications posited nursing as the art and science of human caring. For Watson, nursing is a human science focusing on the study of the relationship of caring to health and healing.[7]

Leaders at the 1989 Wingspread Conference, jointly sponsored by the American Academy of Nursing and Sigma Theta Tau, concurred that caring should be a part of the nursing metaparadigm, replacing the term "nursing" in Fawcett's tetrad of concepts.[8] Since then, other nurse scholars such as Marilyn Ray,[9,10] Simone Roach,[11,12] Sally Gadow,[13,14] Anne Boykin and Savina Schoenafer[15] and Carol Montgomery[16] have contributed to the body of nursing literature on the philosophical and theoretical nature of caring. At this point, nursing has at least 20 years of organized systematic knowledge development related to caring and its relationships to human–environment–health processes, including about 40 books and more than 2,000 articles.[1] The International Caring Conference gathers scholars across the world interested in theory, research, and practice exemplars that illuminate the nature of caring in nursing.

As the caring movement emerged, Rogers was one of the most vociferous opponents of the idea that caring is a defining attribute of the discipline. For her, this idea diminished the focus on the development of the substantive knowledge of nursing, which she defined as the study of unitary human beings and their environment. During a panel discussion, Leininger articulated the uniqueness of nursing as "intimate personalized care within a cultural context that changes the health and well being of an individual," Rogers responded, "I would hate to think that nursing was narrowed to something called intimate personal care. That is a very narrow approach. I don't even know what those words mean."[17(p. 81)]

Mary Jane Smith, a scholar steeped in the unitary worldview, fleshed out this point of view, arguing that caring was a trite, universal expectation of any people who served the public. "Newspaper and television commercials announce that teachers care, physicians care, psychologists care, and even the local plumbers care."[18(p. 54)] She illuminated the ambiguity surrounding the meaning of caring and questioned that such a universal experience could be the core of science. She asserts that if caring is a part of all professional disciplines, then the development of knowledge related to caring "moves us further away from the specificity required of a discipline."[18(p. 54)] Moving it to the abstract, as a way of being, it becomes universal; moving it to the concrete, it becomes a task of caregiving: "Neither direction gives substance to the discipline of nursing."[18(p. 54)] Finally, Smith concedes that "a caring presence where the nurse is knowledgeable in the science and invested in the client's well-being is the desired goal. However, to focus on caring as the essence of nursing sidesteps, the theoretical base conceptualized in nursing frameworks and leads to knowledge development focused on sentiment and tasks."[18](p. 54)

In 1991, Newman, Sime, and Corcoran-Perry issued their critique of the existing metaparadigm. They stated that "there remains the need for more explicit connectedness and social relevance to describe the field of study that constitutes nursing."[19](p. 2) These authors asserted that caring and health are linked within theoretical literature in nursing and that "the essential question of the discipline of nursing has something to do with how nurses facilitate the health of human beings."[19](p. 2) They pose the question "What is the quality of the relationship that makes it possible for the nurse and patient to connect in a transforming way?" and, their well-known focus statement is that nursing is the study of "caring in the human health experience."[19](p. 3)

Fawcett responded to this conceptualization, stating that the focus statement of Newman et al. is flawed because (1) caring is not a dominant theme in all conceptualizations of nursing; (2) it reflects a particular view and kind of nursing; and (3) it may not be conceptualized across cultures.[20](p. vi) Fawcett's critique generated two responses: one from the authors themselves[21] and a second from a group of doctoral students.[22] These respondents argued that (1) the theme of caring is sufficiently dominant and there is sufficient consensus in nursing for its inclusion in the focus statement; (2) caring is a paradigm-free conceptualization in that it may be defined and imagined differently depending on the disciplinary paradigm; and (3) disciplinary definitions are evolutionary and responsive to the patterns of knowledge development in the field of study.

In the panel discussion mentioned earlier, whose proceedings were published, King, Leininger, Parse, Peplau, and Rogers responded to the question, "Is nursing the study of 'caring in the human health experience?'"[1] Only Leininger supported the inclusion of caring as central

to the discipline. The others on the panel rejected its inclusion in the focus statement for various reasons, some of which already have been articulated: It is a process and not a concept; although caring is part of the historical literature, it lacks clear definition; caring is ubiquitous and not a central phenomenon in nursing and in most existing nursing theories; caring is a "scrap basket . . . almost a synonym for nursing practice, not exclusive to nursing; and; caring is associated with women down through the ages, and has not been particularly attuned to the behavior of men."[1](p. 39) Rogers' response was, "I happen to believe that everybody ought to care. But any idea that [caring] is an identifying note for nursing is making us look . . . foolish. Because . . . we all care . . . and I think it's about time that we begin to value knowledge of some sort. . . . What we do is care, but before we can do, we have to know."[1](p. 39–40)

In an illuminating dialogue on the nursing metaparadigm, Fawcett articulated four requirements for a metaparadigm, and in analyzing various alternative representations of the discipline's focus, reasserted her previous positions rejecting caring as central to nursing. "It is not a dominant theme in every conceptualization and, therefore, does not represent a discipline-wide viewpoint, . . . (it) is not uniquely a nursing phenomenon, and may not be generalizable culturally."[23](p. 96)

It is important to note that for Rogers, compassionate care was identified within the realm of nursing art, the creative use of knowledge in service to humankind.[24] Recently, scholars such as Barrett[25] and Malinski[26] have integrated the concept of caring into descriptions of their SUHB science-based practice approaches, with Barrett describing the "caring partnership" and Malinski defining health patterning as "providing knowledgeable caring to assist clients in actualizing potentials for well-being through knowing participation in change."[26](p. 105)

Analysis of the Dialogue on Caring in Nursing

Based on this summary, the concerns surrounding the issues of caring as a defining focus of nursing are

1. *Ambiguity*—that there is a lack of semantic clarity in the use of the term within nursing literature;
2. *Limiting and perspectival*—that the use of the concept to define the focus of nursing is too narrow and its use is reflected only by certain grand theories and not common to all conceptualizations of nursing;
3. *Ubiquitous*—that caring is present in all human service areas and is not unique to nursing;
4. *Nonsubstantive*—that caring relates to an affect or activities with clients and does not connote a substantive body of knowledge for the discipline;
5. *Nongeneralizable*—that caring is different across cultures and national boundaries; and
6. *Feminine*—that caring is associated with women's sensibilities and women's work and reinforces the prejudices associated with nursing in society.

Each of these concerns is addressed in the next sections.

Ambiguity

First, it is true that the nursing literature is rife with multiple meanings of caring, leading to confusion and lack of clarity. Two analyses of caring literature are helpful in discovering the range of meanings of caring in nursing. Boykin and Schoenhofer's[27] analysis queries the caring literature and sorts it into three major categories: (1) the ontological, that is, caring as a manifestation of being in the world; (2) the anthropological, that is, the meaning of being a caring person; and (3) the ethical or the obligation of caring. These authors then suggest issues for knowledge development and education surrounding caring in nursing. Morse and her colleagues[28] completed a content analysis of the work of 35 nursing authors, classifying their work into five major perspectives on caring existing in the nursing literature: (1) caring as human trait, (2) caring as moral imperative, (3) caring as affect, (4) caring as interpersonal interaction, and (5) caring as therapeutic intervention. This analysis lends some clarity to the diversity of perspectives. At its conclusion, Morse and her colleagues offer an instrumental perspective on caring: "It is the authors' opinion, albeit often implicit, that the ultimate outcome of caring is to alter patient responses"[28(p. 10)] and that "If caring changes the course of illness for the patient then the concept may be useful enough to retain its lofty position as the 'essence of nursing.'"[28(p. 12)] They call for a "clear conceptualization of caring that encompasses all aspects of nursing."[28(p. 11)]

A clear conceptualization is indeed necessary, and it is evident that this clarity cannot come from a blending of perspectives on caring. The concept of caring must be conceptualized within the assumptions and worldview or ontology of existing conceptual systems. Each nursing conceptual model or grand theory will have its own definition of caring just as each has its own definitions related to health, human beings, or quality of life. For this reason, Rogerian scholars will require clear conceptualizations of caring within the SUHB.

Limiting and Perspective-Specific

The criticism that caring is limiting and perspective-specific, in that it does not define, in and of itself, the disciplinary perspective of nursing and only appears in certain theoretic perspectives, invites reflection. First, it is true that for most, nursing would not be defined totally as caring. However, for many, the focus of nursing is on the interrelationship of human health, healing, and caring or the study of human–environment–health relationships *and* how these relationships are facilitated through caring.

Unlike some who may argue that nurses are too diverse to have some common ground, it seems essential to articulate for the public and for nursing some core that identifies the discipline. Caring is one element of that core. Caring is in some way a part of the practice tradition of every nursing theory—perhaps not explicitly, but in every intention. Every view, definition, idea, or conception of nursing practice places the nurse with the person–family–community in a relationship with a purpose of fostering the emergence of health, well-being, healing, or quality of life. Is nursing caring? No. But can nursing exist without caring? No. In this way, caring transcends any particular theories (e.g., Leininger, Watson, Boykin, and Schoenhofer) and becomes central to the art or practice of nursing.

Ubiquitous

Next, caring is not unique to nursing, but there is substantive extant and emergent knowledge development within nursing related to this phenomenon. Caring as a concerned, kind, and facilitative stance in human relating should be present in all professional relationships and human encounters. This is certainly true. But this is a superficial representation of caring and one that does not capture the depth of meanings in the theoretical literature on caring. It is analogous to arguing that the SUHB is about taking care of the whole person—and everyone does that. Furthermore, no other discipline is developing knowledge related to how this quality of relationship facilitates health, healing, and the quality of life. This knowledge, generated within nursing, will be essential for other disciplines in which caring relationships are the foundation to their practice. A significant and rich body of scholarship encompassing philosophic, theoretic, empiric, phenomenologic, and literary contributions on caring is growing in nursing.

Caring is the art of nursing, the way of being, and the comportment of the nurse in the sacred dance of healing with the client. In this meaning, caring becomes the ground of practice. Although this may not be the science of nursing, in and of itself, any professional discipline seeks to understand its art of practice. For example, physicians study the art of diagnostic reasoning and attorneys study the art of the argument. There is substantive knowledge related to nursing's art, and this is a legitimate area of scholarship. In this way, the development of the science related to caring is essential to more fully understand the art of nursing.

Nongeneralizable

It is clear that caring is not culturally generalizable, but neither is health, healing, quality of life, or human existence. None of the defining concepts of the discipline of nursing will stand the test of cultural transcendence. The concept of caring will take on shades of meaning, reflected in the specific acts, intentions, or gestures that may be interpreted as caring in different cultures.

Feminine

Finally, rather than eschew and denigrate nursing's feminine heritage or the traits associated with them, it is time to celebrate them. Nursing has been women's work, and the love, caring, sensitivity, and nurturing associated with that work has dyed deeply the fabric of nursing's existence.[29] Certainly, it is not true that men cannot care, for they do and can. Neither does the assertion that the art of nursing incorporates values associated more with the "feminine" mean a devaluing of knowledge development and scientific endeavors. It means that this is a time in evolution when people are moving beyond feminine–masculine dualism. A nurse can have both the passionate commitment to substance and scholarship as well as the appreciation for the love and tenderness that may have emerged from the feminine roots of nursing's practice.

TOWARD CLARIFICATION OF THE CONCEPT OF CARING

A Critique of Concept Analysis

In summary, based on this analysis, caring is a central and significant concept within the discipline; however, there is confusion because of the existing multiple meanings that coexist in the literature. Concept clarification is the process of addressing the ambiguity surrounding concepts. Although there is no doubt that this clarification is important, the process of clarification is at question. Paley[2] criticizes existing methods of concept analysis used in nursing, the most popular being Wilson's analysis as presented and modified by Walker and Avant.[30] Concept analysis that distils a massive array of literature into a list of defining attributes only perpetuates the confusion, for the defining attributes usually reflect the existing semantic disparity. Furthermore, the process for arriving at defining attributes is arbitrary, often based on unstated or differing criteria. Paley argues that the definition of concepts as the building blocks of theories is misleading because it suggests that concepts exist independently before they are cemented into theoretical structures. He proposes that concepts are the niches created by theory because the meaning of the concept comes from its place within the conceptual system. "Concepts are not like bricks; they are more like niches. The only way to clarify a concept is explicitly to adopt a theory that determines what its niche will be. . . . Conceptual clarification, then, is not possible without theoretical commitment . . . and in the absence of theoretical commitment, conceptual clarification is an arbitrary and vacuous exercise."[2(pp. 577–578)]

A Process for Concept Clarification

If one accepts this, the critical question becomes what is caring within SUHB or what is this quality of being in mutual process that is called "caring" within other theoretical contexts? Two assumptions derived from the SUHB guided the inquiry: (1) caring is a way of participating knowingly in human-environmental field patterning; and (2) caring is the manifestation of human-field patterning in this process of participation. The goal of the inquiry was to create constitutive meanings of caring that could be considered pattern manifestations.

Based on Paley's critique, the following process of concept clarification was developed to arrive at the essential meanings of the concept of caring from the unitary perspective.

Identifying the existing meanings of the concept in context: How is caring understood within various paradigmatic and theoretical presentations? Based on the guiding assumptions, the exploration of the caring literature was limited to those authors describing caring as a way of being, a mode of being, or a way of living. This decision eliminated any literature on caring, behaviors or actions, emotions, specific dynamics of the interpersonal process of caring, or antecedents or outcomes of caring. Exemplar sources[5,6,10,11,13,15,16,31–44] that described caring as ontology or way of being were analyzed. Next, semantic expressions from these sources were identified and listed. Semantic expressions were statements or phrases that captured the essence of the meaning of caring as a way of being from these authors' perspectives.

Identifying theoretical niches: Where are concepts with similar meanings to those identified in the first phase residing within the SUHB? Following the review and listing of semantic expressions from the seminal sources on caring, literature[24–26,45–58] from a unitary paradigm was reviewed for the purposes of identifying theoretical niches, or existing concepts that captured the meaning of caring from this perspective. Theoretical niches were listed and related to the clusters of semantic expressions.

Synthesis of the concept through identifying constitutive meanings: The synthesis emerged from the dialogue between the meanings that exist in caring literature and their correspondence to the theoretical niches within the SUHB. Constitutive meanings, phrases that encompassed a cluster of semantic expressions, were developed. When possible, the language of concepts already within the SUHB, that could excellently represent that meaning, was retained in the name of the constitutive meaning.

Instantiation of the concept: What descriptions or exemplars help nurses more fully understand the constitutive meanings of caring? In the phase of instantiation, three narratives were constructed from nursing stories of caring that reflected the constitutive meanings. These narratives were actual events, written in aesthetic form to concretize, illuminate, and evoke the meaning of caring within the SUHB. Although narratives were chosen to provide instances of the concept in this inquiry, other forms such as case study, poetry, music, or visual art may be used.

FINDINGS

Five constitutive meanings emerged from this process. These represent the essential nature of the concept of caring from the perspective of the SUHB. They are not ordered in any way nor are their relationships to each other specified. There may be some overlap of the semantic expressions relating to each constitutive meaning; however, the core of each is distinctive. The live constitutive meanings are (1) manifesting intentions; (2) appreciating pattern; (3) attuning to dynamic flow; (4) experiencing the infinite; and (5) inviting creative emergence. Each of these will be discussed. The shaded boxes in this chapter show selected semantic expressions from the caring literature.

Manifesting Intentions

The first constitutive meaning of the concept of caring from the unitary perspective is manifesting intentions. Manifesting intentions are creating, holding, and expressing thoughts, images, feelings, beliefs, desires, will (purpose), and actions that affirm possibilities for human betterment or well-being. Although not all the semantic expressions from the caring literature that are clustered under manifesting intentions can be listed, selections appear in the box "Semantic Expressions of Caring: Manifesting Intentions." Selected semantic expressions that capture the essence of manifesting intentions include centering on the person,[16] preserving dignity and humanity,[6] commitment to alleviate another's vulnerabilities.[13] providing attention and concern,[34] reverence for each human life,[6] love and copresence,[10] approaching the other in humility,[35] expressing compassion and courage,[31] and being with in authentic presence.[15,38]

From the perspective of the SUHB, intentions are real and powerful within patterning. They are energetic and potentiate dynamic change. The colors of these intentions dye one's world, work, and reality. Manifesting intentions does not refer to having a goal-directed outcome in mind, nor does it mean that the person caring comes to the engagement with a purpose for directing the person in a certain way. Dossey[59] describes it as cooperating with the emerging order instead of trying to change it. Manifesting intention is awareness of what Quinn refers to as being safe, sacred space for the client.[50] This space is characterized by reverence, commitment, genuineness, honesty, attention, and concern, while cherishing values of dignity, love, beauty, peace, and goodness in approaching the purposeful encounter.

Semantic Expressions of Caring:
Manifesting Intentions

- Person-centered intention (Montgomery)
- Preserving dignity and humanity (Watson)
- Committed to alleviating the other's vulnerability (Gadow)
- Giving attention and concern (Gaut)
- Obligations deriving from devotion (Mayeroff)
- Reverence for person and human life (Watson)
- Love and co-presence (Ray)
- Humility, willingness to learn from the other (Mayeroff)
- Authenticity and availability (Montgomery)
- Being with (Swanson-Kaufmann)
- Attention, compassion, focus, courage (Picard)
- Manifestation of ability to feel compassion (Eriksson)
- Honesty and openness to self and other (Mayeroff)
- Regard, fondness, attachment (Gaut)
- Intentional authentic presence (Boykin and Schoenhofer)
- Being with the other in fullness of one's personhood (Boykin and Schoenhofer)
- Intention of knowing, acknowledging, affirming, and celebrating the person (Schoenhofer)

The purpose of engagement is in the interest of the other.[57] Because of this responsibility, self awareness is essential. What thoughts, images, feelings, beliefs, desires, and will are with a person in this process? How does one incarnate these intentions in his or her actions? Growing in the ability to be self-reflective and cultivating stillness, receptivity, imagination, and reverie makes the process of manifesting

intention more conscious, deliberate, and focused. An emergent form of manifesting intentions, one that Newman et al.[55] associates with expanding consciousness, is unconditional love. In unconditional love, one has growing awareness of his or her integral nature, that is, one's connectedness with others and the world.

Appreciating Pattern

The second constitutive meaning of caring was labeled explicitly in the SUHB. It is appreciating pattern. Both Cowling[46–48,60] and Krieger[57] have used the terms "appreciation of pattern." Krieger describes appreciation of the field characteristics in the process of therapeutic touch. Cowling's well-developed praxis method is called unitary pattern appreciation. He defines pattern appreciation as "Discovery in the service of knowing wholeness and essence."[61]

Appreciating pattern captures the essential meaning reflected in the selected semantic expressions from the caring literature listed in the box "Semantic Expressions of Caring: Appreciating Pattern." These include placing value on the other as lovable or being loved;[43] cherishing the wholeness of the human person;[6] valuing and celebrating human wholeness;[15] recognizing the subjectivity and wholeness of the other;[13] acknowledging the emerging pattern without trying to change it;[55] confirming the incalculable worth of the person;[31] seeing the other as perfect in the moment and unfolding possibilities for becoming;[15] and yearning for a deeper understanding and appreciation of the healing resources, life force, pattern, and paradoxes expressed in the relationship.[6]

Semantic Expressions of Caring:
Appreciating Pattern

- Placing value on the other as lovable or worthy of being loved (Rawnsley)

- Cherishing the wholeness of the human being (Watson)
- Valuing and celebrating human wholeness (Boykin and Schoenhofer)
- Assuming the subjectivity of the other is as valid and whole as that of the caregiver (Gadow)
- Acknowledging the emerging pattern without trying to change it (Newman)
- Confirming of human dignity and the incalculable worth of the person (Eriksson)
- Seeing the other as perfect in the moment and unfolding possibilities for becoming (Boykin and Schoenhofer)
- Yearning for a deeper understanding and appreciation of the natural healing resources, life force, pattern, and paradoxes . . . (Watson)
- Having sensitivity to and sensibility of the pattern manifestations that give identity to each person's unique pattern (Cowling)
- Knowing the other (Mayeroff)
- Transcending judgment; no attempt to judge (Montgomery)
- Seeing underneath all that is fragmented to the real existence of wholeness and acknowledging that in appreciation (Cowling)

In his Orienting Features, Cowling[60] describes pattern appreciation as seeking perception of the fullness, the wholeness of the person reflected in the uniqueness of pattern. For Cowling, pattern appreciation requires sensitivity to and sensibility of the pattern manifestations; it implies the sympathetic recognition of excellence of energy field pattern, and it is approached with gratefulness and enjoyment. Pattern appreciation is "seeing underneath all that is fragmented to the real existence of wholeness and acknowledging that in

appreciation."[61(p. 136)] Pattern appreciation is a theoretical niche within the SUHB that exquisitely captures the meaning of a cluster of semantic expressions of caring.

Attuning to Dynamic Flow

Attuning to dynamic flow is the third constitutive meaning of caring in the SUHB. Attuning to dynamic flow is dancing to the rhythms within continuous mutual process. It is a vibrational sensing of where to place focus and attention.

The semantic expressions from the caring literature that reflect the meaning of attuning to dynamic flow appear in the box "Semantic Expressions of Caring: Attuning to Dynamic Flow." These include attuning to the subtleties that present themselves in the moment;[16] being sensitive to self and other;[6] responding to the experience of connectedness;[11] sensing belongingness and interconnectedness;[10] living in the context of relational responsibilities;[15] moving back and forth in the dance of relating;[35] shifting perspectives and patterns of responsiveness;[35] relating in a highly complex synchronization and organismic integration;[44] being with as a well-orchestrated symphony;[44] the magnetic appeal or pull of the universe;[10] experiencing an energetic resonance;[50] and a pattern or vibration of the consciousness that becomes like a tuning fork at a healing frequency.[50]

Semantic Expressions of Caring: *Attuning to Dynamic Flow*

- Attuned to the subtleties that present themselves in the moment (Montgomery)
- Sensitivity to self and other (Watson)
- Response to the experience of connectedness (Roach)
- Sense of belonging and interconnectedness (Ray)

(continued)

- Living in the context of relational responsibilities (Boykin and Schoenhofer)
- Able to detect the person's condition of being and feeling the condition (Watson)
- Alternating rhythms; moving back and forth in the dance of relating: shifting perspectives and patterns of responsiveness (Mayeroff)
- Highly complex synchronization and organismic integration (Gendron)
- Well-orchestrated symphony (Gendron)
- Action of love; the magnet appeal or pull of the universe (Ray)
- Energetic resonance (Quinn)
- Pattern or vibration of nurse's consciousness becoming a tuning fork at a healing frequency while the client has the opportunity to tune or resonate to that frequency (Quinn)

Attuning to dynamic flow is a heightened sensitivity to the rhythmic patterning of relating. Through this attuning, there is a knowing of when and how to move, be still, speak, be silent, laugh, cry, touch, or withdraw.

Experiencing the Infinite

Experiencing the infinite is the fourth constitutive meaning of caring within the SUHB. It is the pandimensional awareness of coextensiveness with the universe occurring in the context of human relating. Within the caring literature, authors such as Watson, Ray, Eriksson, and Montgomery describe this and refer to it in different forms: transcending self, time, and space;[6] a spiritual union;[6] an ontologic mystery;[10] expanding sense of self;[16] and the unfolding of Divine love.[10] Newman

refers to caring as the highest form of knowing;[55] Watson describes this as "the actual caring occasion."[6] Experiencing the infinite is described as those occasions when there is that fullness of being and experience of expansion and connection that defies ordinary language, which is described in the SUHB as pattern manifestations of timelessness, expanding vision, and beyond waking awareness. Ray stated, "The universe is beginning to be recognized as the dwelling place where in everything is to be revered and understood as connected and considered sacred."[10(p. 170)]

Semantic Expressions of Caring:
Experiencing the Infinite

- Transcends the physical and material world bound in time and space (Watson)
- Expanded sense of self; transcendent qualities (Montgomery)
- Highest form of knowing (Newman)
- Unfolding divine love (Ray)
- Inner vision that is apprehended and understood in consciousness as an ontologic mystery (Ray)
- Spiritual union occurring between persons where both are capable of transcending self, time, and space (Watson)
- Actual caring occasion involves the spirit of both, expands the limits of openness: the event has relations between past-present and imagined future (Watson)

Inviting Creative Emergence

The final constitutive meaning of caring in the SUHB is inviting creative emergence. Inviting creative emergence was extracted from Quinn's[50] descriptions of caring in the process of healing and

Newman's descriptions of caring as transforming mutual process.[55] It reflects the
transformative potential of caring for self
and other and the belief in the continuing innovation of emergent patterning.
All exists as possibility, and this way of
being called caring illuminates the vistas
of possibilities. Some semantic expressions that are examples of this meaning are holding a hopeful orientation;[16]
growth in the capacity to express caring;[15]
a transformative experience wherein the
constant birthing of love in caring actions
is the growth of the spiritual life within;[62]
expanding human capacities; and increasing the range of events that can occur in
space and time at the moment and in the
future.[6]

Semantic Expressions of Caring:
Inviting Creative Emergence

- Holding a hopeful orientation
  (Montgomery)
- Growing in the capacity to
  express caring (Boykin and
  Schoenhofer)
- Transforming mutual process
  (Newman)
- Transformative experience
  wherein the constant birthing
  of love in caring actions is the
  growth of the spiritual life within
  (Roach)
- Calling to a deeper life; birthing a
  spiritual life in each person (Ray)
- Expanding human capacities;
  increases the range of events that
  could occur in space and time
  at the moment and in the future
  (Watson)
- Allowing the person to grow in
  own time and in own way; let-
  ting go of the outcome (Mayeroff)
- Facilitating creative emergence
  (Quinn)

INSTANTIATION OF THE CONCEPT THROUGH NARRATIVE

The final phase of this clarification process is instantiation of the concept. Three
narratives were constructed from nursing stories to reflect the identified constitutive meanings. These were narratives
constructed from stories experienced or
shared by others. They are written from
the perspective of the nurse. The first is
called "Ease in Labor" and reflects manifesting intentions.

> The alarms sounded and the three of us
> rushed to the bedside of this laboring
> woman. Her baby was in trouble, heart
> rate disappearing with each contrac-
> tion. Panic gripped the woman and
> she thrashed and cried out in fear for
> her child's life. Her husband walked
> in, sucking in the fear like a sponge.
> I grasped his hand and pulled him
> with me behind her head. I placed
> one hand on her shoulders and the
> other on his. I wanted them to feel my
> strength, to know my hope, to have an
> oasis of peace in this chaos. Although
> she was poked, prodded, flipped, and
> exposed and he was ignored, I whis-
> pered to them, explaining, comforting,
> calming until they moved into the
> delivery room. Afterward, we cried
> together . . . tears of joy and relief for
> the safe passage of Jessica Rose into this
> world.

The next story reflects the constitutive meanings of *appreciating pattern
and inviting creative emergence*. It is called
"Home at the AIDS Center."

> He walked in the door, 6 feet 4 [inches]
> at least, clothes dirty, torn, ripe with
> odor of nights on the street. I embraced
> and welcomed him . . . stiff, still, a tree
> would have given more back. While I
> talked, he looked down and pushed his
> massive hand, cracked, bleeding, ooz-
> ing into my field of vision. I cradled it,
> dressed it as if it belonged to my child.
> He said nothing at all except "John"
> when I asked his name. "Come back,
> John." And he did—again and again—
> always silent. And each time, I greeted

him at the door with an unreturned embrace. Sometimes we'd sit in silence or listen to music, or I'd read a book or some poetry to him. One day, many months after our first meeting, the door opened. "Hi. John! C'mon in," I said. He did, then looked into my eyes and opened his arms.

The constitutive meanings of *attuning to dynamic flow* and *experiencing the infinite* are reflected in this story called, "The Nursing Home."

> I made my rounds, introducing myself, offering my hand to each of them. "I'm the new nurse here. I look forward to knowing you." Mrs. Manelli shook my hand vigorously and recognized me in that moment as her sister Joanie who had died many years earlier. Mr. Carter spoke quietly in phrases I didn't understand and rocked rhythmically in the blue vinyl chair. Mr. Maplethorpe's cool blue eyes followed me as I approached him, then looked down to avoid meeting mine. I was drawn to him like filings to a magnet. Sensing the depth of his sadness, I pulled up the stool and faced him. He never looked up. My eyes met the object of his blank gaze. "Your slippers aren't on—would you like them?" He shook his head. I lifted one foot into my lap and, with lotion, gently rubbed the beautiful gnarled toes and callused heels. I imagined where these feet had been, walking on sandy beaches, running to greet loved ones at the door of his home, pushing the pedals of a piano. . . . And then the next foot. Rhythmically sensing, touching, stroking, and caressing. His muted sobs called me back from that other place and time we shared. "Why are you crying?," I asked. His face glowed softly. "I haven't been touched like that since my wife died." "How long has that been?" "Six years."

In summary, it is true that Martha Rogers did have concerns about caring being named as the essence of nursing. She fought long and hard to advance nursing's identity as a professional discipline. In the

SUHB, she developed a conceptual system that offered a new worldview generating puzzles to be solved and phenomena to be explicated through knowledge development about the nature of the unitary life process.

This worldview has generated a practice tradition that makes a difference in the lives of people. In her eyes, the emergence of the identification of nursing as caring threatened our scientific progress and could be misinterpreted to underscore the anti-intellectualism in nursing[24] and to support the assertion that "there is really nothing to know in nursing." In 1992, she stated, "The nature of caring in a given field depends entirely on the body of scientific knowledge to the field. Caring is simply a way of using knowledge."[51(p. 33)] Although this may be true, nurses have developed and need to continue to develop knowledge of all forms about this way of being. It is part of the essential knowledge of the discipline.

The purpose of this chapter was to clarify the ambiguity surrounding the concept of caring through situating it within one conceptual system, the SUHB. The process of concept clarification attempted to examine points of congruence of existing literature on caring with the theoretical niches in the SUHB where these meanings reside. This process resulted in the identification of five constitutive meanings of caring in the SUHB: manifesting intentions, appreciating pattern, attuning to dynamic flow, experiencing the infinite, and inviting creative emergence. Narratives were developed to ground the abstract meanings in concrete human experience.

In 1966, Rogers wrote: "Nursing's story is a magnificent epic of service to humankind. It is about people: how they are born, and live and die; in health and in sickness; in joy and in sorrow. Its mission is the translation of knowledge into human service. Nursing is compassionate concern for human beings. It is the heart that understands and the hand that soothes. It is the intellect that synthesizes many learnings into meaningful administrations."[63] While distinctive nursing knowledge will provide its form, no one could capture the meaning of caring better than that.

REFERENCES

1. Huch, M. H. (1995). Nursing and the next millennium. *Nursing Science Quarterly, 8*(1), 38–44.
2. Paley, J. (1996). How not to clarify concepts in nursing, *Journal of Advanced Nursing, 24*, 572–578.
3. Leininger, M. (1977). Caring: The essence and central focus of nursing. *American Nurses' Foundation, Nursing Research Report.*
4. Leininger, M. (1978). *Transcultural nursing.* New York, NY: John Wiley & Sons.
5. Watson, J. (1979). *Nursing the philosophy and science of caring.* Boston, MA: Little. Brown & Co.
6. Watson, J. (1985). *Nursing: Human science and human care: A theory of nursing.* Nonwalk, CT: Appleton-Century-Crofts.
7. Watson, J. (1995). Nursing's caring-healing paradigm as exemplar for alternative medicine? *Alternative Therapies, 1*(3), 64–69.
8. Stevenson, J. S., & Tripp-Reimer T (Eds.). (1989, February). Knowledge about care and caring. *Proceedings of a Wingspread Conference.* Kansas City, MO: American Academy of Nursing.
9. Ray, M. A. (1981). A philosophical analysis of caring within nursing. In M. M. Leininger (Ed.), *Caring: An essential human need.* Thorofare, NJ: Slack, Inc.
10. Ray, M. A. (1997). Illuminating the meaning of caring: Unfolding the sacred art of divine love. In M. S. Roach (Ed.), *Caring from the heart: The convergence of caring and spirituality.* New York, NY: Paulist Press.
11. Roach, S. (1987). *The human act of caring.* Ottawa, ON: The Canadian Hospital Association.
12. Roach, S. (1991). The call to consciousness: Compassion in today's health world. In D. A. Gaut & M. M. Leininger (Eds.), *The compassionate healer.* New York, NY: NLN Press.
13. Gadow, S. (1980). Existential advocacy: Philosophical foundations of nursing. In S. Spicker & S. Gadow (Eds.), *Nursing images and ideals.* New York, NY: Springer.
14. Gadow, S. (1988). Covenant without cure: Letting go and holding on in chronic illness. In J. Watson & M. A. Ray (Eds.), *The ethics of care and ethics of cure: Synthesis in chronicity.* New York, NY: NLN.
15. Boykin, A., & Schoenhofer, S. (1993). *Nursing as caring.* New York, NY: NLN Press.
16. Montgomery, C. *Healing through communication: The practice of caring.* Newbury Park. CA: Sage.
17. Smith, M. J. (1988). Perspectives on nursing science. *Nursing Science Quarterly, 1*, 80–85.
18. Smith, M. J. (1990). Caring: Ubiquitous or unique. *Nursing Science Quarterly, 3*, 54.
19. Newman, M. A., Sime, A. M., & Corcoran-Perry, S. A. (1991). The focus of the discipline of nursing. *Advances in Nursing Science, 14*(1), 1–6.
20. Fawcett, J. (1992). [Letter to the Editor]. *Advances in Nursing Science, 14*(3), vi.
21. Newman, M. A., Sime, A. M., & Corcoran-Perry, S. A. (1992). Authors' reply. [Letter to the Editor] *Advances in Nursing Science, 14*(3), vi–vii.
22. Malloch, K., Martinez, R., Nelson, L., Predeger, B., Speak-man, L., Steinbinder, A., & Tracy, J. (1992). [Letter to the Editor]. *Advances in Nursing Science, 15*(2), vi–vii.
23. Fawcett, J. (1996). On the requirements for a metaparadigm: An invitation to dialogue. *Nursing Science Quarterly, 9*, 94–96.
24. Rogers, M. E. (1970). *An introduction to the theoretical basis of nursing.* Philadelphia, PA: FA Davis.
25. Barrett, E. A. M. (1994). Rogerian scientists, artists, revolutionaries. In M. Madrid & E. A. M. Barrett (Eds.), *Rogers' scientific art of nursing practice.* New York, NY: NLN Publishing.
26. Malinski, V. (1994). Health patterning for individuals and families, In M. Madrid & E. A. M. Barrett (Eds.), *Rogers' scientific art of nursing practice.* New York, NY: NLN Publishing.
27. Boykin, A., & Schoenhofer, S. (1990). Caring in nursing: Analysis of extant theory. *Nursing Science Quarterly, 3*, 149–155.
28. Morse, J. M., Solberg, S. M., Neander, W. L., Bottorff, J. L., & Johnson, J. L. (1990). Concepts of caring and caring as a concept. *Advances in Nursing Science, 13*, 1–14.
29. Hughes, L. (1990). Professionalizing domesticity: A synthesis of selected nursing historiography. *Advances in Nursing Science, 12*(4), 25–31.
30. Walker, L. O., & Avant, K. C. (1995). *Strategies for theory construction in nursing.* Norwalk, CT: Appleton & Lange.
31. Eriksson, K. (1997). Caring, spirituality and suffering. In S. Roach (Ed.), *Caring from the heart: The convergence of caring and spirituality.* New York, NY: Paulist Press.

32. Gadow, S. A. (1989). Clinical subjectivity: Advocacy with silent patients. *Nursing Clinics of North America, 24*, 535–541.

33. Gadow, S. A. (1985). Nurse and patient: The caring relationship. In A. Bishop & J. Scudder (Eds.), *Caring, curing, coping: Nurse, physician, patient relationships*. Tuscaloosa, AL: University of Alabama Press.

34. Gaut, D. A. (1983). Development of a theoretically adequate description of caring. *Western Journal of Nursing Research, 5*, 313–324.

35. Mayeroff, M. (1971). *On caring*. New York, NY: Harper & Row.

36. Leininger, M. M. (1990). Historic and epistemologic dimensions of care and caring with future directions. In J. S. Stevenson & T. Tripp-Reimer (Eds.), *Knowledge about care and caring: State of the art and future developments*. Kansas City, MO: American Academy of Nursing.

37. Ray, M. A. (1994). Complex caring dynamics: A unifying model of nursing inquiry. *Theoretic and Applied Chaos in Nursing, 1*, 23–32.

38. Swanson, K. M. Empirical development of a middle range theory of caring. *Nursing Research, 199*(40), 161–165.

39. Watson, J. (1990). Caring knowledge and informed moral passion. *Advances in Nursing Science, 13*, 15–24.

40. Watson, J. (1988). New dimensions in human caring theory. *Nursing Science Quarterly, 1*, 175–181.

41. Eriksson, K. (1997). Understanding the world of the patient, the suffering human being: The new clinical paradigm from nursing to caring. *Advanced Practice Nursing Quarterly, 3*(1), 8–13.

42. Sherwood, G. D. (1997). Metasynthesis of qualitative analyses of caring: Defining a therapeutic model of nursing. *Advances in Nursing Science, 3*(1), 32–42.

43. Rawnsley, M. (1990). Of human bonding: The context of nursing as caring. *Advances in Nursing Science, 13*(2), 41–48.

44. Gendron, D. (1988). The expressive form of caring. *Perspectives in caring monograph 2*, Toronto, ON: University of Toronto Faculty of Nursing.

45. Barrett, E. A. M. (Ed.). (1990). *Visions of Rogers' science-based nursing*. New York, NY: National League for Nursing.

46. Cowling, W. R. (1990). A template for unitary pattern-based practice. In E. A. M. Barrett (Ed.), *Visions of Rogers' science-based nursing*. New York, NY: NLN Publishing.

47. Cowling, W. R. (1993). Unitary knowing in nursing practice. *Nursing Science Quarterly, 6*, 201–207.

48. Cowling, W. R. (1993). Unitary practice: Revisionary assumptions. In M. Parker (Ed.), *Patterns of nursing theories in practice*. New York, NY: NLN Publishing.

49. Madrid, M., & Barrett, E. A. M. (Eds.). (1994). *Rogers' scientific art of nursing practice*. New York, NY: NLN Publishing.

50. Quinn, J. F. (1992). Holding sacred space; the nurse as healing environment. *Holistic Nursing Practice, 6*, 26–36.

51. Rogers, M. E. (1992). Nursing science and the space age. *Nursing Science Quarterly, 5*, 27–34.

52. Rogers, M. E. (1994). Nursing science evolves. In M. Madrid & E. A. M. Barrett (Eds.), *Rogers' scientific art of nursing practice*. New York, NY: NLN Publishing.

53. Rogers, M. E. (1994). Nursing science and art: A prospective. *Nursing Science Quarterly, 1*, 99–102.

54. Rogers, M. E. (1994). The science of unitary human beings: Current perspectives. *Nursing Science Quarterly, 7*, 33–35.

55. Newman, M. A. (1994). *Health as expanding consciousness*. New York, NY: NLN Publishing.

56. Madrid, M. (1997). *Patterns of rogerian knowing*. New York, NY: NLN Publishing.

57. Krieger, D. (1979). *The therapeutic touch: How to use your hands to help or heal*. Englewood Cliffs, NJ: Prentice-Hall.

58. Phillips, J. R. (1997). Martha E. Rogers: An icon of nursing. *Nursing Science Quarterly, 10*(1), 39–41.

59. Dossey, L. (1993). *Healing words*. San Francisco, CA: Harper.

60. Cowling, W. R. (1997). Pattern appreciation: The unitary science/practice of reaching for essence. In M. Madrid (Ed.), *Patterns of Rogerian knowing*. New York, NY: NLN Publishing.

61. Cowling, W. R. (1998). Unitary pattern appreciation. A Presentation at the Seventh Rogerian Conference: Nursing and the Changing Person-Environment: A Rogerian Science View; New York, June 20.

62. Roach, M. S. (Ed.). (1997). *Caring from the heart: The convergence of caring and spirituality*. New York, NY: Paulist Press.

63. Rogers, M. E. (1966). *The education violet*. New York, NY: New York University.

QUESTIONS FOR REFLECTION

Baccalaureate

1. What did you learn about the perspectives of Rogers and other proponents of the Science of Unitary Human Beings and their views on the concept of caring?
2. Why do you think that the proponents of the Science of Unitary Human Beings theory are so opposed to considering caring as a central, significant concept for nursing?
3. How would you define the phrase *concept clarification* as applied by Smith (1999)?

Master's

1. How would you define the phrase *constitutive meaning* as Smith (1999) explained it in her concept clarification process for caring in the context of the Science of Unitary Human Beings?
2. What did you learn from your review of the semantic expressions of caring specific to the constitutive meaning of *manifesting intentions*?
3. How did Smith (1999) use related literature sources on the semantic expressions of caring in the constitutive meaning of *appreciating pattern*? For example: Cowling, Mayeroff, Watson, and so on.

Doctoral

1. What is Smith's (1999) assumption for the concept clarification process used on caring framed by the Science of Unitary Human Beings?
2. What did you observe about the steps that Smith (1999) used to clarify the concept of caring and then positioned it in the context of the Science of Unitary Human Beings? List the steps.
3. Why do you think that Smith (1999) decided on following through on the instantiation process for the concept of caring framed by the Science of Unitary Human Beings?

4

What Is Known About Caring in Nursing Science

A Literary Meta-Analysis

KRISTEN M. SWANSON

Over the past two decades, there has been an escalating interest in the concept of caring, as evidenced in nursing dissertations, publications, investigations, theory debates, curriculum revolutions, conference agendas, and the making of professional policy. At the forefront of these activities are noted nurse theorists and philosophers such as Watson (1985, 1988a), Leininger (1981, 1988), P. Benner (1984), P. Benner and Wrubel (1989), Gaut (1983), Boykin (1994), Boykin and Schoenhofer (1993), Gadow (1980, 1984), and Roach (1984). These scholars remind the profession of nursing and the importance of studying caring because of its pivotal role in the practice of effective nursing as well as its centrality to preserving human dignity and sustaining humankind.

In the early 1990s, based on a review of the publications of 26 nursing authors, Morse, Bottorf, Neander, and Solberg (1991) and Morse, Solberg, Neander, Bottorf, and Johnson (1990) suggested that there were at least five conceptualizations of caring extant in then-current nursing discourse. They concluded that caring had been studied as a human trait, moral imperative, affect, interpersonal relationship, and nursing therapeutic. As this 1997 review of the caring literature was initiated, it became

apparent that nursing dialogue about caring could still best be characterized as a modern-day "Tower of Babel." There were many publications, some data based, some theory based, but few that built on the work of previous investigators. Hence, the *purpose* of this chapter is to summarize a literary meta-analysis of published nursing research on the concept of caring and to propose a framework that adequately integrates the current state of substantive knowledge about caring in nursing. Also, throughout this chapter, issues pertaining to syntax (methodology) are addressed.

At the Wingspread Caring Conference, sponsored by the Robert Wood Johnson Foundation and the American Academy of Nursing, summary papers of the importance of caring were offered by Watson (1990) and Leininger (1990), the philosophic and moral underpinnings were examined by Gadow (1990) and P. J. Benner (1990), and state-of-the-art papers were delivered by Stevenson (1990) and Tripp-Riemer and Cohen (1990). Tripp-Riemer focused on programs of qualitative inquiry pertaining to caring. Stevenson's paper was an extensive review of quantitative studies of therapeutic nursing interventions, in which the term *nursing care* was equated with

From Swanson, K. M. (1999). What is known about caring in nursing: A literary meta-analysis. In A. S. Hinshaw, J. Shaver, & S. Feetham (Eds.), *Handbook of clinical nursing research* (pp. 31–60). Thousand Oaks, CA: Sage. Permission to reprint granted by Sage Publications, Inc.

clinical interventions. The Wingspread Caring Conference is of historic importance to nursing science for several reasons: (a) by virtue of its occurrence, it provided concrete evidence that key professional gatekeepers in the discipline valued the concept of caring to the extent that resources were devoted to scholarly debate of the importance of role of caring in building knowledge for the discipline, profession, and society; (b) it brought together nurse scholars (from empirical, interpretive, and critical postmodern perspectives), consumers and practitioners (individuals were invited because of key familiarity with practicing, receiving, or recognizing the need for caring), and nurse leaders (i.e., from the National Institutes of Health [at that time, the National Center for Nursing Research], the Academy of Nursing, and other professional nursing organizations). Since that time, the visibility of caring in key nursing documents has become more and more commonplace (e.g., the recently revised American Nurses Association Social Policy Statement and current National League for Nursing standards for curriculum evaluation).

This chapter differs somewhat from each of those summaries offered at the Wingspread Conference in that it does not deal with the *philosophic underpinnings* or *importance* of caring to the discipline (the importance is assumed); it reviews *both* quantitative and qualitative published studies and attempts to pull together conclusions about what is known. Furthermore, unlike Stevenson's equating of "nursing care" with "nurse caring," the view taken by this author is that not all of nursing care (practice) necessarily equates with nurse caring (a *way* of practicing). Although many intervention studies (e.g., pain management, pre-op teaching) may be conceptually pulled together under the rubric of caring, unless those studies were published as conceptually grounded in caring, they have not been included in this chapter.

METHODS

Literature reviewed was primarily limited to published, data-based investigations of the concept of caring. Interpretive and empiric-analytic investigations of caring were included in this review. Noticeably lacking is a review of studies that offer a more critical (in the postmodern sense) and/or historic perspective on caring. International publications (English-language only) were retrieved via a computer search of recent nursing literature supplemented with additional studies referenced in those retrieved articles. Having not addressed unpublished theses and dissertations, this chapter is further limited.

Approximately 130 publications (articles, chapters, or books) were reviewed, the preponderance of which were published between 1980 and 1996. Most reviewed investigations focused explicitly on the concept of caring. In those investigations, data were obtained in many ways: from patient charts, observations of practice, and surveys or interviews of patients, families, nurses, students, teachers and other health care professionals. Research participants were observed or queried about their experiences, expectations, preferences, observations, meanings, and/or expressions of caring. Relationships investigated included nurse–colleagues, nurse–patient/family, student–teacher, student–student, student–patients, health care provider–patient/family, and family caregiver–family member. Several articles reviewed actually focused on concepts related to caring (e.g., expert practice or excellence in nursing, reassurance, nursing support, use of nursing intuition, comfort, family caregiving, etc.). These related concepts were included because the researchers' findings ultimately unearthed additional information about the concept of caring (e.g., caring may have been included as a descriptive or essential component of the related concept).

After reading at least half of the articles, a framework for categorizing *findings* from the studies reviewed was inductively derived. Focusing on each study's findings rather than its stated purpose ultimately made more sense. As has oftentimes been this author's experience with qualitative inquiry, the question with which the researchers started out may prove not quite the right direction to have been heading, given what is inductively learned about the phenomenon as it is explored (Swanson-Kauffman, 1986b; Swanson-Kauffman & Schonwald, 1988). In other words, where qualitative inquiry oftentimes takes investigators is not where they thought they were heading—rather, it is where the phenomenon examined takes them. Hence, realizing that findings take pragmatic precedence over questions, *research findings* were categorized into the five hierarchical levels of capacities, commitments/concerns, conditions, caring actions, and consequences.

In Level I, characteristics of persons with the *capacity* for caring are identified. Of interest in Level I findings are questions about whether these traits and characteristics are inherent (nature) or if they may be environmentally enhanced or diminished (nurture). Level II, *concerns/commitments*, focuses on the beliefs or values that undergird caring actions. Categorized in Level III are *conditions*. These are patient-, nurse-, or organization-related circumstances that enhance or diminish the likelihood that caring transactions will take place. Level IV (the bulk of qualitative and quantitative nursing inquiry about caring) describes *caring actions*, behaviors, or therapeutic interventions. Finally, Level V focuses on the positive and negative *consequences* of caring. These are both the intentional and the unintentional outcomes of caring for provider and/or recipient. Also in Level IV, caring actions, inductive findings about the enactment of caring, are categorized under Swanson's five caring categories (Swanson, 1990, 1991, 1993; Swanson-Kauffman, 1986a, 1988), thus providing both a conceptual framework for caring actions and empirical support

for the generalizability of Swanson's middle range theory of caring.

Glaser and Strauss (1967) described two possible levels of theory produced through qualitative inquiry. Theories of the first type, substantive, were considered to be very localized knowledge that is closely tied to the situation, context, or life experience of the limited number of participants included in the investigator's sample. The criteria for "truth" in studies of the substantive theory producing type were that the findings made sense to the people who participated in the investigation and that the researcher rigorously recreated what those participants had in common. Theories of the second type, formal, were considered more general, universal, or abstract and were better understood as descriptions of the structure of a given phenomena, life process, social construction, or concept. Formal theories were not yielded by single, intense, small-n studies; rather, they were the accumulation of a series of investigations about a similar phenomenon. This series could be the work of a given investigator across a variety of samples and settings (e.g., later in this chapter see the discussion of Beck's investigations of caring in academia) or the sum product of a series of investigators working on unearthing the essence of a given phenomena or concept. (This literary meta-analysis might itself be an example of such type.)

The five levels of caring knowledge are considered hierarchical not in order of importance but in the order of level of assumption. For example, an observational study of caring actions (Level IV) assumes that the individual or group studied had the capacity for caring (Level I), the commitment to act in a caring manner (Level II), and the conditions in place that are supportive of caring practices (Level III). Although, for any number of sound reasons, an investigator observing practice may not always administer a "caring capacity inventory" (assuming such an empirical device existed) to the practitioner ahead of time, it is not uncommon for an investigator wishing to study the occurrence of caring to query supervisors and peers for a known-to-be-caring nurse (e.g., as a criteria for recruitment) and to keep careful field notes about what else was going on during the period of observation (to deal with potential Level III historical competing variables). Similarly, if an organizational researcher observed that two separate long-term care facilities differed quite noticeably in contentment level of clients and their families, cleanliness of facilities, and staff retention patterns, the investigator might want to explore potential antecedents to these desirable (Level V) outcomes. The investigator might know personnel at both institutions and feel comfortable assuming that both facilities hire personnel who have the capacity (Level I) for caring and who are committed (Level II) to "doing good." Hence, the investigator may decide to target inquiry at the Level III conditions in place that may or may not support the occurrence of caring, as well as the Level IV caring actions themselves. In both of these examples offered, it is possible that the pragmatic investigators assumed too much and that failure to carefully measure the a priori assumed levels of caring may lead to making faulty or unnecessarily weak conclusions.

LEVEL I: THE CAPACITY FOR CARING

Findings about the characteristics of caring persons were rarely derived from questions directly addressing an individual's capacity to care. Results classified as Level I were more often produced by qualitative investigators posing broad questions such as "What constitutes caring in this critical care setting?" or "What is the experience of participating in a caring encounter for nurses, patients, students, families, and so on?" Typically, these studies yielded two kinds of information: what the nurse *does* and how the nurse *is*. Findings categorized under capacity are from those study results that interpret how a caring person *is*.

Findings from 21 studies that yielded information about caring capacities are listed in Table 4.1. These data were derived from inductive studies employing open-ended questions posed via interviews or written questionnaires. Data were analyzed using a variety of qualitative methods (phenomenology, grounded theory, inductive content analysis). These studies span the years from 1986 to 1996 and involved a total of 718 participants (262 nurses, 174 patients and/or families, 33 health care providers, and 249 nursing students). Findings from these qualitative investigations suggest that the caring nurse is compassionate, empathic, knowledgeable, confident, and reflective.

P. Benner and Wrubel (1989), strongly influenced by the work of Heidigger (1962), postulated that the origins of concern and caring are at the essence of being, a claim that human wholeness is characterized by the capacity for concern, loving, and caring. Similarly, Boykin and Schoenhofer (1993), drawing heavily from the writings of Mayeroff (1971) and Roach (1984), view caring as a human mode of being, a mode that remains with the nurse from moment to moment, hence rendering it possible to enhance the personhood of both client and nurse in any given nursing situation.

M. A. Ray (1987) interviewed eight American critical care nurses and Clarke and Wheeler (1992) interviewed six British nurses. In both of these phenomenologic investigations, questions were raised as to whether the capacity for caring is innate, taught, or due to having been cared for. P. Benner's (1984) phenomenologic investigation of excellence in nursing practice demonstrated that the ability to practice expert caring is enhanced with experience. Suspecting a link between developmental readiness and caring capacity, Soldwisch (1993) hypothesized a positive association between ego stage development and capacity for empathy and congruence. Based on a survey design study of 33 nursing students, she upheld both hypothesized relationships ($p < .03$) and provided evidence that the capacity to care effectively may be linked to maturational readiness.

Future Directions for Level I Inquiry

Similar to the next four levels, knowledge production on the capacity for caring has been quite small, local, and rarely builds on previous studies. The series of substantive investigations have involved small samples, single settings, or limited types of practice (e.g., critical care nurses). Table 4.1 suggests a structure for the capacities of caring providers, but it needs to be tested for utility. Further investigations are needed to develop research

measures with which to quantify caring capacity, explore the origins of caring capacity, examine the effects of nurturing and experience on caring capacity, and examine the relationship between the capacity for caring and the actual occurrence of caring practice. Pragmatically, it is very possible that Level I knowledge about the capacity of individuals (or groups) for caring may most logically be the purview of other disciplines (e.g., developmental psychology, sociology, anthropology), and it would make perfect sense for nurse investigators to build on or adopt outright tools, methods, or theories that adequately deal with this basic level of inquiry about the capacity for caring.

TABLE 4.1 Capacities of Caring Persons

| First Author, Year (Participants) | Caring Capacities | | | | |
	Compassionate	Empathic	Knowledgable	Positive	Reflective
Bäck-Pettersson and Jensen, 1993 (32 nurses)	Compassionate		Competent	Courageous	
Beck, 1991 (47 students)	Compassionate, dedicated	Understanding, empathic	Competent	Confident	Conscience, moral awareness
Beck, 1996 (37 students)	Emotional warmth	Understanding		Has personality	Open, willing to share
Clayton, Murray, Homes, & Greene, 1991 (70 families)	Compassionate	Concerned	Knowledgable	Courageous	Balanced, moral
Coulon, Krause, & Anderson, 1996 (156 students)	Dedicated	Aware, perceptive, intuitive	Knowledgable, competent, skillful	Cheerful, enabling personal qualities	Visionary
Davies & O'Berle, 1990 (1 nurse, 10 cases)	Giving of self, connecting			Self-worth, self-esteem	Looks inward, accepts and acknowledges own responses
Dietrich, 1992 (5 nurses)		Aware of others' needs, sensitive	Knowledgable		

(continued)

TABLE 4.1 Capacities of Caring Persons (*continued*)

First Author, Year (Participants)	Caring Capacities				
	Compassionate	Empathic	Knowledgable	Positive	Reflective
Donoghue, 1993 (82 nurses)		Sympathetic, can take another's perspective, empathic	Knowledgable, skillful		
Drew, 1986 (35 patients)				Self-reliant, adaptive, flexible	Quiet, calm, patient
Euswas, 1993 (30 patients, 32 nurses)	Benevolent		Competent		Constantly present in awareness of self
Farced, 1996 (8 patients)	–	Showing concern, being "in tune"	Knowledgable, skillful	Pleasant, cheerful attitude	
Girot, 1993 (10 nurses)		Concerned, empathic	Appropriately cautious, knows own limits	Good self-concept	Reflective
Halldorsdottir, 1990 (9 students)	Committed	Concerned	Competent	Positiveness	
Jensen, Bäck-Pettersson, & Segesten, 1992 (16 nurses)	Compassionate	Concerned	Knowledgable	Courageous	Reflective
Kahn & Steeves, 1988 (25 nurses)	Compassionate	Empathic			
Miller, Haber, & Byrne, 1992 (16 nurses)	Loving, involved			Feels good within self	
Montgomery, 1992 (35 nurses)	Unconditional love, involved, able to pull from abundance	Receptive to patient experience			Able to transcend ego
Poole & Rowat, 1994 (5 patients)	Patient	Understanding		Good mood	Genuine
Propst, Schenk, & Ciairain, 1994 (9 patients)	Warm	Understanding		Positive manner	
M. A. Ray, 1987 (8 nurses)		Understanding	Achieves mastery, competent	Confident	
Williams, 1992 (17 parents, 33 health care providers)	Have a caring heart		Knowledgable		

LEVEL II: CONCERNS/COMMITMENTS

P. Benner and Wrubel (1989) define concern as

> a way of being involved in one's own world in which people and things matter to one. It describes a phenomenological relationship in which the world is apprehended directly in terms of meaning for the self. Concern is the reason why people act. (p. 408)

Their basic claim is that when something matters to a person, that individual will pay attention to it. What concerns people helps them figure out where their commitments lie.

Level II findings categorized as concerns/commitments were derived from those research studies that focused on the beliefs or values that underlie nurse caring. Watson (1988b) and Noddings (1984) suggest that the source of a provider's values may be his or her compassionate loving essence or possibly adoption of professional values. That is to say, caring could be an act of love, a call to duty, or perhaps both. Similarly, Davies and O'Berle (1990), having closely examined one nurse's supportive encounters with 10 patients, described how having either a global value of the importance of caring or a specific valuing of a given person was essential to motivate the nurse to engage in supportive patient care. Likewise, Boykin and Schoenhofer (1993) claim that "the values and assumptions of nursing as caring can assist the nurse to engage fully in nursing situations with persons where caring is difficult to discover" (p. 37).

Kahn and Steeves (1988) interpreted data from 25 nursing students in a master's degree program in their hermeneutic investigation of the ideologic concepts and principles that nurses bring with them to encounters with patients. Values that undergird practices included professional identity, seeing persons as unique beings, being compassionate and empathic, and believing that their relationships should be therapeutic. Conversely, Kahn and Steeves concluded that a commitment to objectivity oftentimes hampered caring practices.

The results of 18 qualitative investigations that yielded information about the values and beliefs to which nurses are committed are summarized in Table 4.2. These studies included a total of 582 participants (231 students, 309 nurses, 30 patients, and 12 family caregivers). Although it may not have been the stated purpose of many of these investigators to summarize nursing values, their findings (at least in part) are best understood as descriptors of "*why* the nurse does." As outlined in Table 4.2 (and very similar to Kahn and Steeves' conclusions), caring in nursing is based on commitments to recognize the dignity and worth of each person, focus on the needs of the other, connect with the other, do the right thing, and remain present to the nurse's self.

The cultural origins of concerns/ commitments were addressed in Spangler's (1993) ethnonursing investigation of acute care American nurses from two culturally distinct backgrounds. The 22 Anglo-Americans interviewed believed in patients receiving education, being self-caring, and acting in compliance with care recommendations. They expected nurses to be autonomous and in control of situations. The 26 Filipino American nurses valued serious dedication to work, attentiveness to patients' physical comfort (especially cleanliness), and the importance of patience and respect for elders and those in charge. Spangler concluded that Anglo-American nurses reflected Western values of self-reliance, mastery of nature, and primacy of scientific knowledge. The Filipino American nurses reflected more Eastern values of the importance of cleanliness, group orientation, social acceptance, and respect for authority.

TABLE 4.2 Concerns and Commitments

First Author, Year (Participants)	Concerns and Commitments				
	Recognize Dignity and Worth of Each Person	Focus on the Other's Experience	Connect With the Other	Do the Right Thing	Be Present to the Self
Beck, 1991 (47 students)	Value others		Allow participation in another's experiences		Value self
Coulon et al., 1996 (156 students)	Recognize each patient as a person	Holistic approach to care		Care without prejudice, maintain quality standards	Consider nurse's own health
Davies & O'Berle, 1990 (1 nurse)	Value inherent worth of other	Do whatever has to be done to help the other	Establish rapport; give of self	Lend a hand; work on behalf of patient	Find meaning; preserve own integrity
Donoghue, 1993 (82 nurses)				Avoid hurting others	(–) Seeing nursing as just a job
Euswas, 1993 (30 patients, 32 nurses)			Realize intersubjective connectedness		Must be mindfully present and aware
Forrest, 1988 (17 nurses)					Protect self; focus on feeling good about own work
Hughes, 1992 (10 students)		Faculty must place high priority on meeting needs of students			
Kahn & Steeves, 1988 (25 nurses)	See persons as unique individuals		Build therapeutic relationships		(–) Need to maintain objectivity; practice in accordance with professional identity
Kosowski, 1995 (18 students)				Vow to never be noncaring	
McNamara, 1995 (5 nurses)	Value uniqueness of each person	Value spiritual and psychological needs	Must establish nurse-patient relationship		
Miller et al., 1992 (16 nurses)	Respect patient dignity; treat patient as you would like to be treated	Concentrate on patient, even when rushed			Have to feel good within yourself

| | Concerns and Commitments | | | | |
First Author, Year (Participants)	Recognize Dignity and Worth of Each Person	Focus on the Other's Experience	Connect With the Other	Do the Right Thing	Be Present to the Self
Montgomery, 1992 (35 nurses)		Willingly focus on patient, not self; do not try to own patient's experience	Allow for sacredness and interconnectedness of human life; allow self to become part of patient's experience; be willing to fall in love		
Nelms, 1996 (5 nurses)	Seek to create place where other's being can be preserved		Feel for patient; earn leads to more fully feeling self		Call to care = call to conscience = call to authenticity
Parker, 1994 (45 nurses)	Right to be treated as a person; respect for privacy and modesty	Care for whole person; think about how patient feels	Feel for patient; earn and keep patient trust; value compassion	Guard patient's welfare and well-being; know you are responsible; give 100%; willingly fight for patient; be accountable	Know yourself; aim for inner harmony
Powell-Cope, 1994 (12 FCGs)	Must be willing to see gay partner or caregiver as significant other	Phenomenologic orientation to strive to know another's experience	HCP must willingly enter a negotiated relationship with FCG	Shed prejudice	Must willingly confront own sexuality or homophobia
M. A. Ray, 1987 (8 nurses)	Consider "what if it were me or my family member?"	Value understanding the other; value and support patient or family choice	Value trust; giving and receiving leads to bonding	Make patient feel safe; make right decision; weigh in economics	Deal with conflicting values
Spangler, 1993 (48 nurses)	Filipino Americans respect elders	(–) Anglo-Americans expect compliance		Anglo-Americans value patient education and self-care; Filipino Americans value cleanliness and physical comfort	Anglo-Americans value autonomy, control; Filipino Americans value patience, duty, and respect for authority
Swanson, 1990 (19 parents or HCPs)			Attaching is part of care provision	Avoid bad outcomes for others; manage responsibilities	Avoid bad outcomes for self

Note. FCG = family caregiver; HCP = health care provider; (–) = condition that negatively affects caring.

The potential for conflict when a nurse's practice falls short of self-expectations was highlighted in Morrison's (1989, 1990) study of 25 charge-level nurses. Using repertory grid techniques, he asked each participant to generate his or her own list of constructs that characterize ideal nurses. Each nurse was then asked to rate himself or herself on each construct. Potential scores ranged from 0 to 48, and actual scores ranged from 1 to 26, with a mean score of 10.96. Morrison postulated that this gap between the view of self as "carer" and the "ideal carer" could lead to inner conflict wherein the provider might feel never quite good enough.

Finally, Forrest's (1988) phenomenologic investigation of 17 hospital staff nurses demonstrated that their caring actions were affected not just by beliefs but also by their experiences, self-appraisal, and feelings about their work. Unfortunately, as will be discussed in the section on *conditions*, not all nursing contexts are supportive of practicing in accordance with one's capacities or commitments.

Future Directions for Level II Inquiry

Knowledge building pertaining to Level II, commitments and concerns, calls for nursing investigations that rigorously bridge the standards for inquiry in ethics with insights into the everyday experiences of nurses in practice. Care must be taken not to prematurely close on the relevance of classic tenets (e.g., beneficence, justice, autonomy) of biomedical ethics to nursing practice, but nurse investigators are well advised to carefully consider the concerns and commitments that nurses employed in diverse settings (from the bedside to the national political arena) bring to their practice of caring. In addition, from a postmodern critical perspective, nurses must continue to address how the concerns and commitments that the profession holds may serve to inadvertently oppress both its practitioners and care recipients.

LEVEL III: CONDITIONS

Klausner (1971) suggested that any transaction will be affected by the demands, constraints, or resources brought to or evolving from the situation. Findings categorized under *conditions* were most often derived from questions about what affects caring, enhances caring interactions, or inhibits the occurrence of caring. Nurse and patient experiences, backgrounds and/or personalities, society, organizations, health status, and disease complications were all identified as influencing whether or not caring transpired.

Conditions that affect nurse caring could be as powerful and pervasive as homophobic, heterosexist biases (Powell-Cope, 1994), or as happenstance as everyday hassles such as weather or late delivery of supplies. Also important to the occurrence or perceptions of caring are the legal restrictions placed on practitioners. For example, Spangler (1993) noted that in addition to cultural influences on Filipino American nurses, visa restrictions (real or perceived) might also account for the tendency of Filipino American nurses to act in an extremely duty-conscious, dedicated, authority-honoring manner. Legal restrictions (e.g., limitations of licensure) might also account for some circumstances in which patients hold providers accountable for not adequately relieving their pain or completely addressing their immediate concerns.

It would be impossible to account for all conditions that might affect an unfolding nurse–client transaction. However, in Tables 4.3, 4.4, and 4.5, some of the patient- (Table 4.3), nurse- (Table 4.4), or organization- (Table 4.5) related conditions are outlined that may enhance or diminish the occurrence of caring actions. Findings in Table 4.3 were derived from 14 investigations involving 676 participants (177 students, 202 nurses, 72 patients/families, and 225 health care providers). The majority of findings were derived from

TABLE 4.3 Patient-Related Conditions That Affect Caring

First Author, Year (Participants)	Conditions: Patient Related					
	Communication	Personality	Health Problems	Care Needs	Nurse–Patient Relationship	Other
Baer & Lowery, 1987 (140 students)		Cheerful; accepts illness	Has pain	Ambulatory; needs nursing assistance	At least half of the reasons to like or dislike patient care are due to relationship	Tidy; attractive; male
Beck, 1996 (37 students)	(–) Verbally abusive	(–) Combative; (–) distorted self-evaluation	(–) Unpredictable			
Boyd & Munhall, 1989 (15 RN students)		Victimized; vulnerable	Uncertainty in outcomes, treatment diagnoses, distressed	Helpless		
Cohen & Sarter, 1992 (23 nurses)	Patient's gratitude	(–) Patient or family is hard to deal with	Patients becoming well; (–) patient's dying	Physiologic emergencies; psychosocial needs		
Cohen, 1994 (38 nurses)	Patient gratitude; (–) patient or family yelling at nurse	(–) Patient anger	Patients surviving; (–) losing patients	Able to be comforted; (–) no cure available; (–) pain can't be relieved		
Euswas, 1993 (30 patients, 32 nurses)		Vulnerable		Needs nursing assistance		
Forrest, 1988 (17 nurses)	(±) What patient says	(–) Hard-to-care-for patient			(–) Disagreements with patient	
Green-Hernandez, 1991 (12 nurses)	Patient or family responds favorably					
Jenny & Logan, 1996 (20 patients)			Physically and emotionally distressed			

69

(continued)

TABLE 4.3 Patient-Related Conditions That Affect Caring (*continued*)

First Author, Year (Participants)	Conditions: Patient Related					
	Communication	Personality	Health Problems	Care Needs	Nurse–Patient Relationship	Other
Kahn & Steeves, 1988 (25 nurses)	(–) Unwilling to communicate	Alert, personable outgoing; (–) poor self-image; (–) patient's actions cause problems	Many psychosocial problems; dire circumstances	Relies on nurse	"Fits" with nurse's personality; reciprocated friendship	
Leners, 1993 (40 nurses)			Sicker patients bring out stronger use of nurse's intuition.	Nurse is more likely to use intuition in intense relationship		
Peteet, Rose, Medeiros, Walsh-Burke, & Rieker, 1992 (192 HCPs)	Honest about feelings and desires	Spirited; courageous; has will to live; sense of humor; (–) unattractive in personality		Has involved family; (–) unusually demanding	HCP able to identify with patient; patient interested in staff member's life	(–) Unattractive appearance; (–) patient has VIP status
Poole, 1994 (5 patients)			Physiologic concerns	Needs physical care, information, and coordination of services	Reciprocity: contact occurs	
Williams, 1992 (17 parents, 33 HCPs)	(–) Patient or family directly resists support	(–) Manifest anger; (–) denial			(–) Patient or family openly clashes with staff	

Note. (–) = condition that negatively affects caring; (±) = depending on what patient says, could positively or negatively affect caring; HCP = health care provider.

qualitative analyses of written or verbal accounts. One exception is Baer and Lowery's (1987) discriminant analysis of coded and quantified written student narratives of least-versus most-liked patient care situations. Typical studies that produced findings categorized under patient-related conditions focused on providers' preferences for "types" of patients they most liked. It is probably not safe to assume that liking a patient or the enjoyment of caring for a certain kind of patient automatically leads to caring actions (or the converse), but it is highly likely that attraction has at least some part to play in the actions that unfold in the nurse–patient encounter. Patient-related conditions that may influence the occurrence of caring include patient communication, personality, health problems, care needs, relationship with nurse, appearance, and "other."

As will be demonstrated a bit later in this chapter, giving time is frequently referred to as an action that indicates nurse caring. Two investigations provide evidence that patient-related conditions have a key part in soliciting nursing time. Halloran's (1985) exploration of nursing workload involved examining 2,560 patient records. These were the records of every patient admitted to a 279-bed acute care community hospital over a 4-month period. Charts were examined for nursing workload (dependent variable), nursing diagnosis, medical diagnosis, and patient demographics. It was found that 53.2% of the variance in nursing workload was accounted for by the patient's *nursing*-related condition as measured by the index of frequency of each nursing diagnosis. Medical diagnostic-related conditions accounted for 26.3% of the workload variance. When nursing workload was regressed on all independent variables, combined nursing and medical diagnostic indexes accounted for 60% of the variation in daily nursing.

Swan, Benjamin, and Brown (1992) also examined the amount of time it took to provide care. They compared 20 patients with AIDS with 29 patient without AIDS on the variable "daily direct nursing care hours." They documented that patients with AIDS required 6.5 hours per day of direct nursing care; the comparison group took 5.43 hours. Interestingly, both exceeded the state's definitive criteria for a skilled nursing facility, which was 3 hours of direct care per day. Together, Halloran's and Swan et al.'s studies provide evidence that caring—taken in its simplest sense, time—is directly related to patients' needs for supportive or substitutive care.

Table 4.4, Nurse-Related Conditions That Affect Caring, is based on a total sample of 728 participants (322 nurses, 17 patients/parents, 33 health care providers, 258 students, and 98 observations of nursing practice). Once again, the majority of studies leading to the descriptions of nurse conditions affecting caring were derived from qualitative inquiry. Notable exceptions include Weiss' (1984) study of 240 students, wherein 120 males and 120 females were asked to view videotapes of nursing practice and identify instances and antecedents of nurse caring. The results of Weiss' inquiry are listed in Table 4.4.

Young, Koch, and Preston (1989) viewed lack of understanding as a constraint to rural nurses adequately meeting the care needs of persons with AIDS. They offered a 1-day workshop in which they relayed information about HIV/AIDS and provided opportunities to deal with feelings and attitudes toward homosexuality and fears about caring for clients with AIDS. Before the workshop, immediately after, and 3 months after the workshop, participants completed investigator-developed surveys of their knowledge, attitudes, fears, and willingness to care for clients with AIDS. Two hundred nurses attended the workshop, 143 completed

TABLE 4.4 Nurse-Related Conditions That Affect Caring

First Author, Year (Participants)	Conditions: Nurse Related					
	Resources		Constraints		Demands	
	Personal	Professional	Personal	Professional	Personal	Professional
Brown & Ritchie, 1989 (25 nurses)				(–) Lacks communication, conflict management, or family-centered care skills		
Clarke & Wheeler, 1992 (6 nurses)		Talking and sharing with others	(–) Tiredness; (–) unrecognized for their efforts	(–) Frustrations; (–) witnessing patients who can't be cured	(–) Personal problems	(–) Feeling overstretched and too busy; (–) night duty
Cohen & Sarter, 1992 (23 nurses)	Life experience sensitizes and creates empathy	Being able to offer comfort; witnessing miracles and patients surviving	(–) Work evokes old unresolved issues from nurse's life		(–) Difficulties balancing work and home	
Cohen, 1994 (38 nurses)	Having learned from patients about personal priorities	Witnessing survivals due to technological advances; learning new skills; getting through tough times		(–) Having inadequate psychosocial skills; (–) witnessing death, suffering; (–) leaving patients at end of shift who are not well	(–) Bringing work problems home	(–) Balancing many different roles
Donoghue, 1993 (82 nurses)	Caring family upbringing; personal experiences with death and illness; personal satisfaction from caring	Education; more than 1 year experience; observing positive and negative role models				

| | Conditions: Nurse Related | | | | | |
| | Resources | | Constraints | | Demands | |
First Author, Year (Participants)	Personal	Professional	Personal	Professional	Personal	Professional
Forrest, 1988 (17 nurses)	Own experiences; self-appraisal; coping abilities	Learning caring at school; feeling good about work	(–) Personal stress			(–) Dilemmas; (–) conflicts
Green-Hemandez, 1991 (12 nurses)	Caring for self	Education; professional practice; technical competency				
Kahn & Steeves, 1988 (25 nurses)		Can make the temporal investment needed to do the job	(–) Tiredness; (–) animosity; (–) inability to get along with patient	(–) Temporal limits		(–) Can only "spread self so thin"
Kosowski, 1995 (18 students)	Life-learning as background to book learning	Role-modeling; reversing (after seeing bad care modeled); experience leads to awareness				
Leners, 1993 (40 nurses)	Nurse well-being; self-perception	Experience with sensing, identifying, listening to intuition; intense patient relationship				
O'Berle & Davies, 1992 (1 nurse, 10 cases)	Maintains wholeness; deals with stress; self-appraises; assesses personal costs of caring	Feels good about own work				

(continued)

73

TABLE 4.4 Nurse-Related Conditions That Affect Caring (continued)

First Author, Year (Participants)	Conditions: Nurse Related					
	Resources		Constraints		Demands	
	Personal	Professional	Personal	Professional	Personal	Professional
Parker, 1994 (45 nurses)	Experiencing inner harmony	Ability to give knowledgeable care; being accountable for patient's welfare and well-being	(–) Not feeling respected for knowledge; (–) distrust bureaucratic motives	(–) Being unable to tell patient the whole truth; (–) not able to practice according to values		(–) Too many tasks; (–) going along with treatments nurse disagrees with
M. A. Ray, 1987 (8 nurses)		Being comfortable enough with technology to focus on patient				Conflict between use of high-tech care and right to die
Solberg & Morse, 1991 (98 observations)			(–) Detached	(–) Believes infants feel no pain; (–) misses nonverbal cues		
Weiss, 1984 (240 students)		Females attuned to verbal and nonverbal caring; males attuned to technical competency				
Williams, 1992 (17 parents, 33 HCPs)			(–) Personal inabilities; (–) costs of being involved	(–) Not seeing parents as experienced in care of own children		(–) Too intense work; (–) conflict with parents

Note. (–) = condition that negatively affects caring; HCPs = health care providers.

74

the first two surveys, and 56 completed the third survey. On every measure, significant improvements (compared with pre-workshop) were found at the immediate and 3 months postmeasurement times ($p < .01$). Although this study is limited by design, instrumentation, and attrition, it does suggest that knowledge and an opportunity to deal openly with fears may enhance practice in situations in which nurses feel threatened.

Nurse-related conditions that affect caring may be personal (personality, family history) or professional (education, experience) in origin. Conditions may be further broken down into resources, demands, and constraints. An example of a nurse who is "primed" to acting in a caring fashion is one who has the personal resources of a strong, caring family upbringing and who is self-reflective, has limited personal constraints (e.g., is neither tired nor detached) and limited personal demands (e.g., not imbalanced or overburdened), has professional resources such as years of experience and ease with technology, has limited professional constraints (e.g., inadequate psychosocial skills or feeling constricted in how much he or she can disclose to a patient), and experiences minimal professional demands (e.g., feeling overstretched and morally conflicted). As Watson (1988a) has suggested, just as each patient's causal past will affect each caring transaction, so, too, will each nurse's personal and professional demands, constraints, and resources affect the capacity to act in a caring manner.

The organization-related conditions that will affect caring are outlined in Table 4.5. This table is based on a total sample of 543 participants (216 nurses, 65 administrators, 37 patients/family caregivers, 33 health care providers, and 192 individuals affiliated with a given hospital [includes providers and clients]). To date, M. A. Ray (1984, 1989) has published most extensively about characteristics of caring organizations. She strongly emphasizes that what constitutes caring for any individual frequently comes down to his or her role within the organization. Organizationally based factors affecting the occurrence of caring actions include role- and personnel-related demands, constraints, and resources; technologic possibilities and limitations; administrative support, decisions, and expectations; and worksite or practice conditions.

Future Directions for Level III Inquiry

This discussion of Level III conditions has been limited to nurse, patient, and organizational conditions that support the likelihood of caring actions occurring. Staying within this perspective, measures are clearly needed with which to quantify conditions that may serve as competing variables when attempting to investigate links between caring actions and their outcomes. However, there are distinct limits to restrict the measure of environmental conditions to the organizational level. Inquiry pertaining to Level III conditions calls for investigators who carefully consider the unit of analysis as larger than the classic individual nurse–individual patient dyad (practicing within an identified inpatient or community setting) and who recognize the wisdom that can be obtained from the study of aggregates. A more complete understanding of the conditions that affect the practice of caring calls for large-scale studies involving the examination of economic trends, cultural expectations, national policy outcomes, and sociopolitical constructions of what it is to be healthy, who is a patient, and what the criteria and qualifications of providers (nurses included) must be to meet the health care needs of society.

TABLE 4.5 Organization-Related Conditions That Affect Caring

First Author Year (Participants)	Conditions: Organization Related			
	Personnel or Role Related	Technology	Administration	Work or Practice Conditions
J. Brown & Ritchie, 1989 (25 nurses)			(−) No in-service to support parent care; (−) no rewards for parent care	(−) Practice standards do not make nurse accountable for care of parents
Cohen, 1994 (38 nurses)	Sense of community; peer support, respect; (−) poor teamwork; (−) peers critical, dominating, jealous	Learning new technical, psychosocial, or cultural skills; (−) poor equipment; (−) learning the hard way	Encourage development; (−) controlling, unwilling to share authority; (−) limited financial or human resources	(−) Too little time to accomplish all that is required; (−) witnessing poor care; (−) when care seems futile
Cohen, 1992 (23 nurses)	Peer recognition; (−) difficulties with medical staff; (−) peer conflict			(−) Poor staffing, overworked and inadequate time; (−) unexpected crisis
Cooper, 1993 (9 nurses)		Technology can enhance competent care or (−) detract nurse away from patient and to machines		
Dietrich, 1992 (5 nurses)			Promotes communication; visible and available; easy to talk to; allows time to vent concerns; offers recognition; clear organizational mission	(−) Overwhelming workload; (−) lack of time, space, interactions, help, or clear expectations
Duffy, 1995 (56 nurses)			Communicates; creates open, trusting unit culture; share self; invest in staff	
Fareed, 1996 (8 patients)				Reassuring environment is pleasant, unthreatening, and not rigid

76

Conditions: Organization Related

First Author Year (Participants)	Personnel or Role Related	Technology	Administration	Work or Practice Conditions
Forrest, 1988 (12 nurses)	Teamwork; fellow staff support		Supportive unit supervisors; (–) difficult nurse administrators	(–) Poor physical environment; (–) lack of time
Leners, 1993 (40 nurses)		Intuition is used more if there is less equipment to rely on		Intuition is used more if there are fewer others and fewer distractions
Powell-Cope, 1994 (12 FCGs)			Policies must allow FCGs easier access to HCPs	
M. A. Ray, 1984 (192 HCPs, patients, Ad)	Information shared; strong communication; high interactions	Practical and technical skills essential; technology available, maintained, upgraded	Economic welfare considered; coordinating activities and time	
M. A. Ray, 1989 (65 Ad)	Team effort; work divided by roles; care concerns and expressions differ by role	In intensive care and emergency room, use of technology is a way to be caring	Sustain economic viability of organization; garner resources to support care; support patient and nurse; make politically wise decisions	In different units there are differing care concerns (i.e., legal, technical, spiritual)
M. A. Ray, 1987 (8 nurses)		Comfort with technology enables focus on patient and family		
Williams, 1992 (17 P, 33 HCPs)	(–) Politics of nurse–physician communication; (–) inexperience		(–) Inconsistent staffing patterns; (–) cumbersome bureaucracy	(–) Lack of staff; (–) lack of time; (–) too intense workloads

Note. HCPs = health providers; P = parents; Ad = administrators; FCGs = family caregivers; (–) = condition that negatively affects caring.

77

LEVEL IV: CARING ACTIONS

Quantitative Inquiry

There have been two main ways of studying caring actions. First, similar to the previous three levels, involves qualitative analysis of verbal text generated from nurse or client discourse about what caring means to them. Second thrust of caring action investigations involves the use of caring behavior inventories that direct nurses, patients, or students to rank nurse caring behaviors on a least to most important scale. Tables 4.6 and 4.7 briefly summarize research findings pertaining to most highly ranked nurse caring behaviors according to nurses (Table 4.6) and patients (Table 4.7). Table 4.8 focuses specifically on studies that have employed Larson's (1984, 1986, 1987) CARE-Q sort and that published patient- or nurse-ranked behaviors according to Larson's theoretically generated subscales.

Caring behavior ranking studies have employed four different measures. Larson's original CARE-Q sort is the most widely used. It involves 50 nurse caring behaviors and six subscales. Items and subscales were initially generated from the literature. Respondents are directed to sort nurse caring behaviors along a quasinormal distribution ranging from most important (1) to least important (7). Cronin and Harrison's (1988) Caring Behaviors Assessment (CBA) includes 63 behaviors drawn from Watson's (1988) Carative Factors. Items are portrayed on a five-point Likert-type scale. Wolf (1986) generated the Caring Behavior Inventory (CBI) based on the literature and expert input. The original CBI consists of 75 caring words or phrases arranged on a four-point Likert-type scale. Finally, Gardner and Wheeler's (1981, 1987) Supportive Nursing Behaviors Checklist (SNBC) consists of 67 behaviors derived from the literature and expert input. Items are arranged along a seven-point Likert-type scale.

Because Larson's CARE-Q is the most widely used caring behavior measure, Tables 4.6 and 4.7 use Larson's items as the basis for comparison. When other caring measures were employed by investigators, I looked for items similar in meaning to those in the CARE-Q and included them in the comparison. Sometimes, the wordings of the alternative measure were slightly different; hence, noted in the legends under Tables 4.6 and 4.7 are those judgments I made as to which items seemed comparable.

Table 4.6 focuses on nurses' most highly ranked caring behaviors. It is based on a combined sample of 517 nurses. Eight of the samples used Larson's CARE-Q, one sample used Gardner and Wheeler's SNBC, and another used Wolf's CBI. Listed are the top five endorsed caring behavior items per sample. Exceptions are Mangold (1991), who published only the top endorsed behavior, and Gardner and Wheeler, who published only the top three endorsed items. Across all samples, "Listens to the patient" falls within the top five endorsed behaviors. Likewise, 90% of the combined possible sample endorsed "Allows expression of feelings." Seventy-six percent endorsed touching to comfort, 71% favored being perceptive of patient needs, 64% realized the patient knew himself or herself best. These behaviors, which were endorsed as being in the top five–ranked nurse caring behaviors by more than 50% of the total sample, provide strong support for the fact that nurses believe it is important to know the patient well and to offer touch to comfort. Similar to the claim of Tanner, Benner, Chesla, and Gordon (1993), knowing the patient contextually is considered central to providing effective nursing care. Also, nurse touching based on striving to know the patient's feelings and experiences may account for why nurses claim their touching to comfort is therapeutic.

TABLE 4.6 Nurses' Most Highly Rated Nurse Caring Behaviors

Nurses' Most Highly Rated Nurse Caring Behaviors

Caring Behavior Item (Items are Abbreviated)	vonEssen, 1994[a] (19 nurses)	Gooding, 1993 (46 nurses)	Keane 1987 (26 nurses)	Komorita, 1991 (110 nurses)	Larson, 1986 (57 nurses)	Mayer, 1987 (28 nurses)	Mangold, 1991[b] (30 nurses)	Mangold, 1991[b] (30 students)	Gardner, 1981[c] (74 nurses)	Wolf, 1986 (97 nurses)	N/Possible N (Not all scales published comparable items)	Percentage of Possible Subjects
Listens to the patient	1	1	4.5	1	1	1	1	1	3	1	517/517	100
Allows expression of feelings	2	2		2	3	2			2	4 "patience"	412/457	90
Touches when comforting is needed				4	2	4				2 "comforts"	292/383	76
Is perceptive of the patient's needs	4	4		5		5					203/286	71
Realizes patient knows self best		3		3		3					184/286	64
Gets to know patient as a person		5			4				1 "shows interest in patient as person"		177/360	49
Gives the patient treatments and medications on time	2		4.5							5 "respon- sible"	142/383	37

(continued)

79

TABLE 4.6 Nurses' Most Highly Rated Nurse Caring Behaviors (continued)

Caring Behavior Item (Items are Abbreviated)	Nurses' Most Highly Rated Nurse Caring Behaviors										N/Possible N (Not all scales published comparable items)	Percentage of Possible Subjects
	vonEssen, 1994[a] (19 nurses)	Gooding, 1993 (46 nurses)	Keane, 1987 (26 nurses)	Komorita, 1991 (110 nurses)	Larson, 1986 (57 nurses)	Mayer, 1987 (28 nurses)	Mangold, 1991[b] (30 nurses)	Mangold, 1991[b] (30 students)	Gardner, 1981[c] (74 nurses)	Wolf, 1986 (97 nurses)		
Tells patient what is important to know	4									3 "honesty"	116/383	30
Talks to the patient					5						57/286	20
Knows when to call doctor			1								26/286	9
Puts patient first no matter what			3								26/286	9
Gives good physical care			2								26/286	9
Knows how to give shots and manage equipment	3										19/286	7

Note. vonEssen, Larson, Gooding, Mayer = oncology nurses; Keane = rehabilitation nurses; Wolf = mostly adult care nurses; Gardner = medical-surgical and psychiatric nurses; Mangold = faculty and senior nursing students; Komorita = advanced practice nurses and faculty. Measures: Larson's CARE-Q used by Larson, vonEssen, Gooding, Keane, Mayer, Komorita, Mangold, total *n* = 346; Gardner and Wheeler's SNBC used by Gardner, *n* = 74; Wolf's CBI used by Wolf, *n* = 97. Math for combining samples: CARE-Q, SNBC, and CBI users, total *n* = 517; CARE-Q users minus Mangold sample plus CBI and SNBC users, total *n* = 457; CARE-Q users minus Mangold sample plus CBI users, total *n* = 383; CARE-Q users minus Mangold sample plus SNBC users, total *n* = 360; CARE-Q users minus Mangold sample, total *n* = 286; CBI and SNBC users, total *n* = 171.
[a] All references are cited by first author's name only.
[b] Mangold only listed top chosen item.
[c] Gardner only listed top three chosen items.

Table 4.7 outlines the five most highly ranked nurse caring behaviors endorsed by a combined sample of 385 patients drawn from eight separate studies. Once again, Larson's CARE-Q is used as the basis for comparison, as it was used in five of the studies. Two studies used Cronin and Harrison's CBA, and one used Gardner and Wheeler's SNBC. Items were not quite as comparable across these three measures. Hence, the most highly ranked behavior, "Helps me to feel confident adequate care was provided," was only applicable to samples using the CBA and SNBC. This item, along with the second most highly ranked item (93%), "Knows how to give shots and manage equipment," suggest that what patients value most highly is that the nurse is technically competent. The next four most highly endorsed items indicate that the patient wants the nurse to value, know, respect, and relate to them in a positive manner. The last two items endorsed by at least 50% of the combined samples suggest that patients want nurses to respond quickly when called and to know enough to call their doctor when necessary. Clearly, patients want nurses to be competent, focused on their evolving needs, and aware of when it is necessary to garner additional medical support.

It is fascinating to note the apparent divergent values between nurses and patients. Although 100% of the nurses value listening, only 10% of the patients ranked it in their top five behaviors. Likewise, although at least 93% of the patients endorsed the importance of technical skill, only 7% of nurses ranked "Knows how to give shots and manage equipment" in their top five behaviors. The origins of these discrepancies are compelling. Perhaps, the gap lies in the fact that behaviors (not meanings) were solicited. Gaut (1983) stated that "whether certain actions will count as caring is dependent on what the action is, the intent of the doer, and the context in which it is done" (p. 317). It may be that both patients and nurses ultimately intend

to ensure that safe, individualized care is offered, but nurses are challenged by the acts of getting to know each patient's personal needs for safe care, whereas patients are challenged by how the foreign, highly technical equipment surrounding them will be safely used to meet their personal needs.

Table 4.8 lists those studies that published subscale rankings using the Larson CARE-Q. The two overall most highly endorsed grouping of behaviors by nurses are the Comforts and Anticipates subscales. Patients most highly endorsed the Accessible subscale. There was a tie for patients' second most endorsed: Anticipates, and Monitors and Follows Through. Subscale level rankings would suggest that both nurses and patients value accessibility. However, nurses remain challenged to comfort, and patients desire that the nurses anticipate, monitor, and follow through with meeting their needs. Conceivably, nurses view accessibility, anticipating, monitoring, and following through as means to a goal of comforting.

Finally, it must be noted that recently Larson and Ferketich (1993) and Wolf, Giardino, Osborne, and Ambrose (1994) have psychometrically revised their measures. Larson's scale has been factor analyzed and is now a 39-item visual analogue scale called the CARE/SAT (Caring Satisfaction Scale). Based on factor analysis of the revised original scale submitted to 268 hospitalized adults, three subscales were generated: Assistive, Benign Neglect, and Enabling. Surprisingly, the item "Listens to the patient" did not meet requirements for retention. It would be of interest to see if factor analysis of the same revised original scale submitted to nurses would produce similar results. In contrast, Wolf et al. did submit the CBI to a conveniently recruited sample of 278 patients and 263 nurses. The factor analysis yielded a 42-item, four-point Likert-type measure with five factors: respectful deference to

TABLE 4.7 Patients' Most Highly Rated Nurse Caring Behaviors

Caring Behavior Item (Items are abbreviated)	Patients' Most Highly Rated Nurse Caring Behaviors									
	vonEssen, 1994[a] (19 patients)	Gooding, 1993 (42 patients)	Keane, 1987 (26 patients)	Larson, 1984 (57 patients)	Mayer, 1986 (54 patients)	Cronin, 1988 (22 patients)	Mullins, 1996 (46 patients)	Gardner, 1981, 1987 (119 patients)	N/possible N (Not all scales published comparable items)	Percentage of Possible Subjects
Helps me to feel confident adequate care was provided						[b]	2[b]	1	187/187	100
Knows how to give shots and manage equipment		1	3	1	1	3	3		247/266	93
Gets to know patient as a person							1[c]	3[d]	165/187	88
Puts patient first no matter what			2		4	2[e]	4[e]	5[f]	267/385	69
Treats me with respect							5		46/68	68
Is cheerful					2			2[g]	173/317	55
Knows when to call doctor		4	1	2		5			147/266	55
Gives quick response to patient's call		2		3					99/198	50
Is honest with patient	1							4	138/317	44
Gives good physical care		5	5	4					83/198	42

Patients' Most Highly Rated Nurse Caring Behaviors

Caring Behavior Item (Items are abbreviated)	vonEssen, 1994[a] (19 patients)	Gooding, 1993 (42 patients)	Keane, 1987 (26 patients)	Larson, 1984 (57 patients)	Mayer, 1986 (54 patients)	Cronin, 1988 (22 patients)	Mullins, 1996 (46 patients)	Gardner, 1981, 1987 (119 patients)	N/possible N (Not all scales published comparable items)	Percentage of Possible Subjects
Gives the patient treatments and meds on time	3		4	5				X[h]	125/317	39
Anticipates that first times are the hardest	4				5				73/198	37
Knows how to handle equipment						4			22/68	32
Encourages patient to ask questions					3				54/198	27
Is perceptive of patient's needs		5						X	42/317	13
Tells patient what is important to know	2								19/198	10
Listens to patient	5								19/198	10
Helps patient clarify his or her thinking	3							X	19/317	6

Note. vonEssen, Gooding, Larson, Mayer = oncology patients; Keane = rehabilitation patients; Cronin = patients who had a myocardial infarction; Mullins = patients with HIV/AIDS; Gardner = medical-surgical and psychiatric adult patients. Measures: Larson's CARE-Q used by Larson, vonEssen, Gooding, Keane, Mayer, total $n = 198$; Cronin and Harrison's CBA used by Cronin, Mullin, total $n = 68$; Gardner and Wheeler's SNBC used by Gardner, $n = 119$. Math for combining samples: CARE-Q, SNBC, and CBA users, total $n = 385$; CARE-Q and SNBC users, total $n = 317$; CARE-Q and CBA users, total $n = 266$; SNBC and CBA users, total $n = 187$.

a All references are cited by first author's name only.
b "Knows what they're doing" (actual wording of researcher's questionnaire).
c "Treat me as an individual."
d "Showed interest in me."
e "Makes me feel someone is there if I need them."
f "Showed interest in my welfare."
g "Was friendly."
h X = SNBC has a similar item but not rated in top 5.

TABLE 4.8 Larson's CARE-Q Subscale Rankings for Nurses and Patients

CARE-Q Subscale	Nurse Subscale Rankings							Patient Subscale Rankings				
	Mangold, 1991, 1991		Mayer, 1986	Larson, 1986	vonEssen, 1994	Average of Nurse Ranking	Overall Nurse Rank	Mayer, 1986	Larson, 1984	vonEssen, 1994	Average of Nurse Rankings	Overall Nurse Rank
	30 Nurses	28 Students	28 Nurses	57 Nurses	19 Nurses			54 Patients	57 Patients	19 Patients		
Accessible	2	5	5	3	1	3.2	3	1	2	4	2.3	1
Explains	5	2	4	6	6	4.6	6	6	5	3	4.7	4
Anticipates	3	4	1	2	3	2.6	2	4	3	1	2.7	2
Comforts	6	1	2	1	2	2.4	1	3	4	2	3.0	3
Monitors and follows through	4	3	6	5	4	4.4	5	2	1	5	2.7	2
Trusting relationship	1	6	3	4	5	3.8	4	5	5	6	5.3	5

the other, assurance of human presence, positive connectedness, professional knowledge and skill, and attentiveness to the other's experience.

Item-level examination of the revised CBI suggests that Wolf et al. (1994) have quantitatively arrived at a factor structure quite compatible with Swanson's (1990, 1991, 1993) and Swanson-Kauffman's (1986a, 1988) phenomenologically derived five caring categories, Swanson initially derived her categories through phenomenologic inquiry into the caring desires of women who miscarried. She subsequently revised those categories, based on a study of what it is like to provide caring according to 19 care providers (parents or professionals) in a newborn intensive care unit. Finally, the categories were reexamined for their relevance according to eight at-risk new mothers who had received an intensive long-term public health nursing intervention (Swanson, 1991). Each of Swanson's five caring categories is more fully discussed in the next section. Wolf's *attentiveness* parallels Swanson's *knowing*; *human presence* is akin to *being with*; *professional knowledge and skill* is like *doing for*; *respectful deference* echoes *enabling*; and *positive connectedness* has much in common with *maintaining belief.* The similarities between Wolf's and Swanson's findings are at least in part attributable to the fact that their factors or categories were derived from mixed samples of providers and recipients of caring.

Qualitative Inquiry

Initial classification of the qualitatively derived caring actions resulted in a grid of 20 groupings of actions by 67 investigations. This involved a total sample of 2,314 participants (632 nurses, 607 patients/ families, 564 students, 259 health care providers [including nurses], 131 family caregivers, 98 practice observations, and 23 patient charts). Further examination of the 20 action groups led me to realize the utility of using the five caring categories I had previously derived through studies in three separate perinatal contexts. In the end, this effort led to two outcomes: a conceptually based framework for classifying caring actions that were inductively derived across many separate investigations and validation for the generalizability of Swanson's middle-range theory of caring beyond the clinical contexts from which it was originally generated.

Swanson (1991) defines caring as "a nurturing way of relating to a valued other toward whom one feels a personal sense of commitment and responsibility" (p. 162). Similar to the overall framework for this chapter, alluded to in this definition are capacity (capability of valuing another), commitments (personal sense of commitment), role-related condition (responsibility), actions (way of relating), and consequences (nurturing). Categories identified by Swanson and used as an outline for Table 4.9 include *maintaining belief* (sustaining faith in the other's capacity to get through an event or transition and face a future with meaning), *knowing* (striving to understand an event as it has meaning in the life of the other), *being with* (being emotionally present to the other), *doing for* (doing for others what they would do for themselves if it were at all possible), and *enabling* (facilitating the other's passage through life transitions and unfamiliar events). Each of these categories involves subcategories that are italicized in Table 4.9.

Future Directions for Level IV Inquiry

Conceptually caring actions have a lot in common (*universality*, according to Leininger, 1988), but their actual expression will be as different as the individuals involved and the reasons for caring (Leininger's *diversality*). For example, what it takes to enable a single mother with breast cancer to live a quality life versus what it would take to support an elderly person with Alzheimer's to remain with family caregivers would both involve

TABLE 4.9 Inductively Derived Caring Action, Arranged by Swanson's (1990, 1991, 1993) and Swanson-Kauffman's (1986[a], 1988) Caring Categories

	References[a]		References[a]
Maintaining belief			
Believing in or holding in esteem		*Offering realistic optimism*	
1. Holistically viewing the other		1. Having a positive attitude	57,58,59
Recognizing personhood	15,55	2. Offering encouragement	
Acknowledging uniqueness	15	Realistic encouraging	6,19,42,50,57,59
Acknowledging the other	15,49	Bolstering	4,43
Confirming mind, body, and soul	55	Asserting optimism	30
Viewing as whole person	34,36,45,48, 50,55,59	Reassuring	1,6,35,73
		Offering a hope-filled attitude	
(Noncaring) Failing to see uniqueness	31	1. Instilling and sustaining realistic hope	43,50,57,58
2. Unconditionally regarding the other	19,42,65	Seeing future possibilities	40
3. Respecting the other	8,33,38,43, 46,48,57, 60,69	2. Aiming for success	
		Affirming the other's goals and potential	39,59
		Promotes autonomous self-care	44,69
Helping find meaning[b]		Holding high standards for the other	16
1. Affirming experience		*"Going the distance"*	
Affirming meaning	2,19	1. Caring beyond expectations	
Creating memories	46	Risk-taking, courageous	43
Focusing on living, acknowledging dying	26	Going beyond the basics	14,24,36,50,59
2. Finding peace		2. Hanging in there no matter what	
Alleviating guilt	62	Staying until death or well-being	55,70
Considering religious and spiritual needs	17,49	Giving off-duty time	17,50
Knowing			
Avoiding assumptions		*Seeking cues*	
1. Being open to the other's reality		1. Monitoring vigilantly	13,14,17,47
Accepting/open-minded	27,61,65	Keeping watch	13,14,69,73
Being open, receptive	40,52	2. Sensing concerns	25,27
2. Being nonjudgmental	1,27,40	Aware of emotional needs	49
3. Checking back and checking out	50,59,66	Responding to stress	29,40
4. (Noncaring) distorting, minimizing		3. Picking up cues, being sensitive	32,33,68
		Tuning into the nonverbal	50,60
Assessing thoroughly	32,39	*Centering on the one cared for*	
1. Assessing needs	6,12,13,19, 20,31,50, 55,66,70,71	1. Attending to the other	
		Focusing on the other, not self	52
2. Assessing skills and capabilities	1,13,27,40, 48,58,71	Conveying and gaining interest	41,50

(continued)

TABLE 4.9 Inductively Derived Caring Action, Arranged by Swanson's (1990, 1991, 1993) and Swanson-Kauffman's (1986ᵃ, 1988) Caring Categories *(continued)*

	References[a]		References[a]
Centering on the one cared for (cont.)		*Centering on the one cared for (cont.)*	
Concerned	37,42	Ignoring, neglect, being unavailable	12,17,32,37,39, 43,48,66
Individualized/family-centered care	19,23,34,35, 42,46,50, 58,62,70,72	*Engaging the self of both*	
		1. Revealing or sharing self	3,5,42,50, 51,60,61
2. Take the other's perspective	15,36		
Perceiving/intuiting the other's reality	53,70,73	Using self or putting self on the line	17,32,47
3. Listening	6,11,16,27,36, 46,57,65	Being genuine/innermost self	53,57
4. (Noncaring) Focusing away from the other		2. Becoming involved	32,33,36,52,71
		Interpersonal interacting	19,30
Feeling negative about the other	13,32,39,64	Identifying with patient, "This could be me"	20
Performing routinely/ task-oriented	42,44,46	3. Doing more than just a job	39,64

Being with

Being there		*Conveying availability*	
1. Being present/there/with	20,30,33,36,51, 59,63,71,73	1. Reaching out Touching to make a connection	9,65
Supportive/reassuring presence	13,23	Offering help	52
Mindfully present	29,38	2. Following up/following through	6,24
Physically present	58		
Authentic/genuine Preserving	4,5,6,7,11,16,18, 19,46,50,53, 57,60	3. Being accessible or available	27,35,58,72
		Constant presence	59
2. Connecting with the other	2,5,15,19,26,32, 45,50,51	*Enduring with*	
		1. Ongoing relationship	
Intersubjective connecting	29,52	Nurse is part of patient's family	60,70
Not burdening		Involved, extended relationship	15,19,37,63,71
1. Being responsible		Friends, colleagues, comrades	12,24,27,36, 39,42, 44,48,57, 59,62
Considerate/kind/patient	6,16,57,60,69		
Negotiated mutuality/ respectful distance	12,37		
Professional relationship with personal touch	38,50	Bonded, engaged, affiliated	6,14,19,62
(Noncaring) Intrusive/ interfering	39,60	2. Investing time	
		Persistent, timeless, ever changing	39,50,53
2. Building trust	16,27,29,30,37, 43,48,50,60	Spending time	13,15,17,30,34, 36,44,51,57, 61,65,72
3. Preserving self	8,15,62		

(continued)

TABLE 4.9 Inductively Derived Caring Action, Arranged by Swanson's (1990, 1991, 1993) and Swanson-Kauffman's (1986[a], 1988) Caring Categories (*continued*)

	References[a]		References[a]
Sharing feelings		*Sharing feelings (cont.)*	
1. Loving		2. Feeling together	
Demonstrating love or fondness	38,39,43	Sharing/sharing feelings/ beliefs	1,6,7,31,33, 35,45,50
Affection, tenderness	44,48	Reciprocal sharing/ mutuality	4,5,14,40,61,62
Warm attentiveness, pleasantness	35,59	Laughing/crying together	5,11,16,40,50,53
Closeness	33	Social touching to "lighten up"	9
Commitment/compassion	16,37,38,62,66	Expressive caring/responding	13,27

Doing for

Comforting		*Anticipating*	
1. Relieving pain and suffering		1. Being ready	
Pain relief	13,17,23,35, 48,59,62	Anticipating/working in Harmony	10,32,50
		Prepared/organized	16,24,66
Alleviating suffering	43	2. Rapidly responding	
Satiating hunger	23	Handling surprises or emergencies	20
2. Comforting/easing discomfort	17,27,32,35, 41,42,55,68	Swift/spur-of-the-moment response	43,48,50,52
Touching to comfort	6,9,11,32,33, 35,36,44, 45,50,59,62	3. Attending to many things at once	
		Creative/overcoming barriers	12,16,45,60
Performing competently and skillfully		Flexible	8,12,48
1. Technically skilled	13,14,23,25,36, 37,45,48,51, 59,60	Setting priorities/balancing time, energy	20,29
		Protecting	
2. Knowledgable performance	6,19,24,32,33, 35,36,45,46, 60,71,72	1. Guarding safety/privacy	
		Emotional, physical protection	17,32,46,49,62, 70,73
3. Meeting needs	17,23,29,44, 46,50,59,60	2. Modifying the environment	
Preserving dignity		Controlling/modifying environment	17,23,69
1. Doing with	24,29,63	Teaching others how to respond	1
2. Preserving the other's self		Making wise organizational choices	63
Promoting autonomy/ self-esteem	10,13	3. Negotiating the system	
Dignity-preserving acts	46,50,55	Coordinating resources/ systems	19,26,31,38,47,49, 50,51,57,60,65, 70,72,73
Avoiding rudeness or belittling	38,64	4. Advocating for	23,42,43,44,45, 46,55,71
Carrying the load for the other	27		

(*continued*)

TABLE 4.9 Inductively Derived Caring Action, Arranged by Swanson's (1990, 1991, 1993) and Swanson-Kauffman's (1986ᵃ, 1988) Caring Categories (*continued*)

References[a]		References[a]
Enabling		
Informing/explaining		*Supporting/allowing*	
1. Telling it like it is		1. Providing support	23,31,36,42, 46,49,72
Being honest/telling the whole truth	1,27,41,70	Nurturing, consoling	14,31,48
Responding objectively	6,13,16,26,30,31, 33,34,35,41,46 50,57,58,62, 70,72	Enhancing self-esteem	
2. Informing, explaining, coaching 40		2. (Noncaring) Controlling	12,38
		Focusing	
3. Communicating	1,12,16,24,29, 30,36,40,44, 46,47,49,62	1. Focusing, orienting	9,26
		2. Focusing on specific concerns	
4. Many teaching, communicating styles	8	Enhancing maternal-infant attachment	59
Modeling	24,40	Enhancing coping	2,73
Supervising, overseeing	10,31	Resolving fears/tension	23,52,62
Using self as interactive tool	43	*Generating alternatives/ thinking it through*	
Providing opportunities for practice	40	1. Assisting with self-care decisions	19,48,65,70
Validating/giving feedback		2. Empowering/increasing self-efficacy	11,19,26, 57,65,73
1. Confirming/affirming	27,40,43,46,48	3. Counselling/problem solving	16,35
2. Normalizing	11,73		

[a]Numbers refer to references in the Appendix.
[b]New subcategory not previously published by Swanson.

the enabling subcategories of informing/explaining, supporting/allowing, focusing, generating alternatives/thinking it through, and validating/giving feedback. However, the actual content of any of those enabling activities would be based on both knowing the specific client(s) and anticipating the challenges inherent in the relevant disease trajectories. Hence, the implication for designing caring-based intervention studies is that although the investigator may choose a caring framework for the clinical therapeutic, the actual content of the intervention would have to be drawn from knowledge of the health problem, its related symptomatology, and typical human responses to the disease's illness and healing trajectory. The clearest limitation to the study of Level IV caring

actions is the lack of controlled clinical trials wherein protocols for caring-based therapeutic interventions are defined, applied, carefully monitored, and tested for effectiveness in promoting healthy outcomes.

LEVEL V: CARING CONSEQUENCES

Beck (1991, 1992a, 1992b, 1993, 1994) has conducted a program of research examining the experience and outcomes of caring within the academic setting. In her 1994 publication, Beck draws all of her studies together and succinctly and creatively reduces her multiple interpretive studies of caring within academia to the following statement: "Caring is centered in authentic presencing where selfless sharing and fortifying support flourish and lead to uplifting consequences" (p. 115). She further states, "once fortified from being cared-for [people] will, in turn, be better able to nurture their own ability to care for others" (p. 108). Hence, Beck offers phenomenologic validation to the claims of Watson (1988a) that participation in a caring transaction leads to the betterment of both provider and recipient.

Unfortunately, quantitative findings about the consequences of caring are minimal. This fact reflects the limited amount of investigators who have attempted to explicitly link caring-based therapeutic interventions to outcomes. Three exceptions to this claim were found. In the first study, Latham (1996) examined the associations among patient background variables (self-esteem and desire for behavioral and informational control), nurse caring (spiritual caring, supportive caring, physical caring, interpretive caring, and sensitive caring), and patient outcomes (appraisals, psychological distress, coping strategies, and effectiveness). Nurse caring, supportive, was operationalized using Gardner and Wheeler's (1981) SNBC (described previously under "Level IV: Caring Actions"). The other four dimensions of nurse caring were measured using Latham's Holistic Caring Inventory (HCI). The HCI, based on Howard's (1975) holistic dimension of humanistic caring theory, is a 39-item, four-point Likert-type measure. All HCI subscale internal consistencies exceed .90. Although study participants reported experiencing minimal amounts of interpretive, spiritual, and supportive caring, they perceived moderate amounts of physical and sensitive caring. There was a weak (beta weight = .22) but statistically significant ($p \leq .05$) association between desire for cognitive control and perception of receiving supportive caring. Forty percent of the overall variance in coping effectiveness was

accounted for by the combined variables of supportive and sensitive caring, problem and emotion-focused coping, and decreased psychological distress. Post hoc analysis yielded additional information about caring. Those with lower self-esteem perceived more threat (measured as primary cognitive appraisal) from interactions with nurses ($p \leq .05$). Compared with older patients, younger patients were more likely to rate supportive caring behaviors as important ($p \leq .001$). Younger patients also viewed nurses as providing more supportive ($p \leq .001$) and physical caring ($p \leq .01$). Last, those with moderate (versus minimal or no) pain perceived more supportive and physical nurse caring ($p \leq .05$). In summary, Latham's investigation demonstrated that (a) certain patient conditions (self-esteem, age, and pain level) are associated with perceptions of nurses as caring and (b) sensitive and supportive nurse caring contributes to patients' overall coping effectiveness.

In a second quantitative investigation of caring consequences, Duffy (1992) examined the associations between nurse caring and patient satisfaction, health status, length of stay, and health care costs for 86 randomly selected patients. Duffy's Caring Assessment Tool (CAT) was used to quantify nurse caring (10 items, five-point Likert-type scale). The only statistically significant association demonstrated was between the CAT and patient satisfaction, as measured using a 100-mm visual analogue scale ($r = .46$, $p \leq .001$). Caring accounted for 19% of the overall variance in patient satisfaction. The third investigation of caring consequences was also conducted by Duffy (1993). To evaluate the effects of nurse administrators' caring, she developed a measure, based on Watson's (1985) carative factors, known as the CAT-A (94 items, five-point Likert-type scale). Fifty-six nurses participated in Duffy's examination of the relationships between

TABLE 4.10 Consequences of Caring and Noncaring for Clients and Nurses

Consequences of Caring	References[a]	Consequences of Noncaring	References[a]
Client[b] outcomes of caring		**Client outcomes of noncaring**	
Emotional-spiritual		*Emotional-spiritual*	
Enhanced self-esteem/-worth	3,5,6,37,50	Humiliated	64
Enhanced knowledge, coping	37,49,57,65, 67,71	Frightened	64
		Out of control	64
Increased well-being/quality of life	19,61	Despair/helplessness	38
Feeling reassured/confident/ good	4,6,67	Alienation	38
		Vulnerability	38
Gained control/independence	19,30	Lingering bad memories	37
Empowered, sustained, confident	6,19,65		
Positive mental attitude/ uplifting consequences	7,67		
Satisfaction with care/ expectations met	42,67		
Relaxed/happy/merriment	5,50		
Enhanced dignity/personhood	49,61,67		
Fostered spiritual freedom	38		
Enhanced growth and development	5,37,57		
Gratitude/feeling cared-for	4,37,42,67		
Feeling more caring toward others	3,4		
Physical		*Physical*	
Enhanced healing	14,22,42, 47,67	Decreased healing	38
Feeling safe	49		
Life saved	14		
Decreased costs/length of stay	49,65		
Supports current energy	38		
Nurse knows patients' capacities	71		
Increased physical comfort	42		
Better coordination of care	65		
Social			
Meaningful reciprocal relationship	14,19,61		
Family empowered/less dependent	19		
Trust/someone to count on	50,65,67		
Enhanced relationship between patient and FCG	58		
Decreased alienation from HCDS	58		

(continued)

TABLE 4.10 Consequences of Caring and Noncaring for Clients and Nurses (*continued*)

Consequences of Caring	References[a]	Consequences of Noncaring	References[a]
Client[b] outcomes of caring		**Client outcomes of noncaring**	
Nurse outcomes of caring		**Nurse outcomes of noncaring**	
Emotional-spiritual		*Emotional-spiritual*	
Sense of accomplishment, self-satisfaction	28,49,50,52,56	Hardened, oblivious, robot-like	8
Sense of importance/purpose to own life	8,56	Depressed, frightened	8
Experiencing gratitude	21,22,56	Worn down	52
Preserved integrity/well-being	45,54		
Fulfillment/confirmation/ wholeness	15,49,52		
Enhanced self-perception/ self-esteem	5,45,54		
Uplifting consequences/ self-transformation	5,7		
Learning about self/living own philosophy	5,8,15		
Respect for life/aware of own mortality	8		
Looking inward	54		
Professional			
Enhanced intuition/clinical judgment	45,47,71		
Increased skills and knowledge	21,45,71		
Mobilizes more caring	7,54		
Enhanced empathy/ fewer assumptions	8		
Satisfaction with/love of nursing	49,50,65		
Social			
Sense of collegiality	49		
Connecting	52		
Relationship with patient	5,15,56,65		

Note. FCG = family caregiver; HCDS = health care delivery system.
[a]Numbers refer to references in the Appendix.
[b]"Client" can refer to a patient, a family, or a student.

perceptions of administrator nurse caring and staff nurse job satisfaction and turnover rates. The CAT-A had high internal consistency (Cronbach's alpha = 0.99). Mean overall perception of administrator caring was 339.84 and ranged from 196 to 470 (possible range 94–470). The association between the CAT-A and turnover was nonsignificant, but there was a significant association ($r = .36$) with the one-item rating of job satisfaction ($p = .007$).

Table 4.10 summarizes 30 relatively recent (1986–1996) qualitative studies in which potential outcomes of caring were interpreted. The studies used a total sample of 1,185 participants (420 nurses, 203 patients/families, 358 students, 12 family caregivers, and 192 health care providers [including nurses]). Consequences of caring for the one cared for (most often patient or student) were multiple indicators of enhanced well-being, including positive effects on self-esteem, mood, self-efficacy, satisfaction with care, and physical healing. It appears that oftentimes caring is credited with freeing up inner strengths and healing potential. Social benefits of participating in a caring relationship are that the recipient feels he or she can count on the provider, is less dependent, and is better able to navigate the health care system.

The second part of Table 4.10 summarizes the consequences of caring for the one caring (e.g., the nurse). Practicing in a caring manner leads to the nurse's well-being, both personally and professionally. Personal outcomes of caring include feeling important, accomplished, purposeful, aware, integrated, whole, and confirmed. Professionally practicing caring leads to enhanced intuition, empathy, clinical judgment, capacity for caring, and work satisfaction. Social outcomes of caring for nurses include feeling connected both to their patients and to their colleagues.

Also, Table 4.10 very briefly outlines some potential consequences of noncaring. Patients who experience noncaring feel humiliated, out of control, despaired, frightened, and alienated. Sadly, bad memories of the noncaring episode linger. Finally, of greatest concern is the suggestion that participating in a noncaring encounter may lead to prolongation of physical healing. Noncaring also takes its toll on nurses, resulting in nurses becoming worn down, robot-like, depressed, hardened, and frightened.

Future Directions for Level V Inquiry

It is essential that nurse investigators take seriously the need to document the consequences of caring. The term *consequences* is deliberately chosen for two reasons. First, it draws attention to the thought pattern that underlies the thinking of clinical investigators (i.e., the occurrence of "y" is consequent to the earlier occurrence of "x"), and second, it highlights both the intended and unintended outcomes and potential side effects of caring actions. This chapter only highlights "good" from caring and "bad" from noncaring; it does not address the power differences assumed within a caring framework and the personal costs of caring.

Nurse researchers working in a clinical arena need to expand (some may say constrict) their thinking to consider caring as a commodity that may be measured, rigorously applied, and tested for its effectiveness in promoting healing, recovery, or optimal well-being. Such inquiry calls for nurse investigators who value the importance of caring and have clinical insight into the caring needs of a specific clinical group; the resources to design caring-based, clinically relevant controlled studies; and clarity about the intended and potentially unintended measurable consequences of caring protocols. Upon completion of such investigations, nurse scientists need to enter into dialogue about the universal mechanisms by which caring affects well-being. Such conceptual or philosophic debate should highlight the basic structure of caring, its antecedents, and its consequences.

CARING RELATIONSHIPS

Alluded to throughout this chapter has been the fact that some relationships may be considered caring and others are rendered noncaring. L. D. Ray (1995) critically dealt with the concern that for so many studies the range of responses is very narrow and skewed toward positive perceptions when examining patient perceptions of nurse caring or satisfaction with nursing care. Ray questioned whether clients answered positively due to having low expectations, respondent bias, or fear of negative sanctions for speaking frankly. Alternatively, she questioned if the issue lies in concept measurement error; that is, examining caring as though it occurred along a normal distribution versus viewing it as an expected given and measuring it as a norm-referenced criterion (e.g., *safe caring* should be expected at 100% and any deviance from that norm should be the focus of measurement).

Halldorsdottir (1991) interviewed nine patients and nine students about potential modes of being with another person. She proposed a creative framework consisting of five possible ways of characterizing nurse–patient relationships. Type 1, "biocidic" relationships, are defined as life destroying: They are "acid-edged," lead to anger, despair, and alienation, with the ultimate effects of diminishing healing and well-being, leaving the participants vulnerable and haunted by unforgettable bad memories. Type 2, "biostatic" relationships, are life restraining, wherein nurses coldly treat patients as a "nuisance," leading them to believe that the nurse does not care and is blind to them and their situation. Type 3, "biopassive" relationships, are defined as "life-neutral." The relationship is basically apathetic or detached, there is no person-to-person acknowledgment, and lives or energy levels are neither enhanced or diminished. Type 4, "bioactive" relationships, are life sustaining. This is the classic professional nurse–patient relationship, characterized as benevolent, kind, and concerned. The result of this encounter is that energy levels are sustained and good will ensues. Type 5, "biogenic" relationships, involves being fully present, with healing love flowing. Personhood is mutually acknowledged, care is negotiated, and professional intimacy (creative distance with respect and compassion) ensues. This relationship fosters spiritual freedom (Halldorsdottir, 1991).

Tieing together the deliberations of L. D. Ray (1995) with the findings of Halldorsdottir (1991), it is possible that most nurse–patient interactions fall between Types 3 (the "at least" or normative criterion) and 5 (perhaps the "extra credit" expectation). Type 3 relationships might characterize the transaction between a task-oriented nurse (e.g., the "med-nurse" who in a 30-second interaction safely administers 10:00 a.m. medications). A Type 4 interaction might characterize most nurse–patient interactions in which effective psychosocially and physiologically oriented therapeutic interventions transpire (e.g., an ongoing relationship between a school nurse and the group of "regulars" who stop by the health clinic). Type 5 interactions might be those exquisite moments of intimate connection—the occasions in which both nurse and patient feel transformed (even if only for the day) for having made it through a challenging time together (e.g., a midwife's and a couple's exhilaration at bringing forth a new life). Nurse–patient interactions that do not meet the Type 3 criterion would fall into the noncaring or possibly malpractice or abusive range (Type 2 = neglect; Type 1 = direct abuse).

CONCLUSIONS

Over the past few decades, the discipline of nursing has entertained considerable discourse about what constitutes appropriate methods for studying nursing phenomena. Historically, this discourse has been labeled the "qualitative–quantitative debate." It is beyond the scope of this chapter to deal with the limitations of such either–or discussion; however, this debate cannot go unacknowledged in summarizing the state of scientific knowledge about caring. Clearly, scientists interested in the concept of caring have, by and large, stuck with the more interpretive methods of knowledge building. The challenge remains for the discipline to allow for the coexistence of multiple paradigms for inquiry about caring. It is time to build on the rich descriptions and interpretations of caring that have been reviewed through this literary meta-analysis. From a strictly pragmatic stance, caring thoughts, theories, and concepts need to be translated into useful measures and testable protocols that are employed in replicable, generalizable research designs.

In this chapter, an attempt has been made to bring clarity to discourse about the concept of caring in nursing. It has been suggested that disciplinary conversations might best be characterized as having five levels of discussion. When referring to the concept *caring*, there is a need to be clear about whether the discourse is about the capacity for caring, the concerns and commitments that underlie caring, conditions that inhibit or enhance caring, caring actions, or the consequences of caring. Also, a theoretical framework for categorizing therapeutic, caring interventions, based on Swanson's middle range theory of caring was proposed and supported throughout this chapter.

It is safe to say that collectively (across the discipline), at an interpretive level, much is known about caring. However, there remain minimal quantitative empirical studies. Disciplinary challenges that lie ahead include the production of psychometrically sound measures for examining each level of caring; careful examination of associations within, between, and among the five caring levels; and a commitment to framing nursing intervention studies (caring actions) under the language of caring, hence providing a measurable and conceptually congruent framework to tie together the sound science underlying the practice of essential and effective professional nurse caring.

REFERENCES

Aamodt, A. M., Grassl-Herwehe, S., Farell, F., & Hutter, J. (1984). The child's view of chemically induced alopecia. In M. M. Leininger (Ed.), *Care: The essence of nursing* (pp. 217–234). Thorofare, NJ: Slack.

Bäck-Pettersson, S. K., & Jensen, K. P. (1993). "She dares": An essential characteristic of the excellent Swedish nurse. In D. Gaut (Ed.), *A global agenda for caring* (pp. 257–265). New York, NY: National League for Nursing.

Baer, E. D., & Lowery, B. J. (1987). Patient and situational factors that affect nursing students' like or dislike of caring for patients. *Nursing Research, 36*(5), 298–302.

Beck, C. T. (1991). How students perceive faculty caring: A phenomenological study. *Nursing Educator, 16,* 18–22.

Beck, C. T. (1992a). Caring among nursing students. *Nursing Educator, 17,* 22–27.

Beck, C. T. (1992b). Caring between nursing students and physically/mentally handicapped children: A phenomenological study. *Journal of Nursing Education, 31*(8), 361–366.

Beck, C. T. (1993). Caring relationships between nursing students and their patients. *Nurse Educator, 18*(5), 28–32.

Beck, C. T. (1994). Researching experiences of living caring. In A. Boykin (Ed.), *Living a caring-based program.* New York, NY: National League for Nursing.

Beck, C. T. (1996). Nursing students' experiences caring for cognitively impaired elderly people. *Journal of Advanced Nursing, 23*(5), 992–998.

Benner, P. (1984). *From novice to expert.* Menlo Park, CA: Addison-Wesley.

Benner, P., & Wrubel, J. (1989). *The primacy of caring.* Menlo Park, CA: Addison-Wesley.

Benner, P. J. (1990). The moral dimension of caring. In J. S. Stevenson & T. Tripp Reimer (Eds.), *Knowledge about care and caring: State of the art and future developments* (pp. 5–17). Washington, DC: American Academy of Nursing.

Bottorf, J. L. (1993). The use and meaning of touch in caring for patients with cancer. *Oncology Nursing Forum, 20*(10), 1531–1538.

Bowers, B. J. (1987). Intergenerational caregiving: Adult caregivers and their aging parents. *Advances in Nursing Science, 9*(2), 20–31.

Boyd, C. O., & Munhall, P. L. (1989). A qualitative investigation of reassurance. *Holistic Nursing Practice, 4*(1), 61–69,

Boykin, A. (1994). *Living a caring-based curriculum.* New York, NY: National League for Nursing.

Boykin, A., & Schoenhofer, S. (1993). *Nursing as caring: A model for transforming practice.* New York, NY: National League for Nursing.

Brown, L. (1986). The experience of care: Patients' perspectives. *Topics in Clinical Nursing, 8*(2), 56–62.

Brown, J., & Ritchie, J. A. (1989). Nurses' perceptions of their relationships with parents. *Maternal Child Nursing Journal, 18*(2), 79–96.

Burfitt, S. N., Greiner, D. S., Miers, L. J., Kinney, M. R., & Branyon, M. E. (1993). Professional nurse caring as perceived by critically ill patients: A phenomenologic study. *American Journal of Critical Care, 2*(6), 489–499.

Burns, M. (1994). Creating a safe passage: The meaning of engagement for nurses caring for children and their families. *Issues in Comprehensive Pediatric Nursing, 17,* 211–221.

Bush, H. A. (1988). The caring teacher of nursing. In M. M. Leininger (Ed.), *Care: Discovery and uses in clinical and community nursing* (pp. 169–187). Detroit, MI: Wayne State University Press.

Chipman, Y. (1991). Caring: Its meaning and place in the practice of nursing. *Journal of Nursing Education, 30*(4), 171–175.

Clarke, J. B., & Wheeler, S. J. (1992). A view of the phenomenon of caring in nursing practice. *Journal of Advanced Nursing, 7,* 1283–1290.

Clayton, G. M., Murray, J. P., Homes, S. D., & Greene, P. S. (1991). Connecting: A catalyst for caring. In P. Chinn (Ed.), *Anthology on caring* (pp. 155–168). New York, NY: National League for Nursing.

Cohen, M. Z., Haberman, M. R., &, Steeves, R. (1994). The meaning of oncology nursing. *Oncology Nursing Forum,* 21(Suppl. 8), 5–8.

Cohen, M. Z., Haberman, M. R., Steeves, R., & Deatrick, J. A. (1994). Rewards and difficulties of oncology nursing. *Oncology Nursing Forum, 21*(Suppl. 8). 9–17.

Cohen, M. Z., & Sarter, B. (1992). Love and work: Oncology nurses' view of the meaning of their work. *Oncology Nursing Forum, 19*(10), 1481–1486.

Collins, B. A., McCoy, S. A., Sale, S., & Weber, S. E. (1994). Descriptions of comfort by substance using and non-using postpartum women. *Journal of Obstetric and Gynecologic and Neonatal Nursing, 23*(4), 293–300.

Cooper, M. C. (1993). The intersection of technology and care in the ICU. *Advances in Nursing Science, 15*(3), 23–32.

Coulon, L., Krause, K. L., & Anderson, M. (1996). The pursuit of excellence in nursing care: What does it mean? *Journal of Advanced Nursing, 24*(4), 817–826.

Cronin, S. N., & Harrison, B. (1988). Importance of nurse caring behaviors as perceived by patients after myocardial infarctions. *Heart and Lung, 17*(4), 374–380.

Davies, B., & O'Berle, K, (1990). Dimensions of the supportive role of the nurse in palliative care. *Oncology Nursing Forum, 17*(1), 87–94.

Dietrich, L. (1992). The caring nursing environment. In D. A. Gaut (Ed.), *The presence of caring in nursing* (pp. 69–87). New York, NY: National League for Nursing.

Donoghue, J. (1993). Humanistic care and nurses' experience. In D. Gaut (Ed.), *A global agenda for caring* (pp. 267–279). New York, NY: National League for Nursing.

Drew, N, (1986). Exclusion and confirmation: A phenomenology of patients' experiences with caregivers. *Image: The Journal of Nursing Scholarship, 18*(2), 39–43.

Duffy, J. R. (1992). Impact of nurse caring on patient outcomes. In D. A. Gaut (Ed.), *The presence of caring in nursing* (pp. 113–136). New York, NY: National League for Nursing.

Duffy, J. R. (1993). Caring behaviors of nurse managers: Relationships to staff nurse satisfaction and retention. In D. Gaut (Ed.), *A global agenda for caring* (pp. 365–377). New York, NY: National League for Nursing.

Euswas, P. (1993). The actualized caring moment: A grounded theory of caring in nursing practice. In D. Gaut (Ed.), *A global agenda for caring* (pp. 309–326). New York, NY: National League for Nursing.

Fareed, A. (1996). The experience of reassurance: Patient's perspectives. *Journal of Advanced Nursing, 23*(2), 272–219.

Finn, J. (1993). Caring in birthing: Experiences of professional nursing and generic care. In D. Gaut (Ed.), *A global agenda for caring* (pp. 63–79). New York, NY: National League for Nursing.

Flaherty, M. J. (1988). Seven caring functions of Black grandmothers in adolescent mothering. *MCN Journal, 17*(3), 191–207.

Forrest, D. (1988). The experience of caring. *Journal of Advanced Nursing, 14,* 815–823.

Gadow, S. (1980). Existential advocacy: Philosophical foundation of nursing. In S. Spicker & S. Gadow (Eds.), *Nursing images and ideals* (pp. 86–101). New York, NY: Springer.

Gadow, S. (1984). Touch and technology: Two paradigms of patient care. *Journal of Religion and Health, 23*(1), 63–69.

Gadow, S. (1990). The advocacy covenant: Care as clinical subjectivity. In J. S. Stevenson & T. Tripp Riemer (Eds.), *Knowledge about care and caring: State of the art and future developments* (pp. 33–40). Washington, DC: American Academy of Nursing.

Gardner, K. G., & Wheeler, E., (1981). Patients' and staff nurses' perceptions of supportive nursing behaviors: A preliminary analysis. In M. M. Leininger (Ed.), *Caring: An essential human need* (pp. 109–113). Thorofare, NJ: Slack.

Gardner, K. G., & Wheeler, E. (1987). Patient's perceptions of support. *Western Journal of Nursing Research, 9*(1), 115–131.

Gaut, D. (1983). Development of a theoretically adequate description of caring. *Western Journal of Nursing Research, 5,* 313–324.

Girot, E. A. (1993). Assessment of competence in clinical practice: A phenomenological approach. *Journal of Advanced Nursing, 18,* 114–119.

Glaser, B. G., & Strauss, A. L. (1967). *The discovery of grounded theory: Strategies for qualitative research.* New York, NY: Aldine.

Gooding, B. A., Sloan, M., & Gagnon, L. (1993). Important nurse caring behaviors: Perceptions of oncology patients and nurses. *Canadian Journal of Nursing Research, 25*(3), 65–76.

Green-Hernandez, C. (1991). A phenomenological investigation of caring as a lived experience in nursing. In P. Chinn (Ed.), *Anthology on caring* (pp. 111–131). New York, NY: National League for Nursing.

Halldorsdottir, S. (1990). The essential structure of a caring and uncaring encounter with a teacher: The perspective of the nursing student. In M. M. Leininger & J. Watson (Eds.), *The caring experience in education* (pp. 95–108). New York, NY: National League for Nursing.

Halldorsdottir, S. (1991). Five basic modes of being with another. In D. Gaut & M. M. Leininger (Eds.), *Caring: The compassionate healer* (pp. 37–49). New York, NY: National League for Nursing.

Halloran, E. J. (1985). Nursing workload, medical diagnostic related group, and nursing diagnosis. *Research in Nursing and Health, 8,* 421–433.

Heidigger, M. (1962). *Being and time* (J. Macquarrie & E. Roninson, Trans.). New York, NY: Harper & Row.

Hinds, P. S. (1988). The relationship of nurses' caring behaviors with hopefulness and health care outcomes in adolescents. *Archives of Psychiatric Nursing, 2*(1), 21–29.

Howard, J. (1975). Humanization and dehumanization of health care: A conceptual view. In J. Howard & A. Strauss (Eds.), *Humanizing health care* (pp. 57–102), New York, NY: John Wiley.

Hughes, L. (1992). Faculty-student interaction and the faculty perceived climate for caring. *Advances in Nursing Science, 14*(3), 60–71.

Irwin, B., & Meier, J. (1973). Supportive measures for relatives of the fatally ill. *Communicating Nursing Research, 6,*119–128.

Jenny, J., & Logan, J. (1996). Caring and comfort metaphors used by patients in critical care. *Image: The Journal of Nursing Scholarship, 28*(4), 349–352.

Jensen, K. P., Bäck-Pettersson, S. R., & Segesten, K. M. (1992). The caring moment and the green-thumb phenomenon amongst Swedish nurses. *Nursing Science Quarterly, 6*(2), 98–104.

Kahn, D. L., & Steeves, R. H. (1988). Caring and practice: Construction of the nurse's world. *Scholarly Inquiry for Nursing Practice, 2*(3), 201–216.

Keane, S. M., & Chastain, B. (1987). Caring: Nurse-patient perceptions. *Rehabilitation Nursing, 12*(4), 182–185.

Klausner, S. Z. (1971). *On man and his environment.* San Francisco, CA: Jossey-Bass.

Komorita, N. I., Doehring, K. M., & Hirchert, P. W. (1991). Perceptions of caring by nuise educators. *Journal of Nursing Education, 30*(1), 23–29.

Kosowski, M.M.R. (1995). Clinical learning experiences and professional nurse caring: A critical phenomenological study of female baccalaureate nursing students. *Journal of Nursing Education, 34*(5), 235–242.

Larson, P. J. (1984). Important nurse caring behaviors perceived by patients with cancer. *Oncology Nursing Forum, 11*(6), 46–50.

Larson, P. J. (1986). Cancer nurses' perceptions of caring. *Cancer Nursing, 9*(2), 86–91.

Larson, P. J. (1987). Comparison of cancer patients and professional nurses' perceptions of important nurse caring behaviors. *Heart and Lung, 12*(2), 187–193.

Larson, P. J., & Ferketich, S. L. (1993). Patient satisfaction with nurse caring during hospitalization. *Western Journal of Nursing Research, 15*(6), 690–707.

Latham, C. P. (1996). Predictors of patient outcomes following interaction with nurses. *Western Journal of Nursing Research, 18*(5), 548–564.

Leininger, M. M. (1981). The phenomenon of caring: Importance of research and theoretical considerations. In M. M. Leininger (Ed.), *Caring: An essential human need.* Thorofare, NJ: Slack.

Leininger, M. M. (1988, November). Leininger's theory of nursing: Cultural care diversity and universality. *Nursing Science Quarterly, 7*(4), 152–160.

Leininger, M. M. (1990). Historic and epistemologic dimensions of care and caring with future directions. In J. S. Stevenson & T. Tripp Riemer (Eds.), *Knowledge about care and caring: State of the art and future developments* (pp. 19–31). Washington, DC: American Academy of Nursing.

Lemmer, C. M. (1991). Parental perceptions of caring following perinatal bereavement. *Western Journal of Nursing Research, 13*(4), 475–493.

Leners, D. W. (1993). Nursing intuition: The deep connection. In D. Gaut (Ed.), *A global agenda for caring* (pp. 223–240). New York, NY: National League for Nursing.

Lovgren, G., Engstrom, B., & Norberg, A. (1996). Patient's narratives concerning good and bad caring. *Scandinavian Journal of Caring Sciences, 10,* 151–156.

Mangold, A. M. (1991), Senior nursing students' and professional nurses' perceptions of effective caring behaviors: A comparative study. *Journal of Nursing Education, 30*(3), 134–139.

Mayer, D. K. (1986). Cancer patients' and families' perceptions of nurses' caring behaviors. *Topics in Clinical Nursing, 8*(2), 63–69.

Mayeroff, M. (1971). *On caring.* New York, NY: Harper & Row.

McNamara, S. A. (1995). Perioperative nurses' perceptions of caring practices. *Association of Operating Room Nurses Journal, 61*(2), 377–388.

Miller, B. K., Haber, J., & Byrne, M. W. (1992). The experience of caring in the acute care setting: Patient and nurse perspectives. In D. A. Gaut (Ed.), *The presence of caring in nursing* (pp. 137–156). New York, NY: National League for Nursing.

Milne, H. A., & McWilliam, C. L. (1996). Considering nursing resource as caring time. *Journal of Advanced Nursing, 23*(4), 810–819.

Montgomery, C. L. (1992). The spiritual connection: Nurses' perception of the experience of caring. In D. A. Gaut (Ed.), *The presence of caring in nursing* (pp. 39–52). New York, NY: National League for Nursing.

Morrison, P. (1989). Nursing and caring: A personal construct theory study of some nurses' self-perceptions. *Journal of Advanced Nursing, 44,* 421–426.

Morrison, P. (1990). An example of the use of repertory grid techniques in assessing nurses' self-perceptions in caring. *Nurse Education Today, 10,* 253–259.

Morse, J. M., Bottorf, J., Neander, W., & Solberg, S. (1991). Comparative analysis and conceptualizations and theories of caring. *Image: The Journal of Nursing Scholarship, 23*(2), 119–126.

Morse, J. M., Solberg, S. M., Neander, W. L., Bottorf, J. L., & Johnson, J. L. (1990), Concepts of caring and caring as a concept. *Advances in Nursing Science, 13*(1), 14.

Mullins, I. L. (1996). Nurse caring behaviors for persons with Acquired Immune Deficiency Syndrome/Human Immunodeficiency Virus. *Applied Nursing Research, 9*(1), 18–23.

Nelms, T. P. (1996). Living a caring presence in nursing: A Heidiggerian hermeneutic analysis. *Journal of Advanced Nursing, 24*(2), 368–374.

Noddings, N. (1984). Caring.' *A feminine approach to ethics and moral education.* Berkeley, CA: University of California Press.

O'Berle, K., & Davies, B. (1992). Support and caring: Exploring the concepts. *Oncology Nursing Forum, 19*(5), 763–767.

Parker, M. E. (1994). Living nursing's values in nursing practice. In D. A. Gaut & A. Boykin (Eds.), *Caring as healing: Renewal through hope* (pp. 48–65). New York, NY: National League for Nursing.

Peteet, J. R., Rose, D. M., Medeiros, C., Walsh-Burke, K., & Rieker, P. (1992). Relationships with patients: Can a clinician be a friend? *Psychiatry, 55,* 223–229.

Poole, G., & Rowat, K. (1994). Elderly clients' perceptions of caring of a home-care nurse. *Journal of Advanced Nursing, 20,*422–429,

Powell-Cope, G. M. (1994). Family caregiving of people with AIDS: Negotiating partnerships with health care providers. *Nursing Research, 43*(6), 324–330.

Propst, M. G., Schenk, L. K., & Ciairain, S. (1994). Caring as perceived during the birth experience. In D. A. Gaut & A. Boykin (Eds.), *Caring as healing: Renewal through hope* (pp. 252–264). New York, NY: National League for Nursing.

Raudonis, B, M. (1993). The meaning and impact of empathetic relationships in hospice nursing. *Cancer Nursing, 16*(4), 304–309.

Raudonis, B. M., & Kirschling, J. M. (1996). Family caregivers' perspectives on hospice nursing care. *Journal of Palliative Care, 12*(2), 14–19.

Ray, L. D. (1995). Caring in clinical intervention research: Design and measurement issues [Abstract]. *Communicating Nursing Research, 28*(3), 282.

Ray, M. A. (1984). The development of a classification system of institutional caring. In M. M. Leininger (Ed.), *Care: The essence of nursing and health* (pp. 95–111). Thorofare, NJ: Slack.

Ray, M. A. (1987). Technological caring: A new model in critical care. *Dimensions of Critical Care Nursing, 6*(3), 166–173.

Ray, M. A. (1989). The theory of bureaucratic caring for nursing practice in the organizational culture. *Nursing Administration Quarterly, 13*(2), 31–42.

Riemen, D. J. (1986). Non-caring and caring in the clinical setting: Patients' descriptions. *Topics in Clinical Nursing, 8*(2), 30–36.

Roach, S. (1984). *Caring: The human mode of being: Implications for nursing—perspectives in caring* [Monograph 1]. Toronto, Ontario, Canada: Faculty of Nursing, University of Toronto.

Schroeder, C., & Maeve, M. K. (1992). Nursing care partnerships at the Denver Nursing Project in Human Caring: An application and extension of caring theory in practice. *Advances in Nursing Science, 15*(2), 25–38.

Sherwood, G. (1991). Expressions of nurses' caring: The role of the compassionate healer. In D. A. Gaut & M. M. Leininger (Eds.), *Caring: The compassionate healer* (pp. 79–87). New York, NY: National League for Nursing.

Sherwood, G. (1993). A qualitative analysis of patient responses to caring: A moral and economic imperative. In D. Gaut (Ed.), *A global agenda for caring* (pp. 243–255). New York, NY: National League for Nursing.

Solberg, S., & Morse, J. M. (1991). The comforting behaviors of caregivers toward distressed postoperative neonates. *Issues in Comprehensive Pediatric Nursing, 14,* 79–92.

Soldwisch, S. S. (1993). Care, caritas, and ego development. In D. Gaut (Ed.), *A global agenda for caring* (pp. 293–307). New York, NY: National League for Nursing.

Spangler, Z. (1993). Generic and professional care of Anglo-American and Filipino-American nurses. In D. Gaut (Ed.), *A global agenda for caring* (pp. 47–61). New York, NY: National League for Nursing.

Steeves, R., Cohen, M. Z., & Wise, C. T. (1994). An analysis of critical incidents describing the essence of oncology nursing. *Oncology Nursing Forum, 21*(Suppl. 8), 19–25.

Stevenson, J. S. (1990). Quantitative care research: Review of content, process, product. In J. S. Stevenson & T. Tripp Riemer (Eds.), *Knowledge about care and caring: State of the art and future developments.* Washington, DC: American Academy of Nursing.

Swan, J. H., Benjamin, A. E., & Brown, A. (1992). Skilled nursing facility care for persons with AIDS: Comparison with other patients. *American Journal of Public Health, 82*(3), 453–455.

Swanson, K. M. (1990). Providing care in the NICU: Sometimes an act of love. *Advances in Nursing Science, 13*(1), 60–73.

Swanson, K. M. (1991). Empirical development of a middle-range theory of caring. *Nursing Research, 40*(3), 161–166.

Swanson, K. M. (1993). Nursing as informed caring for the well-being of others. Image: *The Journal of Nursing Scholarship, 25*(4), 352–357.

Swanson-Kauffman, K. M. (1986a). Caring in the instance of unexpected early pregnancy loss. *Topics in Clinical Nursing, 8*(2), 37–46.

Swanson-Kauffman, K. M. (1986b). A combined qualitative research methodology for nursing research. *Advances in Nursing Science, 8*(3), 58–69.

Swanson-Kauffman, K.M. (1988). The caring needs of women who miscarried. In M. M. Leininger (Ed.), *Care: Discovery and uses in clinical and community nursing* (pp. 55–70). Detroit, MI: Wayne State University Press.

Swanson-Kauffman, K. M., & Schonwald, E. (1988). Phenomenology. In B. Sarter (Ed.), *Paths to knowledge: Innovative research methods for nursing* (pp. 97–105). New York, NY: National League for Nursing.

Tanner, C. A., Benner, P., Chesla, C., & Gordon, D. R. (1993). The phenomenon of knowing the

patient. *Image: The Journal of Nursing Scholarship, 25*(4), 273–280.

Tripp-Riemer, T., & Cohen, M. Z. (1990). Qualitative approaches to care: A critical review. In J. S. Stevenson & T. Tripp Riemer (Eds.), *Knowledge about care and caring: State of the art and future developments* (pp. 83–96). Washington, DC: American Academy of Nursing.

vonEssen, L., Burstrom, L., & Sjoden, P. O. (1994). Perceptions of caring behaviors and patient anxiety and depression in cancer patient-staff dyads. *Scandinavian Journal of Caring Science, 8*(4), 205–212.

Watson, M. J. (1985). *Nursing: The philosophy and science of caring.* Boulder: Colorado Associated University Press.

Watson, M. J. (1988a). *Nursing: Human science and human care.* New York, NY: National League for Nursing.

Watson, M. J. (1988b). Response to "Caring practice: Construction of the nurses' world." *Scholarly Inquiry for Nursing Practice, 2*(3), 217–221.

Watson, M. J. (1990). Human caring: A public agenda. In J. S. Stevenson & T. Tripp Riemer (Eds.), *Knowledge about care and caring: State of the art and future developments* (pp. 41–48). Washington, DC: American Academy of Nursing.

Weiss, C. J. (1984). Gender-related perceptions of caring in the nurse-patient relationship. In M. M. Leininger (Ed.), *Care: The essence of nursing and health* (pp. 161–181). Thorofare, NJ: Slack.

Williams, H. A. (1992). Comparing the perception of support by parents of children with cancer and by health professionals. *Journal of Pediatric Oncology, 9*(4), 180–186.

Winters, G., Miller, C., Maracich, L., Compton, K., & Haberman, M. R. (1994). Provisional practice: The nature of psychosocial bone marrow transplant nursing. *Oncology Nursing Forum, 21*(7), 1147–1154.

Wolf, Z. R. (1986). The caring concept and nurses' identified caring behaviors. *Topics in Clinical Nursing, 8*(2), 84–93.

Wolf, Z. R., Giardino, E.R., Osborne, P. A., & Ambrose, M.S. (1994). Dimensions of nurse caring. *Image: The Journal of Nursing Scholarship, 26*(2), 107–111.

Young, E. W., Koch, P. B., & Preston, D. B. (1989). AIDS and homosexuality: A longitudinal study of knowledge and attitude change among rural nurses. *Public Health Nursing, 6*(4), 189–196.

Appendix follows on next page.

Appendix: Studies Quoted in Tables 4.9 and 4.10

Reference	Year	Author(s)	Participants	Reference	Year	Author(s)	Participants
1	1984	Aamodt, Grassl-Herwehe, Farell, and Hutter	8 Children	21	1994	Cohen, Haberman, Steeves, and Deatrick	38 Nurses
2	1993	Bäck-Pettersson and Jensen	32 Nurses	22	1992	Cohen and Sarter	23 Nurses
3	1991	Beck	47 Students	23	1994	Collins, McCoy, Sale, and Weber	36 Patients
4	1992a	Beck	53 Students	24	1996	Coulon, Krause, and Andersen	156 Students
5	1992b	Beck	36 Students	25	1993	Cooper	9 Nurses
6	1993	Beck	22 Students	26	1990	Davies and O'Berle	1 Nurse, 10 cases
7	1994	Beck	136 Students, 17 Faculty	27	1992	Dietrich	5 Nurses
8	1996	Beck	37 Students	28	1993	Donoghue	107 Nurses
9	1993	Bottorf	8 Patients	29	1993	Euswas	32 Nurses,
10	1987	Bowers	27 Elders, 33 FCGs	30	1996	Fareed	30 Patients
11	1989	Boyd and Munhall	15 Nurses	31	1988	Flaherty	8 Patients, 12 grandmothers
12	1989	J. Brown and Ritchie	25 Nurses	32	1993	Finn	3 Patients
13	1986	L. Brown	50 Patients	33	1988	Forrest	17 Nurses
14	1993	Burfitt, Greiner, Miers, Kinney, and Branyon	13 Patients	34	1993	Girot	10 Nurses
15	1994	Burns	8 Nurses	35	1987	Gardner and Wheeler	110 Patients
16	1988	Bush	14 Students	36	1991	Green-Hernandez	12 Nurses
17	1991	Chipman	26 Students	37	1990	Halldorsdottir	9 Students
18	1992	Clarke and Wheeler	6 Nurses	38	1991	Halldorsdottir	9 Patients, 9 students
19	1991	Clayton, Murray, Hornes, and Greene	70 Families	39	1988	Hinds	25 Patients
20	1994	Cohen, Haberman, and Steeves	38 Nurses	40	1992	Hughes	10 Students
				41	1973	Irwin and Meier	20 HCPs, 20 FCGs
				42	1996	Jenny and Logan	20 Patients

Reference	Year	Author(s)	Participants	Reference	Year	Author(s)	Participants
43	1992	Jensen, Bäck-Pettersson, and Segesten	16 Nurses	57	1994	Poole and Rowat	5 Patients
44	1988	Kahn and Steeves	25 Nurses	58	1994	Powell-Cope	12 FCGs
45	1995	Kosowski	18 Students	59	1994	Propst, Schenk, and Clairain	9 Patients
46	1991	Lemmer	28 Parents	60	1996	Raudonis and Kirschling	9 FCGs
47	1993	Leners	40 Nurses	61	1993	Raudonis	14 Patients
48	1996	Lovgren, Engstrom, and Norberg	80 Patients, 12 family members	62	1987	M. A. Ray	8 Nurses
49	1995	McNamara	5 Nurses	63	1984	M. A. Ray	192 HCPs
50	1992	Miller, Haber, and Byrne	15 Patients, 16 nurses	64	1986	Riemen	10 Patients
51	1996	Milne and McWilliam	14 HCPs, 6 Patients	65	1992	Schroeder and Maeve	29 Patients
52	1992	Montgomery	35 Nurses	66	1991	Sherwood	10 Patients
53	1996	Nelms	5 Nurses	67	1993	Sherwood	10 Patients
54	1992	O'Berie and Davies	1 Nurse, 10 cases	68	1991	Solberg and Morse	98 Observations
55	1994	Parker	45 Nurses	69	1993	Spangler	48 Nurses
56	1992	Peteet, Rose, Medeiros, Walsh-Burke, and Rieker	192 HCPs	70	1994	Steeves, Cohen, and Wise	38 Nurses
				71	1993	Tanner et al.	130 Nurses
				72	1992	Williams	17 FCGs, 33 HCPs
				73	1994	Winters, Miller, Maracich, Compton, and Haberman	23 Patient charts

Note. FCGs = family caregivers; HCPs = health care providers.

QUESTIONS FOR REFLECTION

Baccalaureate

1. What did you learn about analyzing the concept of caring as you read Swanson's (1999) meta-analysis?
2. What was Swanson's (1999) search strategy as she selected citations to include in her literary meta-analysis?
3. What are the patient-related conditions that affect caring according to the literature sources cited by Swanson (1999)?

Master's

1. What follow-up studies are needed to address the concern raised by Swanson (1999) on noncaring nursing?
2. What are the characteristics of the studies cited by Swanson (1999) in the *Level IV: Caring Actions* section of her literary meta-analysis on caring?
3. How did Swanson (1999) apply the caring categories from her theory of caring to organize caring actions?

Doctoral

1. Analyze Swanson's chapter to answer this question: How did knowledge of the concept of caring evolve in the scholarly literature included in this section, from earliest to latest?
2. What process did Dr. Kristen Swanson use to induce the five hierarchical levels of inquiry she described and used to analyze the caring literature? Describe the process.
3. What was the importance of the persistent themes across Swanson's chapter regarding the outcomes of caring?

5

Metasynthesis of Caring in Nursing

Deborah Finfgeld-Connett

To date, the concept of caring has not been clearly conceptualized (Boykin & Schoenhofer, 2001; Brilowski & Wendler, 2005; Sherwood, 1997; Smith, 1999). For example, caring has been described as a human trait, moral imperative, interpersonal relationship, therapeutic intervention, and an affect (Morse, Solberg, Neander, Bottorff, & Johnson, 1990). Caring has also been cast less favorably as slave morality (Paley, 2002). Along with this lack of clarity, caring has been threatened by financial constraints that have placed greater emphasis on medical diseases, symptoms, diagnoses, and cost-effective treatment protocols (Barker, 2000; Euswas, 1993; Gardner, 1992; Leininger, 1993; Turkel, 2001; Woodward, 1997; Yam, 1999).

Despite these challenges, some nursing scholars contend that caring is the essence of nursing practice (Bishop & Scudder, 1991; Eriksson, 1997; Leininger, 1993; Smith, 1999; Watson, 1985), and it should become part of nursing's paradigm (Sourial, 1997). If this is the case, more clearly explicating the concept is imperative. As such, the purpose of this investigation was to enhance the understanding of the concept of caring.

A search of the nursing literature uncovered many concept analyses and qualitative investigations of caring that were designed to clarify the construct inductively. Until now, however, these findings remained largely isolated, and only one known metasynthesis has been conducted (Sherwood, 1997). Although this work was enlightening, it did not reflect the findings from concept analyses or recently completed qualitative studies. In addition, the results revealed little about the antecedents of caring. In light of the work that remained to be carried out, the research question that was posed for this investigation was how can caring be better understood by using an inductive metasynthesis approach?

METHODOLOGY

Metasynthesis is a method of reinterpreting and reshaping existing qualitative findings (McClean & Shaw, 2005). Metasynthesis was deemed appropriate for this investigation, as its purpose is to formulate an evidence-based interpretation of a phenomenon or process and push theoretical and conceptual understanding forward (Schreiber, Crooks, & Stern, 1997). This method involves the synthesis of isolated findings (vs. raw data) from topically related qualitative research

From Finfgeld-Connett, D. (2008). Metasynthesis of caring in nursing. *Journal of Clinical Nursing, 17,* 196–204. Permission to reprint granted by John Wiley & Sons, Inc.

studies and results in a transformed conceptualization of the construct of interest. Metasynthesis methods for this investigation were adapted from Finfgeld (2003).

Because of the purported importance of caring within nursing (e.g., Bishop & Scudder, 1991; Eriksson, 1997; Leininger, 1993; Smith, 1999; Watson, 1985), the goal of this project was to clarify the concept within the discipline. Moreover, based on the preponderance of literature related to caring in nursing, it was hypothesized from the outset that coding categories could be saturated based on the data (i.e., findings) collected strictly from the nursing literature. It was also deemed appropriate to limit the sample to nursing, as excessively large samples can preclude in-depth data analysis (Sandelowski, Docherty, & Emden, 1997) and result in arrant generalizations that are of little practical value (Kearney, 1998; Paterson, Thorne, Canam, & Jillings, 2001).

SAMPLE

Purposive sampling was carried out. The electronic version of Cumulative Index of Nursing and Allied Health Literature (CINAHL) was searched from 1988 to 2006. The term caring was not included as a search heading in this database until 1988. References were also located by scanning reference lists of relevant articles and book chapters.

Caring was searched in combination with the terms or phrases concept analysis, qualitative studies, phenomenology, grounded theory, and ethnography. The term care was not used to search; as in the CINAHL database, care is associated with specific techniques, treatments and/or therapies, which were not the foci of this investigation. Qualitative studies and concept analyses that explored phrases such as caring presence were also not included, as the sole construct of interest was caring. These combined search strategies resulted in more than 534 qualitative studies and concept analyses of caring. Documents were selected from this collection by using the following parameters:

1. The expressed a priori purpose of the study or concept analysis was to investigate caring.
2. The study or concept analysis was conducted by using predetermined, explicit, and widely accepted concept analysis methods or qualitative research methods.
3. The findings appeared as if they were well-supported by the data.
4. The findings reflected the perspectives of staff, care recipients, and family members of care recipients.
5. The focus of the study was patient-centered caring versus student-centered or colleague-centered caring.
6. Findings from student nurses were excluded, as the perspectives of seasoned nurses are thought to reflect more accurately the experience of caring over time.
7. Articles that consisted of personal narratives, stories, and incidental reports of caring that lacked data analysis were excluded, as they were not considered qualitative research studies. Sandelowski and Barroso (2003) classify them as "no-finding reports" (pp. 909–910).
8. Studies that used content analysis or a variation thereof and presented results in a categorical manner were included. Sandelowski and Barroso (2003) classify these types of studies as "topical surveys" (p. 910). They indicate that findings from topical surveys are "close to the original

data" (p. 908) and have the potential to be valuable and "highly informative" (p. 912).

9. Studies that qualified as "thematic surveys" (p. 912) and conceptual/thematic descriptions (p. 913) according to Sandelowski and Barroso's (2003) typology were included. Findings from these types of studies reflect greater data transformation than those found in the topical survey category.

Sandelowski and Barroso (2003) indicate that their typology of qualitative studies is not intended to be used as a tool for "evaluating the scholarly merits of a study" or for determining if a study is "good enough to be included in a research integration study" (p. 907). Paterson et al. (2001) add that it is not possible to exclude all methodologically flawed qualitative investigations from a metasynthesis, as standards change over time, and researchers' perspectives vary according to their training and preferences. As such, investigations and concept analyses were not excluded from this metasynthesis based on merit, as there are no known unequivocal criteria to assess the quality of qualitative investigations and concept analyses. Finally, analysis of findings from qualitative studies as well as concept analyses is in keeping with emergent concept advancement methods such as those outlined by Hupcey and Penrod (2003).

In total, 49 qualitative reports of caring investigations and 6 concept analyses were included in this study. Combining data from differing epistemological perspectives (i.e., grounded theory, phenomenology, concept analysis, and so on) were deemed strength, as triangulation of findings is achieved by combining data from multiple theoretical and methodological traditions (Finfgeld, 2003).

DATA ANALYSIS

Grounded theory served as a backdrop for this investigation. In particular, the constant comparative method was used to analyze the data, and a process orientation (e.g., causal conditions, context, action/interactional strategies, and consequences) framed the study (Strauss & Corbin, 1998). As noted by Paterson et al. (2001), identification of a theoretical framework is important when conducting a metasynthesis, as it assists in the identification of relevant concepts and constructs, guides sampling, and serves as a basis for interpreting findings. Framing caring within a process also appeared apt, as Sherwood (1997) metasynthesis of caring provided evidence of temporal patterns.

Each qualitative study or concept analysis was carefully read and findings were highlighted. Shortly after beginning to read and study each document, it was possible to categorize data using in vivo and metaphorical codes. As organizing categories began to emerge, the data were placed into an electronic matrix. A transformed conceptualization of caring took shape as codes merged and abstract categories were saturated. Two of the coding strategies that emerged during data analysis are illustrated in Table 5.1.

Toward the end of data analysis, diagrams were used to identify links and interrelationships among categories and a process was articulated. During the final phase of data synthesis, Walker and Avant's (2005) process categories (i.e., antecedents, attributes, and consequences) assisted in transforming the data and building a newly constructed conceptualization of caring. Use of Walker and Avant's (2005) process categories was apt, as they are congruent with the temporal nature of grounded theory (e.g., causal conditions, context, action/interactional

TABLE 5.1 Example of Coding Strategy

Codes	Subcategories	Categories
Skills	Nursing knowledge and skills (competence)	Professional maturity
Decision making		
Interpersonal skills		
Competence		
Knowledge base		
Experience		
Ability to cope	Professional maturity	
Self-confidence		
Co-worker support	Background environment	Conducive work environment
Teamwork		
Supportive management		
Conducive environment		
Learning experience		
Adequate time		

strategies, and consequences) as outlined by Strauss and Corbin (1998).

FINDINGS

Overview

Caring is an interpersonal process (Figure 5.1) that is characterized by expert nursing, interpersonal sensitivity, and intimate relationships. Antecedents to the process include a need for and openness to caring on the part of the care recipient. In regard to the care provider, preconditions consist of professional maturity, moral underpinnings, and a conducive work environment. As a result of caring, nurses' and patients' experience improved the mental well-being. Improvements in physical well-being are reported by patients. In keeping with the nature of a process, the outcomes of caring go on to influence future occurrences. These findings are described in greater depth in the remainder of this chapter.

References in the findings section of this chapter are representative of sources

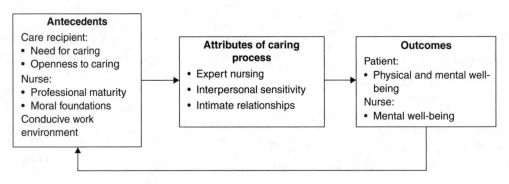

FIGURE 5.1

Process of caring.

that support the results. Because of space limitations and concerns regarding the readability, exhaustive lists of all supporting sources are not included.

Attributes

Process

In keeping with grounded theory (Strauss & Corbin, 1998), the data support that caring consists of a process (e.g., Clarke & Wheeler, 1992; Green-Hernandez, 1991; Leininger, 1981; Swanson, 1990; Turkel, 2001). In particular, Burfitt, Greiner, Miers, Kinney, and Branyon (1993), Sadler (2000), and Wilkin and Slevin (2004) indicate that caring is an interpersonal process. This process may evolve in minutes (Clayton, Murray, Horner, & Greene, 1991; Minick, 1995), over extended periods of time (Burfitt et al., 1993; Clarke & Wheeler, 1992; Clayton et al., 1991; Euswas, 1993; Green-Hernandez, 1991; Leininger, 1981; Turkel, 2001; Wilkin & Slevin, 2004), or not at all (Nikkonen, 1994). Whether caring is actualized depends on the presence or absence of antecedent conditions (Euswas, 1993). The caring process is context specific and continually changes based on the prevailing circumstances (Euswas, 1993; Leininger, 1981).

Expert Nursing

Expert nursing practice is a critical attribute of the caring process. Of great importance is the ability to identify the nuances and meanings accurately of another's situation (Clarke & Wheeler, 1992; Forest, 1989; McCance, 2003; Swanson, 1990, 1991) through well-honed assessment skills (Lucke, 1997; McNamara, 1995; Miller, Haber, & Byrne, 1992; Sherwood, 1991, 1993; Spangler, 1993; Swanson, 1991; Wilkin & Slevin, 2004). This is followed by the execution of expert physical, psychosocial, and spiritually oriented nursing interventions (Green-Hernandez, 1991; Heskins, 1997; Turkel, 2001; Wilkin & Slevin, 2004; Yam & Rossiter, 2000). These interventions include not only doing and advocating for patients, but also empowering them to care for themselves (Clayton et al., 1991; Leininger, 1981; Swanson, 1990, 1991; Swanson-Kauffman, 1986).

Interpersonal Sensitivity

Interpersonal sensitivity is key to the caring process and is characterized by trenchant, intuitive, and empathic insight into another's suffering (Beck, 1995; Eriksson, 1997; Euswas, 1993; Ford, 1990; Forrest, 1989; McNamara, 1995; Montgomery, 1992; Swanson, 1990, 1991; Swanson-Kauffman, 1986). Such insight is made possible by being physically and mindfully present, centering completely on the patient (Eriksson, 1992; Euswas, 1993; Ford, 1990; Forrest, 1989; Leininger, 1993; Sherwood, 1991, 1993, Swanson, 1991), and being emotionally open and available (Forrest, 1989; Swanson, 1991; Wiman & Wikblad, 2004).

Interpersonal sensitivity is demonstrated by going beyond the routine (Beck, 1995; Brown, 1986; Burfitt et al., 1993; Clayton et al., 1991; Eriksson, 1992; Ford, 1990; Morrison, 1991; Propst, Schenk, & Clairain, 1994; Sherwood, 1991), which may involve creativity (Eriksson, 1992; Lucke, 1999) and daring (Back-Pettersson & Jensen, 1993; Lucke, 1997, 1999). In other instances, interpersonal sensitivity may be demonstrated through simple gestures such as attentive listening (Clarke & Wheeler, 1992; Green-Hernandez, 1991; Miller et al., 1992; Wilkin & Slevin, 2004), making eye contact (Eriksson, 1992; Turkel, 2001), touching (Clarke & Wheeler, 1992; Eyles, 1995; Green-Hernandez, 1991; Leininger, 1981, 1993; McNamara, 1995; Miller et al., 1992; Wilkin & Slevin, 2004), and offering verbal reassurances (McCance, 2003; Wilkin & Slevin, 2004). The antithesis of interpersonal insensitivity is nursing practice that is hurried (Burfitt et al., 1993; Forrest, 1989; Riemen, 1986) and mechanical (Forrest, 1989; Halldorsdottir & Hamrin, 1997; Morrison, 1991; Swanson-Kauffman, 1986; Wiman & Wikblad, 2004).

In keeping with the attribute of interpersonal sensitivity, each person is respected

(Beauchamp, 1993; Clarke & Wheeler, 1992; Clayton et al., 1991; Eyles, 1995; Forrest, 1989; Halldorsdottir & Hamrin, 1997; Lucke, 1997; McCance, 2003; McNamara, 1995; Miller et al., 1992; Turkel, 2001; Wilkin & Slevin, 2004), and care is delivered in a nonjudgmental fashion (Clayton et al., 1991; Eyles, 1995; McNamara, 1995). Caring is personalized for each person (Clayton et al., 1991; Ford, 1990; Lucke, 1997; McCance, 2003; McCance, McKenna, & Boore, 1997; Miller et al., 1992; Morrison, 1991; Sherwood, 1991, 1993; Swanson-Kauffman, 1986; Turkel, 2001; Yam & Rossiter, 2000) and cultural differences are taken into consideration (Leininger, 1981; McNamara, 1995; Spangler, 1993; Wilkin & Slevin, 2004).

Intimate Relationships

Caring includes the development of close intimate relationships (Halldorsdottir & Hamrin, 1997; Nikkonen, 1994; Propst et al., 1994) that are characterized as protective (Sherwood, 1991; Swanson, 1991) and trusting (Beeby, 2000; Buchanan & Ross, 1995; Clarke & Wheeler, 1992; Euswas, 1993; Halldorsdottir & Hamrin, 1997; Leininger, 1981; Lucke, 1997; McNamara, 1995; Miller et al., 1992; Sherwood, 1993; Turkel, 2001). Nurses who enact caring are deeply involved (Clarke & Wheeler, 1992; Ford, 1990; Minick, 1995; Montgomery, 1992) such that they grieve with individuals who are grieving and are happy with those who are happy (Eriksson, 1992). At times, this type of intimacy leads to strong emotional feelings such as anger, weariness, irritation, joy (Nikkonen, 1994), and love (Beauchamp, 1993; Nikkonen, 1994; Sherwood, 1991; Swanson-Kauffman, 1986).

Caring develops in relationship to family members as well as patients (Beeby, 2000; Burfitt et al., 1993; Clayton et al., 1991; Finn, 1993; Green-Hernandez, 1991; Heskins, 1997; Leininger, 1993; Miller et al., 1992; Sherwood, 1991; Wilkin & Slevin, 2004; Yam & Rossiter, 2000). In regard to significant others, caring involves listening, providing information, and offering reassurance (Beeby, 2000). It also means encouraging close associates to express their concerns, insuring that they look after themselves (Heskins, 1997), and helping them cope with difficult situations (Beeby, 2000).

Patients and family members feel comfortable sharing personal thoughts and feelings in an open and honest manner (Clarke & Wheeler, 1992; Eyles, 1995; Lucke, 1997; Nikkonen, 1994). In turn, nurses may offer similar information about themselves (Clayton et al., 1991; Lucke, 1997). As such, reciprocity exists between the nurse and the care recipient (Beeby, 2000; Burfitt et al., 1993; Clayton et al., 1991; Green-Hernandez, 1991; Lucke, 1997; McCance et al., 1997; Montgomery, 1997; Nikkonen, 1994; Pollack-Latham, 1991; Wros, 1994), which provides ongoing validation of the caring process (Buchanan & Ross, 1995; Forrest, 1989; Montgomery, 1997; Pollack-Latham, 1991). That said, a professional milieu is maintained throughout the duration of the relationship (Buchanan & Ross, 1995; Burfitt et al., 1993; Miller et al., 1992; Morrison, 1991), as there are times when nurses must be firm, do things the patient does not like, or provide information that is not welcome (Clarke & Wheeler, 1992; Forrest, 1989;). As implied earlier, it is important for nurses to avoid strictly personal relationships to prevent emotional depletion and disengagement (Montgomery, 1997).

Cultural variations in caring relationships are of particular note. For example, findings from a study of caring among Taiwanese nurses and their aging patients suggest that caring exchanges are not reciprocal. Instead, interactions with elders are contextualized by cultural expectations that the nurse will have "the upper hand" and remain "indifferent" (Liu, 2004, p. 149).

Antecedents

Needs and Openness

In order for caring to occur, individuals must present with physical, psychosocial, and/or spiritual needs (Brown, 1986; Sadler, 2000; Turkel, 2001; Yam & Rossiter, 2000). Although patients are usually the focus of caring, psychosocial and spiritual vulnerabilities may also be evident among family members (Clayton et al., 1991; Green-Hernandez, 1991). These needs may be ongoing (Clarke & Wheeler, 1992) or crisis oriented (Wiman & Wikblad, 2004), and caring is adapted to context-specific circumstances.

Findings suggest that caring is very difficult if patients are not consciously aware and open to it (Clayton et al., 1991). Resistant individuals include those who are angry, aggressive (Beeby, 2000; Clarke & Wheeler, 1992), or overly demanding (McCance, 2003; Yam & Rossiter, 2000). Through no fault of their own, patients may also be unable to fully engage in caring because of their age (e.g., newborns) or health problems (e.g., dementia and unconsciousness) (Beeby, 2000; Burfitt et al., 1993; McCance, 2003; Wilkin & Slevin, 2004).

Professional Maturity

Professional maturity is another antecedent to caring. Examples of coding categories that support this finding include knowledge base (Clarke & Wheeler, 1992; Euswas, 1993; Lucke, 1997; Pollack-Latham, 1991), the ability to cope (Clarke & Wheeler, 1992; Forrest, 1989; Green-Hernandez, 1991; Pollack-Latham, 1991), and competence (Euswas, 1993; Forrest, 1989; Green-Hernandez, 1991; Lucke, 1997).

Caring entails nursing competence in the areas of knowledge acquisition, decision-making, and execution of skills (Clarke & Wheeler, 1992; Clayton et al., 1991; Halldorsdottir & Hamrin, 1997; Wilkin & Slevin, 2004; Yam, 1999; Yam & Rossiter, 2000). Professional maturity also involves the learned capacity to cope with the psychic and physical challenges that co-occur with situations in which caring is needed. Nurses who enact caring are able to become deeply involved without succumbing to overemotional (Euswas, 1993),

destructive, controlling, and self-centered forms of helping (Montgomery, 1992, 1997; Wros, 1994). They have cultivated the ability to protect themselves and maintain a healthy emotional balance (Euswas, 1993; Forrest, 1989; Green-Hernandez, 1991; Montgomery, 1997; Morrison, 1991; Nikkonen, 1994; Pollack-Latham, 1991; Yam, 1999). Spiritual and philosophical belief systems, the ability to manage personal vulnerabilities (Montgomery, 1997; Pollack-Latham, 1991), self-awareness (Montgomery, 1997; Pollack-Latham, 1991; Yam & Rossiter, 2000), and self-confidence (Beeby, 2000; Clarke & Wheeler, 1992; Forrest, 1989; Miller et al., 1992) help enhance professional maturity and the ability to sustain caring.

Moral Foundations

Moral foundations are another antecedent to caring and involve a commitment to act benevolently (Buchanan & Ross, 1995; Euswas, 1993; Eyles, 1995). Committed benevolence is comprised of ethical ways of knowing (Euswas, 1993; Wros, 1994) such that caring is enacted in a conscientious (Eyles, 1995; Morrison, 1991;) and responsible manner (Clarke & Wheeler, 1992; Eyles, 1995; Nikkonen, 1994; Wiman & Wikblad, 2004).

Conducive Environment

Although some assert that caring is at least partially innate (Clarke & Wheeler, 1992; Clayton et al., 1991; Pollack-Latham, 1991), there is also evidence to suggest that, for it to be fully expressed, caring must be cultivated. Learning experiences that may hasten the development of caring include previous relationships in which it was evident (Clarke & Wheeler, 1992; Forrest, 1989; Pollack-Latham, 1991), religious training, professional education (Forrest, 1989), and role modeling (Yam & Rossiter, 2000).

In addition, work environments must be conducive to the enactment of caring. Caring is made possible by health care systems and management personnel that value it over simple task completion (Clarke & Wheeler, 1992; Montgomery, 1997; Touhy, Strews, & Brown, 2005; Yam, 1999; Yam & Rossiter, 2000). Essential elements of a conducive working environment include adequate resources (Clarke & Wheeler, 1992; McCance, 2003; Montgomery, 1997; Wilkin & Slevin, 2004; Yam & Rossiter, 2000) and time to carry out caring (Beeby, 2000; Clarke & Wheeler, 1992; Green-Hernandez, 1991; McCance, 2003; Pollack-Latham, 1991; Wilkin & Slevin, 2004).

To maintain caring, nurses must also experience it (Beeby, 2000; Clarke & Wheeler, 1992; Montgomery, 1997; Touhy et al., 2005; Yam & Rossiter, 2000). This involves having reasonable work expectations (Clarke & Wheeler, 1992; Minick, 1995; Montgomery, 1997) and being recognized for significant accomplishments (Beeby, 2000; Pollack-Latham, 1991; Touhy et al., 2005). It also means having support from team members who help validate caring and reduce stressful working conditions (Beeby, 2000; Buchanan & Ross, 1995; Forrest, 1989; McNamara, 1995; Montgomery, 1997; Wilkin & Slevin, 2004; Yam, 1999; Yam & Rossiter, 2000).

Consequences

Patients' Physical and Mental Well-Being

As a result of caring, patients experience improvements in physical and mental well-being. They report a sense of decreased stress (Green-Hernandez, 1991; Leininger, 1981; McNamara, 1995; Miller et al., 1992; Pollack-Latham, 1991; Sherwood, 1993), improvements in self-esteem (Brown, 1986; Eyles, 1995; Halldorsdottir & Hamrin, 1997; Lucke, 1997; Miller et al., 1992), a positive mental attitude (Buchanan & Ross, 1995; Halldorsdottir & Hamrin, 1997; McCance, 2003; Sherwood, 1993; Turkel, 2001), personal growth (Clayton et al., 1991; Eriksson, 1992; Lucke, 1999; Pollack-Latham, 1991; Sherwood, 1993; Smith, 1999; Sourial, 1997), and self-actualization (Euswas, 1993; Green-Hernandez, 1991; Montgomery,

1992). Patients also experience improved physical well-being (Buchanan & Ross, 1995; Burfitt et al., 1993; Clayton et al., 1991; McCance, 2003; McNamara, 1995; Sherwood, 1993; Turkel, 2001), which is due, in part, to an increased ability to care for one's self (Clayton et al., 1991; Eyles, 1995; Halldorsdottir & Hamrin, 1997; Lucke, 1999).

Nurses' Mental Well-Being

Because of the reciprocal nature of caring, nurses report an improved sense of mental well-being. Caring results in feelings of satisfaction (Buchanan & Ross, 1995; Eriksson, 1992; McNamara, 1995; Miller et al., 1992; Montgomery, 1992, 1997; Pollack-Latham, 1991; Sadler, 2000) and renewal (McNamara, 1995; Miller et al., 1992; Montgomery, 1997; Sadler, 2000). Nurses also report personal growth (Eriksson, 1992; Ford, 1990; McNamara, 1995; Montgomery, 1997; Sadler, 2000), especially in the form of self-actualization (Euswas, 1993; Green-Hernandez, 1991; Pollack-Latham, 1991; Sherwood, 1993).

In concordance with a process orientation, the outcomes of caring go on to influence its occurrence in the future. In particular, resultant mental well-being produces openness to caring at a later date. For nurses, feelings of satisfaction and renewal (Miller et al., 1992; Montgomery, 1997) influence the likelihood that caring will be manifested in future. Similarly, a sense of security (Clayton et al., 1991; Halldorsdottir & Hamrin, 1997; Sourial, 1997) and a positive mental attitude (Halldorsdottir & Hamrin, 1997; Lucke, 1999; McCance, 2003; Turkel, 2001) will position patients for caring when a need for it arises at a later date.

DISCUSSION

The conceptualization of caring that emerged from this investigation is consistent with the patterns of caring that

Sherwood (1997) inferred from her meta-synthesis. The results from this work go a step further, however, in that they place caring into a more cohesive process.

The findings are in keeping with the probabilistic view of concepts in which rigid criteria for membership in a category are discarded and contextual variations are possible (Morse, 1995). These variations do not negate the importance of clearly articulated antecedents, attributes, and consequences. Instead, they allow for discrepancies because of cultural or situational circumstances and scholars' best estimates of probable truth (Penrod & Hupcey, 2005).

It is interesting to note that the findings from this metasynthesis are in keeping with results from efforts to delineate caring by using factor analysis. Using the latter methodology, caring is thought to be a four-factor structure consisting of knowledge and skill, assurance, respectfulness, and connectedness (Wu, Larrabee, & Putman, 2006). These factors are consistent with expert practice, interpersonal sensitivity, and intimate relationships. This confluence of findings suggests triangulation of results across methodologies.

Similarities between the results of this metasynthesis of caring and findings from a metasynthesis of nursing presence (Finfgeld-Connett, 2006) are also noteworthy. For this reason, a formal comparison of the two constructs using advanced concept analysis methods (e.g., Morse, 1995) is recommended. Formal comparisons of nursing terminology are important for the development of theoretical frameworks that can be used in practice and research.

Results from this investigation are particularly said in terms of the intellectual, moral, and interpersonal components of caring. That said, the overt actions involved in caring remain somewhat obscure. Skott and Eriksson (2005) suggest that the physical aspects of caring are the hidden work of clinical nursing. They also indicate that the psychomotor and visceral components of caring remain ambiguous because of their connection with the body and the challenges involved in objectifying them.

Consistent with Sherwood's (1997) metasynthesis findings, the results from this investigation do not offer much insight into the nature of care recipients' needs or their openness to caring. Moreover, the findings offer little insight into how to recognize these antecedents. Additional research is needed to better articulate these preconditions, as opportunities to enact caring may not be easily recognized among reticent patients. This is especially true when reticence is conveyed as nonresponsiveness or belligerence. A lingering research question is whether it is possible for expert nurses to overcome patients' reticence to caring.

Despite the fact that caring extends to family members, the data are silent on outcomes related to them. However, based on the patients' outcomes, it is inferred that family members experience improved mental health as a result of caring. Additional research is needed to confirm this hypothesis.

Given that caring is not totally innate, health care agencies and educational institutions are urged to devote more resources to cultivating the caring among employees (Touhy et al., 2005) and students (Coyle-Rogers & Cramer, 2005; Lee-Hsieh & Turton, 2004). On the basis of the findings from this study, this means role modeling caring, valuing caring over simple task completion, establishing reasonable work assignments and expectations, and providing supportive feedback. It also means creating a culture of interpersonal sensitivity in which individual differences are valued and respected.

As for Paley's (2002) assertion that caring is slave morality, findings from this investigation do not support this contention. In particular, nurses who enact caring are portrayed as creative, daring, assertive, and able to empower patients to care for themselves. Moreover, they are professionally mature enough to strike a healthy balance between caring for others and caring for themselves. The findings also suggest that caring is conducive to improved mental health among nurses. As such, nurse managers and administrators have incentive to provide environments that nurture caring.

CONCLUSIONS

Based on the findings of this metasynthesis, a cohesive process of caring has been explicated. Caring is inferred to be a context-specific interpersonal process that is characterized by expert nursing practice, interpersonal sensitivity, and intimate relationships. It is preceded by a recipient's need and openness to caring and the nurse's professional maturity and moral foundations. In addition, a working environment that is conducive to caring is also necessary. Consequences include improved mental well-being among nurses and patients and improvements in patients' physical well-being. It is recommended that health care agencies and educational institutions devote more resources to cultivating the caring among employees and students. In addition, researchers are urged to better clarify selected elements of the caring process.

REFERENCES

Back-Pettersson, S. R., & Jensen, K. P. (1993). 'She dares:' an essential characteristic of the excellent Swedish nurse. In D. A. Gaut (Ed.), *A global agenda for caring* (pp. 257–265). New York, NY: National League for Nursing.

Barker, P. (2000). Reflections on caring as a virtue ethic within an evidence-based culture. *International Journal of Nursing Studies, 37,* 329–336.

Beauchamp, C. J. (1993). The centrality of caring: A case study. In P. L. Munhall & C. O. Boyd (Eds.), *Nursing research: A qualitative perspective* (pp. 338–358). New York, NY: National League for Nursing.

Beck, C. T (1995). Perceptions of nurses' caring by mothers experiencing postpartum depression. *Journal of Obstetric, Gynecologic, and Neonatal Nursing, 24,* 819–825.

Beeby, J. P. (2000). Intensive care nurses' experiences of caring. *Intensive and Critical Care Nursing, 16,* 151–163.

Bishop, A. H., & Scudder, J. R. (1991). *Nursing: The practice of caring.* New York, NY: National League for Nursing.

Boykin, A., & Schoenhofer, S. O. (2001). *Nursing as caring: A model of transforming practice.* Boston, MA: Jones and Bartlett.

Brilowski, G. A., & Wendler, M. C. (2005). A evolutionary concept analysis of caring. *Journal of Advanced Nursing, 50,* 641–650.

Brown, L. (1986) The experience of care: Patient perspectives. *Topics in Clinical Nursing, 8,* 56–62.

Buchanan, S., & Ross, E. K. (1995). A concept analysis of caring. *Perspectives 19,* 3–6.

Burfitt, S. N., Greiner, D. S., Miers, L. J., Kinney, M. R., & Branyon, M. E. (1993). Professional nurse caring as perceived by critically ill patients: A phenomenologic study. *American Journal of Critical Care, 2,* 489–499.

Clarke, J. B., & Wheeler, S. J. (1992). A view of the phenomenon of caring in nursing practice. *Journal of Advanced Nursing, 17,* 1283–1290.

Clayton, G. M., Murray, J. P., Horner, S. D., & Greene, P. E. (1991). Connecting: A catalyst for caring. In P. L. Chinn (Ed.), *Anthology on caring* (pp, 155–168). New York, NY: National League for Nursing.

Coyle-Rogers, P., & Cramer, M. (2005). The phenomenon of caring: The perspectives of nurse educators. *Journal for Nurses in Staff Development, 21,* 160–170.

Eriksson, K. (1992). Different forms of caring communion. *Nursing Science Quarterly, 5,* 93.

Eriksson, K. (1997). Understanding the world of the patient, the suffering human being: The new clinical paradigm from nursing to caring. *Advanced Practice Nursing Quarterly, 3,* 8–13.

Euswas, P. (1993). The actualized caring moment: A grounded theory of caring in nursing practice. In D. A. Gaut (Ed.), *A global agenda for caring* (pp. 309–326). New York, NY: National League for Nursing.

Eyles, M. (1995). Uncovering the knowledge to care. *British Journal of Theatre Nursing, 5,* 22–25.

Finfgeld, D. L. (2003). Meta-synthesis: The state of the art-so far. *Qualitative Health Research, 13,* 893–904.

Finfgeld-Connett, D. (2006). Meta-synthesis of presence in nursing. *Journal of Advanced Nursing, 55,* 708–714.

Finn, J. (1993). Caring in birthing: Experiences of professional nurse and generic care. In D. A. Gaut (Ed.), *A global agenda for caring* (pp. 63–79). New York, NY: National League for Nursing.

Ford, J. S. (1990). Caring encounters. *Scandinavian Journal of Caring Sciences, 4*, 157–162.

Forrest, D. (1989). The experience of caring. *Journal of Advanced Nursing, 14*, 815–823.

Gardner, K. (1992). The historical conflict between caring and professionalization: A dilemma for nursing. In D. A. Gaut (Ed.), *The presence of caring in nursing* (pp. 241–255). New York, NY: National League for Nursing.

Green-Hernandez, C. (1991). Professional nurse caring: A conceptual model for nursing. In R. M. Neil & R. Watts (Eds.), *Caring and nursing: Explorations in feminist perspectives* (pp. 85–96). New York, NY: National League for Nursing.

Halldorsdottir, S., & Hamrin, E. (1997). Caring and uncaring encounters within nursing and health care from the cancer patient's perspective. *Cancer Nursing, 20*, 120–128.

Heskins, F. M. (1997). Exploring dichotomies of caring, gender and technology in intensive care nursing: A qualitative approach. *Intensive and Critical Care Nursing, 13*, 65–71.

Hupcey, J. E., & Penrod, J. (2003). Concept advancement: Enhancing inductive validity. *Research and Theory for Nursing Practice, 17*, 19–30.

Kearney, M. H. (1998). Ready-to-wear: Discovering grounded formal theory. *Research in Nursing and Health, 21*, 179–186.

Lee-Hsieh, J., & Turton, M. A. (2004). Patient experiences in the development of a caring code for clinical nursing practice. *International Journal for Human Caring, 8*, 21–9.

Leininger, M. M. (1981). *Caring: An essential human need*. Thorofare, NJ: Slack.

Leininger, M. (1993). Culture care theory: The comparative global theory to advance human care nursing knowledge and practice. In D. A. Gaut (Ed.), *A global agenda for caring* (pp. 3–18). New York, NY: National League for Nursing.

Liu, S. (2004). What caring means to geriatric nurses. *The Journal of Nursing Research, 12*, 143–151.

Lucke, K. T. (1997). Knowledge acquisition and decision-making: Spinal cord injured individuals perceptions of caring during rehabilitation. *SCI Nursing, 14*, 871–95.

Lucke, K. T. (1999). Outcomes of nurse caring as perceived by individuals with spinal cord injury during rehabilitation. *Rehabilitation Nursing, 24*, 247–253.

McCance, T. V. (2003). Caring in nursing practice: The development of a conceptual framework. *Research and Theory for Nursing Practice: An International Journal, 17*, 101–116.

McCance, T. V., McKenna, H. P., & Boore, J. R. P. (1997). Caring: Dealing with a difficult concept. *International Journal of Nursing Studies, 34*, 241–248.

McClean, S., & Shaw, A. (2005). From schism to continuum? The problematic relationship between expert and lay knowledge—an exploratory conceptual synthesis of two qualitative studies. *Qualitative Health Research, 15*, 729–749.

McNamara, S. (1995). Perioperative nurses' perceptions of caring practices. *AORN Journal, 61*, 377–388.

Miller, B. K., Haber, J., & Byrne, M. W. (1992). The experience of caring in the acute care setting: Patient and nurse perspectives. In D. A. Gaut (Ed.), *The presence of caring in nursing* (pp. 137–156). New York, NY: National League for Nursing.

Minick, P. (1995). The power of human caring: Early recognition of patient problems. *Scholarly Inquiry for Nursing Practice: An International Journal, 9*, 303–317.

Montgomery, C. L. (1992). The spiritual connection: Nurses' perceptions of the experience of caring. In D. A. Gaut (Ed.), *The presence of caring in nursing* (pp. 39–52). New York, NY: National League for Nursing.

Montgomery, C. L. (1997). Coping with the emotional demands of caring. *Advanced Practice Nursing Quarterly, 3*, 76–84.

Morrison, P. (1991). The caring attitude in nursing practice: A repertory grid study of trained nurses' perceptions. *Nurse Education Today, 11*, 3–12.

Morse, J. (1995). Exploring the theoretical basis of nursing using advanced techniques of concept analysis. *Advances in Nursing Science, 17*, 31–46.

Morse, J. M., Solberg, S. M., Neander, W. L., Bottorff, J. L., & Johnson, J. L. (1990). Concepts of caring and caring as a concept. *Advances in Nursing Science, 13*, 1–14.

Nikkonen, M. (1994). Caring from the point of view of a Finnish mental health nurse; a life history approach. *Journal of Advanced Nursing, 19*, 1185–1195.

Paley, J. (2002). Caring as a slave morality: Nietzschean themes in nursing ethics. *Journal of Advanced Nursing, 40*, 25–35.

Paterson, B. L., Thorne, S. E., Canam, C., & Jillings, C. (2001). *Meta-study of qualitative health research: A practical guide to meta-analysis and metasynthesis*. Thousand Oaks, CA: Sage.

Penrod, J., & Hupcey, J. E. (2005), Enhancing methodological clarity: Principle-based concept analysis. *Journal of Advanced Nursing, 50,* 403–409.

Pollack-Latham, C. L. (1991). Clarification of the unique role of caring in nurse–patient relationships. In P. L. Chinn (Ed.), *Anthology on caring* (pp. 183–209). New York, NY: National League for Nursing.

Propst, M. G., Schenk, L. K., & Clairain, S. (1994). Caring as perceived during the birth experience. In D. A. Gaut & A. Boykin (Eds.), *Caring as healing: Renewal through hope* (pp. 252–264). New York, NY: National League for Nursing.

Riemen, D. J. (1986). Noncaring and caring in the clinical setting: Patients' descriptions. *Topics in Clinical Nursing, 8,* 30–36.

Sadler, J. J. (2000). A multiphase approach to concept analysis and development. In B. L. Rodgers & K. A. Knafl (Eds.), *Concept development in nursing: Foundations, techniques, and applications* (pp. 251–283). Philadelphia, PA: Saunders.

Sandelowski, M., & Barroso, J. (2003). Classifying the findings in qualitative studies. *Qualitative Health Research, 13,* 905–923.

Sandelowski, M., Docherty, S., & Emden, D. (1997). Qualitative meta-synthesis: Issues and techniques. *Research in Nursing and Health, 20,* 365–371.

Schreiber, R., Crooks, D., & Stern, P. N. (1997). Qualitative meta-analysis. In J. M. Morse (Ed.), *Completing a qualitative project: Details and dialogue* (pp. 311–326). Thousand Oaks, CA: Sage.

Sherwood, G. (1991). Expressions of nurses' caring: The role of the compassionate healer. In D. A. Gaut & M. M. Leininger (Eds.), *Caring: The compassionate healer* (pp. 79–88). New York, NY: National League for Nursing.

Sherwood, G. (1993). A qualitative analysis of patient responses to caring; a moral and economic imperative. In D. A. Gaut (Ed.), *A global agenda for caring* (pp. 243–255). New York, NY: National League for Nursing.

Sherwood, G. D. (1997). Meta-synthesis of qualitative analyses of caring: Defining a therapeutic model of nursing. *Advanced Practice Nursing Quarterly, 3,* 32–42.

Skott, C., & Eriksson, A. (2005). Clinical caring-the diary of a nurse. *Journal of Clinical Nursing, 14,* 916–921.

Smith, M. (1999). Caring and the science of unitary human beings. *Advances in Nursing Science, 21,* 12–28.

Sourial, S. (1997). An analysis of caring. *Journal of Advanced Nursing, 26,* 1189–1192.

Spangler, Z. (1993). Generic and professional care of Anglo-American and Philippine American nurses. In D. A. Gaut (Ed.), *A global agenda for caring* (pp. 47–61). New York, NY: National League for Nursing.

Strauss, A., & Corbin, J. (1998). *Basics of qualitative research: Techniques and procedures for developing grounded theory.* Thousand Oaks, CA: Sage.

Swanson, K. M. (1990). Providing care in the NICU: Sometimes an act of love. *Advances in Nursing Science, 13,* 60–73.

Swanson, K. M. (1991). Empirical development of a middle range theory of caring. *Nursing Research, 40,* 161–166.

Swanson-Kauffman, K. M. (1986). Caring in the instance of unexpected early pregnancy loss. *Topics in Clinical Nursing, 8,* 37–46.

Touhy, T. A., Strews, W., & Brown, C. (2005). Expressions of caring as lived by nursing home staff, residents, and families. *International Journal for Human Caring, 9,* 31–37.

Turkel, M. C. (2001). Struggling to find a balance: The paradox between caring and economics. *Nursing Administration Quarterly, 26,* 67–82.

Walker, L. O., & Avant, K. C. (2005). *Strategies for theory construction in nursing.* Upper Saddle River, NJ: Pearson/Prentice Hail.

Watson, J. (1985). *Nursing: The philosophy and science of caring.* Boulder, CO: Colorado Associated University Press.

Wilkin, K., & Slevin, E. (2004). The meaning of caring to nurses: An investigation into the nature of caring work in an intensive care unit. *Journal of Clinical Nursing, 13,* 50–59.

Wiman, E., & Wikblad, K. (2004). Caring and uncaring encounters in nursing in an emergency department. *Journal of Clinical Nursing, 13,* 422–429.

Woodward, V. (1997). Professional caring: A contradiction in terras? *Journal of Advanced Nursing, 26,* 999–1004.

Wros, P. (1994). The ethical context of nursing care of dying patients in critical care. In P. Benner (Ed.), *Interpretive phenomenology: Embodiment, caring, and ethics in health and illness* (pp. 255–277). Thousand Oaks, CA: Sage.

Wu, Y., Larrabee, J. H., & Putman, H. P. (2006). Caring behaviors inventory: A reduction of the 42-item instrument. *Nursing Research, 55,* 18–25.

Yam, B. M. C. (1999). Perceptions of caring behaviours among Hong Kong nurses: A preliminary analysis. *Singapore Nursing Journal, 26,* 19–22.

Yam, B. M. C., & Rossiter, J. C. A. (2000). Caring in nursing: Perceptions of Hong Kong nurses. *Journal of Clinical Nursing, 9,* 293–302.

QUESTIONS FOR REFLECTION

Baccalaureate

1. How is the purpose of Finfgeld-Connett's (2008) metasynthesis explained in relation to the concept of caring?
2. What was the sampling approach of Finfgeld (2008)? Explain in detail.
3. How did Finfgeld-Connett (2008) explain the data analysis methods that she used?

Master's

1. How can you apply the findings from Finfgeld-Connett's (2008) metasynthesis to nursing practice situations?
2. What is the contribution of expert nursing to the attributes of the caring process from the perspective of Finfgeld-Connett's study?
3. What are the outcomes of the process of caring according to Finfgeld-Connett's (2008) metasynthesis?

Doctoral

1. How do the findings of Finfgeld-Connett's (2008) metasynthesis relate to Sherwood's methasynthesis (1997)?
2. What is the systematic process used by Finfgeld-Connett (2008) to select citations from the many studies and concept analyses she initially located?
3. How are the methods of grounded theory and Walker and Avant's (2005) process of theory construction applied to Finfgeld-Connett's (2008) data analysis?

III

Theoretical Perspectives on Caring

Marlaine C. Smith

OVERVIEW OF THEORETICAL DEVELOPMENT

*P*art III of this anthology includes classic theoretical publications by the most well-known caring theorists. The theories provide organizing structures that shape our understanding of phenomena.

Madeleine Leininger was the first nursing scholar to assert the centrality of caring in nursing. On the basis of her studies of 30 cultures, she created a taxonomy to classify care behaviors across cultures. Her theory was influenced by her anthropological roots. The fledgling conceptual model evolved over a decade into the theory of cultural care diversity and universality represented by the "sunrise model." One of Leininger's earliest papers is presented in this book.

Jean Watson was on the ground floor of developing caring theory in nursing. In 1979, her book *Nursing: The Philosophy and Science of Caring* was published. In this book, the 10 carative factors (CFs) presented an organizing structure that shaped the way caring was conceptualized and practiced in nursing. The theory reflected humanitarian and relational values, offered an alternative to the medical model, and asserted caring as essential to nursing. Over time, Watson's work changed considerably as she incorporated more substantive transpersonal, metaphysical, and spiritual ideas into her writing. These ideas influenced her concepts of transpersonal caring, the caring occasion, and caring–healing modalities.

Watson's theory of human caring is loosely constructed, and some argue that it is a philosophy, whereas others argue that it is a middle range theory. Watson, herself, eschews these attempts to classify her theory, agreeing that it is philosophy, theory, and ethic. In her latest work, Watson transforms her CFs into Caritas Factors. Watson's Caring Science Institute (WCSI) is educating a growing cadre of nurses in caring theory. In this anthology, four of Watson's publications are included: chapters from two books and two classic articles.

In the late 1970s, Josephine Paterson and Loretta Zderad developed humanistic nursing theory. This theory, influenced by existential-phenomenological philosophy, emphasized the interhuman realm of nursing, the goal of nurturing well-being and more-being, the focus on responding to the call for nursing, and identification of the nursing situation as the between in which nursing is understood. This theory was revolutionary at its time and influenced both Boykin and Schoenhofer and perhaps Watson's theoretical thinking.

In the mid to late 1980s, Sister M. Simone Roach was developing her philosophy or theory of nursing. Sister Roach advanced caring as the human mode of being. She listed a series of caring attributes that she named the "Six Cs." These "Six Cs" of compassion, competence, confidence, conscience, commitment, and comportment provides an organizing framework that is useful to structure the acquisition of these attributes by nurses and students.

Boykin and Schoenhofer's theory of Nursing as Caring was introduced in 1993. This general theory, or grand theory, of nursing is based on a set of six assumptions. The first assumption is that all persons are caring by nature of their humanness. This caring is expressed differently as persons grow in their ability to live caring. Nursing is nurturing the growth of living caring. The nurse comes to know the one nursed by listening to his or her story and understanding what matters most in the moment. The nurse hears the call for nursing from the one nursed and responds to that call. The nurse nurtures the growth of the other in caring. The nursing situation is the shared lived experience between the nurse and the one nursed, in which personhood is enhanced (Boykin & Schoenhofer, 1993, p. 24).

In the 1980s, caring theory grew in countries throughout the world. Katie Eriksson's theoretical work in Finland is one prominent international caring theory included in this anthology. Eriksson focused on compassion for the suffering human being. Her theory was based on eight assumptions that emphasize the humanity and holiness of the human body, soul, and spirit. The caritas motive comes from an ethos of love and responsibility for the other.

The middle range theory of caring developed by Kristen Swanson emerged from the findings of three phenomenological studies within perinatal nursing. Swanson's findings were synthesized into five caring processes with identifiable dimensions. The caring processes are knowing, being with, doing for, enabling, and maintaining belief. This middle range theory provides a guide for making caring visible in nursing practice.

Finally, Sigridur Halldorsdottir related caring behaviors of nurses to health and well-being and situated these behaviors on a continuum. The structure emerged from two studies of caring behaviors, and it is helpful in understanding the consequences of both caring and uncaring for both patients and nurses. The

five modes of being are life destroying or biocidic, life restraining or biostatic, life neutral or biopassive, life sustaining or bioactive, and life giving or biogenic.

Theory development in caring has grown significantly in the 21st century with several middle range theories emerging. The growing interest in theory-guided practice in hospital settings stimulated by the Magnet Hospital criteria has generated the growth of caring theories on multiple levels. These theories are living in practice and being transformed by practice. More research is being framed within caring theoretical perspectives, expanding caring science.

CHAPTER SUMMARIES

Chapter 6: In this chapter, arguably the foundational paper in the development of caring science in nursing, Madeleine Leininger (1978) lays the groundwork for the establishment of caring as a central distinguishing phenomenon in the discipline of nursing. The paper was presented in 1978 at the First Caring Conference in Salt Lake City, Utah. In it, she argues that "caring is the central and unifying domain for the body of knowledge and practices in nursing" (p. 3), and that the systematic scientific study of caring can both advance the discipline and enhance the care of those served by nursing. She argues that very little is known about care and caring, yet care and caring are essential for human growth, development, and survival (p. 4). In addition, she argues that the study of caring is essential for the survival of the human race, and that societal forces such as the increased use of technology in health care are demeaning and depersonalizing human life. She asserts that the trend can be turned around through "those in the nursing profession [providing] a renewed emphasis on human caring . . ." (p. 8).

In this chapter, Leininger presents a synthesis of her thinking and her work of the previous 10 years in which she studied caring in about 30 different cultures. Assumptions, hypotheses, a conceptual framework to guide inquiry, and principles and guidelines form the foundations of transcultural nursing theory. During this era, nursing was striving to differentiate itself from medicine and to lay claim to its distinctive focus as a discipline. Leininger was one of the first nurses prepared through the nurse scientist program, receiving her PhD in anthropology. The intent of this federal program was to infuse nursing with the scientific traditions of other fields by immersing their scholars in doctoral studies in these fields. Leininger's work reflects this immersion in anthropology. She asserts that care and caring are universally human but expressed differently in the lifeways of each culture. Her definitions reflect this emphasis:

> Professional nursing care [is] . . . those cognitively learned humanistic and scientific modes of helping or enabling an individual, family, or community to receive personalized services through specific culturally-defined or ascribed modes of caring processes, techniques, and patterns to improve or maintain favorably healthy conditions for life or death. (p. 135 in this volume)

Eleven assumptions and ten theoretical statements or hypotheses form the foundations of transcultural caring theory. Leininger's Conceptual and Theory-Generating Model to Study Transcultural and Ethnocaring Constructs is presented and explained. The principles or guidelines are offered to assist nurses in practice. These include assertions related to the cultural variations associated with caring and care behaviors and expressions. She concludes that a transcultural nursing approach is promising for the advancement of caring across cultures.

Chapter 7: Like several other nursing theorists of the 1970s, Jean Watson was stimulated to develop her theory through creating an organizing framework for the nursing curriculum. As the director of the undergraduate nursing program at the University of Colorado School of Nursing, Watson developed the organizing framework that evolved over time into her philosophy and theory of caring. In the introductory chapter, she focuses on nursing education within a university and the importance of the liberal arts as a foundation for this education. She contrasts science and humanities, extolling the virtues of both in the study of nursing. This foreshadows her future emphasis on a human science perspective for nursing. "The science of caring combines science with the humanities. The science of caring cannot be completely neutral with respect to human values. It cannot remain detached from or indifferent to human emotions — pain, joy, suffering, fear and anger" (Watson, 1979, p. 5).

The second chapter is CFs in Nursing. Here, Watson states that while curative factors aim at curing the patient of a disease, CFs aim at helping the person attain or maintain health or a peaceful death (p. 7). Seven basic assumptions for the Science of Caring in Nursing are listed. These are a prelude to the future theoretical development in that they include references to the interpersonal nature of caring, the relationship between caring and human health, being nonjudgmental, creating a caring environment, the complementarity of caring and curing, and the centrality of caring to nursing (p. 9). The 10 CFs are listed and the first three are explicated in this chapter. The first is the formation of a humanistic altruistic value system. Watson encourages the nursing student to reflect on personal values and beliefs, and emphasizes the importance of the capacity to "view humanity with love and to appreciate diversity and individuality" (p. 11). She even encourages development of these values through literary immersion, meditation, and therapy, and draws from some of the contemporary psychologists who assert that the sense of self becomes extended with consideration for the welfare of others. In the description of the second CF, instillation of faith-hope,

Watson synthesizes classical philosophy, spirituality, and mind–body psychology to illuminate the importance of faith and hope to human life. "Regardless of what scientific regimen is required for the care of the person, the nurse discovers what is meaningful and important for that particular person" (p. 15). Watson instructs nurses to respect the values and beliefs of others and to consider the whole person. The third CF, cultivation of sensitivity to self and others, is about the acknowledgment of feelings. In the 1970s, nurses were expected to be objective, hiding their own and ignoring their patients' feelings. Watson stated that acknowledging these feelings was essential to caring for the whole person, and that sensitivity to one's own feelings facilitated the development of empathy, the ability to feel with others. This CF was related to promoting actualization of self and others.

Chapter 8: This chapter, "Foundations of Humanistic Nursing," is included in this text (Paterson & Zderad, 1976/1988) because these authors present foundational concepts that appear in other caring theories. Originally, published in 1976, Josephine Paterson and Loretta Zderad created a theory that reflects existential-phenomenological philosophy. They begin by stating that nursing is a response to a human situation in which help is needed and provided (p. 11). They define nursing as a phenomenon related to the health–illness of the human condition, and that "every nursing act has to do with the quality of a person's living and dying" (p. 12). For Paterson and Zderad, nursing is concerned not only with well-being but with more-being, actualizing the fullness of human potential.

The concepts of humanistic nursing theory include human potential, intersubjective transaction, well-being, more-being, being and doing, and choice. Human potential includes being becoming. Intersubjective transaction acknowledges that the nurse and the person

nursed are in a subject-to-subject relationship in which nurturance occurs in "the between" (Paterson & Zderad, 1976/1988, p. 13). In nursing practice, being and doing are inextricably linked. While doing is more emphasized, presence "can be known much more vividly than . . . can be described" (p. 13). The active presence of the nurse or being with is "turning one's attention toward the patient, being aware of and open to the here and now shared situation, and communicating one's availability" (p. 14). Each person is a totality of his or her choices. The nurse engages with the one nursed to increase the possibilities of making responsible choices (p. 16).

Humanistic nursing is defined as "a nurturing response of one person to another in need it aims at the development of human potential, at well-being and more-being" (p. 14). As such, both the nurse and the person nursed are affected. Humanistic nursing is the expression of the authentic commitment of nurturing human potential lived out through an active presence with the whole being of the nurse (p. 15). While this authentic presence may not be lived or experienced in all encounters, "moments of genuine presence in the nurse–patient situation will attest to their reality and to the fact that these beautiful moments give meaning to nursing" (p. 15). The humanistic nurse acknowledges freedom and choice and presents opportunities for the one nursed to exercise this freedom.

The framework for nursing is the nursing situation, the space between the nurse and the one nursed. Paterson and Zderad define the nursing situation as a "particular kind of human situation in which the interhuman relating is purposely directed toward nurturing the well-being or more-being of a person with perceived needs related to the health-illness quality of living" (p. 18). What is explored within this nursing situation follows: the participants (persons and nurse), meeting (being-becoming), the goal (well-being and more-being), and the intersubjective transaction (being with and doing with) (p. 18). Within the nursing situation, the lived experience of both the patient and the nurse and the development of their full human potential are explored. The concepts in Paterson and Zderad's theory of humanistic nursing such as call and response, the nursing situation, intersubjectivity, authentic presence, more-being and well-being, and being with and doing for were foundational to Boykin and Schoenhofer, Watson's, and Swanson's theories of caring.

Chapter 9: Sister Simone Roach's (1987/2002) book is a treatise on caring in nursing. We selected Chapter 3 on selection of caring attributes to include in this anthology because in it she elaborates the "Six Cs" as the essential attributes of caring. These can offer a simple mnemonic that can assist novices in remembering these attributes as they integrate them into their practice in nursing. The Six Cs are compassion, competence, conscience, confidence, commitment, and comportment. Roach defines compassion as "a way of living born out of an awareness of one's relationship to all living creatures" (p. 50). The Latin origin of the word means to suffer with. Compassion involves being moved to action from being able to imagine the other's experience as one's own. "Compassion is a relationship, lived in solidarity with others, sharing their joys, sorrows, pain and accomplishments" (p. 51). Roach draws from a variety of scholars including Henri Nouwen and Matthew Fox, theologians, to grasp the deep spiritual essence of compassion. Competence is defined by Roach as "the state of having the knowledge, judgment, skills, energy, experience and motivation required to respond adequately to the demands of one's professional responsibilities" (p. 54). She says that "while competence without compassion can be brutal and inhumane, compassion without competence may be no more than a meaningless, if not

harmful, intrusion into the life of a person or persons needing help" (p. 54). She refers to the importance of practicing competently with an awareness of power differentials and protecting the dignity and needs of patients. Confidence is "the quality that fosters trusting relationships" (p. 56). Roach emphasizes the importance of establishing trust in the nurse–person relationship. This trust is grounded in nursing's professional codes of ethics, because it is the foundation for fidelity and mutual respect without paternalism. Conscience can be understood as the "morally sensitive self attuned to values" (p. 58). Roach refers to it as the sacred core of self and the center of personal integrity, and she states that conscience grows out of the experience of valuing self and others (p. 61). The fifth C is commitment, and it is defined as "complex affective response characterized by a convergence between one's desires and one's obligations, and by a deliberate choice to act in accordance with them" (p. 62). The final C is comportment or "meaning bearing, demeanor or to be in agreement or harmony with" (p. 64). Roach is using comportment to reflect dress and language that carries message and meaning to those with whom one relates. Comportment means that caring is reflected in one's presentation of self to others. These Six Cs provide a helpful framework for describing professional caring in nursing practice.

Chapter 10: In 1988, Watson's classic paper presented her evolving theory of human caring that incorporated elements of the unitary worldview, Gadow's (1987) preservation of subjectivity, metaphysical and transcendent dimensions reflected through aesthetics, and the holographic and extended science metaphor. She begins by introducing the idea that a new model in health care is needed, one in which caring supersedes curing in importance. In light of the prevalence of chronic disease, understanding caring and its relationship to health and healing becomes more critical. The health care system is in need of reform to reflect the caring values.

In the late 1980s, Sarter identified four contemporary nursing theories that were redefining nursing (Rogers' Science of Unitary Human Beings, Parse's theory of man–living–health, Newman's theory of health as expanding consciousness, and Watson's theory of human caring). Concepts of process, evolution of consciousness, self-transcendence, open systems, harmony, relativity of space-time, pattern, and holism were common across these theories. Gadow (1987) referred to caring as a moral ideal, an end in itself rather than a means to an end. Gadow (1985) stated that when human dignity is diminished, the patient is no longer the center of his or her own experience. When nurses reduce others to the moral status of objects, they likewise objectify themselves, becoming less human (Watson, 1988, p. 176).

Watson describes the metaphysical and transcendent dimensions of human caring theory. The energetic qualities of human relating and the caring consciousness of the nurse are reflected in a poem called "Midwife" written by Marilyn Krysl, who was commissioned by Watson as Dean of the University of Colorado School of Nursing, to capture the majesty and mystery of nursing in poetry. Watson includes holographic principles to represent the nature of caring–healing: the whole of caring–healing consciousness is contained in a single caring moment, the one caring and the one cared for are interconnected to others and to the Universe, the caring consciousness of the nurse is communicated to the one cared for, and caring–healing consciousness is spatially and temporally extended and is dominant over illness (Watson, 1988, p. 179).

The new or extended science views affected Watson's human caring theory and corresponding with the ancient wisdom of Hildegard of Bingen. The physical resides in the spiritual field or the body resides in consciousness. The metaphysical affects the physical rather than the physical creating or containing the spiritual.

Chapter 11: Katie Eriksson is a caring scholar from Finland who developed a theory of caring for the suffering human being. In this article, she is calling for a more humanistic caring science that authentically reflects its ontological core. From a hermeneutic stance, understanding is primary, reflecting a new key in caring science. This notion of hermeneutics is more than methodology; it is a conception of science in which theory is open and co-created through participation and interpretation. In this way, "understanding, interpretation and application is not method, but substance" (Eriksson, 2001, p. 62).

Eight basic assumptions of Eriksson's (2001) theory are presented as follows: (1) the human being is an entity of body, soul, and spirit; (2) the human being is a religious being, but all have not recognized this dimension; (3) the human being is holy, and human dignity means accepting the obligation of serving with love and existing for the sake of others; (4) health is movement in becoming, being and doing, and striving for integrity and holiness, which is compatible with bearable suffering; (5) the basic category of caring is suffering; (6) the basic motive of caring is the caritas motive; (7) caring implies alleviating suffering in charity, love, faith, and hope, and that natural caring is expressed through tending, playing, and teaching in a sustained relationship; and (8) caring relationship forms the meaningful context of caring and derives its origin from the ethos of love, responsibility, and sacrifice that is a caritative ethic (p. 62).

"Compassion and love form the caritas motive, the basic motive of caring. The major idea of caring is to alleviate suffering and to preserve and safeguard human life" (Eriksson, 2001, p. 62). The deepest ethical motive is to respect the dignity of the person (p. 63). Suffering can be alleviated in a responsible relationship in which there is a desire to do good (p. 63). Eriksson draws from Levinas (1988) in asserting the postulate that in caring science, ethics precedes ontology, or being in relationship is primary to being. When this is considered, responsibility to the relationship or ethics is more fundamental than existence itself. Eriksson describes possible paths to the development of caring science as autonomous, a medical science influenced by caring, or an interdisciplinary science.

Chapter 12: Sigridur Halldorsdottir's (1991) article classifies five modes of being with another based on a continuum of caring. The classification came from an analysis of the data from two studies of patients' and students' descriptions of caring and uncaring encounters. The five modes of being are life destroying or biocidic, life restraining or biostatic, life neutral or biopassive, life sustaining or bioactive, and life giving or biogenic.

The biocidic mode is the most inhuman and is characterized by abuse, threats, manipulation, coercion, aggression, humiliation, infantilization, depersonalization, or dominance (Halldorsdottir, 1991, p. 39). The person receiving this treatment experiences initial disbelief, followed by anger that grows into despair and helplessness. The recipient begins to lose identity and feels that he has no value. This leads to vulnerability and can negatively impact well-being. The one engaging in this mode of being is hardened and cold, without regard for justice and suffering of the other.

The biostatic or life-restraining mode of being is being insensitive or indifferent to the other. It can be imposing will or attempting to control the other, and may appear as blaming, accusing, or fault finding. The patient experiences the nurse as insensitive and feels like a nuisance, that he is bothering the nurse. The nurse practicing from this mode objectifies the patient. This results

in feelings of disease or discouragement (Halldorsdottir, 1991, p. 41).

The biopassive or life-neutral mode of being is a detachment from the other. There is no connection, and while there is no destructive behavior, there is no presence at all. The patient is left with a sense of loneliness and experiences a sense of perceived apathy. The nurse may appear to be absentminded, overwhelmed, tired, or dissatisfied with her job.

In the life-sustaining or bioactive mode of being there is benevolence, good will, kindness, and concern from the nurse. The nurse is engaged with the patient, respects, and protects him. The patient feels secure and safe with this mode of being, and the patient's health and well-being are positively affected.

The final mode of being is biogenic or life giving. Here, the nurse is truly present to the other, connecting subject-to-subject. There is an acknowledgment of personhood and the nurse is truly invested in the well-being of the other. This is a healing relationship in which the nurse and the person meet as partners. The patient experiences a sense of optimism, appreciation, encouragement, and reassurance. The person feels cared for and this decreases anxiety and increases a sense of well-being. There is a flow of divine energy from the nurse to the person (Halldorsdottir, 1991, p. 46).

Halldorsdottir's chapter is imbued with spiritual references including a lovely poem called "One Family."

Chapter 13: Kristen Swanson's (1991) middle range theory of caring was developed inductively through three phenomenological studies in perinatal contexts. In this chapter, she introduces the theory through identifying the five caring processes, dimensions of each of these processes, and a definition of caring. Swanson supports the caring processes with excerpts from the three studies as follows: a study of women who had miscarried; a study of care providers in the newborn intensive care nursery; and a study of young mothers who received a public health intervention.

The five caring processes that were common across these studies were knowing, being with, doing for, enabling, and maintaining belief. Knowing was defined as "striving to understand an event as it has meaning in the life of the other" (p. 163). It includes dimensions of avoiding assumptions about the other, centering on the one cared for, assessing, seeking cues, and engaging the self of both. Being with is "being emotionally present to the other" (p. 163). It includes the dimensions of being there, conveying ability, sharing feelings, and not burdening. Doing for is fulfilling the needs of the one cared for through direct ministrations. The dimensions of doing for include comforting, anticipating, performing competently/skillfully, protecting, and preserving dignity. Enabling is nurturing the ability of the other to carry out essential role-related activities. The dimensions of enabling are informing/explaining, supporting/allowing, focusing, generating alternatives/thinking it through, and validating/giving feedback. Maintaining belief is "sustaining faith in the other's capacity to get through an event or transition and face a future with meaning" (p. 165). The dimensions of maintaining belief are believing in/holding in esteem, maintaining a hope-filled attitude, offering realistic optimism, and going the distance. Swanson defines caring as "a nurturing way of relating to a valued other toward whom one feels a personal sense of commitment and responsibility" (p. 165).

Chapter 14: The first two chapters of Boykin and Schoenhofer's (1993) book are included. The first chapter provides the foundation for the general theory of Nursing as Caring. The second chapter elaborates the theory itself. The major assumptions of the theory are persons are caring by virtue of their humanness;

persons are caring, moment to moment; persons are whole or complete in the moment; personhood is a process of living grounded in caring; personhood is enhanced through participating in nurturing relationships with caring others; and nursing is both a discipline and a profession (p. 3). Boykin and Schoenhofer assert that all persons are caring and they grow in their capacity for caring. While not all acts are perceived or experienced as caring, the person acting is inherently caring. Boykin and Schoenhofer draw from Mayeroff, Roach, Watson, Gadow, and Parse in developing the fundamentals of Nursing as Caring. The commitment to know self and other as caring persons is foundational. As one comes to know self as caring, he or she strives to express caring more perfectly. Persons live caring and in relationships there are opportunities to nurture the expression of caring for self and other. The wholeness (fullness of being) of persons is present in the moment (p. 9). "Here, valuing and respecting each person's beauty, worth and uniqueness is lived as one seeks to understand fully the meaning of values, choices, and priority systems through which values are expressed" (p. 9). Nursing is both discipline and profession. It is a field of knowledge and a service to humankind. As a human science, multiple ways of knowing are used to understand nursing phenomena.

The nursing situation is the focus of the second chapter of the book. Nursing is discovered within the context of the nursing situation. Nursing focuses on nurturing the growth of persons living and growing in caring (Boykin & Schoenhofer, 1993, p. 22). The nurse enters into a relationship with the goal of coming to know the other as caring. The nurse listens for the call for nursing and seeks through direct invitation to understand what matters most to the person in the moment. This structures the call for nursing. The nurse responds by nurturing the growth of the other in living caring.

The nursing situation is "the shared lived experience in which the caring between the nurse and nursed enhances personhood" (p. 24). Caring is the authentic and intentional presence of the nurse with another where the nurse seeks to know the other, to respond to the call for nursing in which the other is supported, sustained or strengthened in living and growing in caring (p. 25).

Chapter 15: On the 10th anniversary of *Nursing Science Quarterly*, in 1997, Jean Watson revisited the roots and evolution of her philosophy and theory of human caring and looked to its future development. Watson described her motivation for writing her first book as trying to differentiate nursing from the biomedical science model and to offer an alternative based on the values of personhood, life, health, and healing. She credits the influences of phenomenological psychology and philosophy, the existential work of Yalom, Peplau's interpersonal theory of nursing, and philosophers such as Kierkegaard, Whitehead, de Chardin, Sartre, and Gadow. Watson refers to the 10 CFs as a structure that reflected spiritual, aesthetic, and humanitarian values as the core of nursing. She conceptualized the CFs as the core while the medico-technological work of nursing is the trim. In 1988, Watson began to incorporate concepts related to the unitary-transformative paradigm and in 1997, she advanced the postmodern turn in nursing.

As she reflected on the future of human caring theory, Watson (1997) emphasized the importance of ontological caring competencies and advanced caring–healing modalities, which are the postmodern form of the Nightingale tradition (p. 50). The ontological caring competencies reflect the expanding consciousness of the nurse including intentionality, presence, and the manifestation of mind-body-spirit. "Practices such as centering, meditation, breath work, yoga, prayer, connections with nature and other forms of daily contemplation are essential to living the theory of human caring" (p. 51). Another prospective for the theory is the evolution of caring as a discipline in its own right. The Center for Human Caring at the University of Colorado was a model developed to be a laboratory to advance human caring theory and the values and vision surrounding it. The Denver Nursing Project in Human Caring was an example of a nursing center founded on Watson's caring theory. Finally, Watson calls for a redefinition of nursing guided by a caring–healing–health model that advances nursing qua nursing as a discipline (Watson, 1997, p. 52).

Chapter 16: Thirty years after the publication of her first edition of this book, Jean Watson has preserved the classic elements of her 1979 book and transformed them to reflect her most recent thinking. She begins this new edition with an overview (Watson, 2008) that chronicles the evolution of Watson's philosophy and theory over 30 years. In a personal way, she invites the reader into understanding the inner questions and influences that motivated the development of her life's work. She explains that this motivation came from a commitment to the mission of nursing and to its covenant with the society to preserve human dignity, humanity, and wholeness (p. 2).

Watson summarizes her primary theoretical books: *Nursing: The Philosophy and Science of Caring* (Watson, 1979), *Nursing: Human Science and Human Care: A Theory of Nursing* (Watson, 1985), *Postmodern Nursing* (Watson, 1999), and *Caring Science as Sacred Science* (Watson, 2005). In the first book, Watson (1979) contrasts caring from curing through identifying and elaborating the 10 CFs. These factors are the essential aspects of caring that differentiate professional nursing from a medico-technological practice. In the second book, Watson (1985) enters the transpersonal realm with greater emphasis on the caring occasion or the caring moment, experiences of the art of transpersonal caring. In this book, she articulates her tenets that include human freedom, holism, aesthetic ways of knowing, an ontology of time and space, and a human science perspective. In *Postmodern Nursing*, Watson (1999) more deeply explores the unity of the mind–body–spirit field and its relationship to healing. She embraces caring consciousness and the importance of the spiritual evolution of the practitioner. In her most recent theoretical work, Watson (2005) identifies three assumptions as follows: the infinity of the Human Spirit and evolving universe, the ancient and emerging cosmology of a unity consciousness of relatedness of All, the ontological ethic of Belonging before our Separate Being (Levinas, 1969), facing and deepening our humanity (Levinas, 1969), the ethical demand of responsibility for other's life, and the relationship of intentions, thoughts, and consciousness to the transpersonal field (p. 9).

Chapter 2 is included in this volume because it illustrates the primary difference between the 1979 and 2008 editions of *Nursing: The Philosophy and Science of Caring*, the transformation of CFs to caritas processes (CP). The core aspects of Watson's theory of human caring are relational caring as ethical–moral–philosophical values-guided foundation; caring core: 10 CP; transpersonal caring moment-caring field; caring as consciousness—energy, intentionality, and presence; and caring–healing modalities (p. 30). A table is presented that contrasts the CFs and CP. CP reflected the connection between caring and love (p. 31). Watson lists the core principles/practices from carative to caritas as follows: practice of loving-kindness and equanimity, authentic presence: enabling deep belief

of other, cultivation of one's own spiritual practice—beyond ego, "being" the caring–healing environment, and allowing for miracles (p. 34). The caritas nurse is one who lives the CP "working from a human-to-human connection—working from an open, intelligent heart center rather than the ego center" (p. 35). This must be cultivated through some daily practice.

REFERENCES

Boykin, A., & Schoenhofer, S. (1993). *Nursing as caring: A model for transforming practice* (pp. 3–30). New York, NY: National League for Nursing.

Eriksson, K. (2001). Caring science in a new key. *Nursing Science Quarterly, 15*(1), 61–65.

Halldorsdottir, S. (1991). Five basic mode of being with another. In D. A. Gaut & M. Leininger (Eds.), *Caring: The compassionate healer* (pp. 37–49). New York, NY: National League for Nursing.

Leininger, M. (1978). The phenomenon of caring: Importance, research questions and theoretical considerations. In M. Leininger (Ed.), *Caring: An essential human need: Proceedings of the three national caring conferences* (1988, Foreword, pp. 3–15). Detroit, MI: Wayne State University Press.

Paterson, J. G., & Zderad, L. T. (1988). *Humanistic nursing* (pp. 11–20). New York, NY: NLN Publishing. (Original work published 1976)

Roach, M. S. (2002). *Caring, the human mode of being: A blueprint for the health professions.* (pp. 41–66). Ottawa, Ontario: CHA Press. (Original work published 1987)

Swanson, K. M. (1991). Empirical development of a middle range theory of caring. *Nursing Research, 40*(3), 161–166.

Watson, J. (1979). *The philosophy and science of caring* (pp. 1–21). Boston, MA: Little, Brown & Company.

Watson, J. (1997). The theory of human caring: Retrospective and prospective. *Nursing Science Quarterly, 10*(1), 49–52.

Watson, J. (2008). *The philosophy and science of caring* (Rev ed.). Boulder, CO: University Press of Colorado.

6

Caring—An Essential Human Need

Proceedings of Three National Caring Conferences

Madeleine M. Leininger

A series of interesting historical events led to the development of the National Caring Conferences of which this proceeding contains the first three annual sessions. During the 1976 American Nurses Convention in New Jersey, Dr. Jody Glittenberg and I presented a program on the general subject of caring as the essence of nursing. We found that many nurses in attendance were enthusiastic and eager to address the concept of caring as important to nursing. In subsequent communications, these nurses stated: "Isn't it strange that I have attended these ANA conventions for many years, but this is the *first* time I have heard nurses talk directly about caring as the essence of nursing. It seems that we have talked about everything else but caring attitudes and activities." Another recent graduate said, "This is the first time I have ever heard nurses talk about caring or care as related to nursing care. I had nothing like these concepts in my nursing program, and yet they make sense and seem so logical and essential to nursing. In our classes we were taught about curing medical diseases, understanding medical diagnostic techniques, and everything but caring. Thank you for putting caring into nursing care." These and other comments reaffirmed my belief that nurses would focus on caring and its importance in giving nursing care to people if they had some substantive concepts about caring. The nursing students seemed eager to learn about caring if faculty would address the subject.

My early work on cross-cultural caring done in the Eastern Highlands of New Guinea in 1960–1962 was the first comparative study focused (in part) on caring phenomenon. This work made me realize the paucity of knowledge about caring and the limited research on the subject. Since then, I have been involved in the study of cultures regarding caring and social structure, and I saw the need for the National Caring Conferences for nurses and others interested in caring.

Another major factor that led to the National Caring Conferences and the study of the caring phenomenon was the highly positive response of nursing students to special lectures and seminars on caring I had given over the last 16 years while teaching at the Universities of Colorado, Washington, and Utah. These students seemed to come alive whenever caring ideas, theories, or research areas were discussed with them, and especially from a cross-cultural perspective. But with the

From Leininger, M. M. (1988). *Caring: An essential human need* (Foreword). Detroit, MI: Wayne State University Press. Permission to reprint granted by Wayne State University Press.

limited articles and research studies on caring and its relationship to nursing, the students had a difficult time sustaining their interest; and only a few faculties would discuss caring as well, as most of them concentrated only on medical diseases and curing. Therefore, care was the unknown phenomenon that needed to be explicated, analyzed, and used in nursing care as the distinct essence and unifying focus for the nursing profession.

When plans began to take shape for the National Caring Conferences, I was pleased that several nurse leaders such as Em Bevis, Jean Watson, Marilyn Ray, and another colleague, Ann Hyde, were eager for in-depth exchanges on the subject. These colleagues became active supporters for the National Caring Conferences that began in 1978. Thus, several important historical events contributed to my initial work and leadership to make caring a central focus of nursing research and practice, and to establish National Caring Conferences in this country and abroad.

Encouragingly, there are plans to continue with these yearly national conferences in the future and to build upon the previous conferences. The plan is to hold the national conferences in different places in the United States to stimulate national interest in theoretical, clinical, and research studies related to caring and nursing care. The first three conferences were held at the University of Utah in Salt Lake City. They were of high caliber and had participants with multidisciplinary interests, but predominantly nursing and anthropological backgrounds. These colleagues were genuinely interested in advancing ideas on the theory of and in systematically studying caring as well as identifying therapeutic caring practices. Unfortunately, the number of nurses who have conducted studies focused specifically on components or phenomena of caring are few; and so the research and theory will remain a major emphasis for the national conferences in the future.

Essentially, the national conferences have been directed toward these major goals:

1. Identification of major philosophical, epistemological, and professional dimensions of caring to advance the body of knowledge that constitutes nursing and to help other disciplines use caring knowledge in human relationships.
2. Explication of the nature, scope, functions, and structure of care and its relationship to nursing care.
3. Explication of the major components, processes, and patterns of care or caring in relationship to nursing care from a transcultural nursing perspective.
4. Stimulation of nurses and others to systematically investigate care and caring and to share their findings with other interested colleagues.

Unlike many national meetings in nursing, these conferences were in-depth "think-tank" theory, and research sharing sessions were designed to explore scholarly ideas about caring. The theoretical, research, and clinical aspects of caring have been a central focus of each conference. The participants have met this challenge and remain committed to advance a body of knowledge in nursing about caring. Social scientists and key nurse leaders served as gadflies to sharpen the thinking of the group and to advance ideas beyond local ethnocentric viewpoints. Many nurses who had already participated in the past seven National Transcultural Nursing Conferences were among the most active discussants, and they could use the cross-cultural content for the debates and to explicate caring ideas. This analytical approach to explicate theoretical ideas on caring was crucial to advance ideas about care phenomena. Thus, the participants questioned, theorized, and predicted outcomes of caring for nurses, and for use by other disciplines interested in caring. Unfortunately, many of the productive discussions about caring could not be included in this chapter, but these original papers remain as historical, theoretical, research, and practice documents for future researchers to build upon.

As a consequence of the three National Caring Conferences, there is a growing cadre of nurse scholars and other colleagues who are eager to share, learn, refine, and develop caring content for nursing and for other multidisciplinary uses. The multidisciplinary exchanges were an important outcome of the conferences. For many nurses, it was their "scholarship food." Several nurses said to me: "These conferences are unquestionably helping me develop my professional knowledge and interests." Most importantly, the following trends have clearly become evident from the national conferences:

1. There is definitely more interest and more writings by nurses on the subject of care and caring than in the past, and from all indications, one can predict that more nurses will be writing and doing research on caring in the future.
2. There are several students in master and doctoral programs in nursing eager to study caring behaviors, processes, and outcomes if they can find faculty knowledgeable enough to guide their work on caring. These students seem avid to shift their research from the study of medical diseases, symptoms, and curing to the study of various aspects of caring and its relationship to nursing care.
3. The importance of caring as the heart or central and unifying focus of nursing is *now* being mentioned by nursing leaders at national meetings. Prior to the mid-1970s, there had been virtually no specific focus on caring phenomena and its relationship to nursing care. Instead, topics at most national meetings were about nurse shortages, unions, economic welfare, legislation, and entry into professional practice and related concerns. There

was nothing about the sources of caring knowledge and how caring might distinguish nursing from other disciplines.
4. More nursing faculties are now trying to teach ideas about caring phenomena and to encourage research studies on this subject.
5. Other health disciplines, such as physicians, psychologists, and anthropologists, are also becoming interested in caring behaviors and activities.

In general, there is a cultural movement focusing on caring phenomena in nursing, which is diffusing within and outside the discipline. This movement reflects a new (or renewed) interest in the unknown dimension of care and its relationship to nursing care. It is making us realize how much there is yet to learn about care and caring. Likewise, business and public establishments are speaking about caring services. But more specific to nursing, there is a critical need to establish caring as our *central and unique focus of the discipline*. Scientific and humanistic caring knowledge with related clinical skills could greatly advance the profession and help the public more fully understand nurses' contributions to society. The original content in this book, plus other writings and research on the subject of caring, should help nurses to value and know the concept of caring. It should stimulate nurses to make caring the central and dominant domain of nursing and to pursue further research on caring. It should help to clarify and reduce current ambiguities about such frequently heard questions from students and professional nurses as, "What is nursing?" "What is nursing about?" "How is nursing different from medicine?" In time, I hope we will be able to establish a scientific and humanistic body of knowledge with practices related to generic caring and nursing care which will be nursing's distinctive contribution to society.

As the initiator and chairwoman of these National Caring Conferences, it has been most encouraging to see the above developments transpire, and especially to see nurses excited to discuss and focus on the concept of caring. Already these conferences are having an influence upon nursing leaders, students, and other colleagues. Since the National Caring and Transcultural Nursing Conferences have been initiated during the last decade, leadership is now needed to help nurses learn more about caring and nursing care phenomena. Furthermore, the nursing profession should sponsor and financially support future national and international conferences on caring. Such local, regional, and national conferences are essential to explicate cultural, intellectual, and clinical ideas on caring and nursing care dimensions. The motto of "Caring is the essence of nursing and the unique and unifying focus of the profession" and the logo should serve as a key referent and symbolic guides for the future. The cross-cultural aspects of caring will be a goal for transcultural nurse specialists who are prepared in anthropology and nursing through graduate study.

In summary, I believe that an enlightened era in nursing has occurred in which some highly promising and new areas of research, teaching, and practice have been launched related to caring and nursing care. Caring, I believe, is the sine qua non of the nursing profession, which can make nursing a respected, recognized, and distinct discipline. Understanding scientific and humanistic caring knowledge with clinical skills has the great potential to help individuals know about natural processes and outcomes of human caring, growth, helping processes, and survival. Will the nursing profession take the lead in the pursuit of the study of caring in its fullest dimensions to improve the health and well-being of humans? I hope so.

THE PHENOMENON OF CARING: IMPORTANCE, RESEARCH QUESTIONS, AND THEORETICAL CONSIDERATIONS*

In recent years, a few nurse researchers have directed their work toward theories, models, and research methods to explicate the body of knowledge relevant to the discipline of nursing. Such intellectual activities have been essential and encouraging in order to identify the nature, essence, and domains of inquiry that will help to advance nursing and to distinguish the field from other academic and professional disciplines. Much more rigorous work is needed by nurse scholars to achieve this important goal in nursing.

In the identification of domains of inquiry in nursing, it is an interesting and curious fact that there has been very limited systematic and rigorous study regarding the nature and phenomenon of caring by nurse researchers. Although nurses have linguistically said that they *give care* and they talk about nursing care activities, still there has been virtually no systematic investigation of the epistemological, philosophical, linguistic, social, and cultural aspects of caring, and the relationship of care to professional nursing care theory and practice. Furthermore, care per se is seldom defined in nursing, and yet it is used regularly as the suffix to nursing.

The purpose of this chapter, as introduction to the first National Caring Conference, is to explore some general philosophical, linguistic, cultural, and professional viewpoints, assumptions, questions, and theoretical considerations about caring as the central and unifying domain of inquiry for nursing as a discipline and for professional practices. Studying caring as an area for humanistic and scientific nursing care will also be discussed.

*Leininger, M. M. (1988). *Caring: An essential human need.* (chapter 1, pp. 3–15). Detroit, MI: Wayne State University Press. Permission granted by Wayne State University Press.

Potential of Caring as a Central and Unifying Domain for Nursing

It has long been the author's position *that caring is the central and unifying domain for the body of knowledge and practices in nursing*, and a systematic investigation of caring could advance the discipline of nursing and ultimately provide better nursing care to people.[1] I hold that an in-depth knowledge of caring from diverse perspectives and from a historical, philosophical, and epistemological study will enable nurses and other caregivers to know the full nature of care or caring behaviors, patterns, and processes. Most importantly, as nursing moves toward full disciplinary status, it will be essential for nurses to know the nature, scope, and distinguishing features that characterize nursing from other health disciplines. I hold that caring behavior and practices *uniquely* distinguish nursing from the contributions of other disciplines. Thus, the critical and essential challenge is for nurses to systematically and rigorously explicate and analyze caring phenomena in depth and breadth, and from a cross-cultural viewpoint.

The importance of caring to the nursing profession and to humanity appears evident, but there are many questions yet to be answered:

1. What is the essential nature of care/caring?
2. How is caring expressed among different cultures in the world?
3. What are the philosophical and epistemological arguments for caring and nursing in human cultures?
4. What is the cultural history of caring in nursing from an anthropological viewpoint?
5. What are the essential generic elements of caring?
6. What is the difference between professional and nonprofessional caring attributes, processes, and patterns?
7. What characterizes caring patterns and processes in nursing from other disciplines?
8. What are the cross-cultural differences in human caring and professional caring?
9. What does caring for strangers mean?
10. What is the relationship of care to nursing care?
11. What are the categories of care and nursing care?
12. What theories about care or caring offer promise to know caring phenomena and its fullest dimensions? and
13. Why has nursing failed to study the epistemological, philosophical, and cultural aspects of caring as generic to nursing?

When answers to these and other questions become known, a *body of caring science* will evolve to advance nursing knowledge and other professional aspects about care behaviors and processes in nursing.

Undoubtedly, caring has long been expressed by human cultures throughout the history of humankind. Care, I believe, was *essential* for human growth, development, and survival. This anthropological and nursing position makes one pause to consider the importance and significance of caring for the human race and for the life ways of homo sapiens as a species. If this major assumption can be investigated, then nurses and others should give more attention to this phenomenon. Such research would be especially pertinent to nursing as a profession since they have laid claim to nursing care for many decades. Caring appears to be an extremely important and generic construct in human services. It appears to be at the heart of all health care services. It is the largely unknown ingredient for helping humankind in wellness, illness, and stressful situations. Why then it has so little attention been given to caring by humanistically oriented scientists and caregivers? This question is an intriguing one that has yet to be answered, and one which deserves more thought than it has received in the past. It is a question that could lead to many fascinating research lines of inquiry about human behavior in health and illness states.

Worldview: An Anthropological Approach to Study Care and Caring

During the past decade, I have been active in designing and conceptualizing ways to study caring phenomenon from both nursing and anthropological perspectives.[1,2] The need exists for a broad framework for cross-cultural differences and similarities about patterns, processes, and behaviors related to care and caring. At the same time, a need exists to explore in-depth the multiple aspects of caring from an anthropological viewpoint, including the cultural, linguistic, and professional practices of nursing as a caring profession. To meet these expectations, I have used an ethnoscientific approach to study the perceptions, cognitions, and actions of a designated group of nurses and clients in different cultures (Leininger, 1964–1981). The ethnonursing context and practices of caring were also studied. It was the worldview of the informants that has been extremely helpful to my investigation of caring phenomenon for this view supports and is closely related to ethnocaring and ethnonursing.

It was Redfield who introduced the term, "worldview" to social science many years ago. Worldview refers to the way individuals or cultures grow, perceive, and know their world about them.[3] This concept should be an integral part of *all* nursing practices, teaching, and research work. The worldview approach expects that the nurse would understand the world of the client, and to feel, know, and experience his or her world. The worldview means that one tries to get a broad gestalt of another person's lifeways or a cultural perspective of living. Using this approach, one constantly seeks for insight about many diverse aspects of human living, and yet looks at the unifying values and lifeways of an individual. Sensitivity and attention to the aspects of values and beliefs are important in seeing the worldview of another human being, as well as the context in which that individual lives.

In the use of the worldview and the ethnoscientific approach to caring, one focuses upon linguistic and daily features of caring from the individual's viewpoint as well as group cultural views about caring. Both the *similarities* and *differences* among individuals as they know, perceive, and experience caring are important. The humanistic and scientific aspects of caring are also identified when a worldview approach is used to study caring.

A worldview approach is essential to conceptualize paradigms, theories, and models related to holistic caring. Kuhn has discussed the role and importance of paradigms in the evolution of the body of knowledge of a discipline, and he challenges the belief that knowledge and scientific fields have developed through steady and slow increments of knowledge. He believes that science advances through a revolution in which concepts, theories, and research methods are overthrown by new paradigms that are accepted by the majority of scientists in that discipline.[4] It is my position that advances in knowledge occur both by *revolution* and *evolution*. Nurses must be aware of both processes to develop a body of knowledge about caring and nursing care phenomena. Diverse paradigms about caring are therefore important to revolutionize and to help evolve nursing—especially its distinctive features. Paradigms that move beyond local worldviews to cross-cultural paradigms of caring are essential in order to help nurses discover the universal and specific aspects of caring. Most importantly, worldview paradigms are needed to study the humanistic and scientific aspects of caring in broad dimensions.

Ambiguities About Caring

Vagueness and ambiguities about caring by nurses have been evident for many years. Nurses and other health professionals use the terms *care, caring, health care,* and *nursing care,* but there is virtually no scientific or humanistic knowledge base for these terms. Moreover, there is divergent professional and social usage about care. The effects or consequences of caring behaviors upon individuals, families, and communities by professional caregivers remain limitedly validated or understood to date. The terms *care, caring,* and *nursing care* are often used interchangeably among nurses, and frequently in a loose and nondiscriminatory manner in written and verbal discussion. Many divergent ideas are used by nurses when they talk about care in different settings and with different preparation. So when nursing care is used by nurses, ambiguities exist regarding the meaning, function, and therapeutic usage of nursing care.

Further consideration of the linguistic and functional usages of care reveals that *care* and *nursing care* are something which all nurses are expected to know and to use in practice. The generic use of care and its relationship to nursing care is also unclear in teaching and research. Concepts about caregivers and care recipients remain an area of inquiry, as well as care activities, patterns, and behaviors. Presently, in many schools of nursing, in-depth presentations on the nature of caring behaviors, processes, and patterns remain unexplored. Nursing faculty will speak of *nursing care,* and different ideas about medical care are often discussed. Furthermore, nursing curricula still contain far more content on medical diseases, conditions, and curative treatment regimes than nursing care or caring behaviors.[5] Searching for the essence, nature, expression, and function of caring and its relationship to nursing care remains a major area of investigation. Linguistic, philosophical, and professional usages of care or caring are open areas for teaching and research in nursing. I believe we should not continue to make linguistic usage and professional claims to care and nursing care with so little knowledge about the essential and generic nature of care. Diverse theories and conceptual frameworks (or paradigms) about care/caring would help to explicate caring and care. Again, why such limited attention to caring, when it is claimed by nursing and is of much interest to nurses? It is unfortunate that caring has not been a central theoretical and research area in nursing until very recently. Instead, there are research studies on topics such as time, motion, energy, adaptation, and other concepts. Concepts and theories related to caring appear essential to know and to link with ideas related to nursing care. Thus, it is time to focus on caring in research, teaching, and practice in order to bring credence and legitimacy to a major implied and claimed concept that has been used in nursing for more than 100 years.

Rationale for Studying Caring

To encourage nurse researchers and others to pursue caring research, several major reasons can be offered why this construct appears important to investigate.

First, the construct of **care** *appears critical to human growth, development, and survival for human beings for millions of years.* Caring appears to be the largely unknown ingredient for helping others under the threat of illness in a humanistic and scientific manner. From an anthropological viewpoint, I hold that caring must have been a mode of human action and relatedness from the beginning of humankind. Caring appears to be one of the most human acts and a quality for being human rather than animal-like in behavior. Unfortunately, anthropologists have not explicated caring as essential to human existence; and yet the need seems logical for human survival through the millennia.

One can assume that cultures depended upon care and caring through millions of years for human survival; however, the prehistory and historical aspects of caring have not been identified. How was caring expressed by cultural groups and among individuals? How was caring manifested in the prehistoric days when people lived in changing and precarious environments? What would constitute primitive caring and how would it differ from professional caring today?

I believe that caring was the *critical* and *important factor that* assisted homo sapiens through cultural evolution. I believe that caring was essential to growth and survival of the race amid a variety of stressful environmental changes. I believe that humanistic caring helped people to live and survive under most adverse and changing environments and in relation to changing economic, political, cultural, and social factors.

A second reason to study care is to explicate caregiver and care recipient roles in various living and survival contexts. Presently, we know little about caregiver and care recipient behaviors as well as the ways care is provided by different nurses and non-nurses in diverse cultures. Caregiving behaviors associated with health and illness must have been important in the prehistoric days as well as today to help people overcome trauma and illness states. Who were the early caregivers and how was care given? Have women always been the principal caregivers? How was care given when environmental catastrophies occurred, such as floods, fires, and hurricanes? In diverse societies, human caring modes must have been as significant in the past as they are today. Caring must also have linked people together in patterns of interdependency. One also wonders if caregivers had status in the past, and if not, why? What status or recognition is given to caregivers today? What historical means do we have to study caregiver and care recipient roles? How did caregiver behavior become culturally constituted with explicit

socialization processes in the distant past? These additional questions address important historical and epistemological aspects of care behavior and cultural patterns, and they offer ideas for future research studies.

A third reason for studying caring is to *preserve* and *maintain* this human attribute for current and future human cultures. Today, there are multiple forces that appear to be devaluing and demeaning human life such as the lack of respect for human lives through homocides and suicides. There is the depersonalization of humans with technological equipment. And there are multiple economic, political, and legal constraints that daily threaten humans and reflect a lack of human caring or concern for others. Evidence of war, feuds, violence, and legal threats are the other signs of the less-caring society in which we live. We need to buttress a caring lifeway to ourselves and others to preserve and maintain human societies. Caring processes, patterns, and expressions might well become extinct if we do not recognize caring and value it in our lives. Without caring, one could speculate that the human race could destroy itself. I believe that caring helps to bridge human relatedness, concern, and compassionate help to others. Human care appears to have existed through time and is universal to human existence and helping processes, and therefore, it must be preserved. With the increased use of technology, human caring appears less evident in health and human services, and health professionals such as those in the nursing profession could provide a renewed emphasis on human caring and make known caring attributes.

A fourth reason for studying caring is that since the beginning of modern professional nursing, the nursing profession has not systematically studied caring in relation to nursing care. Although Florence Nightingale used the term *care*, she never explicated, defined, or discussed its function. Her use of care was often noted in relation to helping people live or survive in their physical or natural environment. To Nightingale, care was related to cleanliness, fresh air, good food, rest, sleep, and exercise.[6] Good health care seemed synonymous with good health habits and a healthy environment. According to Nightingale, the goal or task of nursing is "to put the patient in the best condition for nature to act upon him."[7] Her ideas were primarily on environmental and physical care, especially when sick. These ideas were important for nursing and its evolution as a profession, but care per se was not defined.

Definition of Care/Caring

Since the days of Florence Nightingale, the word *care* has been used in nursing as a verb, as in *to be cared for, caring for others*, or *to manifest care* with concern, compassion, and interested in another human being. Care and caring appear to have multiple conceptualizations and characterizations. Although care has a common and recurrent usage by nurses, definitions of care are needed to include strangers who give care by comfort, alleviation of distress, and other human ways. Although definitions of *nursing care* can be found in the literature, there are few that define the *generic concept of care*. For example, in Henderson's work (frequently used by nurses), she speaks of nursing and implies care activities:[8]

> Nursing is primarily helping people (sick or well) in the performance of those activities contributing to health, or its recovery (or to a peaceful death) that they would perform unaided if they had the necessary strength, will, or knowledge.

For heuristic purposes, I define *care/caring* in a generic sense as those *assistive, supportive, or facilitative acts toward or for another individual or group* with evident or anticipated needs to ameliorate or improve a human condition or lifeway. I define *professional caring* as those cognitive and culturally learned action behaviors, techniques, processes, or patterns that enable (or help) an individual, family, or community to improve or maintain a favorable healthy condition or

lifeway. And finally, I define *professional nursing care* as *those cognitively learned humanistic and scientific modes of helping or enabling an individual, family, or community to receive personalized services* through specific culturally defined or ascribed modes of caring processes, techniques, and patterns to improve or maintain a favorable healthy condition for life or death.[9]

In the above definitions, one will note that the emphasis is on *helpful* and *enabling* activities of individuals, social, and community groups based on culturally defined, ascribed, or sanctioned modes of helping people. I believe that caring acts can be culturally identified through the beliefs, values, and practices of cultural groups. From a cross-cultural study of caring behaviors, one can then identify what caring acts, processes, and techniques are culturally specific, and those that are universal. Other theoretical and philosophical positions will be discussed later with the focus on discovering transcultural nursing care phenomenon.

In Mayeroff's work, he speaks about caring with some general attributes:[10]

> Caring is the antithesis of simply using the other person to satisfy one's needs. The meaning of caring I want to suggest is not to be confused with such meanings as wishing well, liking, comforting and maintaining, or simply having an interest in what happens to another. Also, it is not an isolated feeling or a momentary relationship, nor it is simply a matter of wanting to care for some person. Caring, as helping another grow and actualize himself, is a process, a way of relating to someone that involves *development*, in the same way that friendship can only emerge through mutual trust and a deepening and qualitative transformation of the relationship.

Rollo May also offered some ideas about care in his discussion about man living and relating to the world in which he lives:[11]

Care is the necessary source of eros, the source of human tenderness. . . . Care is given power by nature's sense of pain; if we do not care for ourselves we are hurt . . . .

In care one must by involvement with the objective fact, do something about the situation; one must make some decisions. This is where care brings love and will together . . . .

From cursory review of the philosophy and the social, biological, and health science literature, the terms *care* and *caring for others* are frequently used. Many diverse ideas are associated with care, such as being used analogously with love, tenderness, compassion, and empathy. Accordingly, in the dictionary, the verbs *care, caring,* and *cared* mean: to have an interest in, to be concerned for, to provide or look after, and to be disposed to help others.[12] One could then infer that *to not care* for someone would reflect indifference, antipathy, disregard for another, lack of attention, or no interest in helping another human being. Noncaring behaviors are of equal interest to study.

During the past decade, I have found in studying nearly 30 world cultures through interviews, structured questionnaire guides, literature sources, and direct observations that there are many concepts associated with care or caring. Intercultural variations clearly exist with no universal ethnoscience definition or social usage of care by cultural representatives. While the data are still under analysis and being checked for validation of what informants *said* with the *actual* cultural practices, the following constructs are associated closely with care/ caring (varying in cultural usage with respect to which terms are used in different cultures): support, tenderness, touch, compassion, empathy, stress alleviation, presence, loving acts, comfort, direct and indirect helping behaviors, enabling, facilitating, nurturance, succorance, surveillance, protection, restoration, instructive acts, coping, concern, interest in, trusting,

and need fulfillment.[9] With each of these constructs, there are many embedded ideas associated with the concepts of care or caring. And there are some constructs that may not be found in designated cultures. For example, the nurse as a caregiver is not permitted by cultural rules to touch a patient in the Yap culture. How would an Anglo-American nurse provide care to the Yap people in the Micronesian cultural area? Many extremely fascinating data are coming from my investigation, which should throw new light on old conceptualizations of nursing care and the need to use transcultural caring knowledge in culturally specific ways.

Some Assumptions and Beliefs About Human Caring

In pursuit of knowing the nature of humanistic and scientific caring, and based on my preliminary research findings, I have identified several assumptions to guide nurses' deliberations about caring. The following assumptions may challenge nurses to discover in depth the phenomenon of caring:

1. Human caring is a universal phenomenon, but the expressions, processes, and patterns vary among cultures.
2. Every nursing care situation has transcultural caring behaviors, needs, and implications.
3. Caring acts and processes are essential for human development, growth, and survival.
4. Caring should be considered the essence and unifying intellectual and practice dimension of professional nursing.
5. Caring has biophysical, psychological, cultural, social, and environmental dimensions that can be studied, and practices to provide holistic care to people.
6. Transcultural caring behaviors, forms, and processes have yet to be

verified from diverse cultures; when this body of knowledge is procured, it has the potential to revolutionize present-day nursing practices.

7. To provide therapeutic nursing care, the nurse should have knowledge of caring values, beliefs, and practices of the client(s).

8. Caring behaviors and functions vary with social structure features of any designed culture.

9. The identification of universal and non-universal folk and professional caring behaviors, beliefs, and practices will be important to advance the body of nursing knowledge.

10. Differences exist between the essence and essential features of caring and curing behaviors and processes.

11. There can be no curing without caring, but there may be caring without curing.

Some Theoretical Statements and Hypotheses About Caring

The following theoretical statements or hypotheses are offered to stimulate research studies on caring behaviors, processes, and patterns. A few nurses are already investigating aspects of these hypotheses.[9]

1. Intercultural differences in beliefs, values, and practices of caring would reflect differences in nursing care practices.

2. Self-care practices will be valued and practiced in cultures that value individualism and independence in social structure features, whereas group care practice will be valued and practiced in cultures where interdependency and high individualism are *not* espoused.

3. Congruence between caregiver and care recipient's behaviors and goals is important for therapeutic practices to occur.

4. The greater the differences between folk caring values and professional caring values, the greater the signs of cultural conflict and stresses between professional caregivers and non-professional care receivers.

5. Technological caring acts, techniques, and practices differ in cultures and have different outcomes for health and nursing care practices.

6. The greater the efforts of professional nurses to blend the folk caring practices with professional care practices, the greater the signs of clients' satisfactions.

7. The nurse as a professional caregiver may produce unfavorable stresses and conflicts with the client due to lack of knowledge about cultural beliefs, values, and practices of caring.

8. Symbolic forms of nursing care behaviors have referent meanings in different cultural groups and necessitate that nurses study the meaning and functions of symbols in cultures to give efficacious nursing care.

9. The greater the signs of technological caregiving, the less the signs of interpersonal care manifestations.

10. Caring behaviors and patterns are closely linked to social structure features.

A Conceptual Model for Studying Transcultural Nursing Care Theories and Practices

During this time, I have been investigating the definitions, nature, and scope of the care and caring, using an ethnoscientific approach (Leininger, 1964–1981). The study of the cultural usages, meanings, and functions of caring in different cultures appears closely related to the social structure and cultural beliefs of people. Essentially, my research is focused on explicating and, studying caring phenomenon from different cultural viewpoints. A body of ethnocaring knowledge is being sought. I am interested in how people perceive, know, and experience caring behaviors in different cultures so that nurses can use this knowledge in providing both cultural-specific or cultural-universal nursing care practices. *The ultimate goal is to improve health care to people.* Transcultural health care should become more manifest, along with the new generation of nursing care theories and practices.

To date, approximately 30 cultures have been studied by direct interviews, structured questionnaires, library data, and direct observations focused upon beliefs and practices related to caring. From these data, a taxonomy of caring constructs, theories, and hypotheses are being developed. The conceptual framework is given in Figure 6.1.[9] In the model, one can identify a dynamic process to cross-cultural caring phenomenon. It is a process model to show how the knowledge on caring is obtained and validated. On the left side of the model, Phase I, are the major sources from which I derived ethnocaring data that have been identified, namely, by doing an ethnography (or lifeways of the societies), studying the social structure features, cultural values, and in identifying the health-illness caring behaviors and practices in a designated culture. Phase I is followed by Phase II, which focuses upon the identification of the major enthnocaring constructs from data obtained from Phase I domains, and examples of these constructs are offered. Several subsets of ideas are found within each construct. These constructs have been prioritized and defined by the people. Phase III reflects the next step in ethnocare study by analyzing the data and developing theories that will be tested in subsequent research. The model also shows ways to recycle findings to check for reliability and validity of the data.

From the research work to date, there are several common principles or guidelines that have become evident and could be used to help nurses focus on and further refine caring behaviors and processes. They are as follows:

1. Caring behaviors and processes can be identified in cultures to help guide nursing care decisions and actions.
2. Caring behaviors appear closely related to the social structure features of designated cultures and can help to predict nursing care behaviors of the cultural groups.
3. Caring rituals may be therapeutic and non-therapeutic depending upon how closely the caregiver links activities with cultural values and beliefs.
4. Caring behaviors vary transculturally in priorities, expressions, and need satisfactions.
5. Westernized nurses tend to rely heavily on technological and psycho-physiological stress alleviation activities to help clients; whereas nurses in non-Westernized cultures tend to rely more frequently on non-technological and more sociocultural expressions of behaviors.
6. Caring behaviors appear more important than curing in recovery of clients, but receive less economic and social reward than curing by physicians.
7. Efficacious caring tends to be humanistically oriented and reflects professional care concepts of concern, compassion, stress alleviation, nurturance, comfort, and protection, and especially by female caregivers.
8. Caring behaviors have important symbolic referents that need to be identified and used in therapeutic care practices.
9. Caregiving and care receiving behaviors require signs of reciprocal behavior satisfactions for such activities to continue over time.
10. Professional nursing care values, beliefs, and practices tend to follow more medical and curing model attributes in the United States than caring attributes as perceived by the clients.

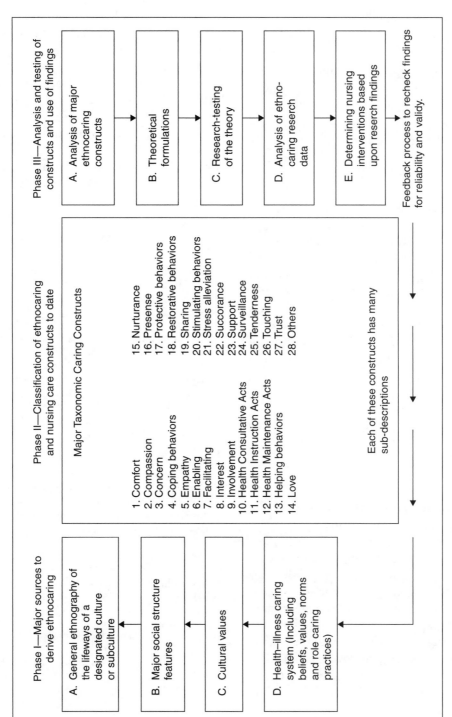

FIGURE 6.1

Leininger's conceptual and theory-generating model to study transcultural and ethnocaring constructs.

Note. The model was developed in 1968 and reflects revisions and additions since that time. (The ethnocaring definitions are not presented here.)

Data come from 30 cultures using a modified ethnoscience and ethnonursing research approach.

11. Self-care is gaining emphasis in the United States, but has less credence and relevance in other parts of the world—especially non-Western cultures—where other care is emphasized.

Such preliminary findings (and others yet to be identified) indicate the enormously rich data found in a cross-cultural focus on caring. Guides to help nurses and others give therapeutic care were obtained from such data. Knowledge of the values, beliefs, and practices of a culture regarding caring opens the door to culture-specific care and universal caring practices. The close interrelationships of care, culture, and social structure are clearly apparent from my cross-cultural work on caring behaviors, patterns, and processes. It appears essential that professional nurses know variations in cultural caring, and the ways caring is linked with specific value systems. Future and ongoing research on caring and its relationship to nursing care appears highly promising and encouraging. I believe a new breakthrough in nursing has occurred with the focus on caring and its relationship to nursing and health care practices. Nurses should build upon such research findings, and other theories and research studies of caring.

In summary, caring should be the central, critical, and unifying domain and focus for nursing care knowledge. The generic construct of caring is essential to explicate nursing. The possibilities for developing a scientific and humanistic body of nursing knowledge related to caring appear favorable. However, too many nurses are still following medicine and focusing on their medical model of diagnosing and curing largely physical illnesses, rather than on the caring

phenomenon. The transcultural nursing approach provides a highly promising mode for studying universal and non-universal aspects of caring in all areas of nursing for all cultures. This knowledge can then be linked to nursing care practices and to make essential changes for a humanistic and scientific body of caring knowledge. This contribution will not only serve nursing but also serve other disciplines and human groups. I believe we are on the threshold of some new discoveries in nursing that will make nursing's contribution visible, substantive, and distinctive in the near future.

REFERENCES

1. Leininger, M. (1977, February). Caring: The essence and central focus of nursing. *American Nurses' Foundation (Nursing Research Report)*, *12*(1), 2.
2. Leininger, M. (1976). Towards conceptualization of transcultural health care systems: Concepts and a model. In *Health care dimensions*. Philadelphia, PA: FA Davis.
3. Redfield, R. (1957). *The little community*. Chicago, IL: University of Chicago Press.
4. Kuhn, T. S. (1970). *The structure of scientific revolutions*. Chicago, IL: University of Chicago Press.
5. Leininger, M. Review of Large Sample of Baccalaureate and Master Degree Programs for NLN Board of Review from 1976–79.
6. Nightingale, F. (1969). *Notes on nursing*. New York, NY: Dover Publications.
7. Nightingale, F. (1964). *Notes on nursing: What it is and what it is not* (p. 3). Philadelphia, PA: B. Lippincott.
8. Henderson, V., & Nite, G. (1978). *Principles and practice of nursing* (6th ed.). New York, NY: Macmillan Publishing.
9. Leininger, M. (1978). *Transcultural nursing concepts, theories, and practices* (pp. 35–38, 39). New York, NY: John Wiley and Sons.
10. Mayeroff, M. (1971). *On caring* (p. 1). New York, NY: Harper & Row Publishers.
11. May, R. (1969). *Love and well* (pp. 286–288). New York, NY: Norton.
12. *Oxford English Dictionary*, p. 339.

QUESTIONS FOR REFLECTION

Baccalaureate

1. What does Dr. Leininger identify as the focus of the discipline of nursing? Does this adequately distinguish nursing from other disciplines?
2. According to Leininger, is touch a universal expression of caring? Why or why not?
3. Provide one example of how Leininger's principles or guidelines can be applied to the care of a patient.

Master's

1. What is the evidence for Leininger's principles and guidelines?
2. Using Leininger's framework, develop an evidence-based practice question using the Population-Intervention-Comparison or Control-Outcomes (PICO) framework.
3. Provide an example of the application of the principles of transcultural caring to your population of interest.

Doctoral

1. How did Leininger's experiences and background shape the development of her theory and research interests?
2. What are theoretical assumptions? What are the origins of Leininger's theoretical assumptions?
3. Select one of the hypotheses that Leininger identifies. How would you test this hypothesis through a research study?

7

Nursing: The Philosophy and Science of Caring

JEAN WATSON

NURSING AS THE SCIENCE OF CARING

In nursing education and practice, change is the order of the day. The goals of nursing education, the means of fulfilling them, and the bases for evaluating them depend almost exclusively on the goals of nursing practice. Even though educational goals may be as different as the students and teachers themselves, "one recurrent educational goal [that is stated] with some consistency is that of equipping the student with the necessary skills to live effectively and productively in the world of tomorrow."[1]

Nursing education was moved from the confines of the hospital to the university to establish nursing as a discipline and to give the nurse greater knowledge and understanding of human behavior. That foundation helps the nurse in caring for other people. A goal of many nursing programs is the pursuit it of self-actualization, as reported in Kramer and Reed's study.[2]

The aim of this curriculum is to educate individuals to be self-directive, to be able to think critically, to be able to realize their fullest potential.

The curriculum is designed to facilitate and create a climate for each student to fully pursue her own process of self-actualization and to foster it in others.

Nurse educators must prepare students to practice in conditions of constant change. At the same time, nurse educators emphasize preparation for future practice.

Therefore, the basic requirement for professional nursing is a liberal education, an education that has nothing—and everything—to do with a professional education. The liberal arts are the arts of communication and the arts of using the mind. They are indispensable to further learning, and they should help the student to pursue a lifelong self-education that is liberal and liberating.

The liberal arts are the bases of teaching people to think clearly and thoroughly—the bases of reading, writing, speaking, listening, and valuing.[3] In the past, it was held that learning was neutral in regard to values. That view is now being challenged. Educators, especially those in nursing, are again seriously concerned with the full range of human development, including the formation of moral and esthetic values.[4]

The liberal arts can give nursing education a timeless quality that is relevant regardless of the changes that occur. The

From Watson, J. (1985). *Nursing: The philosophy and science of caring* (pp. 1–20). Boulder, CO: University Press of Colorado. This is the second printing of this book. The book was first published in 1979. Permission to reprint to print and ebook formats, throughout the world, in all languages by University Press of Colorado. This permission applies only to print and ebook format for the first edition of *Caring in Nursing Classics* to be published by Springer Publishing Company.

liberal arts are the arts of becoming human and of relating to other people. The liberal arts and the humanities belong to the heart of higher education. They provide analytic skills and self understanding. Nursing needs to promote and maintain visions, perspectives, and values that allow for creative possibilities. Such a foundation makes the other kinds of scientific and professional knowledge lasting and significant.

In nursing, it is easy to fall prey to current trends and fads of education and practice. Nursing is becoming established as an academic discipline that requires a liberal arts education, as well as a scientific and professional education. It is, therefore, incumbent on the profession and the academic community to adhere to the purpose of a university education—to gain knowledge and understanding.[3] More energy is now expended in the acquisition of scientific knowledge than of understanding. Nursing tries to understand people and how they cope with health and illness.

Nursing covers an area of knowledge somewhere in the biophysical, behavioral, and social sciences and the humanities. It tries to understand how health and illness and human behavior are interrelated. Nursing education rarely concentrates on that level of understanding. In some ways, nursing schools are still technical, professional schools. Many teachers and schools state attempts to develop self-actualization. However, they end up hidden, primarily teaching specialized terminology, procedures, scientific principles, the basic content of behavior, pathophysiology, and the disease processes.

Teaching mostly the rules and procedures—the "trim"—of nursing does not lead to understanding people and how they cope with health and illness. Even if all the rules and procedures could be taught (they cannot), many things taught today are outdated in a few years.

The way to understand nursing is to understand it in its context and in its relationship to other subjects. Philosophy, the

humanities, history, psychology, physiology, sociology, anthropology, and all the other social sciences affect—and affected by—nursing. That centrality of nursing makes it a field to be studied in the university. The way to understand nursing is to identify, describe, and research those central humanistic-scientific factors that are essential to effecting positive health change. Those factors are primary mechanisms in "caring for" another human being. They lie somewhere between the sciences and humanities. Nursing today is a discipline that interfaces with the academic world and the professional world.

BALANCING SCIENCE WITH HUMANISM—THE SCIENCE OF CARING

As a university subject, nursing must achieve a delicate balance between scientific knowledge and humanistic practice behaviors. It is, therefore, important (if not critical) for nursing to realize the need for both a professional education and a liberal arts education.

A conscious effort on the part of the health profession to control disease, prolong life, and alleviate pain has brought dramatic results. However, the humanities and the behavioral sciences address themselves to deeper values of the quality of living and dying, which involve philosophical, ethical, psychosocial, and moral issues, Because of the differences between science and the humanities, it is now possible to define an outcome of scientific activity (e.g., prolongation of life) without referring to its esthetic-humanistic aspect (e.g., the quality of life and death).

SIMILARITIES AND DIFFERENCES BETWEEN SCIENCE AND THE HUMANITIES

There are differences as well as similarities between science and the humanities. It is crucial to know the important functions that science cannot perform for the practice behavior and the important functions that the humanities cannot perform for the knowledge base. Understanding those differences helps the student and practitioner understand why both perspectives are needed in nursing.

Science is concerned with ordering human behavior and producing detachment from individual experiences. Science is neutral in regard to human values. Science is concerned with methods, generalizations, and predictions.[5, 6] However, there are important functions that science cannot perform, perhaps because it asks different kinds of questions than do the humanities.

The humanities address themselves to the understanding and evaluation of human goals and experiences. They are concerned with people's emotional responses to experiences. The humanities look for individual differences and uniqueness. They examine the diversity and quality of human experiences. In the humanities, imagination and insight are validated from within, without justification by scientific criteria.

Because of the important differences between the sciences and the humanities, the educator must be aware of the strengths and weaknesses of each. Science lacks the capacity for humanistic learning because it is not concerned with human goals and values. Science is not concerned with individual experience. Science cannot be expected to keep alive a sense of common humanity. [6]

The humanities, on the other hand, cannot give predictable solutions to the problems of human nature. The humanities cannot provide the hard database that comprises the intellectual content of nursing and the other health sciences.

The new student in nursing, and even the experienced graduate nurse, may struggle with the differences between the sciences and the humanities. Because of their own value systems, they may emphasize one domain and ignore the other. But both domains are important in nursing and the other health sciences. The nurse must understand what each domain can and cannot contribute to nursing.

In spite of the inherent differences between science and the humanities, there exists the capacity for the science of caring that approaches human problems from both directions. The science of caring combines science with the humanities. The science of caring cannot be completely neutral with respect to human values. It cannot remain detached from or indifferent to human emotions—pain, joy, suffering, fear, and anger. At the same time, as its name indicates, the science of caring is guided by scientific knowledge, methods, and predictions. The scientific base of caring integrates the biophysical sciences with the behavioral sciences, and so necessitates a recognition and utilization of the humanities. A science of caring requires the nurse to examine and try to understand the meaning of human actions and values that determine human choice in health and illness.

An understanding of the essential characteristics of sciences and the humanities—the ways in which they are similar and different—gives nursing and the other health professions a better opportunity to complement and enhance the use and applications of both domains.

The nursing profession must identify, describe, and research the interaction of both domains that form the base of the science of caring.

REFERENCES

1. Harvey, O. J. (1970). Belief systems and education: Some implications for change. In J. Crawford (ed.), *The affective domain* (pp. 67–91). Washington, DC: Communications Service Corporation.
2. Kramer, McD., & Reed, J. L. (1972). Self-actualization and role conception of baccalaureate degree nurses. *Nursing Research, 21,* 111.
3. Hutchins, R. (1977, May 22). Learning the rules is no longer sufficient. (Remarks delivered in 1974 at the Graduate Studies and

Research Center of California State University at Long Beach.) Rocky Mountain News. pp. 1–2.

4. Chandler, J. (1976). Moral values and liberal learning. *The Wake Forest Magazine, 23*, 28.
5. Morganthau, H. J. (1972). *Science: Servant or master?* New York, NY: New American Library.
6. Prior, M. E. (1962). *Science and the humanities.* Evanston, IL: North-western University Press.

CARATIVE FACTORS IN NURSING

The day-to-day practice of professional nursing requires a grounding in a humanistic value system that a nurse continues to cultivate. The humanistic value system must be combined with the scientific knowledge base that guides the nurse's actions. That humanistic-scientific combination underlies the science of caring. In explaining the interaction of humanism and science, this chapter organizes the core of nursing according to carative factors relevant to the science of caring. The term carative is used in contrast to the more common term curative to help the student to differentiate nursing and medicine. The carative factors are the factors that the nurse uses in the delivery of health care to the patient/client. The carative factors are developed from a humanistic philosophy that is central to caring for another human being and that is founded on a steadily growing scientific base.

Curative factors aim at *curing* the patient of disease, whereas *carative* factors aim at the *caring process* that helps the person attain (or maintain) health or die a peaceful death.

The carative factors discussed here present nursing care as a deeply human activity. Those factors are not presented as final, because there may be an unlimited number of ways to characterize and produce a therapeutic result in nursing care. The factors provide a tentative foundation for the science caring that nursing encompasses and need to be further delineated, expanded, and researched. Nevertheless they are the factors that I think form the whole nursing.

To discuss the carative factors in more detail, the basic premises relevant to nursing as the science of caring must be set forth. Nursing is concerned with promoting health, preventing illness, caring for the sick, and restoring health. Nursing has traditionally focused on integrating the biophysical knowledge with the knowledge of human behavior to promote wellness and to care for the sick. In the present (as in the past), the emphasis is on health promotion rather than on specialized treatment of disease. Because of that focus, nursing is concerned with the knowledge and understanding of "care," which is different from but complementary to the knowledge and understanding of "cure," which is in the domain of medicine.[1]

BASIC PREMISES FOR THE SCIENCE OF CARING IN NURSING

The basic premises for a science of caring in nursing are broad and complex ones and provide the foundation for the usefulness of "caring" as a construct in nursing science.

1. Caring (and nursing) has existed in every society. Every society has had some people who have cared for others. A caring attitude is *not* transmitted from generation to generation by genes. It is transmitted by the culture of the profession as a unique way of coping with its environment. Nursing has always held a caring stance regarding other human beings. That stance has been threatened by a long history of procedure-oriented demands and the development of different levels of nursing. However, the opportunities for nurses to obtain advanced education and engage in higher level analyses of problems and concerns in their education and practice have allowed nursing to combine its humanistic orientation with the relevant science.

2. There is often a discrepancy between theory and practice or between the scientific and artistic aspects of caring, partly because of the disjunction between scientific values and humanistic values.

BASIC ASSUMPTIONS FOR THE SCIENCE OF CARING IN NURSING

The following are the basic assumptions for the science of caring in nursing.

1. Caring can be effectively demonstrated and practiced only interpersonally.
2. Caring consists of carative factors that result in the satisfaction of certain human needs.
3. Effective caring promotes health and growth of an individual or a family.
4. Caring responses accept a person not only as he or she is now but as what he or she may become.
5. A caring environment is the one that offers the development of potential while allowing the person to choose the best action for himself or herself at a given point in time.
6. Caring is more "healthogenic" than is curing. The practice of caring integrates the biophysical knowledge with the knowledge of human behavior to generate or promote health and to provide ministrations to those who are ill. A science of caring is therefore complementary to the science of curing.
7. The practice of caring is central to nursing.

It is difficult to understand how "caring" helps people to the extent that positive mental, physical, social, or spiritual health changes result. However, if the basic components of the caring process are identified, studied, and researched, they will be seen to comprise a scientific-humanistic basis for nursing interventions.

OVERVIEW OF THE CARATIVE FACTORS

There are 10 primary carative factors that form a structure for studying and understanding nursing as the science of caring.

Those carative factors are given as follows:

1. The formation of a humanistic-altruistic system of values
2. The instillation of faith–hope
3. The cultivation of sensitivity to one's self and to others
4. The development of a helping-trust relationship
5. The promotion and acceptance of the expression of positive and negative feelings
6. The systematic use of the scientific problem-solving method for decision making
7. The promotion of interpersonal teaching–learning
8. The provision for a supportive, protective, and (or) corrective mental, physical, sociocultural, and spiritual environment
9. Assistance with the gratification of human needs
10. The allowance for existential-phenomenological forces

The first three carative factors interact to establish a philosophical foundation for the science of caring. To a large extent, those factors are interdependent; they function together in a process that promotes positive health changes. Since the first three carative factors are interrelated, they are discussed together in this chapter. They comprise a unified context because of their philosophical-value-laden orientation for care.

The other carative factors are discussed separately—even in separate chapters when the content necessitates an extensive development. These factors, although they are related to values and philosophies, are discussed according to a scientific data base. After the philosophical orientation, the ordering moves from a more basic foundation of absolute values to more scientific factors that are interrelated for nursing education and practice.

FORMATION OF A HUMANISTIC-ALTRUISTIC VALUE SYSTEM

As a given, caring must be grounded on a set of universal human values—kindness, concern, and love of self and others. A humanistic-altruistic value system usually begins early in one's life, and it continues to grow and mature. As one reaches young adulthood, humanizing of values becomes more established, a point that coincides often with a person's decision to become a nurse.

In such a case, the natural development of humanistic values can be facilitated through the exchange of attitudes and beliefs and of the learning and role modeling that occur between the student nurse and the nursing educator.

The maturing person begins to associate the human meaning of values and how they are related to the achievement of social purposes. Likewise, the person begins to draw from personal experiences and motives to affirm and promote values.[2]

A humanistic-altruistic value system is a qualitative philosophy that guides one's mature life. It is the commitment to faction of receiving through giving, and it involves the capacity to view humanity with love and to appreciate diversity and individuality. Such a value system helps one to tolerate differences and to view others through their own perceptual rather than through one's own.

A humanizing of values is derived from one's childhood experiences, including the relationship with one's parents. It is enhanced and expanded from exposure to and the study and of different philosophies, beliefs, and lifestyles.

Studying the humanities encourages the freeing of one's thoughts about and perceptions of people from different cultures. A foundation for empathy is laid as one becomes aware and appreciative of different ideas, tastes, and divergent views of life, death, and the world in general.

Past life experiences, as well as study and exploration, help instill a higher level of feeling, thinking, and behaving toward others. Humanistic values and an altruistic approach to life influence the day-to-day patterns of living.

Caring is based on a guiding force and value system that affect the encounters between the nurse and other persons. Whether one is conscious of one's philosophy and values, they affect one's caring behavior. Humanistic values and altruistic behavior can be developed through consciousness raising and a close examination of one's views, beliefs, and values. They can be further developed through (for example) experiences with different cultures, early experiences that have aroused compassion and other emotions, study of the humanities, literary and artistic experiences, value-clarification exercises, and personal growth experiences (e.g., meditation and therapy).

Any one of these and other experiences may help one recognize and use values to establish a philosophy of life that promotes maturity, satisfaction, and integrity. Altruistic values and behavior bring meaning to one's life through relationships with other people.

Before the nurse can make a social contribution through altruistic service, she or he must resolve some of the problems related to personal and professional identity. Although self-awareness and self-examination are necessary for maturing, the nurse must move beyond them and get outside herself or himself to make the most meaningful contribution to self, others, and society. Adler[3] believed that everyone tends to develop *social interest* as he or she outgrows egotism and strives for superiority over self.

Having a humanistic-altruistic value system in nursing does not mean that the nurse must adopt a sacrificial, all-giving, and self-denying behavior. It means that the self should be developed in such a humanizing way that there is an *extension of the sense of self.* I agree with the view of Adler, Allport, and others that a sense of self becomes extended when the welfare of another person, a group enterprise, or some other valued object has a prominent place in one's life.[2-5] As Allport states:

Maturity advances in proportion as lives are decentered from the clamorous immediacy of the body and of egocenteredness. Self-love is a prominent and inescapable factor in every life, but it need not dominate. Everyone has self-love, but only self-extension is the earmark of maturity.[4]

A humanistic-altruistic value system encompasses Allport's concept of maturity. Caring consists of humanistic-altruistic feelings and acts that promote the best professional care and the most mature social contributions. For those reasons, I consider the formation of a humanistic-altruistic value system the first and most basic factor for the science of caring.

INSTILLATION OF FAITH-HOPE

The instillation of faith-hope is the second carative factor. That factor interacts with the formation of a humanistic-altruistic value system to enhance the other carative factors. The nurse and other health professionals must not ignore the important role of faith-hope in the carative and the curative processes.

The therapeutic effects of faith-hope have been documented throughout history. Hippocrates thought that mind and soul of the ill person should be inspired before his illness was treated. Aristotle was aware that the theater had a therapeutic effect on the person who became psychologically involved with the performance. Asclepius, the Greek god of medicine, was often pictured with his two daughters—Hygiea, the goddess of health, and Panacea, the goddess of healing,

Hygiea guarded health by prescribing self-discipline and a good environment. Panacea used drugs and manipulations to heal.[6]

In ancient Egypt, the priest and the physician were the same person. For many centuries, Egyptian medicine was closely associated with religion and faith.

Faith-hope traditionally has been important in treatment to relieve the symptoms of illness; medicine itself was secondary magic, incantations, spells, and prayers. Miracles of faith appear often in the Bible. Other ancient approaches to treatment, such as the Babylonian's astrological approach, were based on supernatural explanations of the causes of and cures for illnesses. Mesmer, who treated illness through suggestion, explained that when he pointed a rod at sick people, animal magnetism flowed from the rod and healed them.[7]

The earliest attempts at group psychotherapy used inspirational, authoritative approaches.[8] For example, in 1905, Dr. Joseph H. Pratt held group meetings with tuberculosis patients to instruct them in hygienic practices. Encouragement and inspiration were side effects of Pratt's approach, and they had a psychotherapeutic effect.

Adler—and later Dreikurs—considered encouragement the central mechanism in teleoanalytic group counseling. Both men thought that success in group counseling depended largely on the counselor's ability to encourage and that failure was usually due to the inability to encourage.[3, 8]

In the field of psychotherapy, it is established that the therapist plays a critical role.[8-10] Yalom identified instillation of hope as a curative factor in therapy. Yalom's factor is closely related to the carative factor faith-hope.

Lipkin[7] identified two factors that affect the treatment of every patient: the power of suggestion and the power of the relationship. The effects of hypnosis and placebos, both forms of suggestion, range from relief of minor headache pain to removal of the major symptoms of illness. The power of suggestion (the power of positive feeling) is linked to the instillation of faith-hope.

The nurse must instill in the patient a sense of faith-hope in the nurse and in the treatment. Faith-hope may help the patient to accept information from the nurse and to engage in attitude change and health-seeking behavior. Faith-hope is so basic that it can affect the healing process and the outcome of illness. There is sample documentation of the positive effects of treatments based entirely on faith-hope. The effects of the potent drug atropine can be reversed or even abolished by suggestion. ". . . drugs and gadgets come and go, how often it is suggestion that produces the cure . . .".[6]

Today, self-discipline for health is often ignored, and the help of a healing agent—a person, treatment, or drug—is sought.

Many people believe or feel instinctively that illness and death are the results of an evil and invisible destructive force. Many people believe that when everything else fails to cure an illness, something still "needs to be done." In many instances, the something is having faith in a person, or in a health regimen, or in a belief system to "carry them through."

Some people think that the present era is the "beginning of the end of physical medicine." Medicine is only one of a number of ways of treating illnesses. Millions of people believe that movements of the stars, if properly interpreted, can reveal their fates. Traditional medicine and treatment are used as adjuncts to other approaches or at best in conjunction with other practices, such as therapeutic massage, acupuncture, and the psychic revelation of one's former lives.

The recent interest in card reading and in astrological and biorhythmical charts indicates that, for many people, faith in the supernatural plays an important role in their health and well-being. The popular interest in Eastern philosophies and practices also attests to the satisfaction that faith-hope and discipline bring many people. Meditation, behavioral therapy, and biofeedback are modern examples of how some people use faith-hope to improve their state of well-being. Such practices are ancient and they are commonly accepted today. Five or ten years ago they were considered bizarre or not beneficial. Now they are widely used by scientists and lay persons alike.

It is within a scientific framework as well as within a faith-hope–instilling framework that the nurse takes care of others. The interaction within a personal relationship is an important carative factor. Regardless of what scientific regimen is required for the care of a person, the nurse discovers what is meaningful and important for the particular person. The person's beliefs are never disregarded; they are encouraged and respected as significant influences in promoting and maintaining health.

Even when scientific medicine says that nothing can be done for a patient, the nurse can provide care. . . .

Intelligent people have sought non-scientific treatments of and solutions to their psychological and physical problems. Scientific medicine has traditionally held that those nonscientific approaches cannot cure a patient. However, the current response to that attitude is, "If those approaches have nothing to offer, why do they satisfy and help so many people?"

A nurse who practices the science of caring transcends the limitations and restrictions of a scientific approach because of her or his respect for and knowledge and appreciation of the whole person. The nurse knows from studying human behavior and the behavioral sciences that the use of physical medicine is only one way of responding to the health–illness concerns of another person. Instillation of faith-hope—in one's self and one's competence or in another person—is incorporated into the science of caring. The healing power of belief should never be overlooked. The instillation of faith-hope is difficult to define because it is never a finished process. The nurse must always consider that factor to practice the science of caring.

The holistic nature of responding to another person justifies faith-hope as a contributing influence in people's lives.

Faith-hope builds on and draws from a humanistic-altruistic value system to promote holistic professional care and produce positive health. The formation of a humanistic-altruistic value system and the instillation of faith-hope complement each other and further contribute to the third carative factor—the cultivation of sensitivity to one's self and to others.

CULTIVATION OF SENSITIVITY TO SELF AND OTHERS

To be human is to feel. All too often people allow themselves to *think* their thoughts but not to *feel* their feelings. The only way to develop sensitivity to one's self and to others is to recognize and feel feelings—painful ones as well as happy ones.

The development of self and the nurturing of judgment, taste, values, and sensitivity in human relationships evolve from emotional states. The development of feelings is encouraged by the humanities and compassionate life experiences. The recognition and development of feelings lead to self-actualization through self-acceptance and psychological growth.

Most people do not achieve their potential. They tend to look for opportunities outside themselves. But the source for development is within. A starting point is to develop a level of consciousness about one's feelings to look into one's self. People often are afraid to look within because they fear that if they are honest they will see only imperfections. Sensitivity to one's

self and one's feelings can be threatening because it may seem that there is no way to handle feelings or that one is not able to change, Therefore it seems easier to push back feelings, to deny them, to refuse to deal with them, or to become consumed by them.

However, a balanced sensitivity to one's feelings gives one a foundation for empathy with others. One must recognize, accept, and be willing to explore one's own feelings. That allows one to recognize and accept the feelings of others, an ability that is related to the fifth carative factor: the promotion and acceptance of the expression of positive and negative feelings. Those who are not sensitive to their own feelings find it difficult to be sensitive to the feelings of others. People who repress their own feelings may be unable to allow others to express or explore their feelings.

Sensitivity to one's self and to others may determine the extent to which the nurse is able to develop self and fully use self with others.

The educational and practice situations in nursing often prevent or at best discourage the nurse from being too sensitive to or getting too involved with another's feelings. The nurse may overreact to protect her or his own feelings. As a result, the nurse often forms impersonal, detached professional relationships, in which she or he hides behind a so-called professional character armor.[1] The nurse often deals with her or his own feelings by camouflaging potential conflicts between the nurse and the patient/client. However, the conflicts are not resolved for either the nurse or the other person, as the following example shows.

A young woman had a first child who was stillborn. The woman had had a long and painful labor, and during the labor she had learned that her child was dead. Although the woman had participated actively in the labor, at the moment of her child's birth, the woman's face had been covered ostensibly to prevent her from seeing her dead child. Perhaps the real reason for the covering was to protect the staff from their own anxieties and feelings of inadequacy. The staff lacked sensitivity to themselves and to the woman. They did not offer primary care and prevention. Both scientific knowledge and intuition say that in a situation like the one just described, the feelings of the hospital staff and of the patient should be acknowledged and dealt with. If they are not, both the staff and the patient are deprived of a significant experience. In such a situation, both parties are suffering. If the covering up and denial of the suffering continue, pathology results that can affect the nurse's mental health and practice behaviors and the patient's mental health and behavior. The process that is established in a situation such as the one just described can extend to numerous other situations unless nurses continually observe themselves and their relationships with others. If nurses—helping professionals—fail to be human at sensitive or painful times, they fail at helping. They succeed only in hiding behind their role and their insecurities and anxieties; and they contribute nothing to their own health or the health of others.

The morning after the delivery just described, the young mother asked a student nurse, "Do they always cover your face when you deliver a baby?" That innocent and simple question shows that a lack of sensitivity can make a painful experience even more painful.

Nurses must be genuine to themselves and their feelings. Honesty toward self promotes authenticity and sensitivity toward others, and it lays a foundation for primary prevention. A nurse attains and promotes health and higher level functioning only if she or he forms person-to-person relationships as opposed to manipulative relationships.

Primary preventive care occurs when nurses are committed to high-level health and growth for themselves and others. When the carative factor of sensitivity

to themselves and others is operating, nurses function as whole persons and can give holistic care. Both the patients and the nurses retain their separate identities.

Authenticity with self and others is the foundation for integrity. From it, an *I–Thou*[11] relationship can result that an empathetic relationship for acceptance, exploration, and growth.

Practicing sensitivity to self and others becomes "something basic"[1] that is common to all types of nursing. Sensitivity to self and others builds on the formation of a humanistic-altruistic value system and the instillation of faith-hope, and it commits the nurse to helping other people achieve such goals as satisfaction, comfort, freedom from pain and suffering, and level wellness.

The nurse who is sensitive to feelings is able to make another person feel understood, accepted, and capable of moving toward a more mature level of functioning and growth. The nurse who is sensitive is better able to learn another person's view of the world. The culture, language, belief system, and values influence her or his desire for and concern about comfort, recovery, and wellness. People are always growing and maturing. Health–illness problems and interpersonal relationships are valuable aids to growth and maturity—to developing potentialities as well as actualities. In the context of caring, the nurse never assumes that she or he knows the other person, but at each meeting she or he continues to try to get to know the patient/client. That approach requires sensitivity to one's self and to others.

The nurse who recognizes and uses her or his sensitivity and feelings promotes self-development and self-actualization and is able to encourage the same growth in others. Because the carative factor sensitivity to one's self and to others is considered basic to nursing, it may not be explicitly acknowledged, valued, or used. But it cannot be taken for granted, and so it has been discussed in this chapter as a distinct carative factor. Without that factor, nursing care would fail.

REFERENCES

1. Jourard, S. M. (1964). *The transparent self.* Princeton, NJ: Van Nostrand.
2. White, R. W. (1975). *Lives in progress* (3rd ed.). New York, NY: Holt, Rinehart and Winston.
3. Adler, A. (1927). *Understanding human nature.* Philadelphia, PA: Chilton.
4. Allport, G. W. (1961). *Pattern and growth in personality.* New York, NY: Holt, Rinehart and Winston.
5. Maslow, A. H. (1976). *The farther reaches of human nature.* New York, NY: Viking.
6. Ackerknecht, E. H. (1968). A short history of medicine *(p. xvii).* New York, NY: Ronald.
7. Lipkin, M. (1975). *The care of patients.* New York, NY: Oxford University Press.
8. Gazda, G. M. (1975). *Basic approaches to group psychotherapy and group counseling* (2nd ed.). Springfield, IL: Thomas.
9. Bergin, A. C., & Garfield, S. L (Eds.). (1971). *Handbook of psychotherapy and behavior change: An empirical analysis.* New York, NY: Wiley.
10. Rogers, C. R. (1967). *Person to person: The problem of being human.* California, USA: Real People Press.
11. Buber, M. (1937). *I and Thou.* New York, NY: Scribner's.

QUESTIONS FOR REFLECTION

Baccalaureate

1. What is the value of liberal arts to nursing education?

2. Which is most important: sciences or humanities in nursing education? Support your answer with at least two reasons.

3. Select one of the first three CFs and describe the importance of that factor. Provide an example of how it is evident in nursing practice.

Master's

1. You are caring for an elderly man in renal failure who undergoes dialysis three times a week. He tells you that he wants to die, that he has nothing to live for. How would you approach him guided by Watson's second CF?

2. How is nurse practitioner practice different from the medical practice of primary care?

3. You are working with nurses who are rude, insensitive, and hurtful to coworkers and to patients. How can you create a more caring–healing environment by cultivating sensitivity to self and others?

Doctoral

1. Did the CFs adequately distinguish nursing from medicine? How?

2. Do the 10 CFs capture the whole of nursing practice? What is missing?

3. How would you define "human science"? What are the tenets of a human science? Is nursing a human science? Why or why not?

8

Foundations of Humanistic Nursing

JOSEPHINE G. PATERSON AND
LORETTA T. ZDERAD

FOUNDATIONS OF HUMANISTIC NURSING

Nursing is a response to the human situation. It comes into being under certain conditions—one human being needs a kind of help and another gives it. The meaning of nursing as a living human act is in the act itself. To understand it, therefore, it is necessary to consider nursing as an existent, a phenomenon occurring in the real world.

THE PHENOMENON OF NURSING

The phenomenon of nursing appears in many forms in the real lived world. It varies with the age of the patient, the pathology or disability, the kind and degree of help needed, the duration of the need for help, the patient's location and his potential for obtaining and using help, and the nurse's perception of the need and her capacities for responding to it. Nursing varies also in relation to the sociocultural context in which it occurs. Being one element in an evolving complex system of health care, nursing is continuously appearing in new specialized forms. As professionals, we are accustomed to viewing nursing as we practice it within these specialty contexts—for example, pediatric, medical, rehabilitation,

intensive care, long-term care, community. There seems to be no end to the proliferation of diversifications. Even the attempts of practitioners to combine specialties give rise to new specialties, such as community mental health nursing and child psychiatric nursing.

So it is difficult to focus on the phenomenon of nursing as an entity without having one's view colored by a particular clinical, functional, or societal context. Yet, if we can "bracket" (hold in abeyance) these adjectival labels and the preconceived viewpoints they signify, we can consider the thing itself, the act of nursing in its most simple and general appearance.

Well-Being and More-Being

In this most basic sense, disregarding the particular specialized forms in which it appears, the nursing act always is related to the health–illness quality of the human condition, or fundamentally, to a man's personal survival. This is not to say that all instances of nursing are matters of life and death, but rather that every nursing act has to do with the quality of a person's living and dying.

Nursing is related to health and illness is self-evident. How it is related is not so apparent. "Health" is valued as

From Paterson, J., & Zderad, L. (1988). Foundations of humanistic nursing. *Humanistic nursing* (pp. 11–22). New York, NY: National League for Nursing. Permission to reprint granted by the National League for Nursing, New York, NY.

necessary for survival and is often proposed as the goal of nursing. There are, in actuality, many instances of nursing that could be described as "health restoring," "health sustaining," or "health promoting." Nurses engage in "health teaching" and "health supervision." On the other hand, there are instances in which health, taken in its narrowest meaning as freedom from disease, is not seen as an attainable goal, as evidenced, for example, in labels given to patients such as "terminal," "hopeless," and "chronic." Yet in actual practice, these humans' conditions call forth some of the most complete, expert, total, beautiful nursing care. Nursing, as a human response, implies the valuing of some human potential beyond the narrow concept of health taken as absence of disease. Nursing's concern is not merely with a person's well-being but with his more-being, with helping him become more as humanly possible in his particular life situation.

Human Potential

Since nursing involves one human being helping another, the notion of humaneness has been associated traditionally with nursing. Nursing practice is criticized justifiably when it is not humane and is taken for granted or praised when it is. The expectation of humaneness is so ingrained in the concept of nursing that some nurses are surprised when it is acknowledged by patients. If a patient thanks them for their kindness, patience, or concern, these nurses reply, in their embarrassment, "Oh, that's part of my job."

However, to equate nursing's humanistic character solely with an overflowing of the milk of human kindness is a serious error of oversimplification. Such a limited view, in fact, is a dehumanizing denial of man's potentials. As a human transaction, the phenomenon of nursing contains all the human potentials and limitations of each unique participant. For instance, frustration, discouragement, anger, rejection, withdrawal, loneliness, aggression, impatience, envy, grief, despair, pain, and suffering are constituents of nursing, as well as tenderness, caring, courage, trust, joy, hope. In other words, since nursing is lived by humans, the "stuff" of nursing includes all possible responses of man—man needing and man helping—in his situation.

Intersubjective Transaction

Looking again at the phenomenon of nursing as it occurs in the real lived world, obviously it is always an interhuman event. Whenever nursing takes place, two (or more) human beings are related in a shared situation. Each participates according to his own mode of being in the situation, that is, as a person nursing or as a person begin nursed. Since one is nursing and the other is being nursed, it follows that the essential character of the situation is "nurturance." In other words, the phenomenon of nursing involves nurturing, being nurtured, and a relation—the "between" in which or through which the nurturance occurs.

On reflection, it is obvious that nursing is an intersubjective transaction. Both persons, nurse and patient (client, family, group), necessarily participate in the proceedings. In this sense, they are *inter*dependent. Yet, they are both subjects, that is, each is the originator of human acts and of human responses to the other. In this sense, they are *in*dependent. The intersubjective transactional character of nursing cannot be escaped when one is experiencing the phenomenon, either as nurse or as patient. Consider, for example, some of the most common nursing activities such as feeding and being fed, comforting and being comforted, giving and taking medications. Although this intersubjectivity is unmistakably known in experience, it is extremely difficult to conceptualize and convey it to others. It rarely is found in descriptions of nursing, and to the unfortunate extent that it is missing, the descriptions are not true to life.

In real life, nursing phenomena may be experienced from the reference points of nurturing, of being nurtured, or of the nurturing process in the "between." For instance, the nurse may describe comfort as an experience of comforting another person; the patient, as an experience of being comforted. However, while each has experienced something within himself, he also has experienced something of the "between," namely, the message or meaning of the "comforting–being comforted" process. This essential interhuman dimension of nursing is beyond and yet within the technical, procedural, or interactional elements of the event. It is a quality of being that is expressed in the doing.

Being and Doing

As an intersubjective, transactional experience, nursing necessarily involves both a mode of being and a doing of something. The being and doing are interrelated so inextricably that it is difficult, even distorting, to speak of one without the other. Descriptions of nursing, however, often focus primarily (sometimes exclusively) on the doing aspect of the process, on the nursing techniques or procedures. The observable acts are more easily discerned and discussed. They can be measured, counted, and charted. Yet, in the actual interhuman experience of nursing the weight of being is felt. Presence and the effect of one's presence can be known much more vividly than they can be described. Still, not to attempt to describe them is to present only a half, or perhaps less than half, of the nursing picture.

When a nurse refers to a nurse–patient interaction during which a change in the patient's condition or behavior was noted, one hoping to get a description of nursing may ask, "What did you do?" Often the answer is a description of a manual action or a verbal interchange. Sometimes the nurse responds, "Nothing, I was just there." Perhaps it is the question that is wrong. The respondent usually interprets "doing" in a limited sense. In reality, everything the nurse does is

colored by the character of her being in the situation. The nursing act itself is a behavioral expression of the nurse's state of being, for example, concerned, fatigued, hurried, confident, hopeless.

Furthermore, there is a kind of being, a "being with" or a "being there," that is really a kind of doing for it involves the nurse's active presence. To "be with" in this fuller sense requires turning one's attention toward the patient, being aware of and open to the here and now shared situation, and communicating one's availability.

Whether the nursing act is verbal, manual, or both; a silent glance; or physical presence, some degree of intersubjectivity is involved and warrants recognition. To become more aware of and explore more fully this essential constituent of nursing, we need to focus on the participants' modes of being in the situation. Rather than ask the nurse, "What did you do in the nurse–patient situation?" we ought to ask, "What happened between the two of you?"

HUMANISTIC NURSING

When the meaning of nursing is sought by scrutinizing the phenomenon, that is, by examining the nursing event itself as it occurs in real life, one finds nursing embedded within the human context. As a nurturing response of one person to another in need, it aims at the development of human potential, at well-being and more-being. As something that happens between people, it reflects all the human potential and limitations of the persons involved. As an intersubjective transaction, it holds the possibility for both persons to effect and be affected, the possibility for both to become more. At its very base, nursing is humanistic. It is, at once, man's expression of and his striving for survival and further development in community.

In a way, to specify nursing as humanistic seems redundant. In view of its source and goals how could it be otherwise? However, the term "humanistic nursing" was coined thoughtfully and used purposely here to designate a particular nursing approach. Not only does the term signify full recognition of nursing's human foundation and meaning but it also points the direction for nursing's necessary development. What is proposed here is the enrichment of nursing by exploring and expanding its relations to its human context.

Authentic Commitment

When it is genuinely humanistic, nursing is an expression, a living out, of the nurse's authentic commitment. It is an existential engagement directed toward nurturing human potential. The humanistic nurse values nursing as a situation in which the necessary conditions for such human actualization exist and is open to the possibilities in the intimately shared nurse–patient here and now.

Humanistic nursing calls for an existential involvement, that is, an active presence with the whole of the nurse's being. This involved presence is personal and professional. It is personal—a live act stemming from this unique, individual nurse. It is a chosen human response freely given; it cannot be assigned or programmed. The involvement is professional—goal directed. It is based on an art–science; it is held accountable.

Anyone familiar with typical hectic nursing situations could justifiably question the actual attainability of such an existential involvement. It goes without saying that it would be humanly impossible for a nurse to be wholly present to numerous patients for 8 hours a day. But any nurse who has experienced moments of genuine presence in the nurse–patient situation will attest to their reality and to the fact that it is these beautiful moments that give meaning to nursing. In terms of actual practice, it is more realistic to think of humanistic nursing as occurring in various degrees. It may be more useful, in fact, to consider humanistic nursing a goal worth

striving for; an attitude that strengthens one's perseverance toward attaining the difficult goal; or fundamentally, a major value shaping one's nursing practice.

Process—Choice and Intersubjectivity

For the process of nursing to be truly humanistic it must bear out, that is, be a lived expression of, the nurse's recognition and valuing of nursing as an opportunity for the development of the human person. To this end, humanistic nursing process echos existential themes related to a person's becoming through choice and intersubjectivity.

Existentially speaking, man is his choices. This does not mean that a man can be anything he chooses. Naturally, each individual is unique, having his own particular potentials and limitations. Nor is this view a denial of the forces of unconscious motivation and habit. It does not imply that all of a person's actions result from totally conscious deliberations. By saying, "I am my choices," I mean I am this here-and-now person because in my past life I took particular paths in preference to others; of the possibilities open to me, I actualized certain ones.

In this sense, I am my history, I am what I am, what I have become. But I am also what I am not, what I have not become. I am a nurse, this unique here and now nurse with particular experience, knowledge, skills, and values; without other experience, knowledge, skills, and values. Through self-reflection, I know that I have changed and I have experienced growth from within. I know myself as a being capable of becoming more, capable of actualizing my possibilities, my self. So I am my choices not only in terms of my past but also in regard to my future, my possibilities.

Man is an individual being necessarily related to other men in time and space. As every man is beholden to other men for his birth and development, interdependence is inherent in the human situation. In this sense, human existence is coexistence.

The deeper significance of this truth has been recognized and elucidated by many thinkers, especially those in the existential stream. Over and over, their writings reveal the paradoxical tension of being human: Each man is, at once, independent, a unique individual and interdependent, a necessarily related being. As Wilfrid Desan says, referring to man as subsistent relation, "He is towards-the-other but he is not-the-other."[1]

Furthermore, as Martin Buber and Gabriel Marcel maintain, it is actually through his relations with other men that a man becomes, that his unique individuality is actualized. To know myself as "individual" is to experience myself as this particular unique here-and-now person and other than that there-and-now person. Or in other words, to know myself as me is to see myself in relation to and distant from other selves. As Buber so beautifully states, "It is from one man to another that the heavenly bread of self-being is passed."[2]

Logically, it follows that the possibility for self-confirmation exists in any intersubjective situation. However, in everyday life, this self-confirmation is experienced to different degrees or on different levels in interhuman relating. Since both persons are independent subjects acting with their human capacity for disclosing or enclosing themselves, there is no guarantee that the availability and presence necessary for a genuine confirming encounter will come forth. Presence, the gift of one's self, cannot be seized or called forth by demand, and it can only be given freely and be invoked or evoked.

Since man becomes more through his choices and the aim of nursing is to help man toward well-being or more-being, the humanistic nursing effort is directed toward increasing the possibilities of making responsible choices. Such choice involves, in the first place, an openness to and an awareness of one's own situation. A choice is a response to possibility. Therefore, one must first recognize that possibilities or alternatives exist. This openness to options is experienced as a freedom to choose as well as a freedom from the bonds of habit and stereotyped response, from routine, and from the veils of the obvious. It means getting in touch with one's experience and one's subjective–objective world. As one becomes more acutely aware of his personal freedom of choice, there arises concurrently an awareness of the quality of choice and of the responsibility that is always implied in the freedom. Then follows reflective consideration of one's unique situation with its possible alternatives and an examination of the values inherent in them. Finally, the act of choosing is expressed in a response to the situation with a willingness to accept the responsibility for its foreseeable consequences. Through this experience, the person becomes aware of himself as an individual. As a subject choosing freely and responsibly, he knows himself as distinct from and yet related to others.

Nursing, being an intersubjective transaction, presents an occasion for both persons, patient and nurse, to experience the process of making responsible choices. Through living this process in nursing situations, the nurse develops her own potential for responsible choosing. The satisfaction, often in the form of a sense of vitality and strength, that is felt in making responsible competent professional judgments reinforces the habit. In personally coming to experientially appreciate the growth-promoting character of responsible choosing, the nurse may more readily recognize the value of such experiences for any person, including the one currently labeled "patient." The humanistic nurse, therefore, is alert to opportunities for the patient to exercise his freedom of choice within the limits of safe and sound practice. She is constantly assessing his capabilities and needs and encourages his maximum participation in his own health care program. Through coexperiencing and supporting the process in the patient's experience from his point of view, the nurse nurtures his human potential for responsible choosing. Both patient and nurse become more through in making responsible choices in the intersubjective, transactional nursing situation.

Theory and Practice

The term "humanistic nursing" refers to a kind of nursing practice and its theoretical foundations. The two are so interrelated that it is difficult, in fact even somewhat distorting, to speak exclusively of either the practice or the theory of humanistic nursing. When, for the sake of clarity or emphasis, discussion is focused on either the practical or the theoretical realm, thoughts of the other realm cast their shadows on the fringes. For in our view, for the process of nursing to be truly humanistic means that the nurse is involved as an experiencing, valuing, reflecting, conceptualizing human person. From the other side, the theory of humanistic nursing is derived from actual practice, that is, from being with and doing with the patient. "Theory," says R. D. Laing, "is the articulated vision of experience."[3]

Humanistic nursing is not a matter solely of doing but also of being. The humanistic nurse is open to the reality of the situation in the existential sense. She is available with her total being in the nurse–patient situation. This involves a living out of the nurturing, intersubjective transaction with all of one's human capacities which include a response to the experienced reality. Man is able to set his world at a distance as an independent opposite and enter into relation with it. In fact, according to Buber, this is what distinguishes existence as human. It is man's special way of being.[4] For nursing to be humanistic in this full sense of the term requires being and doing in the situation and subsequently setting the experienced reality at a distance (that is, objectifying it) and entering into relation with it. The nurse's reflective response to her lived world may take the shape of any form of human dialogue with reality, such as science, art, or philosophy.

Viewed existentially, every nursing event is unique, a live intersubjective transaction colored and formed by the individual participants. Although the event is ephemeral, the resultant experiential knowledge is lasting and cumulative. So from the nurse's daily commonplace grows a body of clinical wisdom. The need for describing nursing phenomena, for expressing and conceptualizing lived nursing worlds, is basic to the theoretical and actual development of humanistic nursing. In summary, we contend that humanistic nursing practice necessarily involves the conceptualization of that practice and an examination of its inherent values and that humanistic nursing theory must be derived from nurses' lived experience. The interwoven theory and practice are reciprocally enlightening.

Framework—The Human Situation

It is easy to recognize the intrinsic interrelatedness of humanistic nursing theory and practice and the consequent necessity for their concurrent development. It is even quite easy to take the next steps of valuing such development and committing oneself to the task. But then the question arises: Where to begin?

Humanistic nursing is concerned with what is basically nursing, that is, with the phenomenon of nursing wherever it occurs regardless of its specialized clinical, functional, or sociocultural form. So its domain includes any or all nursing situations. And within this domain, since humanistic nursing is an intersubjective transaction aimed at nurturing well-being and more-being, its "stuff" includes all possible human and interhuman responses. To conceive of so limitless a universe for study is at once exhilarating and overwhelming. How can one get a handle on the nursing universe? Is it possible to envision an inclusive frame that would allow an orderly, systematic, and hopefully productive approach to the development of humanistic nursing?

The key is to return again to the source, to look at the phenomenon of nursing as it occurs in real life. From this perspective, the human situation sets the stage where nursing is lived. The major dimensions of humanistic nursing, then, may be derived from this situation. Existentially, man is an incarnate being always becoming in relation with men and things in a world of time and space. The nursing situation is a particular kind of human situation in which the interhuman relation is purposely directed toward nurturing the well-being or more-being of a person with perceived needs related to the health–illness quality of living. The elements of the frame, based on this view of humanistic nursing, would include incarnate men (patient and nurse) meeting (being and becoming) in a goal-directed (nurturing well-being and more-being) intersubjective transaction (being with and doing with) occurring in time and space (measured and as lived by patient and nurse) in a world of men and things. In other words, the inexhaustible richness of lived nursing worlds could be explored freely, imaginatively, and creatively in any direction suggested by the dimensions of this open framework. It allows for a variety of angular views.

For example, in terms of man as incarnate, it is certainly not new for nurses to focus on man's bodily existence. Naturally, one of nursing's basic concerns always has been care of people's physical needs. To view nursing from the perspective of the human situation, however, is to see beyond physical care, beyond the categorization of man as a biopsychosocial organism. The focus is on the person's unique being and becoming in his situation.

Every man is inserted into the common world of men and things through his own unique body. Through it, he affects the world and the world affects

him. Through it, he develops his own unique, personal, private world. When a person's bodily functions change during illness, *the* world and *his* world change for him. The nurse needs to consider how the patient experiences his lived world. Ordinary things which nurses simply take for granted, such as hospital noises or odors, touching, bathing, feeding, sleep or meal schedules, may have very different meaning for individual patients. They may or may not be experienced as nurturing in a particular person's lived world.

In the humanistic perspective, the nurse also is viewed as a human person, as a being in a body rather than merely as a function or a doer of activities. Conscious recognition of this fact opens many areas for exploration. Obviously, the nurse's actions (her being with and doing with), that affect the patient's world, are expressed through her body. How is nurturance communicated and actually affected through nursing activities? From the other side, consider the nurse as being affected by the world through her body. What depths of "nursing content" could we fathom if we accepted the existential dictum that "the body knows?" Would we dismiss so lightly those gems of clinical wisdom nurses attribute disparagingly to "gut reaction," "unscientific intuition," or "years of experience"? Would we value serious exploration and extraction of these natural resources in the nursing world?

The framework suggests, further, the possibilities of exploring the development of human potential, both patient's and nurse's, as it occurs in the unique domain of nursing's intersubjective transactions. What human resources are called forth in the shared situations during which nurses coexperience and cosearch with patients the varied meanings of being and becoming over the entire range of life from birth to death? How does it occur? What is the process? What promotes well-being or becoming more when facing life, suffering, death? For the patient? For the nurse? What knowledge gained through the study of nursing, a particular form of the human situation, could be contributed to the general body of human sciences?

Finally, within this framework, all the phenomena experienced in the nursing situation could be explored in relation to their attributes of time and space. More specifically, from an existential perspective, the focus would be directed toward the significance of lived time and space, that is, time and space as experienced by the patient and/or the nurse and as shared intersubjectively. For example, waiting, silence, chronicity, emergency, positioning a patient in bed, moving through space in a wheelchair, crutch walking, and pacing could be considered from the standpoint of the patient's experienced space and time, or from the nurse's, or as a shared event. Explorations of this kind could provide valuable insights into important nursing phenomena, such as presence, empathy, comfort, and timing.

The human situation, is the ground within which nursing takes form. As such, it provides a framework for approaching the study and development of humanistic nursing. As an angular view, it holds the focus on the basic question underlying nursing practice: Is this particular intersubjective, transactional nursing event humanizing or dehumanizing?

CONCLUSION

This chapter explored the foundations of humanistic nursing. The discussion flowed naturally, perhaps unavoidably, into the realm of meta-nursing. "Naturally," for the humanistic nursing approach is itself an outgrowth of the critical examination of nursing as an experienced phenomenon. From this existential perspective of nursing as a living human act, the meaning of nursing is found in the act itself, in nursing's relation to its human context.

Reflection on nursing as it is lived in the real world revealed its existential, nurturing, intersubjective, and transactional character. The process of humanistic nursing stemming from the nurse's authentic commitment is a kind of being with and doing with. It aims at the development of human potential through intersubjectivity and responsible choosing.

The actualization of humanistic nursing is dependent on the concurrent, development of its practice and theoretical foundations by practicing nurses. An open framework derived from the human situation was offered to suggest possible dimensions of humanistic nursing practice that could be described and articulated into a body of theory.

Nurses who have considered this humanistic nursing approach in terms of their daily practice have felt at home in the ideas. The conceptualizations fit their personal nursing experience. If there is any strangeness in the approach, it is perhaps that it does not follow the contours of the clinical specialties to which we have grown so accustomed that they may be more ruts than roads. This is not to say that humanistic nursing is opposed to clinical specialization in nursing. In fact, clinical nursing, as it exists in any form, is its very heart and base. Humanistic nursing is not compartmentalized into clinical (or functional or sociocultural) specialties because it applies in all clinical areas. It is, in the most basic sense, cross-clinical. This may be the great advantage of humanistic nursing. By orienting its explorations ontologically, it may foster genuine cross-clinical studies of nursing phenomena. If nurses with highly developed abilities in particular forms of nursing would struggle together in collaborative cross-clinical studies of nursing phenomena, specialization would serve to advance rather than fragment all nursing.

REFERENCES

1. Buber, M. (1965). Distance and Relation (R. G. Smith, Trans.). In M. Friedman (Ed.), *The knowledge of man* (p. 71). New York, NY: Harper & Row Publishers.
2. Buber, M. 1965. *The Knowledge of Man* (p. 60). New York: Harper Torchbooks.
3. Desan, W. *The planetary man*, Vol. I: *A Noetic Prelude to a United World* (p. 37). New York, NY: The Macmillan Company.
4. Laing, R. D. (1967). *The politics of experience* (p. 23). New York, NY: Ballantine Books.

QUESTIONS FOR REFLECTION

Baccalaureate

1. What is intersubjectivity? Is it always present? How do we know when it is present?
2. What is the difference between more-being and well-being?
3. Describe a situation in which authentic presence made a difference in your own well-being or more-being.

Master's

1. A family nurse practitioner is conducting a well-baby exam. The mother tells the nurse practitioner that she does not intend to consent for immunizations because of the danger of autism. How might the nurse practitioner respond guided by Paterson and Zderad's concepts of choice and human freedom, well-being, more-being, and intersubjectivity?
2. How would you provide evidence for the value of authentic presence in nursing practice?
3. How does the nurse come to know the one nursed in the fullness of his or her being?

Doctoral

1. How are the concepts of nursing situation similar and different in Paterson and Zderad's and Boykin and Schoenhofer's theories?
2. Evaluate Paterson and Zderad's theory using appropriate criteria. What are the strengths and limitations of the theory?
3. Paterson and Zderad quote R.D. Laing who states, "Theory is the articulated vision of experience." With this definition, what is the difference between theory and practice?

9

Caring: The Human Mode of Being

M. SIMONE ROACH

REFLECTIONS ON CARING ATTRIBUTES

In preparation for the first edition of this work (1987), clarification of the concept of human caring came from many sources—the experience of caregivers in education and practice, the ordering of ideas in curriculum development, and observations about what caregivers do when they are caring. The question, What is a nurse doing when he or she is caring?, elicited a wide range of specific responses. To arrange these responses in a manageable order, the "Six Cs" were structured. The study, however, raised a large number of other questions that needed to be addressed.

THE CARING UNIVERSE

The following categories were chosen to allow for diversity in focus and provide logical areas of inquiry for this work. The use of such categories may be instructive in understanding human caring as it is in itself may facilitate development of models for inquiry into caring actions and may be useful for the articulation of education and learning in the caring sciences generally. Such categories have been helpful for the writer in understanding the originality, as well as the complementarity, of the growing body of literature on caring from various perspectives of research in both education and practice.

1. *Ontological.* Ontology is an inquiry into the being of something and into its range of possibilities and asks the questions: What is the being of caring? What is caring in itself?
2. *Anthropological.* Anthropology poses questions such as, Is caring rooted in and claimed as a value in the cultural identity of people? How is human caring expressed among different peoples and cultures?
3. *Ontical.* Onticology refers to the study of some entity in its actual relation with other entities. Examples of ontic statements include normative statements about how one wishes to live, statements of obligation, factual statements and questions. . . . In this category, I include the functional and ethical aspects of caring. What is a person doing when he or she is caring? What obligations are entailed in caring?
4. *Epistemological.* Epistemology is concerned with ways of knowing. Questions in this category include, What are the different ways in which caring may be known, observed, and expressed?
5. *Pedagogical.* The pedagogical category is concerned with teaching and learning and the strategies used to facilitate specific learning needs and goals. How is caring learned and taught?

From Roach, S. (2002). *Caring, the human mode of being* (2nd ed.) (chapter 3, pp. 41–66). Ottawa, Canada: Canadian Healthcare Association. Permission to reprint granted by the Canadian Healthcare Association.

The purpose of identifying a caring universe as a way of posing questions relevant to areas of study is simply to clarify the approach and focus of this particular work. A comprehensive treatment of each is not intended. While some reflections may relate to all categories—the nature of caring as such; what it means to be a caring person; caring functions and behaviors; the knowing, teaching, and learning of caring—these categories are not dealt with systematically. The main purpose of the work is to engage the reader in a process of reflection and inquiry about caring as the *human mode of being*, about human caring as expressed in virtuous acts and to assist in naming one's identity as a professional person intentionally committed to care.

While caring ontology is the overriding theme throughout this work, this chapter focuses on the ontical category. As noted previously, ontic statements include normative statements about how one wishes to live; statements of obligation; expressions of one's "Weltanschauung"; how one incurs moral guilt; factual statements, questions in science, and factual statements of everyday personal and professional life. Functional and ethical manifestations of caring are included in this category.

THE SIX Cs

The Six Cs of Compassion, Competence, Confidence, Conscience, Commitment, and Comportment evolved over time in response to the question, What is a nurse doing when she or he is caring? At this level, specific manifestations of caring as represented by such behaviors as taking the time to be with, checking factual information, identifying and using relevant knowledge, performing technical procedures, showing respect, maintaining trusting relationships, keeping a commitment and comportment in dress and language were generalized into the Six Cs. These are referred to as attributes of caring

and, while not mutually exclusive, serve as a helpful basis for the identification of specific caring behaviors.

Before beginning this second revised edition, a session was arranged with members of the nursing practice committee of St. Martha's Regional Hospital, Antigonish, Nova Scotia. In consultation with the nurse manager of intensive care, palliative care, and progressive care units, a case study was prepared and presented to a group of seven, ranging in experience from 15 to 30 years. While this case study was not identified exclusively with one particular patient, patients, family, and staff on these units commonly experienced the elements highlighted in the study.

The purpose of meeting with members of the nursing practice committee was to obtain feedback on how they see their nursing role as individuals, as members of a team, and to determine what they considered to be the call it represented to nursing in general. To allow for a spontaneous response to the case study, without the influence of bias from my work, the nurses were not given material on the Six Cs prior to the meeting. To my knowledge, no one had used my work on caring, at least not recently.

Each nurse was asked to read the case study and, without discussing it with anyone else, reflect on what this situation called forth in her personally and from nursing in general. After observations were shared, each nurse was asked to discuss the case with a person next to her. A group response was then solicited and both personal and group responses were recorded. After a short break, a brief overview of the Six Cs from the original work was presented, and the group was then provided with a form on which they would record responses.

THE CASE STUDY

Mrs. D., a 52-year-old woman, is a patient in progressive care unit following admission from emergency 3 days ago. She experienced pain in the upper left quadrant for 4 days prior to admission and has had poor appetite and weight loss for several months. She is experiencing lethargy and nausea and, while the pain is under control, she complains of much abdominal discomfort and has little desire for food. Her husband and three adult children are regular visitors, revealing a closely knit family. A medical consultation with the family has just concluded, and the surgeon has related to them the seriousness of Mrs. D.'s condition, noting she has a malignant, inoperable tumor of the pancreas. He assured them everything will be done to keep her as independent and comfortable for as long as possible. Given the progression of her condition, he advised consultation with palliative care and proposed plans for home care, with pain and symptom control. The nurse attending the conference noted the anxiety of the family and the desperate emotional state of the husband. There is obvious disagreement among family members about disclosing the diagnosis to their mother who has a family history of cancer. However, the oldest daughter, a social worker, insists the mother should be given all the facts about her condition, noting her strength and ability to deal with her illness. The other family members disagree, resisting contact with palliative care and pushing the husband to a more protective role, including nondisclosure. A fourth family member has been away from home for several years and has not maintained contact. The father is attempting to trace his whereabouts. He stated this son was "mother's favorite," and often, recently, Mrs. D. has talked about him.

The process with members of the nursing practice committee was carried out in a limited period of time, approximately 1 hour and 30 minutes. The responses were spontaneous and speak for themselves. While the final group response was undoubtedly influenced by an overview of the Six Cs, it was shaped primarily by their initial reaction to the case study. In a letter of appreciation, participants were given written feedback and a copy of the chapter of the book on the Six Cs. I inquired about the accuracy of my summary and invited their comments on the experience. But I did not make a return visit.

Responses revealed much consistency, highlighting the following issues: family involvement and patient–family interaction, truthfulness, the need for information, patient rights, symptom control, and the need for all involved to have an opportunity to participate and communicate feelings. The response of the group as a whole was characterized by a relational quality, with strong emphasis on health team and patient–family involvement. The following is a verbatim summary of specific responses.

Compassion

- Attempt to experience what patient is experiencing
- Patient and family are experiencing the hardest thing possible—loss of someone they love
- Need of family to adjust—the patient may already know
- Recognize loss of patient and family; respond appropriately
- Recognize patient–family needs to express fears, expectations
- Recognize family–patient needs
- Feel for feelings of family members and patient
- Allow expression of "desperate emotional state;" must be a very difficult thing to hear
- They may not have much time; help them come to terms with reality of situation

Competence

- Must know what the condition is about, how treated, and what is available to the patient
- Know how to orchestrate each program and guide patient and family through it
- Importance of experience, understand this illness to be able to treat symptoms: physical, emotional, and so on

- Be able to assess, plan, implement, and evaluate a plan of care to meet the needs of patient–family
- Be aware of upcoming deterioration of condition; support both patient and family
- Understand what patient–family may need physically, emotionally, etc., over next while
- RNs/team has knowledge and skills, communication in guiding patient–family
- Knowledge and experience relative to this diagnosis

Confidence

- I must instill in the patient and family a feeling of confidence
- They have to trust me to give them good information and advice
- We must show that we have the tools to make Mrs. D. comfortable
- Trusting in my ability as a nurse, based on sound knowledge and experience
- Expressing this confidence enables a trusting relationship between nurse–patient–family
- Instill in patient the awareness that you are there for her and for her family
- Comfortable with self (personal qualities, skills)
- Comfortable and open with family and patient
- Enable freedom and aware of risk of taking over for patient–family
- Inform and encourage support of all aspects of care
- Provide holistic care
- Sensitive to ethics. Truthfulness is a big part of this. If truth is brought forward, it gives a trusting relationship with patient and family
- Confidence in trying to bring family together

Conscience

- Trust self and do what I think is right in this situation
- Always advocate for the patient
- Conscience tells me the patient needs to know about her condition; let her decide how to handle it
- Sensitive, informed sense of right–wrong is important to realize that Mrs. D. has a right to know her condition
- Intuitive knowing of what to do or how to respond appropriately
- Helping patient and family to sort out how they are feeling and what their needs are
- Patient must be allowed to put her needs first
- Morals—fine tuned with knowledge and skills
- Understand patient's rights
- Important to let patient know so she can make decisions re her condition and care
- Patient needs to know at appropriate time
- Know patient's rights and ensure that they are not violated
- Ethical decisions to be made, refer to health care team
- Keep informed of ethics–standards
- Know that everyone deals with grave situations differently; deal with everyone as an individual

Commitment

- Sticking with patients through crisis
- Realize ongoing relationships with family; will be with us until patient dies
- As nurses we can help Mrs. D. and family come to terms with her illness
- Staying for the duration and being available when needed

- Letting them know you are committed to them
- Do not give in to the easy way out
- Be there to allow all to express their fears and be an avenue to unite all in a central focus
- Convergence between what you want to do and what you ought to do
- Being able to help family come to consensus so that you–they can be open to patient
- Commitment first for the comfort of the patient and, second, for the whole family, not excluding the patient

Comportment

- Look and sound like the professional I profess to be
- Be true to myself and to the patient
- Important to portray ourselves in a certain way
- Show patient and family that we respect them
- Show patient and family who you are by your dress, manner, and actions
- Always show respect for patient first, disease second
- Present yourself as someone who demands respect
- Always have a way about you that gives family and patient the ability to respect you and, therefore, be comfortable with your knowledge and skills
- Showing the patient and family that I care how they come together for comfort of patient

In writing the account of my session with members of the nursing practice committee of St. Martha's Regional Hospital, I became conscious of the fact there was no mention of spiritual care, at least, not specifically articulated. I did not build into the process a question relative

to spiritual care per se, and I suggest the apparent absence of their attention to this important facet of care was conditioned by the nature of the process itself. This hospital has a strong commitment to its mission and identity as a Christian institution within the Roman Catholic tradition and has a plan for the integration of mission at all levels of its activity. With a vibrant and active Department of Religious and Spiritual Care, "with staff and volunteers available to persons of all denominations and faith traditions, there is no doubt the spiritual needs of this patient and family would have been a priority."

SUGGESTIONS FOR READER PARTICIPATION

The following reflections are offered to the reader as background for further consideration, noting how caring manifests itself in everyday health service, in practice, education, administration, and research. If one is interested in doing so, it might be helpful to revisit the case study. The following questions are a suggested guide only.

1. What is going on?
   - Identify the issues, problems, and dilemmas (if any).
2. Who is involved?
3. What values are explicit, implicit in the narration?
4. What knowledge, affect, skills are required to care for this patient and family?
5. What knowledge, affect, skills do I bring to this situation?
6. How is caring as virtue—as my way of being with this patient and significant others—in this particular situation called forth?
7. What implicit, explicit boundaries does this case study raise for me? For nursing? For health care in general?

8. What is transpiring within myself?

9. What do I wish to be, to become as a person, in my caring ministry?

A FURTHER ELABORATION OF THE SIX Cs

Compassion

Compassion may be defined as a way of living born out of an awareness of one's relationship to all living creatures. It engenders a response of participation in the experience of another, a sensitivity to the pain and brokenness of the other, and a quality of presence that allows one to share with and make room for the other.

In his writings, Henri Nouwen offers key insights on compassion. Of particular significance are reflections he shared with me in the spring of 1980 and published in a work (Nouwen et al., 1983). The word "compassion" is derived from the Latin words pati and cum, which together mean to suffer with and involve us in going

> where it hurts, to enter into the places of pain, to share in brokenness, fear, confusion, and anguish. Compassion challenges us to cry out with those in misery, to mourn with those who are lonely, to weep with those in tears. Compassion requires us to be weak with the weak, vulnerable with the vulnerable, and powerless with the powerless. Compassion means full immersion in the condition of being human. (4)

The resistance this kind of commitment evokes, notes Nouwen, shows that compassion is a much less obvious human virtue than we might be led to believe. It is in discussing this point that Nouwen parts company with some of the contemporary philosophical discussions of caring. He identifies compassion as the radical quality of the Christian life, the call to "be compassionate as your Father is compassionate" (p. 4). But like contemporary philosophical treatises on caring, Nouwen also asserts that it is ultimately through compassion that our humanity grows into fullness.

While working on one of his books, Nouwen and a number of his colleagues visited U.S. Senator Hubert Humphrey to discuss his views on compassion in public life. Humphrey, considered to be one of the most compassionate men in the political life of his time, was more than a little surprised by the purpose of Nouwen's delegation. When he learned of their mission, Humphrey moved from his large desk to a small coffee table in his office. Suddenly, he walked back to his desk, picked up a long pencil with a small eraser at its end and said,

> Gentlemen, look at this pencil. Just as the eraser is only a small part of this pencil and is used only when you make a mistake, so compassion is only called upon when things get out of hand. The main part of life is competition: only the eraser is compassion. It is sad to say, [Humphrey continued], but in politics compassion is just part of competition. (1980, pp. 5–6)

The being compassionate as your Father is compassionate is translated into a call to imitate God's particular way of being with us, God-with-us. According to Nolan (1978), the New Testament account of the miracles of Jesus is evidence of his identification with the suffering, the poor, and the outcast, and he notes "[A]nyone who thinks Jesus' motive for performing miracles of healing was a desire to prove something, to prove that he was the Messiah or Son of God, has thoroughly misunderstood him. His one and only motive for healing people was compassion" (pp. 35–36).

For the Christian, compassion is participation in the compassion of the Godself. It is this participation that provides an antidote for the kind of competitiveness that reduces compassion to the soft eraser at the end of a long pencil, something used only when we make mistakes. Seen within the context of a radical call to the Christian life, compassion becomes our second nature, our natural way of being in the world.

Compassion is a relationship, lived in solidarity with others, sharing their joys, sorrows, pain, and accomplishments. Compassion involves a simple, unpretentious presence to each other, a gift that we seem to have lost even as we have developed sophisticated techniques in our efforts to acquire it. Thus, we cannot go far with commercialized compassion or calculated kindness. For, as Nouwen insists, we do not acquire compassion by advanced skills and techniques. According to his analysis, we receive compassion as a totally gratuitous gift.

As Nouwen (1980) further observes, one of the most tragic events of our time is that we know more than ever before about the sufferings and tragedies of the world, yet we are less able than ever before to respond to them. Perhaps in reflecting on this disturbing reality, we might ponder his insistence that

> [c]ompassion is not a skill that we can master by arduous training, years of study, or careful supervision. We cannot get a Master's degree or a Ph.D. in compassion. Compassion is a divine gift and not a result of systematic study or effort. In a time of so many programs designed to help us become more sensitive, perceptive, and receptive, we need to be reminded continuously that hard work is the fruit of God's pure grace. Therefore, if there is a discipline of compassion, we must understand it as a human response that makes visible a divine gift that has already been given. In title Christian life, discipline is the human effort to unveil what has been covered, to bring to the foreground I what had remained hidden, and to put on the lampstand what had been kept under a basket .... It is the revelation of God's divine spirit in us. (p. 132)

Matthew Fox (1979) considers compassion to be the "world's greatest energy source" and a way of life. He examines compassion from the perspectives of human sexuality, psychology, creativity, science, economics, and politics, and from its central place in the healing of the global village. He asserts that "compassion has been exiled in the West. Part of the flight from compassion has been an ignorance of it that at times borders on forgetfulness, at times on repression, and at times on a conscious effort to distort it, control it and keep it down" (p. 1).

Introducing his analysis with a reflection on what compassion is not, Fox observes that compassion is not pity but celebration; not sentiment but making justice and doing works of mercy; not private, egocentric, or narcissistic but public; not mere human personalism but cosmic in its scope and divine in its energies; not about ascetic detachments or abstract contemplation but passionate and caring; not anti-intellectual but seeks to know and to understand the interconnections of all things. Compassion, says Fox, is not religion but a way of life, that is, a spirituality; not a moral commandment but a flow and overflow of the fullest human and divine energies; not altruism but self-love and other love at one.

The following summary by Fox is helpful:

> Compassion may be a passionate way of living born of an awareness of the interconnectedness of all creatures by reason of their common Creator. To be compassionate is to incorporate one's own fullest energies with cosmic ones into the twin tasks of (1) relieving the pain of fellow creatures by way of justice-making, and (2) celebrating the existence, time and space that all creatures share as a gift from the only One who is fully Compassion. Compassion is our kinship with the universe and the universe's Maker: it is the action we take because of that kinship. (p. 34)

In reflections on compassion, Gula accents care for self as well as care for others.

> Compassion is the virtue which enables us to value the other for himself or herself and not for some functional or utilitarian means to our end.
>
> The heart of compassion is living patiently with others while seeking their well-being. It begins with heeding our own self-care that

nourishes our physical, emotional, spiritual, and moral health. Staying healthy frees us to accept ourselves so that we can be for others without projecting onto them our own needs, fears, and illusions. . . . The virtuous love of self includes neighbor love because we can only come to fulfillment as part of a community of love. Appropriate love of self frees us to meet the needs and to protect the freedom of the vulnerable. (1996, p. 46)

That compassion is an attribute of caring hardly needs defending. In an age where the science and the technology are weighed heavily and often considered the norm for human progress, there is a need to emphasize the humanizing ingredient of compassion and "for the cold and impersonal world of science and technology to be infused by things of the spirit" (Hellegers, 1975, p. 113).

James Cordon speaks about the spirituality of the earth, the compassion of the earth, and about compassion as woven into the fabric of life. Compassion is about experiencing communion and the energy of interconnectedness, supporting the harmony and balance already woven into earth. "Our open invitation is to experience compassion, to fall in love with ourself, with each other, with Earth and the cosmos, to become vulnerable, open, connected" (1994, p. 54). In contemplating the embrace of the earth, attend to the following exercise suggested by Brian Swimme. On a clear night, lie on the ground and look up toward the stars. Close your eyes and imagine you are looking down on the stars because actually you are. What is holding you to the earth? What is keeping you from falling? What does it mean to be held in the embrace of the earth?

Competence

For purposes of this discussion, I shall define competence as the state of having the knowledge, judgment, skills, energy, experience, and motivation required to respond adequately to the demands of one's professional responsibilities.

Compassion, indispensable to the caring relationship, presupposes and operates from a competence appropriate to the demands of human care. While competence without compassion can be brutal and inhumane, compassion without competence may be no more than a meaningless, if not harmful, intrusion into the life of a person or persons needing help.

There was a time when some people, including individuals within the nursing profession, considered kindness and a strong physique as the major requirements for entrance into the occupation of nursing. If this opinion was ever justified, and I suggest it was not, there is no doubt that the demands of nursing today require more than kindness and a strong constitution. Practice in all service professions requires a high degree of cognitive, affective, technical, and administrative skills, with specific competency requirements in each of these areas. Professional caring demands such competence.

One of the threats to caring competence in our day is the misconception and misuse of power. This threat spells the difference between competence as a manifestation of caring and competence as manipulation—as an expression of human violence. The power that is human violence is symbolized by Fox's reference to the up-the-ladder syndrome. In his terms, this syndrome is manifested by an up-down, Sisyphian, competitive, restrictive, elitist survival of the fittest and hierarchical mentality toward living in a world where there can be only winners and losers. It is this kind of power that stifles our capacity to care. In the words of Fox, "When one is climbing a ladder one's hands are occupied with one's own precarious survival and cannot be extended to assist others without putting one's climb and even one's life—if one is high enough upon the ladder—into jeopardy" (1979, p. 49).

It is a power wielded by compulsive people, driven to power, driven to prestige, driven to possessions. It is a kind of power that reflects a restrictive dualistic way of thinking and seeing life's situations exclusively in terms of black–white, either–or, fixed–mutable, science–religion, male–female, conservative–liberal, and so forth. Fox reminds us that this dualism is the ultimate that undermines all possibilities of compassion in the world. And this threat is experienced at a time when we need, perhaps more than ever before, a greater consciousness of the interconnectedness of all things, of a way of seeking both–and, and of a way of living characterized by a letting be, a letting go, and a letting dialectic happen (pp. 85–103).

But caring does indeed demand competence. The ability to care, and to care appropriately and adequately, requires that we have the freedom to learn and the opportunity to practice in our respective professions in a manner compatible with the dignity and needs of those we serve. We should not have to do this, however, at the expense of someone else. We should not have to do it within a power struggle, which suffocates the very source of caring energy, a power struggle that is exemplified by the drive to be at the top of the pyramid. Are there power struggles in your workplace? What effect do they have on team spirit and on the freedom of caregivers to care?

Being-in-the-world, being-for-others is authentic when it calls the other to freedom; it is inauthentic when characterized by dominance and depersonalization. The mature use of power does not preclude respect for self, nor does it imply the relinquishment of legitimate personal autonomy. It implies an understanding of competence tempered by a compassion that is "the ultimate and most meaningful embodiment of emotional maturity" and through which a person "achieves the highest peak and deepest reach in his or her search for self-fulfillment" (Jersild, 1957, p. 201).

Confidence

The term confidence is defined as the quality that fosters trusting relationships.

It seems impossible to think of caring without, at the same time, thinking about the importance of a trusting relationship. It is equally impossible to imagine achieving the goals of service without, at the same time, assuming that the service will be rendered within an environment and under conditions of mutual trust and respect. Much is being done in professional disciplines to foster trusting relationships. But, while confidence might be considered as a given, its absence in the world of everyday affairs creates the need to examine the quality of its presence in the service fields.

In a work by Sissela Bok, the author speaks about the decline in public confidence in the United States. Bok notes:

> The loss of confidence reached far beyond government leadership. From 1966–1976, the proportion of the public answering yes to whether they had a great deal of confidence in people in charge of running major institutions dropped from 73 percent to 42 percent for medicine; for major companies from 55 percent to 16 percent; for law firms from 24 percent (1973) to 12 percent; and for advertising agencies from 21 percent to 7 percent. (1979, p. xviii)

There does not seem to be strong evidence that this situation has changed much for the better during the time since the last edition of this work was published. Frequent litigation infers a rapidly increasing climate of mistrust within the professions, as well as in society as a whole, and a brief search of material on-line reveals the extent of concern about trust and confidence in public institutions. (Global concerns are raised in Pharr and Putnam [2000].)

Duplicity in public life appears under many guises. Duplicity in health care, according to Bok, is similarly camouflaged, in some cases, with deliberate deception in care, and experimentation and research treated casually or with indifference. In relating to this phenomenon, Bok notes the lack of stress on veracity in medical codes, for example, and examines the arguments used to rationalize and justify lying to clients. Codes of ethics for research, particularly those receiving public funding, do provide a safety net, however, and guidelines are there to increase awareness and sensitivity to the violence of human trespass.

The March 23, 2001 edition of the *Toronto Star*, carried the following headline, "Medical Students Pressured to Be Unethical: Survey." According to this report by Helen Branswell, Canadian Press, a survey of medical students at the University of Toronto Medical School "found nearly half had been put in situations where they were pressured to act unethically by their teachers." The situations, as reported, included doing examinations on comatose or anesthetized patients without their consent; without consent, doing procedures for teaching purposes that did not have to be done; and having patients make unnecessary return visits to clinics for teaching purposes only. The associate dean, responsible for the undergraduate medical training program, responded to the coverage by saying the *British Medical Journal* which published the report had done the profession a service. Noting the University of Toronto was no different and certainly no worse than any other school, the focus was welcomed as a means of drawing attention to the issues, and as a reminder that patients could no longer be taken for granted in teaching hospitals. The university has taken steps to strengthen ethics education.

Fidelity to canons of loyalty, to the ethical standards in teaching situations in teaching hospitals, can be on very fragile ground. The attitude that patients admitted to teaching hospitals *know they will be used for teaching and could go elsewhere* is not uncommonly expressed. The tension between teaching and the learning needs of students in all health disciplines and the service–care requirements of patients and families has been ever present. The issue is not *no more patient-centred learning*

but attentiveness and fidelity to the virtue of caring in all situations, acknowledging the patient–family as partners in the educational enterprise, not objects to be used. This obviously presumes respect and always consent.

It is not within the parameters of this work to do a comprehensive study of health care codes of ethics. But reference will be made in a subsequent chapter to challenges to canons of professional ethics as guarantor of, or even as a reliable norm for, ethical practice (Brockett, 1997; Pellegrino et al., 1991). A brief statement from the Canadian Nurses Association *Code of Ethics for Registered Nurses* is of interest here.

The nurse–client relationship presupposes a certain measure of trust on the part of the client. Care and trust complement one another in professional nursing relationships. Both hinge on the values identified in the code. By upholding these values in practice, nurses earn and maintain the trust of those in their care (1997, p. 5).

The use of deception is one issue that still remains as both a threat and a topic of controversy. Regardless of the weight of the arguments used for distorting the truth or the complexity of the problems with which the caring profession has to deal, I still make the claim that deliberate deception—even the co-called "white lie"—not only shatters the confidence of the client but also damages the integrity of the professional as well. Deception destroys confidence; deliberate deception is the antithesis of caring.

Caring confidence fosters trust without dependency, communicates truth without violence, and creates a relationship of respect without paternalism or without engendering a response born out of fear or powerlessness. Confidence, then, is a critical attribute of professional caring.

Conscience

Conscience, understood as the morally sensitive self attuned to values, is integral to personhood (see Maguire, 1978).

Conscience reflects the sacredness of the person, points to the sacred core of the personality and to the centre of personal integrity. Conscience is the voice where the claim of the one is asserted over the power and the persuasion of the many. Conscience is the medium through which moral obligation is personalized.

This is not to claim that conscience is simply a matter of personal opinion and, as such, supersedes the collective moral perceptions of the group. Individual conscience must be sensitive and informed. Individual and collective consciences are not adversaries; it is not a question of one or the other. Moral judgment requires the wisdom of both.

Conscience is related to the whole structure of one's being—to care. Authentic existence by definition is acting in accord with self and conscious awareness; inauthentic existence is not acting in accord with such awareness. Care, as primordial, is the foundation of moral consciousness (see Heidegger, 1962).

Moral norms, standards, principles, and values, grounded in religious faith, shape our actions by enlightening reason and enable us to reflect on and articulate the values by which we live. A further examination of conscience as an ingredient of our reflection and formative in decision making may help us understand the movements of that process.

Most persons experience conscience: "My conscience tells me." "My conscience bothers me." But, as universal as the experience of conscience may be, individual variation and misperceptions are commonplace. The *Canadian Oxford Dictionary* uses the Latin derivative conscientia (knowledge) and conscire (to know or be privy to) (s.v. "conscience"). When the word is broken down into its two derivatives—cum (together) and scientia, scira (to know)—it includes not only knowledge and awareness but *together* as well. This latter interpretation offers an understanding of conscience as connoting a relationship—persons as

social and communal: "Conscience is the person's moral faculty, the inner core and sanctuary where one knows oneself in confrontation with God and with fellowmen [women]. We can confront ourselves reflexively only to the extent that we genuinely encounter the Other and the others" (Haring, 1978, p. 224).

Psychology helps to clarify the understanding of conscience, particularly in the distinction made between it and the superego. In the Freudian school, the superego is interpreted as the policeman of the personal life, regulating behavior strongly influenced by guilt. Gula (1989) likens the superego to the attic of a house where all the "shoulds" and "have-to's" are stored. Regulating behavior from the fingerpointing authorities of the past, in overdependency on being loved and approved, the individual is moved only by external rules, demands, and guilt fixations. Reductionist views eliminate conscience as a factor in shaping behavior, emphasizing instead conscience dependent on training according to social norms or domination by the superego. "The moral conscience, on the other hand, acts in love responding to the call to commit ourselves to value" (p. 126).

O'Connell (1976) provides three helpful distinctions: Conscience: general sense of value, awareness of personal responsibility, capacity for self-direction, human responsibility for good direction. Despite cultural differences in interpretation, "all human persons share a sense of the goodness and badness of their deeds" (p. 89). Conscience: exercise of moral reasoning; identification and perception of values; involves reflection, discussion, and analysis. At this stage, all that shapes our lives and ways of thinking influence decision making. Even when we bring to this process the sincerity of honest judgment, however, we can be wrong. We need the assistance and insights of others, the wisdom of the past and objective voices from the church and society. To make responsible moral–ethical decisions, our conscience needs to be educated. Conscience: concrete judgment pertaining to immediate action.

Gula (1989) parallels the preceding distinction describing conscience as (1) capacity—one's fundamental ability to discern good and evil, (2) process—as the discovering of what makes for being a good person, what particular action is right or wrong, the process of being formed and informed, and (3) judgment—following inquiry and leading to judgment. And Gula remarks, this will be as reliable as the homework we do to inform it.

The word conscience is defined as a state of moral awareness; a compass directing one's behavior according to the moral fitness of things. As an expression of caring, conscience entails responsivity, expressing itself as a response to something that matters and a response to a value as the important-in-itself. It involves the spiritual power of affectivity.

The writer D.C. Maguire considers affective reaction to value to be the "foundational moral experience" (1978, p. 84). Conscience is "the morally conscious self in his [her] acute state of moral awareness" (p. 371). Affective response is not equated with emotivism or mere feeling states. It is an intentional response, deliberate, meaningful, and rational. In locating moral consciousness in love and caring, Maguire relates the following incident from anthropologist Loren Eisley:

> Anthropologist Loren Eisley, starting from the existence of the one-armed skeletal remains of a Neanderthal man, offers an imaginative reflection that is relevant:
>
> Forty thousand years ago in the bleak uplands of south-western Asia, a man, a Neanderthal man, once labeled by the Darwinian proponents of struggle as a ferocious ancestral beast—a man whose face might cause you some slight uneasiness if he sat beside you—a man of this sort existed with a fearful body handicap in that ice-age world. He had lost an arm. But still he lived and was cared for. Somebody, some group of human things, in a hard, violent and stony world, loved this maimed creature enough to cherish him.
>
> Somewhere there in the period of harsh beginnings, there appeared, in Eisley's words, loving, caring, and cherishing. Concern was born and with it morality. . . . What it was the light of a distinctively human consciousness, animated by the unique energy that we have come to call love. This ability to appreciate and respond to the value of personal life in all its forms is the foundation of moral consciousness. (pp. 85–86)

Conscience is the caring person attuned to the moral nature of things. Conscience is not simply a thing added on at some point in one's experience. Conscience grows out of experience, out of a process of valuing self and others. Conscience is the "call of care and manifests itself as care" (Heidegger, 1962, p. 319).

The particular state of moral awareness that constitutes the self at any given time is fallible; its claim on right and wrong is not absolute. In an experiential sense, no one realizes this fact more than the person who struggles to understand the moral implications of human relationships and the moral status of the actions of human beings on one another. Professional caring demands that our moral awareness be fine-tuned by the discipline of knowledge and moral inquiry. Professional caring is reflected in a mature conscience and is understood to subsume the moral–ethical imperatives and norms of professional life.

Commitment

For purpose of this discussion, commitment is defined as a complex affective response characterized by a convergence between one's desires and one's obligations, and by a deliberate choice to act in accordance with them.

A work on educational objectives—affective domain (Krathwohl et al., 1964)—provides helpful insights on the internalization of values. Of particular significance is its placement of commitment on a continuum where internalization of a particular value is recognized as well established. Commitment presupposes or goes beyond other behavioral responses such as willingness to receive, willingness to respond, an acceptance of a value, and a preference for a value. In this work, commitment is considered to be evident when choice is so firm that what one commits oneself to do is synonymous with what one prefers to do. Commitment becomes part of one's identity as a professional, caring person.

In Mayeroff's philosophical analysis, caring is considered to subsume the quality of devotion. According to this analysis, in devotion, as noted previously, there is convergence between what I want to do and what I am supposed to do. Devotion (commitment) is essential to caring: if devotion (commitment) breaks down, caring breaks down. Commitment is a quality of investment of self in a task, a person, a choice or a career, and therefore a quality that is so internalized as a value that what I am obligated to do is not regarded as a burden. But rather it is a call that draws me to a conscious, willing, and positive course of action.

The everyday experiences of persons in health care are shaped by many forces and conditions; some are obvious while others are not. While it is individuals who make commitments, the latter are always influenced by social factors. The health care person brings to work on a given day concerns of family and of personal relationships. And the ability to care itself may be nurtured or hampered by the work environment and constraints of the system. Perhaps Mayeroff's reminder of the reality of human limitation—there are a limited number of persons, projects, and things to which we can commit ourselves at any given time—helps to take these realities into account. In speaking with groups of nurses, emphasizing this point has often been sufficient to diffuse a false

guilt. To realize one's limits in the ability to care and to be compassionate toward self can create the energy caregivers need to care even more.

A work by Farley (1986) provides a comprehensive study of personal commitments—beginning, keeping, and changing. While Farley's work is beyond the scope of this book, her ideas around commitment, love, promise-keeping and, in the context of faith, of covenant are most helpful. In her discussion of forms of commitment, she identifies what she calls a "'prime case' a central form of commitment—one from which all other forms derive some meaning. Commitment to persons, when it is explicit and expressed offers such a 'prime case'" (p. 15). An ethic of care, caring as relational responsibility, presupposes a commitment to persons.

A further distinction Farley makes about the nature of commitments is also enlightening. There are commitments to truth; to values such as the institution and family life; to justice, beauty, and peace; to plans of action; to be a good parent; and to live in accordance with the Gospel. But the common meaning that keeps these values from becoming empty, abstract ideals is willingness to do something. And then there are commitments that may be total or partial. Total commitments involve the whole person, raise identity issues about who one really is and desires to be, and constitute fundamental life options. These may be marriage and family or a choice of a vowed life in a religious order. Partial commitments may include a professional choice, a job or position. In consideration of such distinctions, perhaps the greatest challenge of persons committed to care is to determine priorities and acknowledge limitations in all of them. No attempt is made here to even suggest solutions to a call that is, in reality, a life task.

At any given moment, we experience different levels of commitment and varying degrees of difficulty in being faithful to the choices we believe we ought to make.

Some responses do not require reflection and are so internalized they are almost automatic. A good parent, for example, does not deliberate at 3:00 a.m. whether he or she should respond to the needs of the sick child. Response is an unquestioned and implicit convergence between what the parent wants to do and what he or she ought to do. It is an expression and a manifestation of who she or he is as a person and as a parent. At other times, whether the matter is trivial or seriously complex, a decision requires deliberate reflection and choice may be more difficult. As with the other Cs, commitment is always the challenge that caring demands.

Comportment

The idea of comportment as an attribute of caring emerged from a discussion with a competent and committed clinical nurse specialist. This person expressed concern and uneasiness over what she observed in the dress and language of nurses while caring for patients. The problems involved sloppy dress and inappropriate language, and the concern and uneasiness came from the unfitness of both to the caring image of a professional caregiver. Comportment, meaning bearing, demeanor, or to be in agreement or harmony with, served as an appropriate attribute to subsume these kinds of concerns. It must be noted, however, that the interpretation and use of the word comportment in this context is more restricted than its meaning of *overall commitment*, as sometimes used.

Dress and language are symbols of communication and can be in harmony or disharmony with a caring presence. When we visit a special person, our mode of dress and choice of language are usually in accord with the regard, esteem, and respect with which the person is held. Without necessarily reflecting on the matter, we usually dress and use language consistent with our attitude toward the person or the occasion. We dress appropriately and observe certain socially accepted

protocols when we accept an invitation to a garden party at Buckingham Palace, the White House, or the residence of the governor general of Canada.

In the past few decades, as a reaction or, perhaps, even a protest against conformity to former rigid standards of dress, there has been a radical change to a more practical choice of uniforms appropriate to different situations. Speaking of nursing, Kaiser refers to studies indicating that by the mid-1970s, "the traditional nurse's uniform had become increasingly ineffective as professional clothing, for several reasons" (1985, p. 372). The reasons included a general decline in the prestige of uniforms and an emphasis on "power" dressing among professionals in the larger culture. Many nonprofessional workers' dress resembled that of nurses—the latter thus losing their sense of identity—and greater numbers of men entering the nursing profession. Increasing numbers of nurses were found in more diverse clinical roles and management positions.

But we also experience the shadow side of change, sometimes with an "everything goes" mentality, and less demonstration of what even social grace might require as "professional attire." In some situations, dress codes seem more difficult to establish and even more difficult to adhere to. I suggest we need to reflect on whether such a trend is consistent with our stated beliefs about the dignity of persons, including ourselves as professional caregivers. How does observance of social etiquette in the situations noted previously transfer into regard for the patient, family, colleagues, and others? Given the nature of current practice, I suggest this question deserves honest reflection at all levels of the health care professions. We might begin by asking, Are dress and language of caregivers consistent with the belief that the patient–client is of incalculable worth, and that the caregiver himself or herself is a person of intrinsic worth and dignity?

Caring is reflected in bearing, demeanor, dress, and language. An inquiry into the symbolism of dress and language and their relationship to professional caring could be an interesting area for research. According to Kaiser's study, appearance continues to be an important sign of "legitimacy" and identity for health care workers. Perhaps, the central question is, What does clothing mean? What signs and symbols does dress communicate? And considering there are other signs that communicate something about who we are, Kaiser continues,

> [Y]et clothing is one of the most eloquent and powerful products we use; it is an expressive medium, or concrete way revealing particular ideas in the mind that cannot be otherwise articulated. The object and sign are linked in a way that is highly visual, connected intimately with the person (owner), and conducive to every social dimension of daily life. (p. 219)

SUMMARY

Reflections on the attributes of professional caring presented in this chapter are intended to cast light on the range of possibilities of human caring from the ontical perspective. They are presented as goals that we are always striving to achieve. Given the woundedness experienced by all persons who desire to live the virtuous life, we are not always where we want to be, and we fall short of the expectations we have of ourselves. Such occasions provide a test for the quality of compassion we have toward ourselves.

The ontic category addresses such questions as, How does one wish to live? What obligations are entailed in particular choices? What constitutes caring in the everyday life of a professional person? What is a person doing when he or she is caring? No attempt is made here, however, to deal with these questions in such a manner as to arrive at precise, specific answers. The exercise of responding to a case study was a simple way of drawing out the caring capacity already present and operative in the nurses who composed a nursing practice committee of a regional hospital. It was not designed as a controlled research study.

The Six Cs are used as a broad framework, suggesting categories of human behavior within which professional caring is to be understood. In compassionate and competent acts; in relationships qualified by confidence; through informed, sensitive conscience; through commitment and fidelity; and in a manner of dress and language in harmony with held beliefs about the dignity of persons, specific manifestations of caring are actualized. Behavior expressed by the Six Cs says a great deal about personal identity. Most importantly, such a way of virtuous acting encompasses much of what a professional person wants to be.

QUESTIONS FOR REFLECTION

Baccalaureate

1. Is a dress code necessary to convey caring to patients? Why or why not?
2. How can the nurse grow in compassion?
3. If confidence is one of the Six Cs how can a novice nurse or student present this attribute with a patient?

Master's

1. Are the Six Cs applicable to advanced practice nursing? How so or why not?
2. What is the evidence for Roach's creation of the Six Cs? How did she develop these caring attributes? How might you validate their relevance to your practice?
3. What caring attribute is most compromised in contemporary nursing practice? Support your response with some rationale.

Doctoral

1. What are the categories of inquiry related to caring that Roach includes in "The Caring Universe"? What is the meaning of each?
2. If you are studying the nature of caring, of what it is in itself, what category of inquiry are you engaged in: Ontological? Ontical? Anthropological? Epistemological? Or pedagogical?
3. How might the Six Cs be tested as a theoretical framework? Suggest a research question and possible design to answer it that might address some aspect of the framework.

10

New Dimensions of Human Caring Theory

JEAN WATSON

DAWNING OF A CARING–HEALING CONSCIOUSNESS

The present and future are requiring radical transformations of worldview, as well as level of consciousness about the nature of the health care delivery system, the nurse–patient caring–healing relationships, and even the nature of the nursing profession. The future of medicine and nursing belongs to *caring* more than *curing*. A more radical thesis is that there is movement out of an era in which *curing* is dominant into an era in which *caring* must take precedence (Callahan, 1987). Accordingly, during the past decade, the concepts of care and caring have gained greater awareness and emphasis in nursing literature and research (Benner, 1984, 1988; Leininger, 1980, 1984; Ray, 1987; Watson, 1979, 1985, in press). This shift has been brought about by the impact of science and technology and outdated views of science, along with trends in the health care delivery system, as well as the nature of caring and curing (e.g., more is known about treatment and cure than about healing and human caring processes). Moreover, the ethical differences between care and cure issues are felt more poignantly by nurses than any other professionals (Gadow, 1987); perhaps this is

contributing to a heightened awareness of the need to change and face ethical responsibilities.

As Moccia (1988a, p. 30) puts it, nursing and the health care system are "at the faultline" regarding social activism and caring, which requires a new consciousness. "The choice facing nursing is whether to work toward a health care system that more closely approximates nursing's (caring) values and concerns or to manipulate itself and its members to reserve a place in a system that is increasingly removed from the profession's concerns and expertise." As a result, nursing is in a major transition; indeed the nursing profession is in the process of being redefined.

REDEFINING CONTEMPORARY NURSING

Sarter (1988) analyzed four contemporary nursing theories and identified commonly shared thinking that is related to nursing's redefinition. She reported such consistent themes in recent writings as process, evolution of consciousness: self-transcendence, open systems, harmony, relativity of space-time, pattern, and holism. Thus, a new consciousness is beginning to emerge, which allows the profession

From Watson, J. (1988). New dimensions of human caring theory. *Nursing Science Quarterly*, 1(4), 175–188. Permission to reprint granted by Sage Publications, Inc.

and the discipline of nursing to raise new questions about what it means to be a nurse, to be ill, to be caring, to be healing.

Because of the changing times and human consciousness, there are some new options. Rather than having to stay within the same debate of detecting or fighting disease and remaining in conflict with the larger and more dominant ideology of the system (which often denies or disregards nurses' caring values), there is another moral, if not ontological course that is positing caring as a moral ideal and an end in and of itself (Gadow, 1985, 1987; Watson, 1985). Further, such thinking introduces new human possibilities that accommodate transcendence and other metaphysical concepts in relation to health and illness. This thinking places human caring, as a moral ideal, in a field consciousness of transpersonal caring–healing that becomes dominant over physical illness, the curing ethic, and the dominant treatment ideology (Newman, 1986; Parse, 1981; Rogers, 1970, 1983; Watson, 1985, in press).

Human caring can now be recognized as a place in which health professionals can do and must live (Gadow, 1987) when the system is in crisis, and the outdated morality of treatment and cure "at all costs" is breaking down financially, morally, scientifically, and spiritually. In the human caring framework, the relationship between cure and care is inverted, thereby designating care/caring as the highest form of commitment to patients (Gadow, 1987). In the usual view, cure is the standard, the overriding goal, and care is nothing but a means toward the end. In this inverted framework proposed by Gadow, which is consistent with human caring theory, care/caring becomes the ethical principle or standard by which treatments and interventions are measured. Gadow further suggests that only in the context of care/caring can the overpowering of one person by another, that cure entails, be redeemed. Moccia (1988a) acknowledges that while a substantial number of individual nurses have and always will

practice from a caring model, they have generally done so as employees of systems created and controlled by medicine. What is now surfacing from nurses and the larger society is a challenge to the values and dominant medical ideology for health and healing. That is not to say that society does not need the best that medicine has to offer. However, with this new view of caring as a moral ideal and end, cure is only a means, indeed as Gadow indicates, often a detour from issues of health and healing, one from which there may be no return.

Human caring theory in practice allows the commitment and consciousness of the nurse to transcend (or at least attempt to transcend) the physical material surface and reach beyond to touch the human center of the person (Watson, in press). Without the moral-transcendent perspective a nonprofessional, noninformed practice perpetuates the current controversy that suggests nurses are not moral agents (Cooper, 1988; Packard & Ferrara, 1988; Yarling & McElmurry, 1986). Some of this controversy is highlighted by Kelly's (1988) recent editorial wherein she says that if nurses do not accept a personal mandate to adopt a caring awareness and ethic, they too will be responsible for discarding the ethic of caring. Cooper (1988) explored the caring consciousness in relation to the covenantal relationship and moral commitment. She references Gadow's position that a covenantal relationship provides a more substantial foundation for the nursing caring ethic. On this same line, Fry (1988) questions whether a caring ethic can survive in nursing.

Perhaps caring cannot survive unless it is upheld as a moral ideal, in theory and practice, and unless it becomes a philosophical basis for nursing to more fully actualize its ideology, knowledge, and practice of caring. As Cooper notes: "The nurse's duty of fidelity to the patient is dictated by his or her choice to become a nurse and thereby to embrace the professional and moral responsibility inherent in such a choice" (Cooper, 1988, p. 58). Such thinking, however, is tied to consciousness. Chinn says:

> In nursing, we cannot practice what we do not know. . . . What possibilities might exist If we were to work with a fuller range of knowledge (transcendent, evolving consciousness, human center view of nursing's transpersonal caring–healing phenomena?) . . . If we can learn to value that which we already know about . . . we certainly will begin to comprehend the urgency of shifting our focus in a direction that is more fully consistent with our intents and values. (Chinn, 1988, p. viii; author's parentheses)

Caring further defined in this philosophical and epistemological sense avoids reducing person to the moral status of object and introduces new caring–healing possibilities associated with both the art and science of transpersonal caring–healing and transcendent views of persons in health and illness. Again as Gadow (1985) points out so eloquently, to the extent that human dignity is diminished, the patient is no longer the center of his or her own experience for meaning and coherence. People are reduced to the moral status of objects. An even greater problem associated with this is that when patients are reduced to objects, then professionals are likewise reduced to objects.

Lewis Mumford in the *Myth of the Machine* says it this way:

> We must both in our thinking and our action come back to the human center; for it is there that all significant transformations begin and terminate. (Mumford, 1970, p. 420)

The notion of human center allows for a transpersonal process to go on between the nurse and the patient, which allows for the spirit or the "geist" of both to be present in the caring moment. Transpersonal caring expands the limits of openness and accesses the higher human spirit or field consciousness; therefore, it has the capacity to expand human consciousness, transcend the moment, and potentiate healing (Watson, 1985, in press). Both the one caring and the one cared for

are influenced through the transaction, for better or for worse.

The human caring process has an energy field of its own, which is greater than either one of the persons. It is part of a human consciousness process that can arise from itself, yet it goes beyond itself and becomes part of the life history of each person, as well as part of some larger, deeper, complex pattern of life (Watson, 1985, in press). Therefore, the human center has energy and power of its own, yet the human caring–healing consciousness can potentiate healing and release one's own inner power and resources by creating the expanded energy field. Restoring and preserving the human center maintains the human spirit in the health care system. It helps to prevent succumbing to object status, which further helps prevent caring from becoming a means to an even more technological end that justifies further reduction of person to moral status of machine. The proposed human-centered, caring–healing consciousness is a call to higher power, with the caring–healing consciousness as an existential turning point in the life of both the nurse and the patient, a moment for a call to a higher consciousness and an authentic choice of living.

NURSING IN RELATION TO TRANSPERSONAL CARING THEORY

Nursing within a transpersonal caring perspective attends to the human center of both the one caring and the one being cared for; it embraces a spiritual, even metaphysical dimension of the caring process; it is concerned with preserving human dignity and restoring and preserving humanity in the fragmented, technological, medical cure-dominated systems (Watson, 1985, in press). When transpersonal caring as a moral ideal becomes the highest form of commitment to patients and therefore the standard for care, as well as an end in itself, then nurses are able to return the profession to Mumford's "human center."

Metaphysical Transcendent Dimensions

To capture some of the metaphysical aspects of such notions as human center and transpersonal caring, new language and symbols are often necessary to convey the depth of such human dimensions that occur in the lived moment of nursing and human caring (Watson, 1987a). Poetry is one form of language that reflects the human depth. One such example is the result of prize-winning poet Marllyn Krysl's commissioned work as a visiting poet in the new Center for Human Caring in the University of Colorado School of Nursing. Some of her comments that emerged from her experiences with nurses capture the metaphysical and higher energy dimensions of transpersonal caring described here.

> Caring takes place, so to speak, in the metaphysical realm. We cannot "see" this realm, but we experience it. Over and over I watched the care giver and the person accepting care as they came to constitute one wholeness.
>
> When two of us enter into each other in this way, willingly and receptively, transformation takes place. The gestalt of our separate beings loosens and vibrates. . . . And we are filled with energy, a living material, palpable, substantial.
>
> This energy is nearly visible in the air around us. It is as though we give off light. . . . I became fascinated by these moments of transcendence. They occur again and again, each time . . . a moment of intense energy . . . I felt I was witnessing the invisible brought to light. I was witnessing the spirit made flesh. (Krysl, 1989)

Her exemplary work titled *Midwife* more fully conveys these expanded metaphysical dimensions of transcendence in human caring.

Midwife
Marllyn Krysl*

Though I seem to wait
I'm moving at the speed of light
Though I seem to stand by
I'm running easily over the
   windswept grasslands to where
   the river divides the plains from
   the mountains
Though I seem to stand by
I'm gathering the sweet and the
   bitter herbs in shade and in
   sunlight
I'm digging out the bones of the
   lost animals embedded in the
   lakes of tar
Though I seem idle
I'm releasing the father's fear into
   the wind,
watching the wind disperse it
Though I seem idle
I'm sending the mother the energy
   of the waves of the deep and of the
   shallow waters
Though I seem idle
I'm traveling by night and by day,
   over earth and over sea to meet
   the new being
When I time the contractions
I'm counting the sheeves of grain
   gathered in the mother's harvest
When I measure the opening
I'm calculating the number of
   followers in the mother's fields
And when I touch the father's
   shoulder
I'm singing the many names of the
   ancestors who overcame fear
When I seem to pause
I send light to the father, to the
   mother, to the older sister
When I seem to pause
I send light to those who will wash
   and wrap the new being

*Reprinted by permission of author, Center for Human Caring University of Colorado School of Nursing (1989).

When I listen to the heartbeat of
the new being coming
I hear the tumbling of water down
a great falls
When I lean forward, hands
cupped for the head
I'm dividing the wind in the four
directions
When I lean forward, hands cupped
for the head
I'm gathering together the rain and
the desert heat
And when at last I hold the head in
my hands
I've hoisted the sun to the pinnacle
of the heavens
When I hold the new being in my
hands
I've brought the mother, father and
child to the center of the eleven
sacred circles
And when I lay the new being on
the mother's breast
I'm sending the flocks of goats out
to graze on the hillsides and in the
valleys
I'm letting the fish loose at the
headwaters of the Rivers
I'm letting the birds go upward and
out into the great migrations
When I clamp the cord in two
places
I'm saying the child's two named,
one from the mother, one from the
father
When I give the father the tool to
cut the cord
I'm binding three people together
until the death of the last of the
three
When I take the print of the new
being's foot
I'm writing on the ancient tablet
the word just uttered
When I wait for the placenta
I'm spreading bleached linen on all
the mattresses of darkness
And when it comes, when I examine the placenta

I'm sorting the particles and waves
in the spectrum of light
And when my work is finished and
I go from the place of birth
I walk out across the fields of the
planets into the spaces between
the furthest stars

Holographic-Extended Science Metaphor

While new esthetic language is needed to reflect some of the metaphysical, human center, transcendent higher dimensions of transpersonal caring–healing, so too is a new perspective of science. One science paradigm that offers a hopeful metaphorical model for these more elusive concepts is commonly referred to as the holographic paradigm (Battista, 1982; Bohm, 1976, 1980; Harman, 1982, 1987a; Pribram, 1971; Wilber, 1982). As Harman explains, the old science attempts to explain away consciousness, rather than understand it. "The holographic theory suggests a pulse of energy which in the physical domain seems to occur at a particular instant in time, in the frequency domain is 'timeless,' 'eternal,' and beyond time and space" (Harman, 1982, p. 139). The holographic perspective suggests a new wholeness in all the parts and a perspective wherein consciousness is more nearly cause than effect.

Recent writings in physics and neuroscience speculate that the brain, and indeed the universe, may be like a hologram. A hologram is described as having a realm of frequencies and potential underlying an illusion of concreteness (Watson, 1987b). Pribram (1971) suggests that humans construct "hard" reality by interpreting frequencies from a dimension transcending time and space. Contemporary nursing theoretical systems (Newman, 1986; Parse, 1981; Rogers, 1970) accommodate the holographic thinking by defining human beings as energy fields, open systems engaged in continual energy exchange with the environment, centers of energy, patterns of consciousness, and so on. An energy field of consciousness is a nonphysical phenomenon. A science of cells, at a less sophisticated stage of evolving science, considers physical causation to be somehow more "real" than the more abstract levels of energy field or field-consciousness. Higher order concepts introduced in transpersonal caring–healing processes invoke an expanded science model (Watson, 1985). Indeed, as Moccia (1988b) recently notes, fundamental issues related to ontologies, epistemologies, values, and intentions are now being questioned and clarified to address future directions for nursing science and debate.

At a new level in nursing's caring–healing consciousness, regardless of one's theoretical inclinations, there is the continual need to search and to acknowledge that the traditional models of health-illness and science are inadequate for the lived world of patients and the lived caring–healing processes nurses experience in transpersonal caring moments. Just as poetry, language, and experiences of aesthetics help in seeing the higher level dimensions of nursing, the metaphor of a hologram provides a new science language as well as a new gestalt for viewing the transpersonal caring–healing human field-consciousness phenomena.

Some of the basic holographic principles are captured in the following points (Watson, 1987b, p. 102, adapted from works of Battista, 1982; Bohm, 1976; Pribram, 1971, 1982; Wilber, 1982; and others):

- The whole is in the part.
- There is an inseparable interconnectedness between humans and between humans and the universe.
- Mind/consciousness is joined; consciousness is communicated.
- Human consciousness is spatially extended; consciousness exists through space.
- Human consciousness is temporally extended; consciousness exists through time.
- Human consciousness is dominant over physical matter.

To apply this hologram metaphor to transpersonal caring–healing, one can possibly consider the following connections: (adapted from Watson, 1987b, p. 102)

- The whole caring–healing consciousness is contained in a single caring moment.
- The one caring–healing and the one-being-cared-for-healed are interconnected; caring and healing are connected to other humans and to the higher energy of the universe.
- Human caring–healing (or noncaring–nonhealing) consciousness of the nurse is communicated to the one being cared for.
- Caring–healing consciousness is spatially extended; such consciousness exists through space.
- Caring–healing consciousness is temporally extended; such consciousness exists through time.
- Caring–healing consciousness is dominant over physical illness and treatment.

Transpersonal caring–healing viewed within a holographic framework can be seen as interpenetrating holographic energies, which can provide an avenue for shared consciousness between the nurse and patient (Overman, 1986). The caring–healing moment transforms from a two- to a one-field consciousness. The shared energy system of caring–healing energy is the greater entity. In the transpersonal caring framework proposed, both the one caring and the one being cared for are coparticipants in the process that can potentiate self-healing, regardless of the medical condition. In such a transpersonal caring moment, both are capable of transcending self, time, and space. As Whitehead (1953) described it, this shared caring experience creates its own field. His notion of concrescence indicates the coming together of many to form one. He explained that all past experiences are brought to bear on present occasions and merge with it to form the current experience (Whitehead, 1953). Concrescence and the notion of transpersonal caring–healing imply a completion or a wholeness in the formation of the one caring and imply the intersubjectivity and interconnectedness of persons and the universe.

While such holographic thinking associated with the nurse's caring–healing consciousness does not dictate specific behaviors or actions, the nurse's caring–healing consciousness held as a moral ideal during a transpersonal caring moment directs the nurse toward new ontologies as well as epistemologies in developing nursing theory and nursing science. Such thinking, derived from new ways of valuing, being, and knowing associated with the holographic principles, directs nursing toward certain action pathways for the future and not toward others.

Extended Science-Upward Causation Perspective

Another recent model (Figure 10.1) for accommodating transpersonal caring–healing within a caring–healing consciousness framework is referred to as an extended science view or a shift from the downward causation model to an upward causation model (Harman, 1987b; Sperry, 1987). Sperry (1987), the Nobel Prize recipient in physiology, references this same science shift as a theory of emergent interactionism, in which inner conscious awareness is explicitly recognized as a cause of behavior and a factor in evolution. Such thinking represents a major challenge to the reductionistic, physicalistic, downward causation philosophies, which deny wholeness, context, consciousness, transcendence, metaphysical phenomena, subjectivity, intersubjectivity, caring, health, and healing (McNeill, 1987). Caring and healing by their very nature are concerned with wholeness. Wholeness by its very nature is concerned with interconnectedness and intersubjectivity.

Harman (1987b) and Sperry (1987) suggest that humans are experiencing a "consciousness revolution in science" wherein they are more able to redefine the possible. As such, science is being restructured wherein descriptions of phenomena at different levels are complementary. Indeed there is now the need to reformulate epistemology by accommodating multiple ways of knowing, including the full spectrum of wholeness and context, including subjective, if not intersubjective, transpersonal, metaphysical experiences that invoke higher order concepts that are nonphysical in nature. Such thinking allows nursing to incorporate metaparadigmatic domains of Bingen's visual art that reveals a universal energy field that can be accessed and that perhaps is at the heart of the human center and resides in an

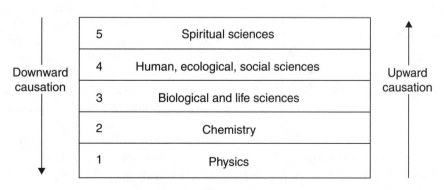

FIGURE 10.1

Upward causation model of science.

Reproduced by permission from Harman (1987).

ever-expanding consciousness; as she conveys, the energy field surrounding the person is in contact with a higher universe, the larger universe, which is shared with others and nature. Such thinking allows nursing to incorporate metaparadigmatic domains such as process, self-transcendence, evolution of consciousness, nonlinear direction, and fluid and relative views of the space-time matrix wherein past and future merge into present (Sarter, 1988). The extended upward looking models of science can more fully and uniquely provide meaningful philosophical, ontological, and epistemological foundations for nursing.

HUMAN DIMENSIONS OF CARING

Clinical health care practices as traditionally defined and practiced with an objective, detached, rationalistic, professional stance are no longer adequate. Nevertheless, it is necessary to acknowledge that the human dimensions of caring are related to what Kierkegaard (1941) suggested as an existential paradox since caring does require a unique combination of closeness and distance. It arises out of the dialectical nature of the genuine human self. Kierkegaard points out that a person must be both a subject (a center of commitment) and an object (an item of analysis), but the actual human experience of a caring moment is beyond the objective-subjective and is indeed intersubjective and transpersonal. The higher consciousness, transcendent potentialities, and real caring–healing possibilities are now being acknowledged in both theory and practice.

As intersubjectivity and a transpersonal caring–healing relationship is further described and studied, a new vision of the human caring healing relationship begins to take shape as both the one caring and the one being cared for become attuned to the caring–healing field consciousness. Such thinking transcends the traditional hierarchical stratification and goes beyond; neither care giver nor care receiver stands

above the other (Gadow, 1985). (Moreover, this view acknowledges that no one health profession stands above the other.) In this new context, a basic humanism emerges in which the human center of both persons is involved. So too can the one caring be a recipient of care and therefore the patient may be a healer.

Dossey (1984) captures some of the dilemma in this way:

> What is the way out (for an alternative to the objective model of medicine)? The admission of both the care provider and care receiver of the murky shadows within each-the woundedness of the healer and the latent healthiness of the (so-called) patient. (Dossey, 1984, p. 204)

An ideal of intersubjectivity and transcendence is based on a belief that people learn from each other how to be human by finding their dilemmas in themselves. What is learned from others is self-knowledge. The self learned from others is self-knowledge. The self learned about or discovered is every self; it is universal, the human self. People learn to recognize themselves in others. The intersubjectivity keeps alive a common humanity (Watson, 1985). Such a perspective transcends parts, physical body, and time-space and acknowledges that a higher energy, consciousness, spirit, or at least some stance with reference to the transcendental is part of the fabric of human existence.

This paper and the theoretical notions behind transpersonal human caring attempt to articulate and elucidate the higher order metaphysical, metaparadigmatic components of nursing and place them within both an esthetic and scientific context. To summarize both the aesthetic and scientific points of view related to new dimensions of human caring, the work of Hildegard of Bingen (Figure 10. 2), a 12th-century scientist, artist, poet, musician, and mystic, is pertinent and instructive. In describing one of her visions that resulted in perhaps her most visually powerful illumination, entitled Compassion,

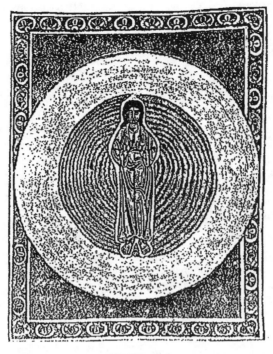

FIGURE 10.2

Art work of Hildegard of Bingen: Study in compassion. *Illuminations of Hildegard of Binger*
text, with commentary by Matthew Fox (1985). Santa Fe, NM: Bear and Company.

she revealed the now acknowledged scientific principle, both artistically and in writing, that "body resides in consciousness, rather than consciousness in body. This powerful healing energy can leave its own field and mix with others and vice versa" (Bingen, by Fox, 1985. p. 23). Such thinking again supports the metaphysical dimensions from the poetry as well as the holographic and upward causation explanation of transpersonal caring–healing, field-consciousness, and the transcendental phenomena discussed. Artistically, one can see that Hildegard of Bingen's visual art reveals a universal energy field that can be accessed and that perhaps is at the heart of the human center and resides in an ever-expanding consciousness; as she conveys, the energy field surrounding the person is in contact with a higher universe, the lager universe, that is shared with other and nature.

SUMMARY

The expanded dimensions of human caring theory presented here are imbedded in an ethic and human value of caring as a moral ideal, with an ontological and epistemological commitment to preserve and restore the human center in theory and practice. In the human center, human caring and healing become transpersonal and intersubjective and open up a higher energy field-consciousness that has metaphysical, transcendent potentialities. These views in turn provide for a new metaparadigm consistent with contemporary nursing theories as well as emergent holographic views of science. Moreover, these dimensions of human caring theory provide some metaphorical and poetic language, as well as ancient artistic visions, of the beauty, mystery, and wonders of the art and science of caring–healing in nursing.

REFERENCES

Battista, J. R. (1982). The holographic model, holistic paradigm, information theory and consciousness. In K. Wilber (Ed.), *The holographic paradigm, and other paradoxes* (pp. 143–149). Boston, MA: New Science Library.

Benner, P. (1984). *From novice to expert.* Menlo Park, CA: Addison-Wesley.

Benner, P. (1998). *The primacy of caring.* Menlo Park, CA: Addison-Wesley.

Bingen, Hildegard of. (1985). In M. Fox (Ed.), *Illuminations of Hildegard of Bingen.* Santa Fe, NM: Bear & Company.

Callahan, D. (1987). *Setting limits: Medical goats in an aging society.* New York, NY: Simon & Schuster.

Chinn, P. (1988). The politics of knowing (editorial), *Advances in Nursing Science, 10*(4), V–VIII.

Cooper, M. C, (1988). Covenantal relationships: Grounding for the nursing ethic. *Advances in Nursing Science, 10*(4), 48–59.

Dossey, L. (1984). *Beyond illness: Discovering the experience of health.* Boulder, CO: New Science Library.

Fry, S. (1988). The ethic of caring: Can it survive in nursing? *Nursing Outlook, 36*(1), 48.

Gadow, S. (1985). Nurse and patient: The caring relationship. In A. H. Bishop & J. R. Scudder (Eds.), *Caring, curing, coping: Nurse-physician-patient relationships* (pp. 31–43). Birmingham, AL: University of Alabama Press.

Gadow, S. (1987). Covenant without cure: Letting go and holding on in chronic illness. Presentation. Ethics of Care, Ethics of Cure Conference (March). Denver, CO: University of Colorado School of Nursing, Center for Human Caring.

Harman, W. (1982). The new science and holonomy. In K. Wilber (Ed.), *Holographic paradigm* (pp. 139). Boston, MA: New Science Library.

Harman, W. (1987a), Toward an extended science. *Noetic Sciences Review, 3,* 9–14.

Harman, W. (1987b). Further comments on an extended science (commentary). *Noetic Sciences Review, 4,* 22–25.

Kelly, L. (1988). Editorial: The ethic of caring: Has it been discarded? *Nursing Outlook, 36*(1), 17.

Kierkegaard, S. (1941). *Concluding: Unscientific post script.* (D. S. Swenson & W. Lowrie, Trans.). Princeton, NJ: Princeton University Press.

Krysl, M. (1989). Midwife and other poems on caring. *Midwife: Poetry on caring.* New York, NY: National League for Nursing.

Leininger, M, (1980). Caring. A central focus of nursing and health care. *Nursing and Health Care, 1*(3), 135–143.

Leininger, M. (1984). *Care: The essence of nursing and health care.* Thorofare, NJ: Charles B. Slack.

McNeill, B. (Ed.) (1987, Fall). Editor's comments. *Noetic Sciences Review, 4,* 19.

Moccia, P. (1988a), At the faultline: Social activism and caring. *Nursing Outlook, 36*(1), 32–33.

Moccia, P. (1988b). A critique of compromise: Beyond the methods debate. *Advances in Nursing Science, 10*(4), 1–9.

Mumford, L. (1970). *The myth of the machine: The pentagon of power* (pp. 420). New York, NY: Harcourt Brace Jovanovich.

Newman, M. (1986). *Health as expanding consciousness.* St. Louis, MO: Mosby.

Overman, B. (1986). *The potentiation of healing: Nursing's healing art.* Unpublished manuscript. N711 theory course, University of Colorado Health Sciences Center, School of Nursing, Denver, CO.

Packard, J. S., & Ferrara. M. (1988). In search of the moral foundation of nursing. *Advances in Nursing Science, 10*(4), 60–71.

Parse, R. (1981). *Man-living-health: A theory of nursing.* New York, NY: Wiley.

Pribram, K. H. (1971). *Languages of the brain: Experimental paradoxes and principles in neuropsychology.* Englewood Cliffs, NJ: Prentice-Hall.

Pribram, K. H. (1982). What the fuss is all about. In K. Wilber (Ed.), *The holographic paradigm.* Boston, MA: New Science Library.

Ray, M. (1987). Technological caring: A new model in critical care. *Dimensions in Critical Care Nursing, 6*(3), 166–173.

Rogers, M. (1970). *An introduction to the theoretical basis of nursing.* Philadelphia, PA: Davis.

Rogers, M. (1983). Science of unitary human beings: A paradigm for nursing. In I. Clements & S. Roberts (Eds.), *Family health: A theoretical approach to nursing care.* New York, NY: Wiley.

Sarter, B. (1988). Philosophical sources of nursing theory. *Nursing Science Quarterly, 1*(2), 52–59.

Sperry, R. (1987). Downward causation: The consciousness revolution in science. *Noetic Sciences Review, 4,* 18–21.

Watson, J. (1979). *Nursing: The philosophy and science of caring.* Boston, MA: Little, Brown. (1985). Boulder, CO: Colorado Associated University Press.

Watson, J. (1985). *Nursing: Human science and human care.* Norwalk, CT: Appleton-Century-Crofts. (1988). Boulder, CO: Colorado Associated University Press.

Watson, J. (1987a). Nursing on the caring edge. Metaphorical vignettes. *Advances in Nursing Science, 10*(1), 10–18.

Watson, J. (1987b). *The dream curriculum. Patterns on nursing: Strategic planning for nursing education.* New York, NY: National League for Nursing Publication.

Watson, J. (in press). Human caring: A subjective model for health sciences. In J. Watson & R. Taylor (Eds.), *They shall not hurt; Human suffering and human caring.* Boulder, CO: Colorado Associated University Press.

Whitehead, A. N. (1953). *Science in the modern world*. Cambridge, UK: Cambridge University Press.

Wilber, K. (1982). *The holographic paradigm and other paradoxes*. Boston, MA: New Science Library.

Yarling, R., & McElmurry, B. (1986). The moral foundation of nursing. *Advances in Nursing Science, 8*(2), 53–73.

QUESTIONS FOR REFLECTION

Baccalaureate

1. What are the implications related to considering caring as an "end in itself" rather than a "means to an end"?
2. Read the poem "Midwife" by Marilyn Krysl. How does that poem represent the metaphysical/transcendent dimensions of caring?
3. Reflect on what Watson means by: "The whole caring–healing consciousness is contained in a single caring moment." What do you think Watson means by a caring-consciousness and caring–healing energy?

Master's

1. Watson describes the importance of an intersubjective relationship as the foundation of transpersonal caring. How would a nurse enter into this kind of relationship?
2. Examine the art work of Hildegard of Bingen called "Study in Compassion." What do you see in this work that informs you about caring?
3. What are the nursing practice implications of Watson's assertion that: "Human caring–healing consciousness of the nurse is communicated to the one being cared for"?

Doctoral

1. What were the consistent themes that Sarter (1988) identified in the redefinition of nursing emerging in the literature of that time?
2. How does the holographic-extended science metaphor described by Watson differ from the dominant traditional science model? What research approaches might honor this new model of science?
3. How is art related to caring ontology and epistemology? Is art a potential method of inquiry for the discipline of nursing?

11

Caring Science in a New Key

Katie Eriksson

*I*t is obvious that there has been a reorientation in caring science in the 1990s toward a more distinctly humanistic way of thinking. In Bernstein's (1983) words, it could be said that the hermeneutic dimension, with its implied emphasis on understanding and interpretation, has been regained. The necessity of a humanistically oriented caring science was pointed out much earlier in the United States as well as in the Nordic countries (see, for example, Eriksson, 1981, 1988; Parse, 1981; Parse, Coyne, & Smith, 1985; Qvarnström, 1978; Watson, 1988), but the time was not yet ripe for its open admission. Those who do research in caring science acknowledge a common core of caring and support the striving for holistic care of the patient but are, on the other hand, not ready to work in a scientific tradition that creates the prerequisites for a deeper understanding of caring in all its complexity. Regaining the hermeneutic dimension and bringing out a humanistic way of thinking means going beyond the immediate experiences and penetrating into the core of caring. It means having the courage to release ourselves from the traditional way of thinking (Parse et al., 1985) and to strike a new note. The aim of this chapter is to discuss some of the preconditions for this reorientation and to present a model (Eriksson, 1988, 1990, 1994, 1997b) for development of humanistic thinking in caring science.

A NEW KEY

Regaining the humanistic dimension can be compared to a new key (Langer, 1942) that is appearing in caring science. As this key is becoming more prominent, the basic premises of caring science thinking tend to be brought into harmony with the new keynote. We get a new ethos, which is capable of bringing out the value of caring in the spirit of the present time. Langer says that every change of key gives a new meaning to the preceding bars and opens up new perspectives on past ideas and arguments. Starting in a new key means bringing to life what has already been said, animating dead words (Lévinas, 1988). It is a reorientation in time with the prevailing context, without leaving the core of caring out of sight. The keynote is found in the ontological core, the inmost being of caring, and every reorientation deepens and brings to the fore this core.

NEW QUESTIONS AND A NEW CONCEPTION OF REALITY

The new key and reorientation imply the formulation of new questions on the

From Eriksson, K. (2001). Caring science in a new key. *Nursing Science Quarterly, 15*(1), 61–65. Permission to reprint granted by Sage Publications, Inc.

basis of the fundamental premises. Reformulating the questions may bring deeper motives to light. Every age has its questions that most profoundly reflect the ripeness of the science that poses the questions and the underlying conception of reality. The depth of the questions is determined by the basic concepts we have at our command (Langer, 1942). Our questions are always restricted in relation to their direction, whereas the direction of the question at the same time constitutes the precondition for arriving at meaningful answers (Gadamer, 1960/1988b). An honestly formulated question, one that seeks the truth, is open and prevents us from being swayed by conventional patterns of thought. Our present language and concepts are insufficient to describe reality, and the task of science is to refine our concepts.

A science loses its vitality when no more questions can be asked, when we run out of new ideas. Asking questions is an art. The development of a humanistic research program could be started by formulating fundamental questions from the standpoint of basic scientific assumptions (Eriksson, 1988, 1990). The task of basic research is to devise new questions. The limit to our thinking is not determined from outside, but from our own inner ability to widen our intellectual horizon and create new ideas. A new note, an original idea, is a vision that always first appears as a metaphor before subsequently assuming a more concrete linguistic form.

THE HERMENEUTIC DIMENSION

The hermeneutic dimension is more than a methodology. It involves a new scientific conception, and sooner or later, we are all obliged to discover it or as Kuhn (1977) says, "In my case the discovery of hermeneutics nevertheless implied something more than that history came to stand out as meaningful. The most immediate and decisive effect concerned my view of science" (p. xiii). Humanism represents a concept of

knowledge that comprises culture and an open concept of theory. According to the original Greek concept of theory, *theory* is an open view of reality and participation in it (Gadamer, 1988a). Hermeneutics forces us to make up our minds about different basic questions in science as follows: What do we mean by science, truth, text, reading, and method? Through hermeneutics, we gain access to new knowledge in the form of historical, philosophical, and other sources dealing with human life.

Introducing the hermeneutic dimension in caring science implies that language, metaphors, words, concepts, and texts are given a central place in the formation of knowledge. In the basic concepts of symbolism, we have the key to all humanistic problems (Langer, 1942). To Gadamer (1960/1988b), understanding is always language-based interpretation, the finding of one's own words. Interpretation is about all the description and naming of events in the world. Understanding, interpretation, and application should not, according to Gadamer, be seen as method, but as substance. In distinction from other hermeneutic theorists, Gadamer does not think that specific methods will bring us closer to truth in the humanistic sciences. Instead, he stresses that humanistic culture derives its origin from rhetoric, which aims at conferring culture and not merely knowledge in a theoretical sense on a person. Understanding is ontology, Gadamer argues, and thus hermeneutics takes us deeper into reality and into the world of the patient.

A NEW CARING SCIENCE DEVELOPS

A brief description of the leading ideas in Eriksson's theory (1987, 1988, 1997a, 1998) and in the discipline of caring science, which have developed since the 1970s and which are being further developed today at the Department of Caring Science at Åbo Akademi University in Finland is given in Table 11.1.

TABLE 11.1 Basic Assumptions of Eriksson's Theory

1. Human being is fundamentally an entity of body, soul, and spirit.

2. Human being is fundamentally a religious being, but all human beings have not recognized this dimension.

3. Human being is fundamentally holy. Human dignity means accepting the human obligation of serving with love and of existing for the sake of others.

4. Health means a movement in becoming, being and doing, and striving for integrity and holiness that is compatible with bearable suffering.

5. The basic category of caring is suffering.

6. The basic motive of caring is the *caritas* motive.

7. Caring implies alleviating suffering in charity, love, faith, and hope. Natural basic caring is expressed through tending, playing, and teaching in a sustained caring relationship.

8. Caring relationship forms the meaningful context of caring and derives its origin from the ethos of love, responsibility, and sacrifice, that is, a caritative ethic.

Viewing the world, we have chosen the term *caring* to emphasize that the focus is on the phenomenon of caring, not on the profession. We call this field of science *caring science*, not *nursing science* (Eriksson, 1997b). The concepts *caring* and *nursing* are notoriously ambiguous. Our idea of caring science is closely related to Parse's (1981, 1995) approach in developing nursing science.

Our vision has been to revive the leading idea of caring, the idea of love and compassion, and to incorporate it once more into the core of caring science. The aim has been to create a humanistically oriented caring science. Our attachment to the challenge can be best captured in the words of Langer (1942) as follows:

> Most new discoveries are suddenly-seen things that were always there. A new idea is a light that illuminates presences which simply had no form for us before the light fell on them. We turn the light here, there and everywhere, and the limits of thought recede before it. A new science . . . is generated by such a basic innovation. (p. 30)

THE ONTOLOGICAL CORE

We started from the assumption that caring science is basically humanistic in nature. The ontological questions, that is, the questions about what the innermost

being of caring reality is actually like, came to the fore in our search for knowledge. It is the questions of "what" rather than "how" that lead to the scientific formation of concepts and theories. In search for the fundamental category of caring, that is, the basic concept or the idea behind all forms of caring, we have used different approaches such as historical research and motive research (Nygren, 1972).

From the standpoint of concepts and the history of ideas, two leading conceptions of caring come to the fore, that of compassion and that of human love, that is, the *caritas* motive, which we see as the basic motive of caring. At the same time, the caritas motive expresses the basic value of caring science and the ethical inducement to all forms of caring. The leading idea of caring is to alleviate human suffering and to preserve and safeguard life and health (Eriksson, 1992a, 1992b, 1992c, 1994, 1997a, 1997b; Lindholm & Eriksson, 1993, 1998).

BASIC ASSUMPTIONS OF ERIKSSON'S THEORY

Ontology is reflected in various basic assumptions, which are made concrete in a multifaceted view and profound understanding of human being, health, suffering, caring, and the world, as well as in our attitude toward these entities. The basic assumptions have been developed since the 1980s and tested theoretically and empirically (Eriksson, 1988, 1997b; Fagerström, Eriksson, & Engberg, 1999; Fredriksson & Eriksson, 2001; Lindholm & Eriksson, 1998; von Post & Eriksson, 1999).

Our ontology (see Table 11.1) is anchored in a conception of human being as an entity of body, soul, and spirit and as basically religious and in suffering as the fundamental category of caring, which can be seen as radically different from a generally accepted perspective primarily based on the natural sciences. This confronted us with the task of creating an epistemology and some general methodological points of departure as a basis for the further development of caring science.

In accordance with the fundamental assumptions of caring science, caring is basically seen as something natural and primordial. Caring has a specific meaning context of its own—a caring relationship that arises in an unselfish relationship with another and from a genuine desire to alleviate suffering. The basic motive of caring, the caritas motive, invites us to caring. The deepest ethical motive in all caring involves respect for the absolute dignity of human being. Holiness is part of human life. Human dignity implies inner freedom and responsibility for one's own and others' lives. The mission of human being is to serve, to exist for the sake of others. The profoundest significance of caring has been reached when a human being has been restored to his or her mission. Starting from the caritas motive, compassion for a fellow human being arises when meeting a suffering human being. Suffering can be alleviated in a relationship characterized by responsibility and a desire to do good. All caring is formed in the relationship between patient and caregiver. In this relationship, the patient is seen as a unique human being, an entity of body, soul, and spirit. This spiritual dimension is stressed as spiritually existential, spiritually religious, and spiritually Christian. Ontologically, every human being, every patient, is fundamentally seen as someone who longs for something beyond their own selves, a God or abstract other (Eriksson, 1992a, 1992b, 1993, 1994; Lindholm & Eriksson, 1998).

Epistemological Standpoints

The most characteristic feature of a young caring science is its endeavor to form itself in terms of its own historical and ontological conditions, which implies that questions of method stay in the background in the initial phase. By expressly formulating the theoretical terms on which the knowledge is enhanced, the preconditions for the generation of theory based on the ontological core can be created. It is necessary for the theoretical core to be made explicit enough before clinical research is launched, which always diffuses the core. Basic knowledge of a field can be achieved without knowing the concrete characteristics, the absolute qualities (Lindström & Eriksson, 1999).

The aim of science is to attempt to create some form of order and intelligibility in our world. It involves a search for some form of a basic pattern, or a theory. The supreme purpose of science is its search for the truth and the evident. The humanistic conception of truth includes the true, the beautiful, and the good (Gadamer, 1960/1988b). The unity of caring, evident caring, is manifested as true, good, and beautiful caring.

Our ontology and basis of value presuppose an open view of knowledge, which implies humility before the limitations of knowledge—the realization that absolute truths cannot be attained even if there is the greatest possible precision and exactness. The understanding attained is only a step forward and a challenge for a continued search for knowledge. Interest in knowledge can be characterized as hermeneutic—emancipatory with an emphasis on the inner understanding of meaning and the formation of ideas, which is seen as constituting the basic precondition for change with fresh ideas. In such a distinctive image of knowledge, both traditions and visions are allowed free scope and can be seen to enrich our understanding of the world of caring (Eriksson, 1998). The open view of knowledge is also an endeavor to understand what is unknown and difficult to capture and is based on confidence in the human capacity for innovative and creative thinking and new ways of doing research. Such search for knowledge also implies something like an archaeological approach. This can be seen as the most important tool of discursive thinking. Awareness of language and handling of concepts are of decisive importance for our development of knowledge.

ETHICS PRECEDES ONTOLOGY

A caring science theory of human relevance is by its nature ethical, and it will be necessary to formulate an epistemological postulate as follows: Ethics precedes ontology. Lévinas (1988) thinks that ethics precedes ontology. In his opinion, an ontology that is not subordinated to ethics is next to impossible, because the understanding of being in general cannot indicate and control the genuine relationship to another person, but it is this relationship that must determine the understanding of being. "The objectivity of sciences which presupposes their inter-subjectivity, i.e., their validity for everyone who tests their results, is based on ethics, not the other way round. Ethics is not an addition to our knowledge, but the basis of knowledge" (Kemp, 1992, p. 48).

Because ethics precedes ontology, the situation is subordinated to ethics. In a concrete sense, this implies that the thought of human holiness and dignity is always kept alive in all phases of the search for knowledge. Ethics precedes ontology in theory as well as in practice. The fact that ethics precedes ontology implies that we assume an attitude to the reality we want to study and influence through caring. It is through understanding and adopting an ethos, that is, the values we embrace or, in the words of Lévinas (1988), "passionate metaphysics" (p. 182), that we indicate the mood and key that accompany our development of knowledge.

DISCUSSION

Caring science and caring as a whole today require humanistic knowledge and the hermeneutical dimension to achieve real progress. Caring is becoming more and more complex, and the patient is standing at the intersection between an increasing number of sciences that attempt to describe and explain him or her and influence the situation. It will be interesting to see in what way the knowledge of care based on human science will be integrated in the formation of knowledge and in nursing care. I see the following three possible ways for the development of humanistic caring science: an autonomous caring science, a medical science more and more influenced by caring, and an interdisciplinary influenced science.

The greatest challenge of all is to develop an autonomous caring science, and it presupposes the development of a caring science body of knowledge from the core of caring not primarily tied to a specific profession. Whether a caring science will be successful in the academic world as well as in clinical practice is to a great extent a question of power and authority. It is a question as to whether the practitioners of caring science are daring enough to assert their own knowledge and its intrinsic value, but it is above all a question of believing in it ourselves and acquiring a caring science identity.

Every theory and new scientific idea has its own career or, to quote James (1975), "At first, as we know, a new theory is attacked as absurd; then it is recognized as true but self-evident and unimportant, and eventually it is considered so important that its opponents themselves claim to have discovered it" (p. 18). Many caring scientists who have launched some bold novelty probably recognize this. The strength of an idea, a theory, or a whole scientific structure lies in its theoretical core and in how well it has been expressed. An epoch comes to an end when the concepts it produced are exhausted. Today, do we have enough originality, courage, and creative zest to develop a humanistic caring science? A decisive precondition is our own bid for basic research.

Another possible line of development is that medical science and research will be more and more concentrated on caring and a human science perspective, because this knowledge is needed and there are questions to be answered. Caring scientists are still engaged in developing this knowledge, but they do not have the official authority to support their own discipline. Caring science knowledge is more and more integrated into medical science, but different concepts are used. From an ethical standpoint, this development can be defended because the knowledge will benefit the patient. As far as caring science is concerned, it implies a disintegration of the discipline. Medical science shows an evergrowing interest in humanistic medical research, and professorial chairs of medicine based on human science are established in the Nordic countries. It will be interesting to see what such knowledge will be called.

A third possible line of development is that caring science ideas will have a stronger impact in interdisciplinary contexts, in which researchers representing different sciences will meet to discuss some concrete problems of caring. The risk is that the caring science thinking will be blurred, mainly because the concepts will be used with different meanings. The knowledge will be more pragmatically oriented and the need for an independent caring science will be questioned. This will be the case especially if caring science will not manage to establish a clear enough identity of its own.

The starting point of this contribution was that there is a new key in caring science, a key that carries the sound of a long tradition and a historical development characterized by the ethos of compassion and love. This is an ethos and a key that is so fundamental to human life that it will always endure and survive in some form. It is my hope that this key will continue to exist in caring and that researchers in caring science all over the world will meet the challenge, making caring science and its intrinsic value recognized. For a science to be taken seriously and to be able to make an impact on society and culture, it must manifest itself as truthful, heuristic, and innovative.

Caring science as an academic discipline has its intrinsic value, which means that scientific progress and development are assessed in terms of their own internal criteria and their generation of substance. A caring science that lacks its own intrinsic value and serves more in the capacity of a *techne* has its role assigned and is molded by other authorities. It will then find it difficult to operate for the benefit of caring. In caring science, the pursuit of knowledge is compatible with the task of exploring the idea of good care and with indicating possibilities of implementing it, independently of professional considerations. The transferring of caring science knowledge and the application of it to professional ends will be a task for academic education. A caring science theory that is successful sheds light on both the successes and the failures of caring or, to finish with a quotation from Langer (1942), "Freedom of thought cannot be reborn without throes; language, art, morality, and science have all given us pain as well as power" (p. 318).

REFERENCES

Bernstein, R. J. (1983). *Beyond objectivism and relativism: Science, hermeneutics and praxis.* Oxford, UK: Oxford Blackwell.

Eriksson, K. (1981). *Vårdprocessen—en utgångspunkt för låroplanstänkande inom vårdutbildningen. Utvecklande av en vårdprocessmodell samt ett läroplanstänkande utgående från vårdprocessen* [The patient care process—An approach to curriculum construction within nursing education. The development of a model for the patient care process and an approach for curriculum development based on the process of patient care] (Unpublished doctoral dissertation). Helsinki University, Pedagogiska Institutionen, Helsinki, Finland.

Eriksson, K. (1987). *Pausen. En beskrivning av vårdvetenskapens kunskapsobjekt* [The pause: A description of the knowledge of caring science]. Stockholm, Sweden: Almqvist & Wiksell.

Eriksson, K. (1988). *Vårdvetenskapen som disciplin, forsknings-och tillämpning-område* [Caring science as a discipline, a field of research, and application]. Vasa, Finland: Åbo Akademi University, Department of Caring Research.

Eriksson, K. (1990). Nursing science in a Nordic perspective. Systematic and contextual caring science. A study of the basic motive of caring and context. *Scandinavian Journal of Caring Sciences, 4*(1), 3–5.

Eriksson, K. (1992a). The alleviation of suffering—The idea of caring. *Scandinavian Journal of Caring Sciences, 6*(2), 119–123.

Eriksson, K. (1992b). Different forms of caring communion. *Nursing Science Quarterly, 5*, 93.

Eriksson, K. (1992c). Nursing: The caring practice "being there." In D. Gaut (Ed.), *The practice of caring in nursing* (pp. 201–210). New York, NY: National League for Nursing.

Eriksson, K. (1994). Theories of caring as health. In D. Gaut & A. Boykin (Eds.), *Caring as healing: Renewal through hope* (pp. 3–20). New York, NY: National League for Nursing.

Eriksson, K. (1997a). Caring, spirituality and suffering. In S. M. Roach (Ed.), *Caring from the heart: The convergence between caring and spirituality* (pp. 68–81). New York, NY: Paulist.

Eriksson, K. (1997b). Understanding the world of the patient, the suffering human being: The new clinical paradigm from nursing to caring, *Advanced Practice Nursing Quarterly, 3*, 8–13.

Eriksson, K. (Ed.). (1993). *Möten med lidanden* [Encountering suffering]. Vasa, Finland: Åbo Akademi University, Department of Caring Research.

Eriksson, K. (Ed.). (1998). *Jubileumsskrift 1987–1997* [Jubilee publication 1987–1997]. Vasa, Finland: Åbo Akademi University, Department of Caring Science.

Fagerström, L., Eriksson, K., & Engberg, I. (1999). The patient's perceived caring needs: Measuring the unmeasurable. *International Journal of Nursing Practice, 5*, 199–208.

Fredriksson, L., & Eriksson, K. (2001). The patient's narrative of suffering—A path to health? An interpretative research synthesis on narrative understanding. *Scandinavian Journal of Caring Sciences, 15*, 3–11.

Gadamer, H. G. (1988a). *Förnuftet vid vetenskapens tidsålder* [Sense in the age of science]. Göteborg, Sweden: Daidalos.

Gadamer, H. G. (1988b). *Truth and method* (2nd ed., J. Weinsheimer & D. G. Marshall, Trans.). London, England: Sheed and Ward Stagebooks. (Original work published 1960)

James, W. (1975). *Works: Pragmatism*. Cambridge, MA: Harvard University Press.

Kemp, P. (1992). *Lévinas, En introduktion* [Lévinas. An introduction]. Göteborg, Sweden: Daidalos.

Kuhn, T. (1977). *The essential tension: Selected studies in scientific tradition and change*. Chicago, IL: University of Chicago Press.

Langer, S. K. (1942). *Filosofi i en ny tonart* [Philosphy in a new key]. Stockholm, Sweden: Geber.

Lévinas, E. (1988). *Etik och oändlighet* [Ethics and endlessness]. Stockholm, Sweden: Symposion.

Lindholm, L., & Eriksson, K. (1993). To understand and to alleviate suffering in a caring culture. *Journal of Advanced Nursing, 18*, 1354–1361.

Lindholm, L., & Eriksson, K. (1998). The dialectic of health and suffering: An ontological perspective on young people's health. *Qualitative Health Research, 8*, 513–525.

Lindström, U. Å., & Eriksson, K. (1999). The fundamental idea of quality assurance. *International Journal for Human Caring, 3*(3), 21–27.

Mauss, M. (1938). Une categorie de l'esprit human: La notion de personne. *Journal of the Anthropological Institute, 68*, 262–281.

Mead, G. H. (1959). Mind, self and society. In A. Strauss (Ed.), *The social psychology of George Herbert Mead* (3rd ed.). Chicago, IL: University of Chicago Press.

Noddings, N. (1984). *Caring: A feminine approach to ethics & moral education*. Berkeley, CA: University of California Press.

Nygren, A. (1972). *Meaning and method*. London, England: Epworth Press.

Orem, D. E. (1971). *Nursing: Concepts of practice*. New York, NY: McGraw-Hill.

Parse, R. R. (1981). *Man-living-health: A theory of nursing*. New York, NY: John Wiley & Sons.

Parse, R. R. (Ed.). (1995). *Illuminations. The human becoming theory in practice and research*. New York, NY: National League for Nursing.

Parse, R. R., Coyne, A. B., & Smith, M. J. (1985). *Nursing research: Qualitative methods*. Bowie, MD: Brady.

Peplau, P. E. (1952). *Interpersonal relations in nursing*. New York, NY: Putnam.

Piaget, J. (1962). *Play, dreams, and imitation in child-hood*. London, UK: Routedge and Kegan Paul.

Piaget, J., & Inhelder, B. (1966). *The psychology of the child*. New York, NY: Basic Books.

Qvarnström, U. (1978). *Patients' reactions to impending death: A clinical study* (Unpublished doctoral dissertation). University of Stockholm, Stockholm, Sweden.

Roach, S. (1984). *Caring. The human mode of being: Implications for nursing.* Perspectives in Caring. Monograph, 1, Toronto Faculty of Nursing, University of Toronto.

Rogers, M. E. (1986). Science of unitary human beings. In V. M. Malinski (Ed.), *Explorations on Martha Roger's science of unitary human beings* (pp. 3–8). Norwalk, CT: Appleton-Century-Crofts.

Schlotfeldt, R. M. (1975). Research in nursing and research training for nurses: Retrospect and prospect. *Nursing Research, 24*, 117–183.

Sullivan, H. S. (1953). *The interpersonal theory of psychiatry.* New York, NY: Norton.

Taylor, C. (1985). *The concept of person in human agency and language: Philosophical papers 1* (pp. 97–114). Cambridge, UK: Cambridge University Press.

Tillich, P. (1952). *The courage to be*. New Haven, CT and London, UK: Yale University Press.

van Kaam, A. (1982). *The emergent self*. Denville, NJ: Dimension Books.

von Post, I., & Eriksson, K. (1999). A hermeneutic textual analysis of suffering and caring in the peri-operative context. *Journal of Advanced Nursing, 30*, 983–989.

Watson, J. (1985). *Nursing. Human science and human care: A theory of nursing.* Norwalk, CT: Appleton-Century-Crofts.

Watson, J. (1988). *Nursing: Human science and human care. A theory of nursing.* New York, NY: National League for Nursing.

QUESTIONS FOR REFLECTION

Baccalaureate

1. Identify and explain one of the assumptions of Eriksson's theory.
2. How will you relate this assumption to nursing care? Provide an example.
3. What is caring science?

Master's

1. Does caring always involve the alleviation of suffering? Why or why not?
2. Compare Eriksson's theory of caring with Watson's theory of caring. How are they alike and different?
3. How might Eriksson's theory guide nursing care with your population of interest? Provide an example.

Doctoral

1. What is the difference between nursing science and caring science?
2. What is the implication of the postulate: "Ethics precedes ontology"?
3. How does Eriksson define theory? How is this different from other conceptualizations?

12

Five Basic Modes of Being With Another

SIGRIDUR HALLDORSDOTTIR

When the weak and the orphaned
are deprived of justice all the foundations of the earth are shaken.

Ps. 82.3–5

Leininger (1988) maintains that caring is
the essence of humanity and is essential
for human growth and survival. She contends that care is one of the most powerful and elusive aspects of our health and
identity and must be the central focus
of nursing and the helping and healing professions. Similarly, Roach (1987)
claims that care is the basic constitutive phenomenon of human existence
and thus ontological in that it constitutes
man as man. She points out that all exis-
tentials used to describe Dasein's self
have their central locus in care. Roach
states, "When we do not care, we lose our
being and care is the way back to being.
Care is primordial, the source of action
and is not reducible to specific actions"
(1987, p. 15).

Although Roach (1984) claims that
caring is the human mode of being, she
wonders how convincing the view is that
caring is the natural expression of what
is authentically human when there is so
much evidence of lack of caring, both

within our personal experiences as well
as in the society around us. Roach points
out that we live in an age where violence
is commonplace and where atrocities are
committed against individuals and communities everywhere. To compound the
effect of such violence on the broader
social body, many incidents enter our living rooms through the press, radio, and
television often as quickly as they occur.

As a result, modes of being with
another in our world involve both caring
and uncaring dimensions. What, then, are
the basic modes of being with another?
By analyzing two of my own studies on
clients' (patients' and students') perceptions of caring and uncaring encounters
(Halldorsdottir, 1989, 1990), as well as
related literature, I have determined that
there are five basic modes of being with
another as follows: life-giving (biogenic),
life-sustaining (bioactive), life-neutral (biopassive), life-restraining (biostatic), and life-
destroying (biocidic) (see Figure 12.1 and
Table 12.1).

In this chapter, I describe the
five basic modes of being with another
through examples of caring and uncaring encounters in hospitals as experienced
by former patients, my co-researchers

From Halldorsdottir, S. (1991). Five basic modes of being with another. In D. A. Gaut & M. Leininger (Eds.), *Caring: The compassionate* (pp. 37–49). New York, NY: National League for Nursing.
Permission to reprint granted by the National League for Nursing, New York, NY.

TABLE 12.1 Five Basic Modes of Being With Another

Life-destroying (biocidic) mode of being with another is a mode where one depersonalizes the other, destroys the joy of life, and increases the other's vulnerability. It causes distress and despair and hurts and deforms the other. It is transference of negative energy or darkness.

Life-restraining (biostatic) mode of being with another is a mode where one is insensitive or indifferent to the other and detached from the true center of the other. It causes discouragement and develops uneasiness in the other. It negatively affects existing life in the other.

Life-neutral (biopassive) mode of being with another is a mode where one does not affect life in the other.

Life-sustaining (bioactive) mode of being with another is a mode where one acknowledges the personhood of the other, supports, encourages, and reassures the other. It gives the other security and comfort. It positively affects life in the other.

Life-giving (biogenic) mode of being with another is a mode where one affirms the personhood of the other by connecting with the true center of the other in a life-giving way. It relieves the vulnerability of the other and makes the other stronger and enhances growth, restores, reforms, and potentiates learning and healing.

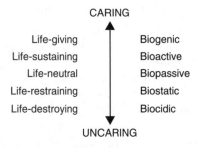

FIGURE 12.1

The caring/uncaring dimension
or continuum.

in the former study (Halldorsdottir, 1989). The phenomenological perspective of qualitative research theory guided the methodological approach to the studies analyzed, involving the use of theoretical sampling, intensive unstructured interviews, and constant comparative analysis.

Nine former patients participated in the former study and data were collected through 18 in-depth, open-ended interviews. Nine former nursing students participated in the latter study and data were collected through 16 in-depth, open-ended interviews. In both studies, interviews were tape-recorded and transcribed verbatim for each participant.

The excerpts used from the former study will be referred to as "modes of being

with a patient," and for the sake of clarity, the feminine will be utilized in reference to the nurse and the masculine in reference to the co-researcher/patient/client. In the text, however, "nurse" and "co-researcher/ patient/client" can refer to both males and females. Evidence from literature, that has a bearing on this matter, will also be given.

The *life-destroying*, or *biocidic*, mode is the most inhumane mode of being with another in the list as given and is represented by violence in all its forms. It means hurting, harming, or deforming the other. This destructive mode manifests in numerous ways as follows: making people dependent or fostering infantilism; being threatening; involving manipulation, coercion, hatred, aggression, and humiliation; involving various kinds of abuse; and often involving an evident lust for power, followed by dominance and depersonalization of the other. Hardheartedness or coldheartedness also may be present here. This mode of being with another most often changes the other to the worse, the harm done depending on the other's strength to endure. It involves the transference of negative energy or darkness to the other. It is the frost the human flower has a hard time enduring without loosing its luster, petals, leaves, and life.

In many respects, the history of humankind is not a positive affirmation of the sanctity of human life as Roach (1987) has rightly pointed out. There seems to be no end to how destructive and brutal the human being can be. Roach also argues that perhaps the greatest threat against human life in our age lies in the erosion of sensitivity toward its value, particularly where the taking of human life becomes part of everyday experience. Roach claims that the public at large has become less and less sensitive to all overt killings—genocide, fratricide, homicide, suicide, and feticide.

As described, the *life-destroying*, or *biocidic, mode of being with a patient* is the most severe form of indifference to the patient as a person, involves harshness and inhumanity, and is characterized by various forms of inhumane attitudes. Although I will not tell their entire stories here, four out of the nine co-researchers in the study under discussion had a biocidic experience. Of those four co-researchers, three asked me whether I had seen *One Flew over the Cuckoo's Nest* and claimed that their nurse was very much like nurse Rachet, as portrayed in that film. None of the co-researchers knew each other.

Although all co-researchers held a unanimous perception that uncaring encounters with nurses were very discouraging and distressing experiences for them as patients, their reactions to such encounters were many sided. Several major themes were identified in their accounts as follows: *initial puzzlement and disbelief*, which is followed by *anger and resentment*. Because of the patient's vulnerable circumstances, however, the patient is most often unable to act out the feelings of anger and resentment, and these strong negative feelings seem to develop into *despair and helplessness*.

Being uncared for in a dependent situation develops feelings of impotence, a sense of loss, and a sense of having been betrayed by those counted on for caring. If, on top of that, the patient is treated by the nurse as somewhat less than human, the patient's feelings soon develop into feelings of *alienation and identity loss*. The patient feels he has no value as a person, that he is indeed less than a person— "a side of beef," "an object," or "a machine." Furthermore, experiencing uncaring increases the patient's own feelings of *vulnerability* within the hospital setting.

Numerous co-researchers alluded to the threat of dehumanization within today's hospitals. It was their unanimous perception that they felt vulnerable and in need of caring when they were in the hospital. Some suggested that this makes patients more sensitive to caring and uncaring. One such former patient stated that,

> I would expect that people being ill makes them vulnerable, so that when they have an uncaring transaction, like someone treats them rudely, they are more *deeply wounded* in that circumstance than if they were healthy and walking the street and someone on the corner said something stupid or insulting. I mean *that* they can shrug off and ignore, but here they are *sick* and in *need*, and probably feel weak in spirit, and weak in body, and so it hits home harder, any such transaction hurts them more.

Other co-researchers related that they perceived uncaring as a transference of negative energy that affected their well-being and delayed or even prevented their recovery. This perceived *negative effect on well-being and healing* is illustrated in time and again in their accounts. Furthermore, it was their unanimous perception that the uncaring encounters made such an indelible impression on them and had a longer lasting effect than caring encounters that they tended to be both *acid edged and memorable experiences*.

Some co-researchers referred to the "memories of uncaring encounters" as scars, and although they seem to be trying to understand or make sense of the experience, they are most often still angry and even have nightmares about the nurses perceived to be uncaring. Some co-researchers identified how the uncaring experience prompted them to think about ultimate realities vis-à-vis death, affected their view of the hospital, and how it continued to even dictate their decisions within the health care system today.

Although most co-researchers had tried to forgive the uncaring nurse, some co-researchers related that that was probably more a result of forgetfulness than forgiveness. These co-researchers sometimes expressed a longing to return and confront the uncaring nurse, if, for nothing more, than to relieve themselves of their anger. At the same time, however, they realized that the nurses perceived to be uncaring were probably unaware of their influences on the patients and would, therefore, not recognize their stories.

Hildegard of Bingen, a remarkable 12th-century abbess, scientist, artist, poet, musician, and mystic, talks about the dryness of carelessness and injustice. She claims that dryness and coldness together make hardness of heart and that drying up destroys our creative powers, marking the end of all good works, and the beginning of laziness and carelessness. She maintains that if we lack an infusion of heavenly dew, we will be turned into dryness and our souls will waste away. From Hildegard's point of view, the ultimate uncaring occurs when we become cold and hardened to injustice. Hildegard (1985) wrote to one churchman: "When a person loses the freshness of God's power, he is transformed into the dryness of carelessness. He lacks the juice and greenness of good works and the energies of his heart are sapped away" (p. 64).

The *life-restraining*, or *biostatic, mode* of being with another involves negatively affecting life in the other by restricting or disturbing the energy already existent in the other. It means being insensitive or indifferent to the other, causes discouragement, and develops uneasiness in the other. It often involves imposing one's own will upon the other, dominating, and controlling the other. It sometimes appears as fault finding, anger, blaming, accusing, and being unfriendly. It is that very coldness and strong wind the human flower has a hard time enduring.

The *life-restraining*, or *biostatic, mode of being with a patient* involves the patient feeling strongly that the nurse does not care and is blind to his feelings by way of negative feedback from nurse to patient. Here, the nurse often treats the patient as a nuisance, that is, if it were not for the patient, the nurse's life would be a lot easier. The patient starts to feel that he is bothering the nurse when asking for help, finds the nurse often cold and unkind, and the nurse's presence destructive in some way. This nurse approach is partly illustrated in the following accounts.

> The second one [uncaring nurse] was *cold*, and I can at least give her that much because I interacted with her enough. The first one, I would just say I was . . . what?, I don't know, a piece of dust on the floor, I mean, I can't, I was a *bother* . . . The people in that room were *just beds*, that's all, you know, beds. She had prescriptions, she had a checklist of what she had to do, you know, your heart, etc., and that's all it was, for everybody, not just for me, you know.

> I had experiences of being in another ward for three days, and there was a tremendous high percentage of noncaring nurses. Actually, this is a nice description saying noncaring nurses, they were completely like . . . cold . . . cold human beings, like *computers*. It's like, sometimes I was worried, I was . . . was wondering if they really even noticed that I was there.

Dossey (1982) asserts that a patient-as-object approach to care delivery is destructive because it violates the oneness and wholeness that are necessary for healthy, viable living systems. Similarly, Gadow (1985) has pointed out that in addition to the domination by apparatus and by experts that can accompany the use of technology, patients can be reduced to objects in a more fundamental way than by the use of machines in the view of the body as a machine. Gadow states, "such reduction occurs because regard for the body exclusively as a scientific object negates the validity of subjective meanings of the person's experience. Those meanings are categorically nonexistent in the scientific object" (p. 36). Furthermore, Gadow (1988) has pointed out that the exercise of power always increases the vulnerability of the one over whom it is exercised, no matter what benevolent purpose the power serves.

The *life-neutral*, or *biopassive, mode* of being with another occurs when one is detached from the true center of the other and when there is no effect on the energy or life of the other. This lack of response, interest, and affect derives from inattentiveness or insensitivity to the other. It refers to the lack of a positive or caring approach rather than the presence of something destructive. Although it has no real effect on the life in the other, it sometimes creates a feeling of loneliness, because there is no mutual acknowledgment of personhood, no person-to-person contact. Furthermore, many seem to experience this apathetic inattention not only as lack of care but as noncaring or uncaring.

The fundamental characteristic of the *life-neutral*, or *biopassive, mode of being with a patient* is perceived apathy, which refers to the approach in which the nurse is perceived to be inattentive to the patients and their specific needs. The co-researchers emphasized that the nurse seemed to care about the routine, the tasks she was supposed to perform, but not about the patient as a person. The nurse is sometimes perceived by the patient as insensitive, absentminded, tired, dissatisfied in her job, or lacking in some caring quality, for example, warmth of voice. Furthermore, the co-researchers perceived these nurses as either unwilling or unable to connect with, or develop attachment to, the patient. The co-researchers' perceptions of detachment

are seen clearly in their accounts. In fact, one co-researcher stated,

> Aahm . . . the way she looked at you . . . like you are not a part of her world . . . or that she doesn't want to attach—you can feel that there is no emotional attachment there.

Bermejo (1987) asserts that a person is essentially characterized by a necessary openness to another. He contends that a person closed in upon and withdrawn into his or her self, hardly deserves the status of person, for this withdrawal, he argues, goes counter to the very core of man's being, which is clamoring first for an opening, and then, based upon that opening, for a total gift of self to another. Bermejo states, "A rejection of this essential, radical opening and the ensuing personal communion would unavoidably have a crippling effect on the fulness of the human person. A man half open is only half a man" (p. 46).

Hildegard of Bingen (1985) states in one of her many books that too often human actions are weak and lukewarm and emerge from people who are more asleep than awake. She claims that in this way people "make themselves weak and poor who do not wish to be busy about justice or about rubbing out injustice or about paying back their debts." Commitment to justice, she insists, would wake people from their sleep and would put zeal back into their lives and work.

Similarly, Matthew Fox (1985) has pointed out that the theme of spiritual maturity as wakefulness has been expressed in religious literature throughout the world. Hildegard also makes a connection between wisdom as wakefulness and folly as sleepfulness. In the Gospel parable, the wise virgins stayed awake and the foolish fell asleep. In Hildegard's terms, we can never climb the mountain of healing, celebration, justice making, and compassion if we do not care, are not committed, are indifferent, and do not fight injustice.

The *life-sustaining,* or *bioactive, mode* of being with another involves benevolence, good will, genuine kindness and concern, beneficence, and kindheartedness. It is protecting life, relieving suffering, keeping promises, respecting the other, and acknowledging the other's humanhood. Thanking and praising and a contrary dislike of constraining others are involved here. Indeed, there exists the heartfelt wish to do no harm. Comforting, encouraging, consoling, strengthening the other, and continuing to support the energy already present in the other adds other dimensions to the bioactive mode.

The *life-sustaining,* or *bioactive, mode of being with a patient* means that the nurse is skillful, knowledgeable, committed to the provision of personalized care, and knows how to safeguard the personal integrity and dignity of the patient. This special kind of nurse approach, which includes *compassionate competence, genuine concern for the patient as a person, undivided attention when the nurse is with the patient, and sober cheerfulness,* is what I call *professional nurse caring* (Halldorsdottir, 1990).

When the nurse succeeded in giving this kind of professional caring, it promoted the feelings of trust in patients, which facilitated the development of attachment between patients and nurses. It is precisely this attachment that forms the basis of a life-giving presence where openness and the transference of positive energy, which affects the other in a profound way, predominates.

This *life-giving,* or *biogenic, mode* of being with another is the truly human mode of being and is represented by healing love. This mode involves loving benevolence, responsiveness, generosity, mercy, and compassion. A truly life-giving presence offers the other interconnectedness and allows for the expansion of the other's consciousness and fosters spiritual freedom. It involves being open to persons and giving life to the very heart of man as a person, creating a relationship of openness and receptivity, yet always keeping a creative distance of respect and compassion. The truly life-giving or biogenic presence restores well-being and human dignity. It is transforming personal presence that deeply changes man. For the recipient, there is an experienced inrush of compassion, often like a current.

Regarding the *life-giving,* or *biogenic, mode of being with a patient*, one co-researcher said this about the fundamental difference between caring and uncaring:

> I'm not sure how to put it other than "personal relationship," the sense is somehow that your spirit and mine have met in the experience. And the whole idea that there is somebody in that hospital who is *with* me, rather than working *on* me.

Another co-researcher explained it this way:

> You know, there is that kind of bonding, that kind of feeling of . . . not intimacy but at least *connection*, there has been a connection made with that person, a connection which I could then follow-up on, you know, I would feel free to do so.

From co-researchers' accounts, it is apparent that this bonding or connection also involves a *creative distance of respect and compassion*, a dimension of professional attachment that has to be present to keep caring in the professional domain. It is also clear that dimensions in true professional caring depend on the depth of attachment developed. Professional attachment development can be conceptualized as a process involving the following five phases: *initiating attachment*, or reaching out; *mutual acknowledgment of personhood*; *acknowledgment of attachment*; *professional intimacy*; and *negotiation of care* (Halldorsdottir, 1990).

This professional nurse–patient relationship is in many ways unusual. The following two accounts provide poignant illustrations:

> She fostered a working relationship between the two of us, as I said importantly as equals, and fostered a sense of

independence for your own growth, your personal growth to the point where you didn't need her in that role anymore.

In most other relationships what you want is some sort of deepening of the ability to communicate or the commitments so that the relationship is ongoing, that is, you want to perpetuate the relationship whereas in nursing and teaching the ideal thing is like parenting, what you want to do is to enable the client to graduate, that is, to leave. The best thing that could happen is that the patient is able enough to stop being a patient. Well, that is a peculiar thing in a relationship, that is, you are hoping for it to stop, for it to be no reason to continue, and then to be able to say goodbye with blessings, so that makes it unusual, I think, as a relationship.

The co-researchers' accounts illustrate clearly their conceptions of how caring positively influences the patient's ability to recover. Some co-researchers articulated the relief that they sensed when they felt cared for and how that diminished anxiety and gave them time to concentrate on getting better. Some co-researchers actually referred to caring as medicine of sorts. One said,

The purpose of the friendliness and the caring is focused on a particular professional activity and a particular very short period in the life of the patient and designed to . . . it's another form of medication of sorts. It's part of the healing, part of the getting the patient better, and it's creating the climate for the patient getting better.

Some co-researchers emphasized that caring affected healing through the psyche of the person. One said,

I think the effect on the psyche of a person is very much a part of the healing, because I believe in treating the whole person, treating them as body, mind, and spirit, not just the body alone but the three of them combined, and if their psyche is being damaged or uncared for, then how can their body get well?

It is apparent from the data that the nurse–patient attachment is perceived by the patient as a therapeutic or healing relationship. It seems that professional caring makes healing more profound, more rapid, and better internalized if it is provided, and it definitely makes the patient feel better healed.

In addition, the data make evident that the patient's reactions to professional caring are quite positive. The professional nurse gets to know the patient as a unique individual and treats that individual accordingly. She communicates to the patient in a way that makes him feel fully accepted as a normal human being and legitimized as a person and as a patient. This helps the patient to feel all right about himself and his hospital stay. Professional caring also seems to give the patient a sense of hope and optimism, encouragement, and reassurance. To feel cared for also gives the patient a sense of security. All this decreases the patient's anxiety, increases the patient's confidence, and positively affects the patient's sense of well-being and healing. From co-researchers' accounts, it is evident that they were, and still are, very grateful for their caring encounters; even if the only one, it is a pleasant memory that they carry away from their hospital stay.

Life flows through the life-giving person like a river and there is a transference of positive energy, strengthening, inspiring, comforting, enlightening, and invigorating the other, bringing joy, hope, trust, confidence, and peace. This life-giving presence is greatly edifying for the soul of the other. It involves dynamism, movement, and growth. It is a healing energy of unconditional love. It is the heavenly sunshine and nourishment the human flower needs to grow and develop, learn, and heal.

Examined in theological perspective, this growth-promoting flow of positive energy from the very center of the life-giving person is a "divine" energy of love and light, which has its source in a personal, living, and life-giving God. Fox

(1979) contends that compassion is a flow and overflow of the fullest human and divine energies born of an awareness of the interconnectedness of all creatures by reason of their common creator. The preciousness of the human being and the inherent dignity of each person is explained by Archimandrite Sophrony (1977) who states, "When our spirit contemplates in itself the 'image and likeness' of God, it is confronted with the infinite grandeur of man, and not a few of us—the majority, perhaps—are filled with dread at our audacity" (p. 44). He further contends that in the Divine Being, the hypostasis constitutes the innermost esoteric principle of Being.

Similarly, in human being, the hypostasis is the most intrinsic fundamental. As Sophrony states,

> *Persona* is the hidden man of the heart, in that which is not corruptible . . . which is in the sight of God of great price (I Peter 3:4)—the most precious kernel of man's whole being, manifested in his capacity for self-knowledge and self-determination; in his possession of creative energy; in his talent for cognition not only of the created world but also of the Divine world. Consumed with love, man feels himself joined with his beloved God. Through this union he knows God, and thus love and cognition merge into a single act. (1977, p. 44)

Again from a theological perspective, those who have gained perfection in caring are called saints. Dumitru Staniloae (1987), a professor of dogmatic theology, provides a closer look at saints. He explains how the gentleness and firmness of the man of God, his power to comfort and incite, his nearness and yet his distance, are all things rooted in the transcendent love of God, which comes close to us in him. Staniloae claims that in the person of the saint, because of his availability, extreme attention to others, and by the alacrity with which he gives himself to Christ humanity is healed and renewed. Staniloae states,

The saint always radiates a spirit of generosity, of forbearance, of attention and willingness to share, without any thought for himself. His warmth gives warmth to others and makes them feel they are regaining their strength, and lets them experience the joy of not being alone . . . the saint immediately creates an atmosphere of friendliness, of kinship, and indeed of intimacy between himself and others. In this way he humanizes his relationships and leaves on them a mark of genuineness, because he himself has become profoundly human and genuine. (p. 3)

Staniloae concludes,

The saint shows us a human being purified from the dross of all that is less than human. In him we see a disfigured and brutalised humanity set to rights; a humanity whose restored transparency reveals the limitless goodness, the boundless power and compassion of its prototype—God incarnate. It is the image of the living and personal absolute Being who became man that is re-established in the person of the saint. By being so truly human, he has reached a dizzy height of perfection in God, while remaining completely at home with men. The saint is one who is engaged in ceaseless, free dialogue with God and with men. His transparency reveals the dawn of the divine eternal light in which human nature is to reach its fulfilment. He is the complete reflection of the humanity of Christ. (p. 7)

This life force, or heavenly sunshine, creates the ideal conditions for the human flower to germinate, sprout, bloom, and bear fruit. It is a positive creative energy through which humanity is healed and renewed.

ONE FAMILY
Father of love
fountain of life and source of light
A dry seed that I am
give that I may dwell in you
and moistened by the dew from heaven
become a fruit of your ever-living love.

Mother of love
venerable rose and queen of
tenderness
A hungry child that I am
give that I may rest against your
breast
and nourished by your cherishing
love
become filled with loving kindness.
Brother of love
divine partner, guide and companion
An unworthy sinner that I am
flood my senses with the light of
your love
and sanctified by your gracious
brotherliness
give that I may flourish in you
my most dulcet morning.
Sister of love
white lily in the cloister of kindness
A mature woman that I am
with love let me serve you
and in our long white gowns
let us in joy and purity of heart
celebrate our sisterhood.

Sigridur Halldorsdottir

REFERENCES

Bermejo, L. M. (1987). *The spirit of life*. Chicago, IL: Loyola University Press.

Dossey, L. (1982). Care giving and natural systems theory. *Topics in Clinical Nursing, 3*(4), 21–27.

Fox, M. (1979). *A spirituality named compassion*. Minneapolis, MN: Winston Press.

Fox, M. (1985). *Illuminations of Hildegard of Bingen*. Santa Fe, NM: Bear and Company.

Gadow, S. (1985). Nurse and patient: The caring relationship. In A. H. Bishop &. J. R. Scudder Jr. (Eds.), *Caring, curing, coping: Nurse, physician, patient relationships*. Tuscaloosa, AL: The University of Alabama Press.

Gadow, S. (1988). Covenant without cure: Letting go and holding on in chronic illness. In J. Watson & M. A. Ray (Eds.), *The ethics of care and the ethics of cure: Synthesis in chronicity*. New York, NY: National League for Nursing.

Halldorsdottir, S. (1989a). *Caring and uncaring encounters in nursing practice: The patient's perspective*. Paper presented at the International Nursing Research Conference, Nursing Research for Professional Practice, held by Workgroup of European Nurse Researchers (WENR), Frankfurt/Main, Germany.

Halldorsdottir, S. (1989b). The essential structure of a caring and an uncaring encounter with a teacher: The nursing student's perspective. In J. Watson &. M. Ray (Eds.), *The caring imperative in education*. New York, NY: National League for Nursing.

Halldorsdottir, S. (1990). *Caring and uncaring encounters in nursing practice: The patient's perspective*. Unpublished manuscript.

Hildegard of Bingen (1985). In M. Fox (Ed.), *Illuminations of Hildegard of Bingen*. Santa Fe, NM: Bear and Company.

Leininger, M. M. (1988). *Caring: An essential human need*. Detroit, MI: Wayne State University Press.

Roach, M. S. (1984). *Caring: The human mode of being, implications for nursing* (Perspectives in Caring Monograph 1). Toronto, Ontario, Canada: University of Toronto, Faculty of Nursing.

Roach, M. S. (1987). *The human act of caring: A blueprint for the health professions*. Ottawa, Ontario: Canadian Hospital Associations.

Sophrony, A. (1977). *His life is mine* (R. Edmonds, Trans.). Crestwood, NY: St. Vladimir's Seminary Press.

Staniloae, D. (1987). Tenderness and holiness. In D. Staniloae (Ed.), *Prayer and holiness: The icon of man renewed in God*. Fairacres, Oxford, UK: SLG Press.

QUESTIONS FOR REFLECTION

Baccalaureate

1. Consider your last health care encounter with a nurse. What mode of being was present? How did you experience this encounter? Was it consistent with the characteristics of this mode of being?
2. List the five modes of being from uncaring to caring.
3. How do patients experience a nurse with a biopassive mode of being?

Master's

1. The advanced practice nurse asks the patient about his "chief complaint" with eyes on the computer screen as she enters data into the electronic health record (EHR). What mode is reflected in this behavior and what might the patient experience as a consequence of mode of being?
2. What is the evidence for Halldorsdottir's classification? Describe and critique these research studies.
3. How can the nurse sustain a biogenic practice?

Doctoral

1. Does the research conducted by Halldorsdottir provide sufficient evidence for her theoretical formulation?
2. How could you further test the modes of being with another through research?
3. Using criteria for evaluating a theory, identify the strengths and limitations of this theory.

13

Empirical Development of a Middle Range Theory of Caring

KRISTEN M. SWANSON

*A*s evidenced by our history, practice, and scholarship, caring has long been recognized as central to nursing. Nursing's service to humanity is to care for the client experiencing actual or potential health deviations until the client (individual or aggregate) is able to independently care for the self. Whether caring is self or other directed, the meaning of caring and the essential components of caring remain unclear.

Noddings (1984) analyzed caring from a philosophical standpoint and noted that the one caring is motivated to resolve or ameliorate the discomfort of the other as a result of having let the self become engrossed in the other's plight. Noddings' use of the term *engrossment* incorporates being able and willing to perceive the other's reality in an "as if" fashion, as if the other's reality were one's own. Benner and Wrubel (1989), like Nodding, propose that caring is central to assessing and intervening on behalf of another. They claim that the focus of a nurse's caring actually defines the areas in which attention is paid to a client's stress and coping needs.

Gilligan (1982) and Ray (1987) place caring in an ethical framework. Gilligan (1982), in her examination of women's development, noted that caring and connectedness are central to a woman's sense of morality and ethics. Ray (1987), in a phenomenological investigation of eight critical care nurses' expressions of caring, identified five caring themes: maturation, technical competence, transpersonal caring, communication, and judgment/ethics. The pervasiveness of an ethic of caring led Ray (1987) to conclude that "the ability of these critical care nurses to apply ethics and morality in distinguishing right from wrong in the attitudes and behaviors associated with the uses of technology was the common denominator of their experiences as a whole" (pp. 167–168).

Several nurse investigators have focused on identifying caring acts. Leininger's (1988) ethnoscientific studies in 52 different cultures led her to conclude that "cultural care has more diverse than similar meanings, and the patterns of care expression, have major implications for building an extensive body of nursing knowledge" (pp. 158–159). Brown (1986), Riemen (1986), and Larson (1984) have examined nurse caring behaviors and descriptions from the perspective of those cared for. Clients perceive caring as those nursing ministrations that are person-centered, protective, anticipatory, physically comforting, and that go beyond routine care. Larson (1984) noted a difference between nurses' and clients'

From Swanson, K. M. (1991). Empirical development of a middle range theory of caring. *Nursing Research*, *40*, 161–166. Permission to reprint granted by Wolters Kluwer.

perceptions of which caring behaviors were the most important. Although clients tended to value physical nursing ministrations, nurses believed they were most valued for their psychosocial supportive interventions.

Watson (1988), who views caring as a moral ideal, suggested that both nursing and medicine are moving out of an era in which cure is dominant and into one in which care takes precedence. However, she noted that more is known about treatment and cure than about healing and caring processes. Watson (1985) claims that nurses practicing, researching, and educating from a stance of caring will ultimately lead to "the promise of human preservation in society" (p. 29).

A universal definition or conceptualization of caring does not exist. Controversy exists within and outside of nursing as to the role of caring in personal and professional relationships. Is caring a process observable only in the context of two or more persons relating? Is it an intent embedded in the behavior of a caregiver? Or is it a perception identifiable only through the eyes of a care recipient? Can caring be taught? Is it a moral ideal? Or is it a way of being in the world? Caring has been discussed and described from each of these perspectives; yet, little inquiry exists from a phenomenological inductive stance whereby caregivers, care receivers, and care observers are queried for their perceptions of caring.

The purpose of this study is to describe the inductive development and refinement of a factor-naming theory of the middle range, an empirically derived descriptive theory pertaining to the characteristics of a specified phenomenon (Dickoff & James, 1968; Merton, 1957).

The theory, derived from phenomenological studies in three perinatal nursing contexts, provides a definition of caring and the five essential categories or processes that are proposed to characterize caring. Discussion proceeds from a

description of the empirical development of the theory to a contrast of the overall definition of caring with Cobb's (1976) definition of social support and concludes with a comparison of the caring processes, Watson's (1979, 1985) carative factors, and Benner's (1984) description of the helping role of nurses.

THEORY DEVELOPMENT

Overview

Caring was studied in three separate perinatal contexts: as experienced by women who miscarried (Study I) (Swanson-Kauffman, 1986a, 1988b), as provided by parents and professionals in the newborn intensive care unit (NICU) (Study II) (Swanson, 1990), and as recalled by socially at-risk mothers who had been the recipients of a long-term, intensive public health nursing intervention (Study III) (Swanson-Kauffman, 1988a). The phenomenological method described by Swanson-Kauffman and Schonwald (1988) was used in all three investigations. Institutional review board approval for protection of human subjects was granted for each project, confidentiality was assured, and informed consent of participants was obtained.

Method

Phenomenology involves four basic steps: bracketing, intuiting, analyzing, and describing (Oiler, 1986; Omery, 1983; Swanson-Kauffman & Schonwald, 1988). Bracketing is a conscious attempt by the investigator to remain critical and aware of the potential for personal bias and a priori assumptions that may skew the meanings intended by study participants. Intuiting is the result of the investigator's remaining open to the meanings attributed to a phenomenon by those who have lived the phenomenon. The investigator need not have experienced the phenomenon per se; however, having solicited many personal accounts of the phenomenon's existence, the investigator experiences the meanings as if the informants' reality were his or her own. Intuiting engages the investigator's self with the existence of those being investigated. Analysis involves the methods by which empirical accounts of a phenomenon are elicited (interviews and/or observations), documented (transcribed tape recordings and field notes), coded (sorted by topics addressed), and categorized into essential meaning components or processes (Swanson-Kauffman, 1986b). In the final phase of phenomenology, the phenomenon is described as the investigator has come to understand it. The description includes definitions of the essential meaning components (processes) and presentation of sufficient data to support the investigator's conclusions. The findings are internally validated through the quotes of the study participants and externally validated through comparison with the literature. The ultimate test of validity of phenomenological inquiry is concept recognition on the part of research consumers. The validity of the investigation is supported if those who have experienced the phenomenon can recognize their own reality in the phenomenological description.

Study I: Caring and Miscarriage

Study I (Swanson-Kauffman, 1986a, 1988b) began with the question "What are the caring behaviors of others that are identified as helpful by women who have miscarried?" Twenty women who had recently miscarried were interviewed on two occasions. About two thirds of the way through data collection and phenomenological analysis, however, it became apparent that focusing on acts and behaviors was not only premature to understanding the conceptual processes of caring but also a naive application of the phenomenological method—a method meant to interpret the meaning of lived experiences. Therefore, the research question that ultimately guided analysis was "What constitutes caring in the instance of miscarriage?" As

summarized in Table 13.1 (first column), the outcome of the miscarriage study was the identification of the five caring processes and their preliminary definitions. These definitions were substantively tied to the clinical context of miscarriage and were awkwardly worded from the perspective of the ones cared for.

Study II: Caring in the Newborn Intensive Care Unit

In Study II (Swanson, 1990), the question posed was "What is it like to be a provider of care in the Newborn Intensive Care Unit (NICU)?" Data were gathered over the course of 1 year through participant observation of care provision, attendance at biweekly ethical grand rounds, and a total of 33 interviews with 19 care providers. Care providers interviewed included one nurse administrator, one biomedical ethicist, one social worker, five mothers, two fathers, four continuity physicians, and five primary nurses. Each of these informants was either a parent or a professional caregiver to at least one of six very low-birth-weight infants. One of the outcomes of this NICU-based investigation was confirmation of the five caring processes and refinement of their definitions to more generalizable, less context-connected meanings that were worded from the perspective of the one caring. The refined definitions are listed in Table 13.1.

Study III: Caring and the Clinical Nursing Models Project

In Study III (Swanson-Kauffman, 1988a), 8 of the 68 young mothers initially enrolled in the Mental Health Intervention Group in conjunction with Barnard et al.'s Clinical Nursing Models Project (1988) were interviewed.

The purpose of the 18-month-long public health nursing intervention was to enable pregnant women who were at high social risk to take control of their lives and ultimately the care of their infants. Despite the highly transient lifestyle of

TABLE 13.1 Definitions of the Five Caring Processes

Study I: Women Who Miscarried[a]	Study II: NICU Caregivers[b]	Study III: At-Risk Mothers[c]
		Caring
		Is a nurturing way of relating to a valued other toward whom one feels a personal sense of commitment and responsibility.
Knowing	Knowing	Knowing
Identifies the woman's desire to be understood for her experience.	Striving to understand and event as it has meaning in the life of the other.	Striving to understand an event as it has meaning life of the other.
Being With	Being With	**Being With**
Illustrates the woman's need to have others feel with her—not necessarily as her, but with her.as her. but with her.	Being emotionally present to the other.	Being emotionally present to the other.
Doing For	Doing For	**Doing For**
Describes the need to have others do for her (i.e., physical care).	Doing for the other as he/she would do for the self if it were at all possible.	Doing for the other as he/she would do for the self if it were at all possible.
Enabling	Enabling	**Enabling**
Depicts the need to have her grieving facilitated.	Facilitating the other's passage through life transitions and unfamiliar events.	Facilitating the other's passage through life transitions and unfamiliar events.
Maintaining Belief	Maintaining Belief	Maintaining Belief
Focuses on the need to have others maintain belief in her capacity to get through the loss and to eventually give birth.	Sustaining faith in the other's capacity to get through an event or transition and face a future of fulfillment.	Sustaining faith in the other's capacity to get through an event or transition and face a future with meaning.

Note. Underlined = proposed; Normal = refined; Bold = confirmed.

[a]*n* = 20; 40 interviews.
[b]*n* = 19; 33 interviews.
[c]*n* = S; S interviews.

many of these young women, 4 years after their participation in the intervention protocol, it was possible to contact and interview eight of the mothers. The research question posed was "How do recipients of a long-term intensive nursing intervention recall and describe the nurse–patient relationship 4 years postintervention?" Through this study, the five caring processes were confirmed, or in one category (maintaining belief), slightly refined; subdimensions of each process were identified; and ultimately, an empirically derived definition of the overall concept of caring was proposed. The processes and overall definition are summarized in Table 13.1 (third column). The subdimensions of the caring processes are listed in Table 13.2.

THE THEORY OF CARING

In the theory's most recent form, caring consists of five categories or processes. They are as follows: (a) *knowing*, (b) *being*

TABLE 13.2 Subdimensions of the Five Caring Processes

Knowing	Avoiding assumptions
	Centering on the one cared-for
	Assessing thoroughly
	Seeking cues
	Engaging the self of both
Being with	Being there
	Conveying ability
	Sharing feelings
	Not-burdening
Doing for	Comforting
	Anticipating
	Performing competently/skillfully
	Protecting
	Preserving dignity
Enabling	Informing/explaining
	Supporting/allowing
	Focusing
	Generating alternatives/thinking it through
	Validating/giving feedback
Maintaining belief	Believing in/holding in esteem
	Maintaining a hope-filled attitude
	Offering realistic optimism
	"Going the distance"

with, (c) *doing for,* (d) *enabling,* and (e) *maintaining belief.* Although each of these categories is presented separately, the categories are not mutually exclusive.

Knowing

Knowing is striving to understand an event as it has meaning in the life of the other. When one is operating from a basis of knowing, the careprovider works to avoid a priori assumptions about the meaning of an event, centers on the one cared for, and conducts a thorough, ongoing cue-seeking assessment of the experience of the one cared for. The provider begins with the premise that the desire is to understand the personal reality of the one cared for. Integral to knowing is the provider's philosophy of personhood and the willingness to recognize the other as a significant being. When knowing occurs, the selves of both provider and recipient are engaged.

One of the mothers from the Clinical Nursing Models Project described how the nurse worked with her to get to her true feelings:

> When things weren't right, I could say that things were fine and it was only a matter of time. I mean the nurse would ask certain questions and there would be no way that I could be consistent without telling the truth. And then we would talk, and pretty soon instead of saying it was fine, I would start out with what was really wrong.

In the NICU study, one group of parents described how much they wanted to be recognized for their experience and needs in the NICU. With the birth of their twin sons, the mother and father were in the unit for the third time. On two previous occasions, in the same hospital, they had experienced the deaths of children born prematurely. In the following quote, the father describes how the staff knowing their experience was essential to meeting their needs:

> They thought at first that we were being like resistive to learning . . . and it wasn't until they found out that this was the "third time in three years we're been here . . . [that] they started to figure out that the most important thing we wanted to find out immediately was the major things. We weren't so concerned about movement and that kind of stuff, the major things we were concerned with was the oxygen, the respirators, and how they were doing feeding . . . I was going in there daily. We'd wash up, she'd reach in and touch them first and I'd go right to the charts and start reading.

External validity for the inductively derived category of knowing is found in the philosophical work of Noddings (1984) who examines caring in the contexts of teaching and parenting. In her book, *Caring: A Feminine Approach to Ethics and Moral Education*, she states that "Apprehending the other's reality, feeling what he feels as nearly as possible, is the essential part of airing from the view of the one-caring" (p. 16).

Being With

The second caring process, being with, is being emotionally present to the other. It involves simply "being there," conveying ongoing availability and sharing feelings, whether joyful or painful. Yet, the presence and sharing are responsibly monitored so that the one caring does not ultimately burden the one cared for. Being with goes one small step beyond knowing. It is more than understanding another's plight; it is becoming emotionally open to the other's reality.

The message conveyed through being with is that the other's experience matters to the one caring.

A woman from the miscarriage study described how the nurse who cared for her during her dilatation and curettage was able to be with her:

> The male nurse—I think he helped me quite a bit because he tried to comfort me as much as possible . . . he tried to be as gentle as possible . . . he even cried a little bit. He made me feel more like he cared. When they were using the vacuum cleaner, the little suction thing—that hurt quite a bit. I was gritting my teeth, waiting for it to be over, and he tried to comfort me and tell me that it was just about finished. . . . He didn't break down and not be able to do his job. . . . He just kept saying, "It's a matter of time." You know, he was so sorry. (Swanson-Kauffman, 1986a, p. 42)

In the NICU study, one nurse described how important it was to be with the infants she cared for:

> Barrett was a chronic baby who died recently. I was one of his consistent people. I loved him and I really liked his parents. He went through everything, a terrible lung disease, he was blind, and then he died of SIDS. . . . Some of these kids have such a short time and it isn't appropriate to say, "Well, if they make it to two years old, we'll start loving them." They need it now. . . . At least before that baby died he knew what it was like to be loved.

Noddings (1984) also provides validation of the being with category. She states that presence can occur even in physical absence. Engrossment in the other, regard, and desire for the other's well-being are signs of presence (p. 19).

Doing For

The third caring category is doing for. This entails doing for the other what he or she would do for the self if it were at all possible. Care that is doing for is comforting, anticipatory, protective of the others needs, and performed competently and skillfully. As Larson (1984) and Riemen (1986) have described, clients will often-times identify nurses' doing for as those acts which are most appreciated. When a person is in a state of being that requires another to do for them, it can be very embarrassing. Consequently, the caregiver must consciously act to preserve the dignity of the other. As Gadow (1984) states, "Dependence upon another for care of the body constitutes an indignity only when the person cared for becomes an object for the caregiver"(p. 67).

Oftentimes, this type of dignity-preserving doing for must be delivered in an unobtrusive, easily forgotten manner. Bowers (1987) beautifully illustrated the dignity preservation inherent in doing for in her discussion of family caregivers' well-thought through schemes to maximize their aging parents' capacity to practice self-care. Similar to the subdimensions of doing for, Bowers has identified five categories of caregiving: anticipatory, preventive, supervisory, instrumental, and protective.

The following quote is a description of doing for on the part of a husband whose wife just miscarried. She stated:

> Tim went to the store and got me some sanitary napkins, which I hadn't used in years . . . and he came home with every style that there is out there, it was like every kind in the world. I still have some! I was so hungry. And he was just real sweet . . . fixed me poached eggs, brought them to me in bed. We didn't even really talk about it. We were both thankful I was OK. He said, "All I really care about is that you're all right." (Swanson-Kauffman, 1986a, p. 43)

Once again, support for doing for as a caring category may be found in the work by Noddings (1984): "When we see the other's reality as a possibility for us, we must act to eliminate the intolerable, to reduce the pain, to fill the need, to actualize the dream" (p. 14).

Enabling

The fourth caring category, enabling, means facilitating the other's passage through life transitions and unfamiliar events. An enabling caregiver is one who uses his or her expert knowledge to the betterment of the other. The purpose of enabling is to facilitate the other's capacity to grow, heal, and/or practice self-care. Enabling involves providing information and explanations as well as offering emotional support in the form of allowing and validating the other's feelings. Enabling often includes assisting the ones cared for to focus on their concerns, generate alternatives, and think through ways to look at or act on a situation.

One mother from the Clinical Nursing Models Project described how tired nurse validated her unsure beliefs about parenting:

> Like I said I was really nervous after Tracy was born. So, I called the nurse up several times. My mother did not believe in breast-feeding. We had many heated arguments over it. My husband, he was like, "Nothing's too good for my baby and doctors say that the breast is best." So my mom and husband got into a few fights. But the nurse, she was always agreeable with everything that I felt and she could always back it up with her research.

Mayeroff (1971) supports the importance of enabling another's passage through transition times. He states: "To care for another, in the most significant sense, is to help him grow and actualize himself" (p. 1).

Maintaining Belief

The final caring process, maintaining belief, is sustaining faith in the other's capacity to get through an event or transition and face a future with meaning. This definition used to conclude with the words "of fulfillment." However, in Study III (Swanson-Kauffman, 1988a), interviews with women whose lives were riddled with challenges to mere survival revealed that fulfillment may be one step beyond reality for some human experiences. Caring that is maintaining belief involves holding the other in esteem and believing in them. The one caring maintains a hope-filled (as opposed to hopeless) attitude and offers realistic optimism as they "go the whole distance with the other person." In nursing, maintaining belief is a pervasive part of our profession; nurses approach human responses as meaningful aspects of their clients' realities. Nurses seek to assist clients to attain, maintain, or regain meaning in their experiences of health and illness.

A young mother from the Clinical Nursing Models Project described how the nurse was there with her all the way:

> I was not only pregnant, I felt very unattractive and I had the boyfriend or the partner to prove that you know that he wanted nothing to do with me, and I got a lot of negative feedback from him. All the while I'm trying to keep real positive and yet feeling I'm failing and then Cindy would put me back up and I would keep going. And I did, I kept going.

In maintaining belief, the goal is not to give the others life meaning. Rather the one caring strives to know, be with, do for, and enable the other so that within the demands, constraints, and resources of the other's life, a path filled with meaning will be chosen. According to Noddings (1984), although we cannot define others' perfection, we must be "exquisitely sensitive" to their ideal of perfection and must act to promote that ideal (p. 102).

CARING: DEFINITION AND DISCUSSION

Through three phenomenological studies, the five caring processes, knowing, being with, doing for, enabling, and maintaining belief, were empirically identified and described. Ultimately, the following definition of caring was inductively derived: *Caring* is *a nurturing way of relating to a valued other toward whom one feels a personal sense of commitment and responsibility.*

Caring as defined through these three perinatal studies is very compatible with Gaut's philosophical analysis of caring. Gaut (1983) has stated that caring, at its very least, involves individual attention to and concern for another, individual responsibility for or providing for at some level, and individual regard, fondness, or attachment.

Although caring is most likely an aspect of all socially supportive relationships, not all caring relationships are experienced as social support. The proposed definition of caring may be contrasted with Cobb's (1976) definition of social support: "Information that one is cared for and loved; that one is valued and esteemed; and that one belongs to a network of mutual obligation" (pp. 300–301). The caveat between caring, as defined through these investigations, and social support, as defined by Cobb, is at the point of mutual obligation. For example, mutually obligating, socially supportive relationships might include new mothers exchanging babysitting, neighbors borrowing sugar, classmates taking notes for each other, or coworkers sharing rides. In each of these instances, although a sense of caring might motivate the willingness to assist another, the assistance is offered with the implicit or tacit agreement that "you would do the same for me if I needed it." In contrast, if one considers the primary caring relationship—the parent–child relationship—the parent cares the child from a sense of responsibility and love, not from the expectation that the child will pay back in kind for services rendered. The child may love back; however, the parent does not care with the expectation that the child will reciprocate. Similarly in nurse–client relationships, the nurse cares without obligating the client to reciprocate. As Norbeck (1984) has proposed, it is possible that the reason patients generally do not list health care providers as members of their social support networks is that patients do not (and hopefully should not) feel a sense of mutual obligation when professional caring is provided.

Leininger (1981) claims that "Caring is the central and unifying domain for the body of knowledge and practices in nursing" (p. 3). Yet, caring is not uniquely a nursing phenomenon. However, there may be characteristic behavior patterns that are universal expressions of nurse caring. For example, Watson (1979, 1985) has identified 10 carative factors and Benner (1984) has delineated eight dimensions of the helping role of the nurse. The factors and role dimensions are nursing acts that universally cut across client health conditions and developmental levels. The theory of caring, carative factors, and helping role provide cross-validation for each other. Table 13.3 facilitates comparison and contrast among the caring processes, carative factors, and helping

TABLE 13.3 Conceptual Cross-Validation of the Caring Processes With Watson's Carative Factors and Benner's Helping Role of the Nurse

The Helping Role of Nursing (Benner, 1984, p. 50)	Caring Process			Carative Factors (Watson, 1985, p. 75)
1. Creating a climate for establishing a commitment to-healing.	Benner 1, 5	Knowing	Watson 1, 3,10	1. Humanistic altruistic system of values.
2. Providing comfort measures and preserving personhood in the face of pain and extreme breakdown.				2. [Instillation of] faith-hope.
3. Presenting	Benner 3, 6.7	Being with	Watson 1, 3, 10	3. Sensitivity to self and others.
4. Maximizing the patient s participation and control in his/her recovery.	Benner 2, 5, 6	Doing for	Watson 4, 8, 9	4. Helping-trusting, human care relationship.
5. Interpreting kinds of pain and selecting appropriate strategies for pain management and control.	Benner 4, 8, 7	Enabling	Watson 6, 5, 7, 4	5. Expressing positive and negative feelings.
6. Proving comfort and communication through touch.	Benner 1, 4	Maintaining belief	Watson 2, 10	6. Creative problem solving caring process.
7. Providing emotional/ informational support to patient families.				7. Transpersonal teaching-learning.
8. Guiding patients through emotional and developmental changes.				8. Supportive, protective, and/or corrective, mental, physical, societal, and spiritual environment.
				9. Human needs assistance.
				10. Existential-phenomenological-spiritual forces.

role. Because the carative factors and helping role are conceptually grounded in the caring processes, the theory of caring provides a meaning base for why the carative factors and helping role may be perceived as nurturing or helpful by nursing clients. The convergence of the caring processes with Watson's factors and Benner's helping role supports the claim that caring is a central and unifying nursing phenomenon; however, it does not render the concept of caring as unique to nursing knowledge or practice.

FUTURE DIRECTIONS

A theory of caring has been derived through studies in three perinatal situations; now, it needs to be examined for its applicability in other nursing and non-nursing contexts. The congruence of the caring processes with Watson's carative factors and Benner's description of the helping role of the nurse provide evidence that the proposed theory of caring may have validity in nursing beyond the perinatal contexts from which it was derived. Furthermore, the data derived from other health professionals and parents in the NICU study and the congruence of the theory with some of the nonnursing literature (Gilligan, 1982; Mayeroff, 1971; Noddings, 1984) suggest that the proposed theory of caring may generalize to relationships other than those occurring just in nursing.

At present, a caring-based nurse counseling program for women who miscarry is being developed and tested (National Center for Nursing Research, R29 NR01899-04). Hopefully, this deductive application of the theory of caring will demonstrate the effectiveness of a caring-based intervention on women's health and, ultimately, document the capacity for caring to enhance healing and the potential to find meaning in human experiences of health and illness.

ACKNOWLEDGMENTS

Grateful acknowledgments are extended to Kathryn Barnard, PhD, RN, FAAN (post-doctoral sponsor) and Jean Watson, PhD, RN, FAAN (dissertation chair), both of whom mentioned the investigator throughout the conduct of these studies.

Funding for the three projects were provided through several sources: Sigma Theta Tau Alpha Kappa Chapter-at-Large; a grant from the McArthur Family Foundation, and an anonymous gift in memory of Panlina Hoff Carey: NCNR individually awarded NSRA Postdoctoral Fellowship 5 F32NR05927; and University of Washington School of Nursing Biomedical Research Support Crust 280 TRR05078.

REFERENCES

Barnard, K. E., Magyary, D., Sumner, G., Booth, C. L., Mitchell, S. K., & Spieker, S. (1988). Prevention of parenting alterations for women with low social support. *Psychiatry, 51*, 248–253.

Benner, P. (1984). *From notice to expert.* Menlo Park, CA: Addison-Wesley.

Benner, P., & Wrubel, J. (1989). *The primacy of caring stress and coping in health and illness.* Menlo Park, CA: Addison-Wesley.

Bowers, B. J. (1987). Intergenerational caregiving: Adult caregivers and their aging parents. *Advances in Nursing Science, 9*(2), 20–31.

Brown, L. (1986). The experience of care: Patient perspectives. *Topics in Clinical Nursing, 8*(2), 56–62.

Cobb, S. (1976). Social support as a moderator of life stress. *Psychosomatic Medicine, 38*, 300–314.

Dickoff, J., & James, P. (1968). A theory of theories: A position paper. *Nursing Research, 17*, 197–203.

Gadow, S. (1984). Touch and technology: Two paradigms of patient care. *Journal of Religion and Health, 23*(1), 63–69.

Gaut, D. (1983). Development of a theoretically adequate description of caring. *Western Journal of Nursing Research, 5*, 313–324.

Gilligan, C. (1982). *In a different choice.* Cambridge, MA: Harvard University Press.

Larson, P. (1984). Important nurse airing behaviors perceived by patients with cancer. *Oncology Nursing Forum, 11*(6), 46–50.

Leininger, M. M. (1988). Leininger's theory of nursing: Cultural care diversity and universality. *Nursing Science Quarterly, 1*(4), 175–181.

Leininger, M. M. (1981). The phenomenon of caring: Importance, research questions, and theoretical considerations. In M. M. Leininger (Ed.), *Caring: An essential human need* (pp. 3–15). Thorofare, NJ: Charles B. Slack.

Mayeroff, M. (1971). *On caring.* New York, NY: Harper & Row.

Merton, R. F. (1957). *Social theory and social structure* (Rev. ed.). New York, NY: Free Press.

Noddings, N. (1984). *Caring: A feminine approach to ethics and moral education.* Berkeley, CA: University of California Press.

Norbeck, J. (1984). Discussion. In K. E. Barnard, P. A. Brandt, B. S. Raff, & P. Carroll (Eds.), *Social support and families of culnerable infants* (pp. 35). New York, NY: March of Dimes Birth Defects Foundation.

Oiler, C. J. (1986). Phenomenology: The method. In P. L. Munhall & C. J. Oiler (Eds.), *Nursing research: A qualitative perspective* (pp. 69–84). Norwalk, CT: Appleton-Century-Crofts.

Omery, A. (1983). Phenomenology: A method for nursing research. *Advances in Nursing Science, 5*(2), 49–63.

Ray, M. A. (1987). Technological caring: A new model in critical care. *Dimensions of Critical Care Nursing, 6,* 166–173.

Riemen, D. (1986). The essential structure of a caring interaction: Doing phenomenology.

In P. L. Munhall & C. J. Oiler (Eds.), *Nursing research A qualitative perspective* (pp. 85–108). Norwalk, CT: Appleton-Century-Crofts.

Swanson, K. M. (1990). Providing care in the NICU: Sometimes an act of love. *Advances in Nursing Science, 13*(1), 60–73.

Swanson-Kauffman, K. M. (1986a), Caring in the instance of unexpected early pregnancy loss. *Topics in Clinical Nursing, 8*(2), 37–46.

Swanson-Kauffman, K. M. (1986b). A combined qualitative methodology for nursing research. *Advances in Nursing Science, 8*(3), 58–69.

Swanson-Kauffman, K. M. (1988a, July). *Caring as a basis for nursing practice.* Paper presented at the NCAST Institute, Seattle, WA.

Swanson-Kauffman, K. M. (1988b). Caring needs of women who miscarried. In M. M. Leininger (Ed.), *Care: Discovery and uses in clinical and community nursing* (pp. 55–69). Detroit, MI: Wayne State University Press.

Swanson-Kauffman, K. M., & Schonwald, E. (1988). Phenomenology. In B. Sarter (Ed.), *Paths to knowledge: Innovative research methods for nursing* (pp. 97–105). New York, NY: National League for Nursing.

Watson, J. (1979). *Nursing: The philosophy and science of caring.* Boston, MA: Little, Brown and Company.

Watson, J. (1985). *Nursing: Human science and human care.* Norwalk, CT: Appleton-Century-Crofts.

Watson, J. (1988). New dimensions of human caring theory. *Nursing Science Quarterly, 2*(4), 175–181.

QUESTIONS FOR REFLECTION

Baccalaureate

1. Name the five caring processes in Swanson's middle range theory of caring.
2. Select one of these processes and provide an example of how you have come to know this process in the care of your patients.
3. What is Swanson's definition of caring?

Master's

1. Select one of Swanson's caring processes and using the dimension of the process explain how you would apply this with your population of interest.
2. What does Swanson mean by the dimension "avoiding assumption" related to the caring process of Knowing?
3. What is the evidence that supports Swanson's middle range theory of caring?

Doctoral

1. Describe the process of building a middle range theory through induction.
2. How is this middle range theory of caring different from a grand theory or conceptual model?
3. Evaluate Swanson's middle range theory of caring using the criteria for evaluating middle range theories.

14

Nursing as Caring: A Model for Transforming Practice
(Chapters 1 and 2)

ANNE BOYKIN AND SAVINA O. SCHOENHOFER

FOUNDATIONS OF NURSING AS CARING

In this chapter, we present the fundamental ideas related to person as caring and nursing as a discipline and profession that serves as the perspectival grounding for the theory Nursing as Caring. We offer our perspective of these ideas as influenced by the works of various scholars, so that the grounding for Nursing as Caring will be understood. We do not intend to offer a novel perspective of the notion of person or a new generic understanding of caring or of discipline and profession, but to communicate some of the ideas basic to Nursing as Caring.

Major assumptions underlying Nursing as Caring include the following:

- persons are caring by virtue of their humanness
- persons are caring, moment to moment
- persons are whole or complete in the moment
- personhood is a process of living grounded in caring
- personhood is enhanced through participating in nurturing relationships with caring others
- nursing is both a discipline and a profession

PERSPECTIVE OF PERSONS AS CARING

Throughout this chapter, the basic premise presides as follows: *All persons are caring*. Caring is an essential feature and expression of being human. The belief that all persons, by virtue of their humanness, are caring establishes the ontological and ethical ground on which this theory is built. Person as caring is a value that underlies each of the major concepts of Nursing as Caring and is an essential idea for understanding this theory and its implications. Being a *person* means living caring, and it is through caring that our "being" and all possibilities are known to the fullest. Elaboration on the meaning of this perspective will provide a necessary backdrop for understanding ideas in subsequent chapters.

Caring is a process. Each person, throughout his or her life, grows in the capacity to express caring. In another way, each person grows in his or her competency to express self as caring person. Because of our belief that each person is caring and grows in caring throughout his or her life, we will not focus on behaviors considered noncaring in this book. Our assumption that all persons are caring does not require that every act of a person necessarily be

From Boykin, A., & Schoenhofer, S. (1993). *Nursing as caring: A model for transforming practice* (pp. 3–30). Sudbury, MA: Jones & Bartlett. Permission to reprint granted by Jones & Bartlett.

caring. There are many experiences of life that teach us that not every act of a person is caring. These acts are obviously not expressions of self as caring person and may well be labeled noncaring. Developing the fullest potential for expressing caring is an ideal. Notwithstanding the abstract context of this ideal, it is *knowing* the person as living caring and growing in caring that is central to our effort in this book. Therefore, even though an act or acts may be interpreted as noncaring, the person remains caring.

Although this assumption does not require that every act be understood as an expression of caring, the assumption that all persons are caring does require an acceptance that fundamentally, potentially, and actually each person is caring. Although persons are innately caring, actualization of the potential to express caring varies in the moment and develops over time. Thus, caring is lived moment to moment and is constantly unfolding. The development of competency in caring occurs over a lifetime. Throughout life, we come to understand what it means to be a caring person, to live caring, and to nurture each other as caring.

Roach and Mayeroff provide some explanation as to what caring involves. Roach, in her works (1984, 1987, 1992), has asserted that caring is the "human mode of being" (1992, p. ix). As such, it entails the capacity to care, the calling forth of this ability in ourselves and others, responding to something or someone that matters and finally actualizing the ability to care (192, p. 47). Since caring is a characteristic of being human, it cannot be attributed as a manifestation of any single discipline. These beliefs have directly influenced our assumption that all persons are caring. Mayeroff, a philosopher, in his 1971 book *On Caring*, discusses caring as an end in itself, an ideal, and not merely a means to some future end! Within the context of caring as process, Roach (1992, 1984) says that caring entails the human capacity to care, the calling forth of this ability in ourselves and others, the responsivity to something or someone that

matters, and the actualizing of the power to care. Even though our human nature is to be caring, the full expression of this varies with the lived experience of being human. The process of bringing forth this capability can be nurtured through concern and respect for person as person.

Mayeroff suggests that caring "is not to be confused with such meanings as wishing well, liking, comforting, and maintaining . . . it is not an isolated feeling or a momentary relationship" (p. 1). He describes caring as helping the other to grow. In relationships lived through caring, changes in the one who cares and the one cared for are evident.

Mayeroff tells us how caring provides meaning and order as follows:

> In the context of a man's life, caring has a way of ordering his other values and activities around it. When this advising is comprehensive, because of the inclusiveness of his caring, there is a basic stability in his life; he is "in place" in the world instead of being out of place, or merely drifting on endlessly seeking his place. Through caring for certain others, by serving them through caring a man lives the meaning of his own life. In the sense in which a man can ever be said to be at home in the world, he is at home not through dominating, or explaining, or appreciating, but through caring and being cared for. (1971, p. 2)

Mayeroff expressed ideas about the meaning of being a caring person when he referred to trust as "being entrusted with the care of another" (p. 7). He spoke of both "being with" the other (p. 43) and "being for" (p. 42) the other, experiencing the other as an extension of self and at the same time "something separate from me that I respect in its own right" (p. 2). To be a caring person means to "live the meaning of my own life" (p. 72), having a sense of stability and basic certainty that allows an openness and accessibility, experiencing belonging, living congruence between beliefs and behaviors, and expressing a clarity of values that enables living a simplified rather than a cluttered life.

Watson, a nursing theorist and philosopher, offers insight into caring. In her theory of Human Care, she examines caring as an intersubjective human process expressing respect for the mystery of being-in-the-world, reflected in the three spheres of mind–body–soul. Human care transactions based on reciprocity allow for a unique and authentic quality of presence in the world of the other. In a related vein, Parse (1981) defines the ontology of caring as "risking being with someone toward a moment of joy." Through being with another, connectedness occurs and moments of joy are experienced by both.

If the ontological basis for being is that all persons are caring and by our humanness caring *is*, then I accept that I am a caring person. This belief that all persons are caring, however, entails a *commitment* to know self and other as caring person. According to Trigg (1973), commitment "presupposes certain beliefs and also involves a personal dedication to the actions implied by them" (p. 44). Mayeroff (1981) speaks of this dedication as devotion and states "devotion is essential to caring . . . when devotion breaks down, caring breaks down" (p. 8). Mayeroff also states that "obligations that derive from devotion are a constituent element in caring" (p. 9). Moral obligations arise from our commitments; therefore, when I make a commitment to caring as a way of being, I have become morally obligated. The quality of the moral commitment is a measure of being "in place" in the world. Gadow (1980) asserts that caring represents the moral ideal of nursing wherein the human dignity of the patient and nurse is recognized and enhanced.

As individuals, we are continually in the process of developing expressions of ourselves as caring persons. The flow of life experiences provides ongoing opportunities for knowing self as caring person. As we learn to live fully each of these experiences, it becomes easier to allow self and others the space and time to develop innate caring capabilities and authentic being. The awareness of self as caring person calls to consciousness the belief that caring is lived by each person moment to moment and directs the "oughts" of actions. When decisions are made from this perspective, the emerging question consistently is, "How ought I act as caring person?"

How one is with others is influenced by the degree of authentic awareness of self as caring person. Caring for self as person requires experiencing self as other and yet being one with self, valuing self as special and unique, and having the courage, humility, and trust to honestly know self. It takes courage to let go of the present, so that it may be transcended and new meaning be discovered. Letting go, of course, implies a freeing of oneself from present constraints so that we may see and be in new ways. One who cares is genuinely humble in being ready and willing to know more about self and others. Such humility involves the realization that learning is continuous and the recognition that each experience is unique. As my commitment to persons as caring moves into the future, I must choose again and again to ratify it or not. This commitment remains binding and choices are made based on devotion to this commitment.

Personhood is the process of living grounded in caring. Personhood implies living out who we are, demonstrating congruence between beliefs and behaviors and living the meaning of one's life. As a process, personhood acknowledges the person as having continuous potential for further tapping the current of caring. Therefore, as person, we are constantly living caring and unfolding possibilities for self as caring person in each moment. Personhood is being authentic, being who I am as caring person in the moment. This process is enhanced through participation in nurturing relationships with others.

The nature of relationships is transformed through caring. All relationships between and among persons carry with them mutual expectations. Caring is living in the context of relational responsibilities. A relationship experienced through caring holds at its heart the importance of person-as-person. Being in the world also mandates participating in human relationships that require responsibility—responsibility to self and other. To the extent that these relationships are shaped through caring, they are consistent with the obligations entailed in relational responsibility, and the "person-al" (person-to-person) relationships. When being with self and others is approached from a desire to know person as living caring, the human potential for actualizing caring directs the moment.

All relationships are opportunities to draw forth caring possibilities, opportunities to reinforce the beauty of person-as-person. Through knowing self as caring person, I am able to be authentic to self and with others. I am able to see from the inside what others see from the outside. Feelings, attitudes, and actions lived in the moment are matched by an inner genuine awareness. The more I am open to knowing and appreciating self and trying to understand the world of other, the greater the awareness of our interconnectedness as caring persons. Knowing of self frees one to truly *be with* other. How does one come to know self as caring person? Mayeroff's (1971) caring ingredients are useful conceptual tools when one is struggling to know self and other as caring. These ingredients include the following: honesty, courage, hope, knowing (both knowing about and knowing directly), trust, humility, and alternating rhythm.

The idea of a hologram serves as a way of understanding self and other. Pribram (1985) offers us an interesting view on relationships in his discussion of hologram. He states that the uniqueness of a hologram is such that if a part (of the hologram) is broken, any part of it is capable of reconstructing the total image (p. 133).

Using this idea, if the lens for "being" in relationships is holographic, then the beauty of the person will be retained. Through entering, experiencing, and appreciating the world of other, the nature of being human is more fully understood. The notion of person as whole or complete expresses an important value. As such, the respect for the total person—all that is in the moment—is communicated. Therefore, from a holographic perspective, it is impossible to focus on a part of a person without seeing the whole person reflected in the part. The wholeness (the fullness of being) is forever present. Perhaps in some context, the word *part* is incongruent with the notion that there is only wholeness. The term *aspect*, or *dimension*, may be a useful substitute.

The view of person as caring and complete is also intentional; it offers a lens for a way of being with another, which prevents the segmenting of that other into component parts (e.g., mind, body, and spirit). Here, valuing and respecting each person's beauty, worth, and uniqueness is lived as one seeks to understand fully the meaning of values, choices, and priority systems through which values are expressed. The inherent value that persons reflect and to which they respond is the wholeness of persons. The person is at all times whole. The idea of wholeness does not negate an appreciation of the complexity of being. However, from the perspective of the theory Nursing as Caring, to encounter person as less than whole involves a failure to encounter person. Until our view is such that it includes the whole as complete person and not just a part, we cannot fully know the person. Gadow's (1984) contrasting paradigms, empathic and philanthropic, are relevant to this understanding. The philanthropic paradigm enables a relationship in which dignity is bestowed as a "gift from one who is whole to one who is not" (p. 68). Philanthropy marks the person as other than one like me. Gadow's empathic paradigm, on the other hand, "breaches objectivity" (p. 67) and expresses participating in the experience of another. In the empathic paradigm, the subjectivity of the other is "assumed to be as whole and valid as that of the caregiver" (p. 68). These paradigm descriptions facilitate our knowing how we are with others. Is the attitude expressed through nursing one person as part or whole? How do these perspectives direct nursing practice?

Our understanding of person as caring centers on valuing and celebrating human wholeness, the human person as living and growing in caring, and active personal engagement with others. This perspective of what it means to be human is the foundation for understanding nursing as a human endeavor, a person-to-person service, a human social institution, and a human science.

CONCEPTION OF NURSING AS DISCIPLINE AND PROFESSION

Our second major perspectival grounding involves a social conception of nursing as a discipline and a profession. Here, ideas such as *social contract* and *human science* are important to understand the scope and significance of this new and developing general theory of Nursing as Caring. Since the theory evolved from a stance that nursing is both a discipline and a profession, a discussion of characteristics of both social structures lays crucial groundwork.

The discipline of nursing and the profession of nursing are inextricably bound and exquisitely interwoven aspects of the single unity of nursing. Each aspect illuminates particular duties, privileges, and realms of activity relevant to nursing as an entity. The discipline of nursing has its origins in the unique social call upon the world to which the practice of nursing is a response. The profession of nursing involves professing an understanding of both the social need from which the calls

for nursing arise and the body of knowledge drawn upon in creating the nursing response.

In this regard, the nature of nursing takes on new dimensions as the domain of nursing knowledge gains clear articulation. As mentioned, our work is predicated on the understanding that nursing is a discipline—a way of knowing, being, valuing, and living. This conception transcends the somewhat artificial divisions between science, ethic, and art as distinct entities and unifies nursing as a practiced discipline. Our understanding of nursing as a discipline has been enriched by our use of the works of Phenix (1964), King and Brownell (1976), and the Nursing Development Conference Group (1979). Further, building on Carper's (1978) application of Phenix to nursing knowledge, it has become clear that addressing nursing as science, ethic, or art, or partitioning nursing into those dimensions, is not adequate for the development of nursing as a unique discipline. Instead, we envision nursing as a unity of knowledge within a larger unity. Knowing nursing, therefore, means knowing the realms of personal, ethical, empirical, and aesthetic—all at once. When that which is known as nursing is known solely as science, or as art, the knowing is not adequate to the requirements of nursing practice, nursing education, or nursing scholarship.

King and Brownell (1976) have ably described the essential characteristics that define disciplines. In this regard, the discipline of nursing is represented by a community of scholars dedicated to developing a particular field of knowledge representing a unique view of humankind and human endeavor. Of course, the domain of any discipline, including nursing, is that which its members assert. The domain embodies the valuative and affective stance taken and implies acceptance of responsibility for the discourse of the discipline. In its most fundamental sense then, a discipline is understood as a pathway of knowing and being in the world. We do not intend that our view of nursing as a discipline denigrate the efforts of the past or present. Rather, we believe our view enables the development of nursing as a discipline of constant discovery and new knowing.

Like disciplines, professions have unique characteristics, as defined by Flexner. Flexner (1919) initially identified the most basic characteristic of a profession that addresses a unique and urgent social need through techniques derived from a tested knowledge base. Professions have their historical roots in those human services that people provided for each other within the existing social institutions (e.g., tribe, family, or community). Thus, each profession, including nursing, has its origins in everyday human situations and the everyday contributions people make to the welfare of others. Flexner's founding conditions for the designation *profession* are reiterated in the American Nursing Association's 1980 Social Policy Statement, in which the idea of a social contract is addressed.

Nursing: A Social Policy Statement was intended to provide nurses with a fresh perspective on practice while providing the society with a view of nursing for the 1980s. The overall intent of this document was to call to consciousness the linkages between the profession and society. While the *Social Policy Statement* is considered by many (see, for example, Allen, 1987; Packard & Polifroni, 1991; Rodgers, 1991; White, 1984) to be outdated; we find the concept of the social contract to be useful when studying the relationship of nurse to nursed. As the foundation for professions, the social contract, although understood to be a "hypothetical ideal" (Silva, 1983, p. 150), is also an expression of people recognizing (1) the presence of a basic need and (2) the existence of greater knowledge and skill available to meet that need than can be readily exercised by each member of the society. Society at large then calls for commitment by a segment of society to the acquisition and use of this knowledge and

skill for the good of all. Social goods are promised in return for this commitment.

Today, the profession of nursing is moving from a social contract relationship toward a covenantal relationship between the nurse and nursed. Although the social contract implies an impersonal, legalistic stance, the covenantal relationship emphasizes personal engagement and ever present freedom to choose commitments. Cooper (1988), for example, discusses her ideas on the relevance of covenantal relationships for nursing ethics. She states "the promissory nature of the covenant is contained in the willingness of individuals to enter a covenantal relationship" (p. 51) and it is within this context that obligations arise. As caring persons, we "see" relationship (covenant) and honor the bond between self and other. The ultimate knowledge gained from this perspective is that we are related to one another (and to the universe) and that harmony (brotherhood and sisterhood) is present as we live out caring relationships.

Concepts of discipline and profession have been dismissed by critical theorists as oppressive, anachronistic, and paternalistic (Allen, 1985; Rodgers, 1991). However, in our study, as we have explored essential meanings of these concepts, we have found that they express fundamental values congruent with cherished nursing values. Although we can agree with critical theorists that discipline and profession have been misused, perhaps too frequently, as tools of social elitism and oppression, this misuse remains inappropriate because it violates the covenantal nature of discipline and profession.

The discipline of nursing attends to the discovery, creation, structuring, testing, and refinement of knowledge needed for the practice of nursing. Concomitantly, the profession of nursing attends to the use of that knowledge in response to specific human needs. Certainly, the basic values communicated in the concepts of discipline and profession are resonate with fundamental nursing values and contribute to a fuller understanding of Nursing as Caring. Included among those shared values are commitment to something that matters, sense of persons being connected in oneness, expression of human imagination and creativity, realization of the unity of knowing with possibilities unfolding, and expression of choice and responsibility.

We have deliberately used the term *general theory of nursing* to characterize our work. The concept of a general theory is particularly useful in the context of levels of theory. Other authors have addressed what they see as three levels of nursing theory as follows: general or grand, midrange, and practice (Chinn & Jacobs, 1987; Fawcett, 1989; Nursing Development Conference Group, 1979; Walker & Avant, 1988). What we intend by the use of the term *general theory* is similar to "conceptual framework," "conceptual model," or "paradigm." That is, a general theory is a framework for understanding any and all instances of nursing and may be used to describe or to project any given situation of nursing. It is a system of values ordered specifically to reflect a philosophy of nursing to guide knowledge generation and to inform practice.

The statement of focus of any general nursing theory offers an explicit expression of the social need that calls for and justifies the professional service of nursing. In addition, the statement of focus expresses the domain of a discipline as well as the intent of the profession, and thus directs the development of the requisite nursing knowledge. Activity to develop and use nursing knowledge has its ethical ground in the idea of the covenantal relationship as expressed in the specific focus of the profession. Fundamental values inherent in the discipline and profession of nursing derived from an understanding of the focus of nursing.

The conception of nursing that we have used in this book views nursing science as a form of human science. Nursing as Caring focuses on the knowledge needed to understand the fullness of what it means to be human and on the methods to verify this knowledge. For this reason, we have not accepted the traditional notion of theory that relies on the "received" view of science and depends on measurement as the ultimate tool for legitimate knowledge development. The human science of nursing requires the use of all ways of knowing.

Carper's (1978) fundamental patterns of knowing in nursing are useful conceptual tools for expanding our view of nursing science as human science here. These patterns provide an organizing framework for asking epistemological questions of caring in nursing. To experience knowing the whole of a nursing situation with caring as the central focus, each of these patterns comes into play. Personal knowing focuses on knowing and encountering self and other intuitively, the empirical pathway addresses the sense, ethical knowing focuses on moral knowing of what "ought to be" in nursing situations, and aesthetic knowing involves the appreciating and creating that integrates all patterns of knowing in relation to a particular situation. Through the richness of the knowledge gleaned, the nurse as artist creates the caring moment (Boykin & Schoenhofer, 1990).

Nursing, as we have come to understand our discipline, is not a normative science that stands outside a situation to evaluate current observations against empirically derived and tested normative standards. Nursing as a human science takes its value from the knowledge created within the shared lived experience of the unique nursing situation. Although empirical facts and norms do play a role in nursing knowledge, we must remember that the role is not one of the unmediated application. Knowledge of nursing comes from within the situation. The nurse reaches out into a body of normative information, transforming that information as understanding is created from within the situation. The same can be said for personal and ethical knowing. Each serves as a pathway for transforming the knowledge in the creation of aesthetic knowing within the nursing situation. The view we have taken unifies previously dichotomized notions of nursing as science and nursing as art and requires a new understanding of science.

Nursing as Caring reflects an appreciation of persons in the fullness of personhood within the context of the nursing situation. This view transcends perspectives adopted in an earlier period of nursing science philosophy. Examples of the earlier view include the notions of basic versus applied science and metaphysics versus theory. The idea of a basic science of nursing disconnects nursing from its very ground of ethical value. Without grounding in praxis, the content and activity of nursing science becomes amoral and meaningless. Similarly, this view transcends an earlier view of nursing theory that treated the unitary phenomenon of nursing as being composed of concepts that could be studied independently or as "independent and dependent variables." Nursing as Caring resists fragmentation of the unitary phenomenon of our discipline. In the subsequent chapter, we will more fully explore implications of this view of nursing as a human science discipline and profession.

REFERENCES

Allen, D. G. (1985). Nursing research and social control: Alternative models of science that emphasize understanding and emancipation. *Image, 17*(2), 59–64.

Allen, D. G. (1987). The social policy statement; A reappraisal. *Advances in Nursing Science, 10*(1), 39–48.

American Nurses Association. (1980). *Nursing: A social policy statement*. Kansas City, MO: American Nurses Association.

Boykin, A., & Schoenhofer, S. (1990). Caring in nursing: Analysis of extant theory. *Nursing Science Quarterly, 4*, 149–155.

Carper, B. (1978). Fundamental patterns of knowing in nursing. *Advances in Nursing Science, 1*, 13–24.

Chinn, P., & Jacobs, M. (1987). *Theory and nursing*. St. Louis, MO: Mosby.

Cooper, M.C. (1988). Covenantal relationships: Grounding for the nursing ethic. *Advances in Nursing Science, 10*(4), 48–59.

Fawcett, T. (1989). *Analysis and evaluation of conceptual models of nursing*. Philadelphia, PA: F.A. Davis.

Flexner, A. (1910). *Medical education in the United States and Canada*. New York, NY: Carnegie Foundation.

Gadow, S. (1980). Existential advocacy: Philosophical foundations of nursing. In S. Spicker & Gadow, S. (Eds.), *Nursing: Images and ideals* (pp. 79–101). New York, NY: Springer.

Gadow, S. (1984). Touch and technology: Two paradigms of patient care. *Journal of Religion and Health, 23*, 63–69.

King, A., & Brownell J. (1976). *The curriculum and the disciplines of knowledge*. Huntington, NY: Robert E. Krieger Publishing.

Mayeroff, M. (1971). *On caring*. New York, NY: Harper & Row.

Orem, D. E., & Nursing Development Conference Group. (1979). *Concept formalization in nursing: Process and product*. Boston, MA: Little, Brown.

Packard, S. A., & Polifroni, E. C. (1991). The dilemma of nursing science: Current quandaries and lack of direction. *Nursing Science Quarterly, 4*(1), 7–13.

Parse, R. (1981). Caring from a human science perspective. In M. Leininger (Ed.), *Caring: An essential human need*. Thorofare, NJ: Slack. (Reissued by Wayne State University Press, Detroit, 1988).

Phenix, P. (1964). *Realms of meaning*. New York, NY: McGraw Hill.

Pribram, K. H. (1971). *Languages of the brain: Experimental paradoxes and principles in neuropsychology*. Englewood Cliffs, NJ: Prentice-Hall.

Roach, S. (1984). *Caring: The human mode of being, implications for nursing*. Toronto, Ontario, Canada: Faculty of Nursing, University of Toronto.

Roach, S. (1987). *The human act of caring*. Ottawa, Ontario: Canadian Hospital Association.

Roach, S. (1992 Revised). *The human act of caring*. Ottawa, Ontario: Canadian Hospital Association.

Rodgers, B. L. (1991). Deconstructing the dogma in nursing knowledge and practice. *Image, 23*(2), 177–81.

Silva, M. C. (1983). The American Nurses' Association position statement on nursing and social policy: Philosophical and ethical dimensions. *Journal of Advanced Nursing, 8*(2), 147–151.

Tillich, P. (1952). *The courage to be*. New Haven, CT: Yale University Press.

Trigg, R. (1973). *Reason and commitment*. London: Cambridge University Press.

Walker, L., & Avant, K. (1988). *Strategies for theory construction in nursing*. Norwalk, CT: Appleton & Lange.

Watson, J. (1988). *Nursing: Human science and human care, a theory of nursing*. Norwalk, CT: Appleton-Century-Crofts. (Original work published in 1985)

White, C. M. (1984). A critique of the ANA Social Policy Statement . . . population and environment focused nursing. *Nursing Outlook, 32*(6), 328–331.

FOUNDATIONS OF HUMANISTIC CARING

In this chapter we present the general theory of Nursing as Caring. Here, the unique focus of nursing is posited as *nurturing persons living caring and growing in caring*. While we will discuss the meaning of that statement of focus in general terms, we will also describe specific concepts inherent in this focus in the context of the general theory.

. . . the several major assumptions that ground the theory of Nursing as Caring [are] as follows:

- persons are caring by virtue of their humanness
- persons are whole or complete in the moment
- persons live caring, moment to moment
- personhood is a process of living grounded in caring
- personhood is enhanced through participating in nurturing relationships with caring others
- nursing is both a discipline and profession

In this chapter, we develop the nursing implications of these assumptions.

All persons are caring. This is the fundamental view that grounds the focus of nursing as a discipline and a profession. The unique perspective offered by the theory of Nursing as Caring builds on that view by recognizing personhood as a process of living grounded in caring. This is meant to imply that the fullness of being human is expressed as one lives caring uniquely day to day. The process of living grounded in caring is enhanced through participation in nurturing relationships with caring others, particularly in nursing relationships.

Within the theoretical perspective given herein, a further major assumption appears as follows: persons are viewed as already complete and continuously growing in completeness, fully caring and unfolding caring possibilities moment to moment. Such a view assumes that caring is being lived by each of us, moment to moment. Expressions of self as caring person are complete in the moment as caring possibilities unfold; thus, notwithstanding other life contingencies, one continues to grow in caring competency, in fully expressing self as caring person. To say that one is fully caring in the moment also involves a recognition of the uniqueness of person with each moment presenting new possibilities to know self as caring person. The notion of "in the moment" reflects the idea that competency in knowing self as caring and as living caring grows throughout the life. Being complete in the moment also signifies something more as follows: There is no insufficiency, no brokenness, or absence of something. As a result, nursing activities are not directed toward *healing* in the sense of making whole; from our perspective, wholeness is present and unfolding. There is no lack, failure, or inadequacy that is to be corrected through

From Boykin, A., & Schoenhofer, S. (2001). *Nursing as caring: A model for transforming practice.* Sudbury, MA: Jones & Bartlett. Permission to reprint granted by Jones & Bartlett.

nursing—persons are whole, complete, and caring.

The theory of Nursing as Caring, then, is based on an understanding that the focus of nursing, both as a discipline and as a profession, involves the nurturing of persons living caring and growing in caring. In this statement of focus, we recognize the unique human need to which nursing is the response as a desire to be recognized as caring person and to be supported in caring.

This focus also requires that the nurse know the person seeking Nursing as Caring person and that the nursing action be directed toward nurturing the nursed in their living caring and growing in caring. We will briefly discuss this theory in general terms here and more fully illuminate it in subsequent chapters.

Nurturing persons living caring and growing in caring at first glance appears broad and abstract. In some ways, the focus is broad in that it applies to nursing situations in a wide variety of practical settings. On the other hand, it takes on specific and practical meaning in the context of individual nursing situations. As the nurse attempts to know the nursed as caring person and focuses on nurturing that person as he or she lives and grows in caring.

When approaching a situation from this perspective, we understand each person as fundamentally caring, living caring in his or her everyday life. Forms of expressing one's unique ways of living caring are limited only by the imagination. Recognizing unique personal ways of living caring also requires an ethical commitment and knowledge of caring. In our everyday lives, failures to express caring are readily recognized. The ability to articulate the instances of noncaring does not seem to take any particular skill. However, when nursing is called for, it is necessary that nurses have the commitment, knowledge, and skill to discover the individual unique caring person to be nursed. For example, the nurse may encounter the one who may be described as despairing.

Relating to that person as helpless recalls Gadow's (1984) characterization of the philanthropic paradigm that assumes "sufficiency and independence on one side and needy dependence on the other" (p. 68). The relationship grounded in Nursing as Caring would enable the nurse to connect with the hope that underlies an expression of despair or hopelessness. Personal expressions such as despair, or fear, or anger, for example, are neither ignored nor discounted. Rather, they are understood as the caring value that is in some way present. An honest expression of fear or anger, for example, is also an expression of vulnerability, which expresses courage and humility. We reiterate that our approach is grounded in the fundamental assumption that all persons are caring and the commitment that arises from this basic value position.

It is this understanding of person as caring that directs professional nursing decision making and action from the point of view of our Nursing as Caring theory. The nurse enters into the world of the other person with the intention of knowing the other as caring person. It is in knowing the other in their "living caring and growing in caring" that calls for nursing are heard. Of equal importance is our coming to know *how* the other is living caring in the situation and expressing aspirations for growing in caring. The call for nursing is a call for acknowledgment and affirmation of the person living caring in specific ways in this immediate situation. The call for nursing says "know me as caring person now and affirm me." The call for nursing evokes specific caring responses to sustain and enhance the other as they live caring and grow in caring in the situation of concern. This caring nurturance is what we call the nursing response.

NURSING SITUATION

The *nursing situation* is a key concept in the theory of Nursing as Caring. Thus, we understand *nursing situation as a shared lived experience in which the caring between nurse and nursed enhances personhood.* The nursing situation is the locus of all that is known and done in nursing. It is in this context that nursing lives. The content and structure of nursing knowledge are known through the study of the nursing situation. The content of nursing knowledge is generated, developed, conserved, and known through the lived experience of the nursing situation. Nursing situation as a construct is constituted in the mind of the nurse when the nurse conceptualizes or prepares to conceptualize a call for nursing. In other words, when a nurse engages in any situation from a nursing focus, a nursing situation is constituted.

In the Scandinavian countries, for instance, all the helping disciplines are called *caring sciences.* Professions such as medicine, social work, clinical psychology, and pastoral counseling have a caring function; however, caring per se is not their focus. Rather, the focus of each of these professions addresses particular forms of caring or caring in particular ranges of life situations. In nursing situations, the nurse focuses on nurturing person as they live and grow in caring. Although caring is not unique to nursing, it is uniquely expressed in nursing. The uniqueness of caring in nursing lies in the intention expressed by the statement of focus. As an expression of nursing, *caring is the intentional and authentic presence of the nurse with another who is recognized as person living caring and growing in caring. Here, the nurse endeavors to come to know the other as caring person and seeks to understand how that person might be supported, sustained, and strengthened in his or her unique process of living caring and growing in caring.* Again, each person in interaction in the nursing situation is known as caring. Each person grows in caring through interconnectedness with other.

Calls for nursing are calls for nurturance through personal expressions of caring and originate within persons who are living caring in their lives and hold dreams and aspirations of growing in caring. Again, the nurse responds to the call of the caring person, not to some determination of an absence of caring. The contributions of each person in the nursing situation are also directed toward a common purpose, the nurturance of the person in living and growing in caring.

In responding to the nursing call, the nurse brings an expert (expert in the sense of deliberately developed) knowledge of what it means to be human, to be caring, as a fully developed commitment to recognizing and nurturing caring in all situations. The nurse enters the other's world to know the person as caring. The nurse comes to know how caring is being lived in the moment, discovering unfolding possibilities for growing in caring. This knowing clarifies the nurse's understanding of the call and guides the nursing response. In this context, the general knowledge that the nurse brings to the situation is transformed through an understanding of the uniqueness of that particular situation.

Every nursing situation is a lived experience involving at least two unique persons. Therefore, each nursing situation differs from any other. The reciprocal nature of the lived experience of the nursing situation requires a personal investment of both caring persons. The initial focus is on knowing the person as caring, both nurse and nursed. The process for knowing self and other as caring involves a constant and mutual unfolding. To know the other, the nurse must be willing to risk entering the other's world. For his or her part, the other person must be willing to allow the nurse to enter his or her world. For this to happen, the acceptance of trust and strength of courage needed by the person in the nursing situation can be awe-inspiring.

It is through the openness and willingness in the nursing situation that presence with other occurs. The presence develops as the nurse is willing to risk entering the world of the other and as the other invites the nurse into a special, intimate space. The encountering of the nurse and the nursed gives rise to a phenomenon we call *caring between*, within which personhood is nurtured. The nurse as caring person is fully present and gives the other time and space to grow. Through presence and intentionality, the nurse is able to know the other in his or her living and growing in caring. This personal knowing enables the nurse to respond to the unique call for nurturing personhood. Of course, responses to nursing calls are as varied as the calls themselves. All truly nursing responses are expressions of caring and are directed toward nurturing persons, as they live and grow in the caring in the situation.

In the situation, the nurse draws on personal, empirical, and ethical knowing to bring to life the artistry of nursing. When the nurse, as artist, creates a unique approach to care based on the dreams and goals of the one cared for, the moment comes alive with possibilities. Through the aesthetic, the nurse is free to know and express the beauty of the caring moment (Boykin & Schoenhofer, 1991). This full engagement within the nursing situation allows the nurse to truly experience Nursing as Caring and to share that experience with the one nursed.

We have noted that each profession arose from some everyday service given by one person or another. Nursing has long been associated with the idea of mothering, when mothering is understood as nurturing the personhood of another. The ideal mother (and father) recognizes the child as caring person, perfect in the moment and unfolding possibilities for becoming. The parent acknowledges and affirms the child as caring person and provides the caring environment that nurtures the child in living and growing in caring. The origins of nursing may well be found in the intimacy of parental caring. The roles of both the parent and the nurse permit and at times even expect

that one be involved in the intimacy of the daily life of another. The parent is present in all situations to care for the child. Ideally, the parents know the child as eminently worthwhile and caring, despite all the limitations and human frailties. As we recognized in Chapter 1, professions arise from the special needs of everyday situations, and nursing has perhaps emerged in relation to a type of caring that is synonymous with parenthood and friendship. The professional nurse, schooled in the discipline of nursing, brings expert knowledge of human caring to the nursing situation.

In the early years of nursing model development, nursing scholars endeavored to articulate their discipline using the perspective of another discipline, for example, medicine, sociology, or psychology. One example of this endeavor is the Roy Adaptation Model, in which scientific assumptions reflect von Bertalanffy's General Systems Theory and Helson's Adaptation Level Theory (Roy and Andrews, 1991, p. 5). Parson's theory of Social System Analysis is reflected in Johnson's Behavioral System Model for Nursing and Orem's Self-Care Deficit Theory of Nursing (Meleis, 1985). A second trend involved declaring that the uniqueness of nursing was in the way in which it integrated and applied concepts from other disciplines. The emphasis in the 1960s on nursing model development came as an effort to articulate and structure the substance of nursing knowledge. This work was needed to enhance nursing education, previously based on rules of practice, and to provide a foundation for an emerging interest in nursing research. Nursing scholars engaged in model development as an expression of their commitment to the advancement of nursing as a discipline and profession, and we applaud their contributions. It is our view, however, that these early models, grounded in other disciplines, do not directly address the essence of nursing.

The development of Nursing as Caring has benefited from these earlier efforts as well as from the work of more recent scholarship that posits caring as the central construct and essence (Leininger, 1988) and the moral ideal of Nursing (Watson, 1985).

The perspective of nursing presented here is notably different from most conceptual models and general theories in the field. The most radical difference becomes apparent in the form of the call for nursing. Most extant nursing theories, modeled after medicine and other professional fields, present the formal occasion for nursing as problem, need, or deficit (e.g., Self-Care Deficit Theory [Orem, 1985], Adaptation Nursing [Roy & Andrews, 1991], Behavioral System Model [Johnson, 1980], and Neuman, 1989). Such theories then explain how nursing acts to right the wrong, meet the need, or eliminate or ameliorate the deficit.

The theory of Nursing as Caring proceeds from a frame of reference based on interconnectedness and collegiality rather than on esoteric knowledge, technical expertise, and disempowering hierarchies. In contrast, our emerging theory of nursing is based on an egalitarian model of helping that bears witness to and celebrates the human person in the fullness of his or her being, rather than on some less-than-whole condition of being.

REFERENCES

Boykin, A., & Schoenhofer, S. (1991). Story as link between nursing practice, ontology, epistemology. *Image, 23,* 245–248.

Gadow, S. (1984). Touch and technology: Two paradigms of patient care. *Journal of Religion and Health, 23,* 63–69.

Johnson, D. E. (1980). The behavioral system model of nursing. In J. Riehl & C. Roy (Eds.), *Conceptual models for nursing practice* (2nd ed.). New York, NY: Appleton-Century-Crofts.

Leininger, M. M. (1988). Leininger's theory of nursing: Cultural care diversity and universality. *Nursing Science Quarterly, 1,* 152–160.

Meleis, A. (1985). *Theoretical nursing: Development & progress.* Philadelphia, PA: J.B. Lippencott.

Neuman, B. (1989). *The Neumans systems model.* Norwalk, CT: Appleton & Lange.

Orem, D. E. (1985). *Nursing: Concepts of practice* (3rd ed.). New York, NY: McGraw Hill.

Roy, C., & Andrews, H. (1991). *The Roy Adaptation Model: The definitive statement.* Norwalk, CT: Appleton & Lange.

Watson, J. (1985). *Nursing human science and human care. A theory of nursing.* Norwalk, CT: Appleton-Century-Crofts.

QUESTIONS FOR REFLECTION

Baccalaureate

1. The first assumption of Nursing as Caring is that persons are caring by virtue of their humanness. How would you explain atrocities perpetrated against humanity if this assumption is true?
2. The nurse encounters a person who is in despair. How might she approach him from the perspective of Nursing as Caring?
3. How does the nurse come to know the other as caring person?

Master's

1. A person with diabetes has not been "complying" with his medical regime. The assumption from Nursing as Caring is that this person is living caring for self. How is this so?
2. Describe a nursing situation that includes a nurse and person from the population group of interest to you.
3. If the person is whole and perfect in the moment, what is the focus of nursing from the perspective of Nursing as Caring?

Doctoral

1. Nursing as Caring is advanced as a general theory of nursing. What is a general theory of nursing? Do you agree with this? If so, why? And if not, why not?
2. What research methods are appropriate to study caring from the perspective of Nursing as Caring?
3. What are the strengths and limitations of Nursing as Caring based on the criteria for evaluating theories?

15

The Theory of Human Caring: Retrospective and Prospective

JEAN WATSON

Nursing: The Philosophy and Science of Caring was first published in 1979, before there was any formal movement in nursing related to nursing theory per se. It emerged from my quest to bring new meaning and dignity to the world of nursing and patient care—care that seemed too limited in its scope at the time, largely defined by medicine's paradigm and traditional biomedical science models. I felt a dissonance between nursing's paradigm (yet to be defined as such) of caring–healing and health, and medicine's paradigm of diagnosis and treatment, and concentration on disease and pathology.

The concepts I defined to bring new meaning to nursing's paradigm were derived from clinically inducted, empirical experiences, combined with my philosophical, intellectual, and experiential background; thus, the early work emerged from my own values, beliefs, and perceptions about personhood, life, health, and healing, and how they manifest clinically and empirically. Further, my work was guided by my commitment to nursing's collective caring–healing role and mission in society as attending to and helping to sustain humanity and wholeness as foundation to health and nursing's purpose for existence.

The original work was further shaped by phenomenological psychology and philosophy, for example, the work of Carl Rogers, the existential work of Yalom, and the interpersonal focus gained from psychiatric-mental health nursing graduate studies. Retrospectively, I can also see how I was almost unconsciously influenced by Peplau's interpersonal domain and the notion of "therapeutic use of self," which later manifested in my work as *presence, authentic caring relationship* (Watson, 1988). Other philosophical and intellectual traditions were Kierkegaard, Whitehead, de Chardin, and Sartre.

My use of the term transpersonal caring in my second book, *Nursing: Human Science and Human Care* (1985), is closely related to the meaning of the term in transpersonal psychology. However, originally my use of the term was inspired by Lazarus as a way to expand the field of meaning associated with a human-to-human caring relationship. Another nursing scholar who, later in my career (mid to late 1980s onward) further inspired and affirmed my thinking was Dr. Sally Gadow; her influence shows up later in my second book. Specifically, the notions of moral ideal and preservation of dignity were consistent with her work and already in her writings.

These early intellectual forces were enlarged, enriched, and inspired

From Watson, J. (1997). The theory of human caring: Retrospective and prospective. *Nursing Science Quarterly*, 10(1), 49–52. Permission to reprint granted by Sage Publications, Inc.

by diverse experiences with nurses and indigenous peoples and cultures of New Zealand, Australia, Indonesia, The Republic of China, Thailand, India, and Egypt. More recently, these influential cultural experiences have been expanded to include Scandinavia, England, Scotland, Canada, Portugal, Kuwait, Brazil, Japan, Korea, and Micronesia, among others. All of my travels and personal and work experiences have confirmed my sense of witnessing a convergence and expansion of Eastern and Western beliefs, worldviews, and values that affect aspects of humanity, life, death, suffering, caring, healing, and health. Thus, my work seeks to confirm that we are all part of the global human–planet–universe condition and connection—all are part of what I consider both universal and specific nursing phenomena of caring and healing, regardless of setting or country. These ideas are embedded in nursing and my world of nursing, but also at this moment in our history, paradoxically, transcend nursing.

OVERVIEW OF ORIGINAL WORK

The original work was organized around *10 carative factors* as a framework for providing a structure and order for nursing phenomena. The carative factors were embedded in a philosophy and value system, which was humanitarian, aesthetic, and spiritual, attempting to honor the human dimensions of nursing's work and the inner life world and subjective experiences of the people we serve.

The *carative factors* in the first work served as a guide to frame what I referred to as the *"core of nursing,"* in contrast to nursing's *"trim."* Core refers to those aspects of nursing that actually potentiate therapeutic healing processes and relationships; they affect the one caring and the one-being-cared-for. Further, the basic core was grounded in what I referred to as the philosophy, science (and art) of caring (which later is posited to be intrinsically

related to healing). The trim referred to the practice setting, the procedures, the functional tasks, the specialized clinical focus of disease, technology, and techniques surrounding the diverse orientations and preoccupations of nursing.

The trim, however, is in no way expendable; it is just that it cannot be the center of a professional model of nursing. Trim exists in relation to something larger and deeper. That something deeper and larger is the caring relationship, the health and healing processes that nurses attend to within a larger professional ethic. Such an ethic and ethos of caring, healing, and health comprises nursing's professional context and mission—its raison d'étre to society. This caring ethic and ethos later becomes the framework to clarify what I think of as a *nursing qua nursing* paradigm, in contrast to a *nursing qua medicine* paradigm (Watson, 1995).

The carative factors are not complete without attending to the second work (Watson, 1985, 1988), which outlines the worldview and philosophical context, for example, oneness of being, with outlines the worldview and philosophical context, for example, oneness of being with respect to person, phenomenal field transpersonal caring relationship, caring occasion, and a caring moment. This wider aspect serves to remind that any nurse–patient encounter can be considered a caring occasion wherein a caring moment can be created and experienced depending upon the consciousness and philosophical (theoretical orientation, which is guiding the nurse consciously or unconsciously). This dynamic aspect of the theory is made more explicit in *New Dimensions of Human Caring Theory* (Watson, 1988), and caring consciousness and caring field are linked, allowing the theory to evolve toward the simultaneity/unitary-transformative paradigms now in the nursing literature. However, some aspects of the work contain components that could be critiqued as being located in the totality, framework.

Nevertheless, in contemporary nursing practices and education, the carative factors are being used, or envisioned, as a bridge that helps a nurse cross over from a traditional nursing-qua-medicine framework, to a more advanced nursing-qua-nursing practice model; a theory if you like that can help to transport nursing from the totality, particularistic paradigm to a simultaneity–unitary–transformative paradigm. This formation leads to further development of both the discipline and the professional practice of nursing. (However, I am aware of inherent contradictions to this way of thinking; one is either in one paradigm or in the other, however, as ideas grow and evolve, one outgrows where one started.)

For this postmodern era, the carative factors provide a language for caring that is linked to nursing and core processes of professional practice. The carative factors and general caring language help to release nursing from its political and practice history of medical language dominance and orientation. The attention to language is especially critical to an evolving discipline, in that during this postmodern era, one's survival depends upon having language; writers in this area remind us "if you do not have your own language you don't exist."

Throughout nursing's history, to this time at the turn of the century, nursing continues to struggle with adopting or adapting others' language for our phenomena. The carative factors thus serve to help define nursing knowledge, practices, and phenomena as distinct from, but complementary with, curing knowledge and practices associated with modern medicine.

CONTEMPORARY STATUS OF WATSON'S CARING THEORY AND A PROSPECTIVE

As this work continues to unfold, it is viewed simultaneously as both theory and beyond theory. Both retrospectively and prospectively, it can be read as philosophy, ethic, or even paradigm or worldview. Regardless of how it is treated, the evolving work continues to make explicit that humans cannot be treated as objects and that humans cannot be separated from self, other, nature, and the larger universe. This caring–healing paradigm is located within a cosmology that is both metaphysical and transcendent with the coevolving human in the universe. The context calls for a sense of reverence and sacredness with regard to life and all living things. It incorporates both art and science, as they are also being redefined, acknowledging a convergence between the two.

The transpersonal caring relationship and authentic presencing translate into *ontological caring competencies* of the nurse, which intersect with *technological medical competencies*. These ontological caring competencies translate even further into advanced caring–healing modalities, nursing therapeutics, healing arts, and so on. These modalities also reconnect nursing with the finest tradition of Florence Nightingale.

Within this evolving perspective of transpersonal caring, new levels of ontological caring competencies arise as foundational to nursing's full emergence and actualization as a mature health profession and distinct discipline within its own paradigm. Transpersonal caring calls forth an authenticity of being and becoming, an ability to be present, to be reflective, to attend to mutuality of being, and centering one's consciousness and intentionality toward caring, healing, wholeness and health, rather than disease, problems, illness, and technocures.

These so-called *ontological caring competencies* become as essential as the *technological medical competencies*, which have largely defined and directed nursing during this century. This area intersects with the latest developments on mind–body medicine, while being rooted in nursing history.

The caring theory and the evolution of the notion of transpersonal caring ultimately evokes and invites ontological development, a transformation of self, a new sense of seeing beyond mere intellectual words—an alignment of intentionality consciousness and one's being-in-action, seeking an authentic presence, an integration of mind–body–spirit which is healing. This mind–body–spirit oneness of being, which is connected with all, elicits the spiritual and expanded views of what it means to be human: embodied spirit, both immanent and transcendent, whole, and connected, in right relation.

This model now more explicitly acknowledges that the nurse, or practitioner, who is working within this theory and its underlying philosophy, needs to cultivate a daily practice for self. Practices such as centering, meditation, breath work, yoga, prayer, connections with nature, and other such forms of daily contemplation are essential to the theory's authenticity and success. In other words, if one is to work from a caring–healing paradigm, one must live it out in daily life. This living authentically requires a commitment to self-care at that deep level of personal practice and discipline, which in turn is honoring one's own embodied spirit, taking time for soul care.

SUMMARY AND PROJECTIONS

The theory of human caring continues to have both a direct and indirect influence on nursing and health science curricula, pedagogy, research, and practice both here and abroad. (*Nursing: Human Science and Human Care*, Watson, 1985, has been translated into Chinese, German, Japanese, Korean, and Swedish.) The theory has been part of the movement of pursuing human science and new paradigm science methodologies for inquiry. The value-based approach and worldview has intersected with the fields of feminist studies, humanities, philosophy, critical scholarship, and caring ethics, as well as postmodern thinking with respect to poststructuralist thinking, social action research, and other contemporary critical approaches in academe.

The newly released, updated *Social Policy Statement* by the American Nurses Association (1995) attests to the influence of nursing caring scholarship in general and its influence upon the field. This revised document acknowledges the general impact in the following statement:

Since 1980, nursing philosophy and practice have been influenced by a greater elaboration of the science of caring and its integration with the traditional knowledge base for diagnosis and treatment of human responses to health and illness. As such, definitions of nursing more frequently acknowledge four essential features of contemporary nursing practice [one of which is]:

> provision of a caring relationship that facilitates health and healing. (ANA, 1995, p. 6)

While it is still debated at the theory and paradigm level, caring remains an ethic, ethos, and foundation for relationship-centered care for nursing and other health professionals. Moreover, it is increasingly emerging as a distinct field of scholarship. For example, there are emerging academic departments in universities in different parts of the world, which are named "Department of Caring Science" or have similar terminology (for example, in Finland, Australia, and Sweden). In this sense, caring is emerging as a disciplinary science focus in its own right, which stems largely from the field of nursing.

There are many exemplars of Watson's human caring theory and its influence in nursing education, practice, and research around the world. The most prominent representation of the work is through the University of Colorado Center for Human Caring. The Center, founded in 1986 in the School of Nursing, was created as the first of its kind. It is an interdisciplinary center for the discipline of nursing, which hosts public and professional programs and sponsors in-resident faculty and scholars and clinicians from around the world. The Center remains committed to exploring new ways to advance the art and science of human caring; some of the efforts have been conceptualized as "ontological design projects" and have ranged from specific curricular activities, piloting new courses, to initiating and supporting nontraditional educational, research, and practice (praxis) models with clinical agencies and academic systems.

The Center fosters epistemological, ontological, methodological, and praxis inquiries that draw upon all ways of knowing, being, and doing with respect to knowledge, practice, and teaching of caring. The Denver Nursing Project in Human Caring is the most prestigious example of a clinical demonstration project where the theory-philosophy paradigm is operating in action. This work has generated international scholarship and affiliations, which are grounded in the theory but also transcend the original work.

To fully actualize this theory requires new ways of thinking and being and acting that converge. At one level, the work is concrete and obvious, but for some it is considered remote, abstract, and ethereal. At whatever level it is approached, it is always fragile and threatened. It requires a personal, social, moral, and spiritual engagement of self—thus a radical transformation of traditional ways of thinking about nursing that no longer hold. The transpersonal aspect of the work invites participants to cocreate the model's further emergence.

Lastly, traditional nursing will need to be redefined within a nursing caring–healing health model as advanced practice nursing becomes more prevalent in the future. Advanced caring–healing modalities within this model are already emerging as untapped nursing arts. The future invites such advancement for nursing qua nursing to come of age as a mature health profession and distinct discipline.

REFERENCES

American Nurses Association. (1995). *Social policy statement*. Washington, DC: Author.

Watson, J. (1985). *Nursing: Human science and human care*. Norwalk, CT: Appleton-Century-Crofts/New York, NY: National League for Nursing.

Watson, J. (1988). New dimensions of human caring theory. *Nursing Science Quarterly, 1*, 175–181.

Watson, J. (1995). Nursing's caring-healing paradigm as exemplar for alternative medicine? *Journal of Alternative Therapies, 1*(3), 64–69.

Watson, M. J. (1979). *Nursing: The philosophy and science of caring*. Boston, MA: Little, Brown and Company/Boulder, CO: Colorado Associated University Press.

QUESTIONS FOR REFLECTION

Baccalaureate

1. Name three philosophers who influenced the development of Jean Watson's theory of human caring.
2. What values are core to the theory of human caring?
3. From Watson's perspective, what is the trim of nursing?

Master's

1. What does Watson mean by a caring consciousness and a caring field?

2. Why are daily self-care practices of centering, meditation, breath work, yoga, prayer, and so on, important for nurses to engage in?
3. What does the ANA *Social Policy Statement* of 1995 say about caring?

Doctoral

1. How are caring–healing modalities related to the tradition of Florence Nightingale?
2. What ideas from Watson's theory are consistent with the unitary-transformative paradigm in nursing?
3. What health policies would be consistent with Watson's human caring theory?

16

Nursing: The Philosophy and Science of Caring (Revised Edition)

Jean Watson

BACKGROUND

Nursing: The Philosophy and Science of Caring (1979) was my first book and my entrance into scholarly work. This book was published before formal attention was being given to nursing theory as the foundation for the discipline of nursing and before much focus had been directed to a meaningful philosophical foundation for nursing science, education, and practice.

The work "emerged from my quest to bring new meaning and dignity to the work and the world of nursing and patient care" (Watson, 1997, p. 49). The theoretical concepts were derived and emerged from my personal and professional experiences; they were clinically inducted, empirically grounded, and combined with my philosophical, ethical, intellectual, and experiential background (Watson, 1997). My quest and my work have always been about deepening my own and everyone's understanding of humanity and life itself and bringing those dimensions into nursing. Thus, the early work emerged from my own values, beliefs, perceptions, and experience with rhetorical and ineffable questions. For example, what does it mean to be

human? What does it mean to care? What does it mean to heal? Questions and views of personhood, life, the birth–death cycle, change, health, healing, relationships, caring, wholeness, pain, suffering, humanity itself, and other unknowns guided my quest to identify a framework for nursing as a distinct entity, profession, discipline, and science in its own right—separate from, but complementary to, the curative orientation of medicine (Watson, 1979). My views were heightened by my commitment to (1) the professional role and mission of nursing; (2) its ethical covenant with society as sustaining human caring and preserving human dignity, even when threatened; and (3) attending to and helping to sustain human dignity and humanity and wholeness in the midst of threats and crises of life and death. All these activities, experiences, questions, and processes transcend illness, diagnosis, condition, setting, and so on; they were, and remain, enduring and timeless across time and space and changes in systems, society, civilization, and science.

The original (1979) work has expanded and evolved through a generation of publications, other books, videos,

From Watson, J. (2008). *Nursing: The philosophy and science of caring* (Rev. ed., pp. 1–11). Boulder, CO: University Press of Colorado. Permission to reprint granted by the University Press of Colorado. Permission to reprint to print and ebook formats, throughout the world, in all languages by University Press of Colorado. This permission applies only to print and ebook format for the first edition of *Caring in Nursing Classics* to be published by Springer Publishing Company.

and CDs, along with clinical-educational and administrative initiatives for transforming professional nursing. A series of other books on caring theory followed and have been translated into at least nine languages. The other major theory-based books on caring that followed the original work include the following:

- *Nursing: Human Science and Human Care. A Theory of Nursing* (1985). East Norwalk, CT: Appleton-Century-Crofts. Reprinted/republished (1988). New York NY; National League for Nursing. Reprinted/republished (1999). Sudbury, MA: Jones & Bartlett,
- *Postmodern Nursing and Beyond* (1999). Edinburgh, Scotland: Churchill-Livingstone. Reprinted/republished New York NY: Elsevier.
- *Assessing and Measuring Caring in Nursing and Health Science* (Ed.) (2002). New York NY: Springer (AJN Book of Year award).
- *Caring Science as Sacred Science* (2005). Philadelphia: F. A. Davis (AJN Book of Year award).

Other caring-based books I coedited or coauthored are extensions of these works but are not discussed here (see, e.g., Bevis & Watson, 1989, *Toward a Caring Curriculum*, New York NY: National League for Nursing [reprinted 1999, Sudbury MA: Jones & Bartlett]; Watson & Ray, 1998 [Eds.], *The Ethics of Care and the Ethics of Care*, New York NY: National League for Nursing; Chinn & Watson, 1994, *Art and Aesthetics in Nursing*, New York NY: National League for Nursing). See also Web site (Watson, 2004a) for complete citations of books and publications.

Nursing: The Philosophy and Science of Caring (1979) provided the original core and structure for the Theory of Human Caring: 10 Carative Factors. These factors were identified as the essential aspects of caring in nursing, without which nurses may not have been practicing professional nursing but instead they were functioning as technicians or skilled workers within the dominant framework of medical techno-cure science. This work has stood as a timeless classic of sorts on its own. It has not been revised since its original publication; only reprints have kept it alive, thanks to the University Press of Colorado.

The 2008 edition was an expanded and updated supplement of the original test, with completely new sections replacing previous sections while other sections that remain relevant are included with only minor revisions. I have been advised to retain the original text in this revision so essential parts of it remain alive, since the original 1979 version may eventually go out of print. Thus, this work retains core essentials of the original text while updating that text with new content, bringing the original book full circle with my own evolution and changes in the work across an almost 30-year span.

To provide the context for this evolution (before I address revisions of the original text), I provide a brief overview of the focus and content of the other books that serve as a background for my evolving work, all of which emerged from the original text of *Nursing: The Philosophy and Science of Caring*.

My second book, *Nursing: Human Science and Human Care, A Theory of Nursing*, was first published in 1985 and has been republished by the National League for Nursing (1988) and Jones and Bartlett (1999). It expands on the philosophical, transpersonal aspects of a caring moment as the core framework. This focus places the theoretical ideas more explicitly within a broader context of ethics, art, and even metaphysics as phenomena within which nursing dwells but often does not name, articulate, or act upon.

As has been pointed out in contemporary postmodern thinking, if a profession does not have its own language, it does not exist; thus, it is important to name, claim, articulate, and act on the phenomena of nursing and caring if nursing is to fulfill its mandate and raison d'être for the society; this second theory text seeks to make more explicit the reality that if nursing is to survive in this millennium, it has to sustain and make explicit its covenant with the public. This covenant includes taking mature professional responsibility for giving voice to, standing up for, and acting on its knowledge, values, ethics, and skilled practices of caring, healing, and health.

What was/is prominent in the second "theory" book is the explicit acknowledgment of the spiritual dimensions of caring and healing. There is further development of concepts such as the transpersonal, the caring occasion, the caring moment, and the "art of transpersonal caring" (Watson, 1985, p. 67). Furthermore, in this work, as reflected in the title, distinctions are made with respect to the context of human science in which nursing resides: for example,

- A philosophy of human freedom, choice, and responsibility.
- A biology and psychology of holism.
- An epistemology that allows not only for empirics but also for the advancement of aesthetics, ethical values, intuition, personal knowing, spiritual insights, along with a process of discovery, creative imagination, and evolving forms of inquiry.
- An ontology of time *and* space.
- A context of inter-human events, processes, and relationships that connect/are one with the environment and the wider universe.
- A scientific worldview that is open (Watson, 1985, p. 16).

Thus, a human science and human caring orientation differs from conventional science and invites qualitatively different aspects to be honored as legitimate and necessary when working with human experiences and human caring–healing, health, and life phenomena.

In this work, one finds the first mention of "caring occasion," "phenomenal field," "transpersonal," and the "art of transpersonal caring" inviting the full use

of self within a "caring moment" (Watson, 1985, pp. 58–72). The caring occasion/caring moment becomes transpersonal when "two persons (nurse and other) together with their unique life histories and phenomenal field (of perception) become a focal point in space and time, from which the moment has a field of its own that is greater than the occasion itself. As such, the process can (and does) go beyond itself, yet arise from aspects of itself that become part of the life history of each person, as well as part of some larger, deeper, complex pattern of life" (Watson, 1985, p. 59).

The caring moment can be an existential turning point for the nurse in which it involves pausing, choosing to "see"; it is an informed action guided by an intentionality and consciousness of how to *be* in the moment—fully present, open to the other person, open to compassion and connection, beyond the ego-control focus that is so common. In a caring moment, the nurse grasps the gestalt of the presenting moment and is able to "read" the field, beyond the outer appearance of the patient and the patient's behavior. The moment is "transpersonal" when the nurse is able to see and connect with the spirit of others, open to expanding possibilities of what can occur. The foundation for this perspective is the wisdom in knowing and understanding that "[w]e learn from one another how to be more human by identifying ourselves with others and finding their dilemmas in ourselves. What we all learn from it is self-knowledge. The self we learn about or discover is every self: it is universal. We learn to recognize ourselves in others" (Watson, 1985, p. 59).

This human-to-human connection expands out compassion and caring and keeps alive our common humanity. All of this process deepens and sustains our shared humanity and helps to avoid reducing another human being to the moral status of object (Watson, 1985, p. 60).

This second work concludes with a sample of human science methodology as a form of caring inquiry. Transcendental phenomenology is discussed as one exemplar of a human science–Caring Science experience of loss and grief experienced and researched among an Aboriginal tribe in Western Australia. Poetry and artistic, metaphoric expressions emerge within the "outback" research experience, using this extended methodology. Such an approach was consistent with the findings and experiences in this unique setting, in which this methodology allowed for a "poetic" effect in articulating experiences as felt and lived, transcending their facts and pure descriptions (descriptive phenomenology).

Thus, the transcendent views were consistent with transpersonal dimensions and provided space for paradox, ambiguity sensuous resonance, and creative expressions, going beyond the surface phenomenology (Watson, 1985, pp. 90–91). For example: "In other words, how could cold, unfeeling, totally detached dogmatic words and tone possibly teach the truth or deep meaning of a human phenomenon associated with human caring, transpersonal caring and grief, and convey experiences of great sorrow great beauty, passion and joy. We cannot convey the need for

compassion, complexity, or for cultivating feeling and sensibility in words that are bereft of warmth, kindness and good feeling" (Watson, 1985, p. 91). The result is poetizing; "it cannot be other than poetic" (Heidegger quoted in Watson, 1985, p. 98).

Such an exemplar of methodology invites a union between the humanities and art with science, one of the perennial themes of my work. Finally, this second book launched my ideas and set the foundation for the next evolution of my work on Caring Science that followed.

The third book, *Postmodern Nursing and Beyond* (1999), brought focus to the professional paradigm that is grounded in the ontology of relations and an ethical–ontological foundation before jumping to the epistemology of science and technology. The focus of this work was the need to clarify the ontological foundation of Being-in-Relation within a caring paradigm, the unity of mind–body–spirit/field, going beyond the outdated separatist ontology of modern Era I medical–industrial thinking. In this chapter, the spiritual and evolved energetic aspects of caring consciousness, intentionality, and human presence and the personal evolution of the practitioner became more

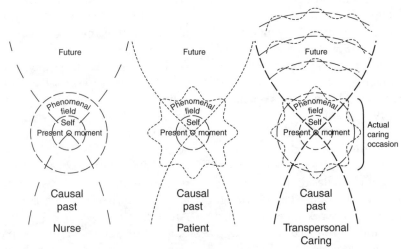

Illustration by Mel Gabel, University of Colorado, Biomedical Communications
Department, Reprinted, with permission, from Watson (1985/1999).

FIGURE 16.1

Dynamics of human caring process, including nurse–patient transpersonal dimension.

developed. This evolution was placed within the emerging postmodern cosmology of healing, wholeness, and oneness that is an honoring of the unity of all.

This postmodern perspective, as developed in the third book, attempts to project nursing and health care into the mid-twenty-first century, when there will be radically different requirements for all health practitioners and entirely different roles and expectations between and among the public and health care systems (Watson, 1999, p. xiii). Prominent in this text is an emphasis on the feminine yin energy needed for caring and healing, which nursing, other practitioners, and society alike are rediscovering because the dominant system is imbalanced with the archetypal energy of yang, which is not the source for healing. Nursing itself serves as an archetype for healing and represents a metaphor for the deep yin healing energy that is emerging within an entirely different paradigm. What is proposed is a fundamental ontological shift in consciousness, acknowledging a symbiotic relationship between humankind–technology–nature and the larger, expanding universe. This evolutionary turn evokes a return to the sacred core of humankind, inviting mystery and wonder back into our lives, work, and world. Such views reintroduce a sense of reverence for and openness to infinite possibilities. Emphasis is placed on the importance of ontological caring–healing practices, grounded in an expanded consciousness and intentionality that intersect with technological treatments of advanced medicine. In this work, Florence Nightingale's original blueprint for nursing is evident and embodies all the caring–healing nursing arts and rituals, rediscovered and honored for new reasons. Metaphors of *ontological archetype, ontological artist, and ontological architect* are used to capture the roles and visions for nursing into this millennium/Era III medicine and nursing (Watson, 1999, pp. xiv–xv).

My most recent theoretical book, *Caring Science as Sacred Science* (2005) (which received an *American Journal of Nursing* [AJN] Book of the Year award in 2006 in the category of research), expands further on the earlier works on raring. This work places Caring Science within an ethical–moral–philosophically evolved, scientific context, guided by the works of Emmanual Levinas (1969, French) and Knud Logstrup (1997, Danish).

This latest work on Caring Science seeks a science model that reintegrates metaphysics within the material physical domain and reinvites ethics-of-belonging (to the infinite field of Universal Cosmic Love) (Levinas, 1969) as before and underneath *being-by-itself* alone—no longer separate from the broader universal field of infinity to which we all belong and to which we return from the earth plane.

Levinas' "ethics of face"—as in facing our own and others' humanity—is explored as a metaphor for how we deepen and sustain our humanity for survival of the human in contrast to "totalizing" the human condition and cutting us off from the infinite source of life and the great cosmic field that unites us all. Logstrup's "ethical demand" brings forth the notion of "ethics of hand," in that he reminds us of the sovereign, unarticulated, and often anonymous ethical demand that "we take care of the life which trust has placed in our hands" (Logstrup, 1997, p. 18).

Caring Science as Sacred Science text identifies these basic assumptions (Watson, 2005, p. 56):

- The infinity of the human spirit and evolving universe.
- The ancient and emerging cosmology of a unity consciousness of relatedness of All.
- The ontological ethic of *Belonging before Our Separate Being* (Levinas, 1969).
- The moral position of sustaining the infinity and mystery of the human condition and keeping alive the evolving human spirit across time, as in *facing and deepening our own and others' Humanity* (Levinas, 1969).

- The ethical demand that acknowledges that we hold another person's life in our hands; this sovereign expression of life is given to us, before and beyond our control with expressions of trust, love, caring, honesty, forgiveness, gratitude, and so on, beyond ego fixations and obsessive feelings that are negative expressions of life (Logstrup, 1997).
- The relationship between our consciousness, words, and thoughts and how they positively or negatively affect our energetic-transpersonal field of being, becoming, and belonging; thus, our consciousness affects our ability to connect, to "be-in-right-relation" with source: the infinite universal cosmic field of love.

In this evolved context of Caring Science, we can appreciate, honor, and face the reality that life is given to us as a gift; we are invited to sustain and deepen our own and others' humanity as our moral and ethical starting point for professional caring–healing, In Levinas' view, "ethics of belonging" (to this universal field of Cosmic Love) becomes the first principle and starting point for any science, allowing ethics and metaphysics to be reunited with conventional science.

These views are not unlike Nightingale's notion of natural healing processes, which draw upon spiritual dimensions that are the greatest source of healing (1969). Indeed, it has been acknowledged in perennial philosophies and Wisdom Traditions across time, cultures, and a diversity of belief systems that the greatest source of healing is love.

Thus, my book on Caring Science brings a decidedly sacred dimension to the work of caring, making more explicit that we dwell in mystery and the infinity of cosmic love as the source and depth of all of life.

We come from the spirit world and return to the spirit source when vulnerable, stressed, fearful, ill, and so forth. This is comparable to Nightingale's notion of putting the patient in best condition for nature to heal, acknowledging that healing draws on nature and natural processes. In this framework, it is acknowledged that we are working with the inner life forces, life energy, and the soul, if you will, of self and other and that we need to connect with the universal infinite field.

> A human being is a part of the whole called the "universe," a part limited in time and space. He [sic] experiences [self], thoughts and feelings, as something separated from the rest, a kind of optical illusion . . . of consciousness. . . . Our task must be to free ourselves from this prison [of illusion] by widening our circle of compassion [love and caring] to embrace all living creatures and the whole of nature in all its beauty. Nobody is able to achieve this completely, but the striving for such achievement is in itself part of the liberation. (Albert Einstein quoted on title page of Williamson, 2002)

When we are conscious of an expanded cosmology and an expanded, deeper moral–ethical foundation, we gain new insights and awakenings; we open to the sense of humanity-in-relation-to-the-larger-universe, inspiring a sense of wonder, wisdom, awe, and humility. We are invited to accept our need for wisdom, beyond information and knowledge alone, and to surrender to both that which is greater than our separate ego-self and the outer world we think we have control over and seek to manipulate.

In the present work, I reassert the emerging, evolving wonder at and appreciation for viewing the human–universe as One. The holographic view of caring mirrors the holographic universe, that is, the whole is in each part and each part affects the whole.

So, in developing concepts and practices, theories and philosophies of caring–healing that intersect with love, we invoke Caring as part of our consciousness and intention to affect the whole with practical engagement from our own unique gifts and talents. In doing so, our part of personal and professional work is contributing to and making a difference in the moment but is also affecting the holographic universal field that surrounds us and to which we all belong.

In other words, through modern science as well as through ancient wisdom traditions, we realize that what we do for ourselves benefits others and what we do for others benefits us. If one person is healed, it is helping to heal all. If others are healed, it helps us to heal. The mutuality of caring affects the universal field to which we all belong, and we energetically affect it with our consciousness and our concrete acts. We all are candidates for awakening a compassionate heart (Chödrön, 2005), the deeper foundation for *caritas nursing*.

I now, 30 years later, after offering an overview and update of the previous texts of my evolved work in Caring Science and the Theory of Human Caring, turn back to the original text and offer revisions and current perspectives for the new edition. Ironically and perhaps not surprisingly, the original text held the blueprint for the evolution of these ideas that have both sustained and expanded over these years.

CARING SCIENCE AS CONTEXT

Nursing: The Philosophy and Science of Caring

The original text begins with a discussion of nursing as the Philosophy and Science of Caring. I now ponder suggesting that today, almost 30 years later, it perhaps could equally be framed as *Caring: The Philosophy and Science of Nursing*. Discussions and ambiguity remain as to the nature of Caring Science and its relation to nursing science. Rhetorical questions arise, such as, are there distinct differences between the two? Do they overlap? Do they intersect? Are they one and the same? These questions perhaps

remain, but the present work offers a distinct position. By transposing the order of nursing and caring, it invites a new discourse and context.

My position is this: Caring Science as a starting point for nursing as a field of study offers a distinct disciplinary foundation for the profession; it provides an ethical, moral, values-guided metanarrative for its science, its human phenomena, and its approach to caring-healing-person-nature-universe. It reintroduces spirit and sacred dimensions back into our work, life, and world. It allows for a reunion between metaphysics and the material-physical world of modern science.

In positing Caring Science as the disciplinary context and matrix that guides professional development and maturity, I acknowledge that there is a difference between the discipline of nursing and the profession of nursing. It is widely known that the discipline (of any field) should inform the profession. The disciplinary matrix of caring carries the metaparadigm, the values, the metaphysics, the philosophical-moral metanarrative with respect to what it means to be human, honoring unity of Being, and the oneness of mind–body–spirit/universe; the discipline offers subject matter foci and a distinct perspective on the subject matter. The profession, without clarity of its disciplinary context, loses its way in the midst of the outer-worldly changes and forces for conformity to the status quo of the moment.

The discipline of nursing, from my position, is/should be grounded in Caring Science; this, in turn, informs the profession. Caring Science informs and serves as the moral-philosophical-theoretical-foundational starting point for nursing education, patient care, research, and even administrative practices.

If nursing across time had been born and matured within the consciousness and clarity of a Caring Science orientation, perhaps it would be in a very different evolved place today: a place beyond the struggles with conventional biomedical-technical science that linger still, beyond the crisis in care that haunts hospitals and systems today, beyond the critical shortage of nurses and nursing that society is experiencing at this turn in history, and beyond the noncaring communities in our life and world. Our world is increasingly struggling with wars, violence, and inhumane acts—be they human-to-human, human-to-environment, or human-to-nature.

In spite of an evolved cosmology for all disciplines today, including physics and basic sciences and other scientific fields, we still often find ourselves locked in outdated thinking within a separatist-material-physical world ontology and an outer-worldview as our starting point. Caring Science, in contrast, has as its starting point a relational ontology that honors the fact that we are all connected and Belong to Source—the universal spirit field of infinity (Levinas, 1969)—before and after the human plane of worldly experiences. Caring Science makes more explicit that unity and connectedness exist among all things in the great circle of life: change, illness, suffering, death, and rebirth. A Caring Science orientation moves humanity closer to a moral community, closer to peaceful relationships with self–other communities–nations, states, other worlds, and time.

Basic Assumptions of Caring Science (Adapted with Minor Modifications from Watson, 1979, pp. 8–9)

- Caring Science is the essence of nursing and the foundational disciplinary core of the profession.
- Caring can be most effectively demonstrated and practiced interpersonally; however, caring consciousness can be communicated beyond/transcends time, space, and physicality (Watson, 2002a).
- The intersubjective human-to-human processes and connections keep alive

a common sense of humanity; they teach us how to be human by identifying ourselves with others, whereby the humanity of one is reflected in the other (Watson, 1985, p. 33).
- Caring consists of Carative Factors/ *Caritas Processes* that facilitate healing, honor wholeness, and contribute to the evolution of humanity.
- Effective caring promotes healing, health, individual/family growth, and a sense of wholeness, forgiveness, evolved consciousness, and inner peace that transcends the crisis and fear of disease, diagnosis, illness, traumas, life changes, and so on.
- Caring responses accept a person not only as he or she is now but also as what he or she may become/is becoming.
- A caring relationship is one that invites emergence of human spirit, opening to authentic potential, being authentically present, allowing the person to explore options—choosing the best action for self for "being-in-right relation" at any given point in time.
- Caring is more "healthogenic" than curing.
- Caring Science is complementary to Curing Science.
- The practice of caring is central to nursing. Its social, moral, and scientific contributions lie in its professional commitment to the values, ethics, and ideals of Caring Science in theory, practice, and research.

Premises of Caring Science (Adapted from Watson, 2005, pp. 218–219)

- Knowledge of caring cannot be assumed; it is an epistemic-ethical-theoretical endeavor that requires ongoing explication and development.
- Caring Science is grounded in a relational, ethical ontology of unity within the universe that informs the

epistemology methodology, pedagogy, and praxis of caring in nursing and related fields.

- Caring Science embraces epistemological pluralism, seeking to understand the intersection and underdeveloped connections between the arts and humanities and the clinical sciences.
- Caring Science embraces all ways of knowing/being/doing: ethical, intuitive, personal, empirical, aesthetic, and even spiritual/metaphysical ways of knowing and Being.
- Caring Science inquiry encompasses methodological pluralism, whereby the method flows from the phenomenon of concern—diverse forms of inquiry seek to unify ontological, philosophical, ethical, and theoretical views while incorporating empirics and technology.
- Caring (and nursing) has existed, in every society. Every society has had some people who have cared for others. A caring attitude is *not* transmitted from generation to generation by genes. It is transmitted by the culture of a society. The culture of nursing, in this instance the discipline and profession of nursing, has a vital social-scientific role in advancing, sustaining, and preserving human caring as a way of fulfilling its mission to society and broader humanity.

Working Definition of Caring Science (Extracted/Modified from Watson, 2004a; Watson and Smith, 2002)

Caring Science is an evolving philosophical-ethical-epistemic field of study, grounded in the discipline of nursing and informed by related fields. Caring is considered as one central feature within the metaparadigm of nursing knowledge and practice. Caring Science is informed by an ethical-moral-spiritual stance that encompasses a humanitarian, human science orientation to human caring processes, phenomena, and experiences. It is located

within a worldview that is nondualistic, relational, and unified, wherein there is a connectedness to All: the universal field of infinity: cosmic love. This worldview is sometimes referred to as

- A unitary transformative paradigm (Newman, Sime, & Corcoran-Perry, 1991; Watson, 1999)
- Nonlocal consciousness (Dossey, 1991)
- Era III medicine/nursing (Dossey, 1991, 1993; Watson, 1999).

Caring Science within this worldview intersects with the arts and humanities and related fields of study and practice.

Caring: Science–Arts–Humanities

To understand nursing as a discipline and a distinct field of study is to honor it within a context of art, the humanities, and expanding views of science. As a distinct discipline, it is necessary to acknowledge that nursing and Caring reside within a humanitarian as well as a scientific matrix; thus, there is an intersection among the arts, humanities, philosophy, science, and technology. The discipline encompasses a broad worldview that honors evolving humanity and an evolving universe that is full of wonder and unknowns as well as known set expectations about our world.

Just as the profession may detour at times from its disciplinary heritage, so too we often forget that an equal need exists for humanistic-aesthetic views of a similar phenomenon. Humanities and the arts seek to answer different questions than science does. It continues to be important to understand the essential characteristics they all bring and the ways in which they are similar and different and in which they also converge.

For example, conventional science is concerned with order, prediction, control, methods, generalizations, detachment, objectivity, and so on. The three classical assumptions that have shaped modern conventional science are *objectivism, positivism, and reductionism* (Harman, 1990–1991;

Watson, 2005). Science in this context cannot answer certain questions about humanity, about caring and what it means to be human. Science generally is not concerned with specific individual responses but more with prediction and generalizations about anonymous others. It cannot be expected or called on to keep alive a sense of common humanity (Watson, 1979, p. 4). It does not offer insights into depth of human experiences such as pain, joy, suffering, fear, forgiveness, love, and so on. Such in-depth exploration of humanity is expressed and pondered through study of philosophy, drama, the arts, film, literature, humanistic studies in the liberal arts, humanities proper, and so on. This perspective is learned through self-knowledge, self-discovery, and shared human experiences, combined with the study of human emotions and relations that mirror our shared humanity.

In spite of inherent differences between science and the humanities, both fields and, in fact, all fields of study are changing, expanding, growing into new dynamic intersections between and among each other. There is a convergence between and among art, science, and spirituality; this convergence is becoming more prevalent among emerging models of mind–body–spirit medicine, so-called complementary–alternative–integrative medicine, and new understandings of the physics of science, energy medicine, spirituality and healing, and so on.

The intersections between art and science help reveal what is beyond the confines and contingencies of the visible world, to "see" that which is deeper, glimpsing the human spirit, the human soul, and its beauty and loveliness, whatever its shape or form (Housden, 2005, p. 3). As Housden put it, art helps our eyes see more than they usually do: about life in general but also about ourselves. The same can be said for the humanities, drama, and also for science, opening up a new horizon of meaning and possibilities. However, art helps us "to bear witness to eternal joy, suffering, pain, and struggle of our own human soul and to feel the poignant, bittersweet reality of our physical mortality" (Housden, 2005, p. 3). In their own ways, art and science remind us that we are "both finite and infinite and everything in between" (Housden, 2005, pp. 10–11). In considering Caring Science, art, the humanities, and the beauty of science and life itself all come into play. When one is engaged in human caring and healing, one cannot ignore the element aesthetics and beauty and the spiritual domain of life's journey.

In Emerson's words: "This dement [beauty] I call an ultimate end. No reason can be asked or given why the soul seeks beauty Beauty in its largest and most profound sense is one expression of the universe" (Emerson, 1982, p. 48). In this sense, then, art transforms us and helps us to see our everyday world differently, in that arts move us into a space where we can create visions of other ways of Being/doing/knowing and ask what it might signify to realize them (Greene, 1991). It is this engagement in art and a sense of beauty that gives rise to wonder, to questioning, and to pondering our Being.

The art and science of caring–healing is emerging in mainstream medicine and nursing, as the public has a hunger for the intersection among art, science, beauty, and spiritual dimensions of the healing arts and health and also has a greater sense of self-knowledge, self-control, and well-being. As Kandinsky (1977) understood it, "the spiritual resides in art" (just as Emerson viewed nature as spirit); perhaps, they are one and the same, tapping into the human spirit of humanity and the universal source of infinity in which we dwell.

In any event, in nursing and caring–healing work, we draw on healing arts in a more expanded way that integrates science, art, beauty, and spirituality. These are manifest in unlimited potential for areas such as visual arts, music, sound, aroma, dance, movement, theater, drama, storytelling, design, psycho-architecture/sacred healing architecture, and a variety of tactile-touch and noncontact, energetic modalities.

Diverse categories of healing arts are emerging. At least four types have been identified:

- Art intended to heal directly, using symbols, images that calm and center.
- Art created by artists to facilitate their own healing; for example, auto-biographical art, representational art depicting incidences of treatment, illness, and change.
- Art about specific aspects of the healing process—pain, loss, body image changes, loss, grief, death, as well as hope, change, joy, insights, and so on.
- Artist-designed psycho-architecture; healing spaces/healing architecture—this art/architecture makes a conscious, intentional, even a technical, precise scientific effort to integrate symbol, myth, archetype, mystery, and legend into architectural and environmental themes. Such art can be considered "ontological design," an integration of sacred geometry into architectural structures so humans can "be" and feel differently as a way of experiencing self-in-harmony, with the sacred universal field of life's energy for healing, wholeness, alignment, and so on. (Lafo, Capasso, & Roberts, 1994, p. 9)

Caring Science seeks to combine science with the humanities and arts. Caring Science is not neutral with respect to human values, goals, subjective individual perceptions, and meanings. It is not detached from human emotions and their diverse expressions, be they culturally bound or individually revealed.

The discipline of nursing—guided by a Caring Science orientation—seeks to study, research, explore, identify, describe, express, and question the relation and intersection between and among the ethical, ontological, epistemological, methodological, pedagogical, and praxis aspects of nursing, including health policies and administrative practices. Thus, a Caring Science orientation seeks congruence between and among clinical nursing science, humanities, the arts, and the human subject matter and phenomena of caring knowledge and practices.

Ontological "Competencies": Caring Literacy[1]

In moving from a discussion of art, beauty, humanities, and science, perhaps there is more awareness of the connection between this integrated way of thinking about Caring Science and human artistry. Such notions translate into what I have previously referred to as *"ontological competencies,"* reframed as *"caring literacy,"* or *"caritas literacy."*

Although the meaning of literacy is associated with the abilities to read and write, the notion of having fluency in caring at both personal and professional levels introduces new meaning to deepen our ways of attending to and cultivating how to *be-deeply human/humane* and *be-caring* and having a healing presence. This form of *being is* a form of human literacy human artistry.

Such literacy includes an evolved and continually evolving emotional heart intelligence, consciousness, and intentionality and level of sensitivity and efficacy, followed by a continuing lifelong process and journey of self-growth and self-awareness. Such an awakening of ones being and abilities cultivates skills and awareness of holding, conveying, and practicing communicating thoughts of caring, loving, kindness, equanimity and so on as part of one's professional being.

This level of evolved being/ontological presence is now ethically required for any professional engaged in caring–healing. Perhaps, this requirement was and has always been present in the tradition of healing professions, but somewhere along the way, professional education and practices took a detour from the very foundation of our shared humanity. A return to a focus on ontological competencies, within the evolved notion of Caring Literacy, seems essential to balance and carry out the pervasive technological competencies, helping to make these skills and forms of Being part of the requirements for nursing education and practice.

Examples of (Ontological) Caring Literacy

I have only begun to identify some of these so-called ontological competencies for cultivating caring literacy (Watson, 1999). (For more exploration of these ideas within the context of Nightingale, see Watson, 1999, Chapter 14.) In addition, an emerging project from the International Caritas Consortium (ICC) is focused on caring literacy and *caritas* literacy, seeking more and more specificity in the knowledge, skills, and ways of being to manifest such literacy. A working document is found in the Addenda as well as on the Web site—www.caritasconsortium.org.[2]

In the meantime, I have identified the following general guideline dimensions as examples of "ontological competencies" that facilitate caring literacy. These directions have emerged from my work over the past decade or so and need to continue to unfold with more specificity—something related to the ICC project—ultimately leading to better documentation and assessment of caring/*caritas*.

I invite readers to identify the ontological–literacy processes they bring to their caring–healing practice and to continue to contribute to more specificity; so, these practices can be taught, documented, researched, and practiced.

Watson's *Caritas* Literacy Dimensions: A Work in Progress

- Cultivate caring consciousness and intentionality as a starting point.
- Ability to "center"—quiet down, pause before entering patient's room or be still in the presence of the other.

- Ability to "read the field" when entering into the life space or field of another.
- Ability to *be present*—*be with* other as well as *do for* other.
- Accurately identify and address person by name.
- Maintain eye contact as appropriate for person/cultural meaning and sensitivity.
- Ability to ground self and other for comforting, soothing, and calming acts.
- Accurately detect other's feelings,
- Stay within the other's frame of reference,
- Invite and authentically listen to the inner meaning, the subjective story of other,
- Authentically listen/hear behind the words,
- Hold other with an attitude of unconditional loving–kindness, equanimity, dignity, and regard,
- Ability to be with "silence," waiting for other to reflect before responding to questions, allowing other's inner thoughts to emerge.
- Respond to the other's feelings and mood verbally and nonverbally, with authentic affective congruence.
- Cultivate and create meaningful caring–healing rituals; translate conventional nursing tasks into purposive healing acts.
- For example, hand washing as purification, cleansing psychically as well as physically; use as opportunity to "center," release, and bless patient/situation while preparing oneself to enter into next moment.
- Incorporate, translate, and expand nursing skills/tasks into nursing arts/caring–healing modalities; for example, intentional use of music-sound, touch, aroma, visual-aesthetic-beauty, energetic approaches, and so on.
- Carry out conventional nursing tasks and procedures, such as basic needs

and physical care acts, as intentional, reverential, and respectful caring–healing arts.

- Cultivate own practices for spiritual growth and evolution of higher/deeper consciousness.
- Others—yet to be identified (see www.caritasconsortium.org).

We need to continue to explore models for cultivating Caring Literacy and skill in attending to our human presence in "Being-in-caring-healing-relationships." These directions incorporate aspects of caring such as silence, song, music, poetry physical and nonphysical touch, centering practices of "presencing"; the use of art, nonverbal expressive forms, spirit-energy-filled conscious affirmations; holding intentions of wholeness, calmness, healing, and so on.

Within this framework of caring literacy, it is important to realize that the nurse is not only *in* the environment, able to make significant changes in the ways of Being/doing/knowing in the physical environment, but that the *nurse IS the environment* (Quinn, 1992; Watson, 2005). Thus, the nurse is invited to engage in significant insight into the *Nurse-Self* as an energetic–vibrational field of consciousness and intentionality (Quinn, 1992), affecting the entire environment for better or for worse. The nurse's (caring–loving) consciousness radiates higher vibrational effects. A nurse without an informed, "literate" caring consciousness can actually be "biocidic"—that is, toxic, life destroying, and destructive to the experience of others (Halldorsdottir, 1991). On the other hand, a nurse who is cultivating ontological competendes in caring literacy is more likely to be "biogenic"—that is, life giving and life receiving for self and other and thereby more likely to engage in and experience a transpersonal caring–healing moment. As the nurse cultivates these ontological literate abilities and sensitivities of caring, there is an invitation to open to inner healing processes that expand to infinite new possibilities.

Ontological–Caring Literacy directions serve only as examples of the intersection between technological competencies and emotional–intellectual literacy of human caring skills of *Being-Caring*. Such exploration into the literacy of caring incorporates the ethical, philosophical, and theoretical foundations of professional caring–healing. This view of Caring Literacy serves as core knowledge that leads directly back to the original Carative Factors and the evolution toward *Caritas Consciousness* and *Caritas Processes*. . . .

CARATIVE FACTORS/*CARITAS PROCESSES:* ORIGINAL AND EVOLVED CORE FOR PROFESSIONAL NURSING

The background on my major books on Caring Theory, Philosophy, and Caring Science helps us see the evolution of my original work. This revised, updated edition builds on the primary source material from the 1979 text and its evolution from what is known as the 10 Carative Factors (CFs) toward ten *Caritas Processes* (CPs). Likewise, this revision incorporates ideas from my previous published works. . . .

Table 16.1 includes the original 1979 Carative Factors (with minor edits from the 1985 book). The original 10 Carative Factors, juxtaposed against the emerging *Caritas Processes*, are summarized in Table 16.2.

Core Aspects Theory of Human Caring

- Relational caring as ethical–moral–philosophical values-guided foundation.
- Caring core: 10 carative factors/*Caritas Processes*.
- Transpersonal *Caring Moment–Caring Field*.
- Caring as consciousness—energy-intentionality–human presence.
- Caring–healing modalities.

TABLE 16.1 Original 10 Carative Factors, Original (1979) Text

1. Formation of a humanistic-altruistic system of values
2. Instillation of faith–hope
3. Cultivation of sensitivity to oneself and others
4. Development of a helping-trusting relationship
5. Promotion and acceptance of the expression of positive and negative feelings
6. Systematic use of the scientific problem-solving method for decision making (refined in 1985 as use of creative problem-solving caring process)
7. Promotion of interpersonal teaching–learning
8. Provision for a supportive, protective, and (or) corrective mental, physical, sociocultural, and spiritual environment
9. Assistance with gratification of human needs
10. Allowance for existential-phenomenological forces (refined in 1985 as existential-phenomeno-logical spiritual dimensions)

Reprinted with permission from (1979). *Nursing: The philosophy and science of caring* (pp. 9–10). Boston, MA: Little, Brown.

TABLE 16.2 Original Carative Factors and Evolved *Caritas Processes*

Carative Factors, 1979	*Caritas Processes*, 2002–2007
1. Humanistic-altruistic values	1. Practicing loving–kindness and equanimity for self and other
2. Instilling/enabling faith and hope	2. Being authentically present; enabling/sustaining/honoring deep belief system and subjective world of self/other
3. Cultivating sensitivity to oneself and other	3. Cultivating one's own spiritual practices; deepening self awareness, going beyond "ego-self"
4. Developing a helping-trusting, human caring relationship	4. Developing and sustaining a helping-trusting, authentic caring relationship
5. Promoting and accepting expression of positive and negative feelings	5. Being present to, and supportive of, the expression of positive and negative feelings as a connection with deeper spirit of self and the one-being-cared-for
6. Systematic use of scientific (creative) problem-solving caring process	6. Creative use of self and all ways of knowing/being/doing as part of the caring process (engaging in artistry of caring–healing practices)
7. Promoting transpersonal teaching–learning	7. Engaging in genuine teaching–learning experiences within context of caring relationship—attend to whole person and subjective meaning; attempt to stay within other's frame of reference (evolve toward "coaching" role vs. conventional imparting of information)
8. Providing for a supportive, protective, and/or corrective mental, social, spiritual environment	8. Creating healing environment at all levels (physical, nonphysical, subtle environment of energy and consciousness whereby wholeness, beauty, comfort, dignity, and peace are potentiated (Being/Becoming the environment)
9. Assisting with gratification of human needs	9. Reverentially and respectfully assisting with basic needs; holding an intentional, raring consciousness of touching and working with the embodied spirit of another, honoring unity of Being; allowing for spirit-filled connection

(continued)

TABLE 16.2 Original Carative Factors and Evolved *Caritas Processes (continued)*

Carative Factors, 1979	Caritas Processes, 2002–2007
10. Allowing for existential phenomenological dimensions	10. Opening and attending to spiritual, mysterious, unknown existential dimensions of life–death–suffering; "*allowing for a miracle*"[a]

Sources: Watson, J. (1979). *Nursing: The philosophy and science of caring.* Boston, MA: Little, Brown; www.uchsc.edu/nursmg/caring.

[a]Idea courtesy Resurrection Health, Chicago IL.

The 10 original Carative Factors remain the timeless structural core of the theory while allowing for their evolving emergence into more fluid aspects of the model captured by the 10 *Caritas Processes.*

In introducing the original concept of Carative Factors as the core for a nursing philosophy and science, I was offering a theoretical counterpoint to the notion of Curative, so dominant in medical science. Thus, the Carative Factors provided a framework to hold the discipline and profession of nursing; they were informed by a deeper vision and ethical commitment to the human dimensions of caring in nursing—the art and human science context. I was seeking to address those aspects of professional nursing that transcended medical diagnosis, disease, setting limited and changing knowledge, and the technological emphasis on very specialized phenomena.

I was asking, What remains as core? My response in 1979 was "The Ten Carative Factors" (embellished in 2007 by the philosophical–ethical value of *Caritas-loving* consciousness).

The CFs were identified as the essential core of professional nursing practice, in contrast to what I called the "trim," that which is constantly changing and cannot be the content or the criteria with which to describe, identify, and sustain professional nursing and its timeless disciplinary stance with respect to caring in society.

As indicated in the original (1979) work, "carative" was a word I made up to serve as a counterpoint to the "curative" orientation of medical science. I identified these 10 factors as the core activities and orientations a professional nurse uses in the delivery of care. They are the common and necessary professional practices that sustain and reveal nursing as a distinct (caring) profession, not as comprising a group of technicians. Nurses apply the CFs constantly but are not aware of them nor have they necessarily named them. Thus, nurses, generally, are not conscious of their own phenomena; they do not have the language to identify; chart, and communicate systematically and so on. This is a result of both a lack of awareness and terminology of caring and of recognized knowledge of those everyday practices that define their work. Without an awareness, additional education, and advancement of professional caring in nursing, these factors are likely to occur in an ad hoc, rather than a systematic, fashion.

Nurses will not be aware or realize the importance of using them/*becoming* them to guide their professional caring practices. Furthermore, without a context to hold these practices, nurses have often devalued their caring work, taking it for granted, without a common language to "see," articulate, act on, reinforce, and advance that work.

If nurses are committed to a model of professional caring–healing, going beyond conventional medicalized-clinical routines and industrial product-line views of nursing (and humanity), yet do not have a theoretical guide to honor, frame, discuss, develop, and advance their profession, a demoralized experience and despair set in over time (Swanson, 1999). If this continues, there is little hope for the survival of professional nursing and its caring–healing practices. Similarly, without furthering this work, there is little to no hope for advancement of Caring Science as the disciplinary foundation for nursing (and other health sciences), little hope for a foundation that guides and contains the values, ethics, moral foundation, and philosophical directions for caring for human beings. Without honoring and attending to Caring Science knowledge and practices, nursing will not be fulfilling its scientific, ethical, professional covenant with its public, or even with itself.

Moving from Carative to *Caritas*

From an academic standpoint related to knowledge development and theory evolution, one can consider that I used the technical process of concept derivation (Walker & Avant, 2005) and extension in transposing and redefining Carative Factors to *Caritas Processes*. That is, in working within the original field of Nursing and Carative thinking, I sought to redefine carative from the parent field, nursing, to the new field of Caring Science with its explicit ethic, worldview, and so on.

Thus, once the carative concept was transposed from nursing per se to Caring Science, *Caritas/Caritas Processes* emerged as a more meaningful concept, generating new connections between Caring and Love. The broader field of Caring Science and its expanded cosmology of unity, belonging, and infinity of the universal field of Love allowed for a more meaningful redefinition for the phenomenon of *caritas nursing* to result. As the transposition from carative nursing to

caritas Caring Science occurred, a new vocabulary for an ontological phenomenon was revealed, allowing for new ways of thinking about caring and inviting a new image, even a metaphor, of caring–healing practices to develop. Furthermore, the new notion of *caritas* offers a new vocabulary/phenomenon for an area of inquiry, leading to additional theorizing and knowledge development at the disciplinary level of nursing and Caring Science.

Table 16.3 is a visual depiction of the process of Concept derivation for extending the theory of human caring from carative nursing to *caritas* within a Caring Science context.

Although each of the original Carative Factors has been transposed and extended into the new language of *caritas*, several core principles are the most essential with respect to a change in consciousness. These five cultivated areas of *caritas* are those that help distinguish the core differences between the notions of carative and *caritas*.

Core Principles/Practices: From Carative to *Caritas*

- Practice of loving–kindness and equanimity
- Authentic presence: enabling deep belief of other
- Cultivation of one's own spiritual practice—beyond ego
- "Being" the caring–healing environment
- Allowing for miracles.

In moving from the concept of carative to *caritas*, I am overtly evoking love

TABLE 16.3 Visual Representation of Concept Derivation and Extension from Carative Nursing to *Caritas Processes* in Caring Science

Concept I:	*Transposed to*	Concept I:	*Redefined*	Concept II:
Carative Factors		Carative		Field II:
Field I: Nursing		New Field II: Caring Science		*Caritas Processes* in Caring Science

and caring to merge into an expanded paradigm for the future. Such a perspective, ironically, places nursing in its most mature paradigm while reconnecting with the heritage and foundation of Nightingale. With *Caritas* incorporated more explicitly, it locates the theory within an ethical and ontological context as the starting point for considering not only its science but also its societal mission for humanity. This direction makes a more formal connection between caring and healing and the evolved human consciousness. The background for this work is available in Watson (2004a).

Emergence of *Caritas Nursing* and the *Caritas Nurse*

My evolution toward *Caritas Processes* is intended to offer a more fluid language for understanding a deeper, more comprehensive level of the work, as well as guidance toward how to enter into, interpret, sustain, and inquire about the intention and consciousness behind the original Carative Factors. Moreover, *caritas* captures a deeper phenomenon, a new image that intersects professional–personal practices while opening up a new field of inquiry for nursing and Caring Science.

However, as one steps into this new work, it is important to consider both the original CFs and the evolved CPs holographically, in that the whole is in any and every part. So, all the factors/processes are simultaneously present; they are either foreground or background when practicing within a professional caring model. Furthermore, the consciousness/intentionality of caring–healing and wholeness is held by the nurse as part of his or her presence in the moment.

What is emerging throughout this shift to *Caritas Processes* is an acknowledgment of a deeper form of nursing: *Caritas Nursing and the Caritas Nurse.* As the work evolves and as each nurse evolves, we learn throughout this book that the more evolved practitioner (working from the higher/deeper dimensions of humanity and evolving consciousness) can be identified as a *caritas nurse,* or one who is practicing or at least cultivating the practices of *caritas nursing.* Another way to identify a *caritas nurse* is as one who is working from a human-to-human connection—working from an open, intelligent heart center[3] rather than the ego-center. This caring consciousness orientation informs the professional actions and relationships of a *caritas nurse,* even while she or he is engaged in the required routine or dramatic, practical–technical world of clinical practices.

For example, in considering CF 1: Humanistic, altruistic value systems, one may wonder what is behind and underneath such a value system that allows it to manifest professionally in one's actions. How is such a value system to be cultivated and sustained for professional caring practices? What personal practices can prepare one for entering into and manifesting this value system throughout one's career?

My response is that this value system comes to life when one cultivates the ongoing practice of loving–kindness and Equanimity, a form of cultivated mindfulness awareness/meditation, a practice that opens and awakens the compassionate, forgiving love of the heart center. This preparation can take the form of daily practice of offering gratitude and connecting with nature; the practice of silence, journaling, and prayer; asking for guidance to be there for another when needed; and developing a practice of forgiveness, silently citing positive affirmations, and opening to blessings in the midst of difficulties, whereby one's consciousness is expanded through all these practices. These are only some examples of how to enter into and sustain this professional ethic of altruism and loving–kindness. This work is related not only to caring but also to the health and healing of practitioner as well as patient.

If "health is expanded conscious-ness," as Newman posits (Newman, 1994), then what is the highest level of consciousness? *It is love* in the fullest uni-versal, cosmic sense. What is the greatest source of healing? It, too, is love. So, in cul-tivating the practice of loving–kindness toward self and other, one is opening his or her heart; one is heightened to give and receive, to be present to what is present-ing itself in one's life, to open to exercising and receiving grace, mercy, forgiveness, and so on. Thus, one can better appreci-ate the gifts of giving and receiving, being there for another person to offer presence, loving consciousness, and informed moral caring actions in the midst of suffering, despair, love, hate, illness, sorrow, ques-tions, trauma, unknowns, fears, hopes, and so on, In this personal/professional caring work, one cultivates an acceptance, a level of humility, before the mystery of it all—opening to it with equanimity com-passion, and mercy as part of the human condition. This level of consciousness with which to enter and sustain profes-sional caring in nursing, while honoring our deep humanity, is founded on a very different model than conventional nursing and medicine.

This mode of *caritas* thinking invites a total transformation of self and sys-tems. In this model of Caring Science, the changes occur not from the outer focus on systems but from that deep inner place within the creativity of the human spirit. Here is where the deep humanity, the individual heart and con-sciousness of practitioners, evolves and connects with the ultimate source of all true re-formation/transformation.

Although the original Carative Factors remain relevant and accessible for first-level concrete entry into the work, once one grows with the ideas and their evolution, it is hoped that one moves more fully into a knowing that is behind the orig-inal material and enters a more profound level of insight, personal/professional growth, understanding, and wisdom. At the same time, the shift allows for nurses and nursing to evolve toward accessing a more fluid, expressive language for com-prehending and articulating the deeper meaning behind the original factors.

CARITAS PROCESSES: *EXTENSION OF CARATIVE FACTORS*

Caring and Love

One day, after we have mastered the winds and the waves, gravity and the tides, we will harness for God the energies of love.

Teilhard De Chardin

Caritas comes from the Latin word mean-ing to cherish, to appreciate, to give special, if not loving, attention to. It repre-sents charity and compassion, generosity of spirit. It connotes something very fine, indeed, something precious that needs to be cultivated and sustained.

Caritas is closely related to the word "carative" from my original (1979) text on Caring Science. However, now, using the terms *caritas* and *Caritas Processes*, I invoke intentionally the "*l*" *word: love*, which makes explicit the connection between caring and love: Love in its fullest univer-sal infinite sense developed in the philos-ophy of Levinas (1969) and explored in my 2005 text *Caring Science as Sacred Science*.

Bringing Love and Caring together this way invites a form of deep transper-sonal caring. The relationship between love and caring creates an opening/alignment and access for inner healing for self and others. Although health may be considered to represent expanding consciousness, love is the highest level of consciousness and the greatest source of all healing in the world. This connec-tion with love as a source for healing extends from the individual self to nature and the larger universe, which is evolv-ing and unfolding. This cosmology and worldview of caring and love—*caritas*—is both grounded and metaphysical; it is immanent and transcendent with the co-evolving human in the universe (Watson, 1999, 2004a).

It is when we include and bring together caring and love in our work and our lives that we discover and affirm that nursing, like teaching, is more than a job. It is a life-giving and life-receiving career for a lifetime of growth and learning. It is maturing in an awakening and an awareness that nursing has much more to offer humankind than simply being an extension of an outdated model of medicine and medical-techno-cure science. Nursing helps sustain human dignity and humanity itself while contributing to the evolution of human consciousness, helping to move toward a more humane and caring moral community and civilization.

As nursing more publicly and professionally asserts these positions from a Caring Science context for its theories, ethics, and practices, we are invited to relocate ourselves and our profession away from a dominant medical science mind-set. Furthermore, we are asked to reconnect nursing's disciplinary source to its noble heritage, within both an ancient and an emerging cosmology—a cosmology that invites and welcomes the energy of universal caring and love back into our lives and world. Such thinking calls forth a sense of reverence and sacredness with regard to our work, our lives, and all living things. It incorporates art, science, and spirituality as they are being redefined.

As we enter into a maturing of Caring Science and evolved *Caritas Processes* as a professional-theoretical map and guide, we are simultaneously challenged to relocate ourselves in these emerging ideals and ideas and question for ourselves how this work speaks to us as a discipline and a practice profession. Each person is asked, invited, if not enticed, to examine, explore, challenge, and question for self and for the profession the critical intersections between the personal and the professional.

This revised work calls each of us into our deepest self to give new meaning to our lives and work, to explore how our unique gifts, talents, and skills can be translated into compassionate human caring–healing service for self and others and even the planet Earth. It is hoped that at some level this work will help us all, in the caring–healing professions, to remember who we are and why we have come here to do this work in the world.

Value Assumptions of *Caritas* (Adapted from Watson, 1985, p. 32)

- Caring and love are the most universal, tremendous, and mysterious cosmic forces; they comprise the primal and universal source of energy.
- Often this wisdom is overlooked, or we forget, even though we know people need each other in loving and caring ways.
- If our humanity is to survive and if we are to evolve toward a more loving, caring, deeply human and humane, moral community and civilization, we must sustain love and caring in our life, our work, our world.
- Since nursing is a caring profession, its ability to sustain its caring ideals, ethics, and philosophy for professional practices will affect the human development of civilization and nursing's mission in society.
- As a beginning, we have to learn how to offer caring, love, forgiveness, compassion, and mercy to ourselves before we can offer authentic caring and love to others.
- We have to treat ourselves with loving–kindness and equanimity, gentleness and dignity before we can accept, respect, and care for others within a professional caring–healing model.
- Nursing has always held a caring stance with respect to others and their health-illness concerns.
- Knowledgeable, informed, ethical caring is the essence of professional

nursing values, commitments, and competent actions; it is the most central and unifying source to sustain its covenant to society and ensure its survival.

- Preservation and advancement of Caring Science values, knowledge, theories, philosophies, ethics, and clinical practices, within a context of an expanding *Caritas* cosmology, are ontological, epistemological, and clinical endeavors; these endeavors are the source and foundation for sustaining and advancing the discipline and profession.

Return to Love as the Basis for *Caritas Consciousness* and Gratitude Toward Self-Others

In a world like ours, where death is increasingly drained of meaning, individual authenticity lies in what we can find that is worth living for. And the only thing worth living for is love. Love for one another. Love for ourselves. Love of our work. Love of our destiny, whatever it may be. Love for our difficulties. Love of life. The love that could free us from the mysterious cycles of suffering. The love that releases us from our self-imprisonment, from our bitterness, our greed, our madness-engendering competitiveness. The love that can make us breathe again. Love a great and beautiful cause, a wonderful vision. A great love for another or for the future. The love that reconciles us to ourselves, to our simple joys, and to our undiscovered repletion. A creative love, A love touched with the sublime. (Okri, 1997, pp. 56–57)

Caritas Process—Cultivating the Practice of Loving Kindness and Equanimity Toward Self and Other as Foundational to *Caritas Consciousness*

When love moves through us it inspires all we do.

Love and compassion must begin with kindness toward ourselves.

One of the greatest blocks to loving kindness is our own sense of unworthiness.

Kornfield (2002, pp. 95, 101, 100)

The Carative Factor: Formation of Humanistic-Altruistic Values system continues to lay the foundation as a starting point for Caring Science. As a given, caring must be grounded within a set of universal human values—kindness, concern, and love of self and others. As one matures into a professional model that focuses on caring–healing and health in its broadest and deepest dimensions, such as the timeless mission of nursing, one must cultivate an awareness and intentionality to sustain such a guiding vision for one's life and work. This factor in its original and evolved sense honors the gift of being able to give and receive with a capacity to love and appreciate all of life's diversity and its individuality with each person. Such a system helps us to tolerate difference and view others through their subjective worldview rather than ours alone.

Regardless of whether one is conscious of one's own philosophy and value system, it is affecting the encounters, relationships, and moments we have with our self and others. These humanistic-altruistic values can be developed through a variety of life experiences: early childhood, exposure to different languages and cultures, history, as well as film, drama, art, literature, and other creative expressions of humanity and personal growth experiences.

These emotions of love, kindness, gentleness, compassion, equanimity, and so on are intrinsic to all humans. These emotions and experiences are the essence of what makes us human and what deepens our humanity and our connection with the human spirit. This awareness is what connects us with the "source" from which we draw our sacred breath for life itself. It is here where we access our energy and creativity for living and being; it is here, in this model, that we yield to that which is greater than our individual ego-self, reminding us that we belong to the universe of humanity and all living things.

For this original Carative Factor (CF) to evolve and mature in its manifestation, we are now called, invited, and challenged to take it to a deeper level in our maturity, our awareness, our experiences, and our expressions. This is a path of deepening who and what we are that prepares us for a lifelong commitment to caring–healing and compassionate human service. Thus, the evolution/extension of the original CF has been both sustained and transcended. The original CFs and evolved *Caritas Processes* are considered the bedrock and most basic foundation for preparing practitioners to engage in and practice the philosophy, science, (and ethic) of caring.

NOTES

1. The movement from the notion of "ontological competencies" to the concept of "Caring Literacy" is influenced by Joan Boyce, Victoria University British Columbia, PhD dissertation: Nurses Making Caring Work: A Closet Drama, and the discussion during her PhD final examination, June 2007.

2. A subgroup from the ICC has a current, ongoing working draft of Caring/*Caritas* Literacy. It is found in Addendum III.

3. This latest ICC document on Caritas Literacy is based on meetings, dialogue, and previous works among the subgroup members: J. D'Alfonso, Scottsdale Health, Scottsdale, Arizona; J. Duffy, The Catholic University of America, Washington, D.C.; Gene Rigotti, InovaHealth, Fairfax, Virginia; J. Watson, University of Colorado–Denver and Health Sciences, Denver, Colorado; and Terri Woodward, The Children's Hospital, Denver, Colorado. The items marked with a check on this document represent items on the Caring

Assessment Tool ©-Version IV (Duffy, Hoskins, & Seifert 2007).

4. As a prelude, *Caritas Nursing* requires cultivation of higher, deeper consciousness, working more and more to awaken the heart-centered chakra upward to the crown chakra in bringing one's full and open self into any caring occasion.

REFERENCES

Bevis, E. & Watson, J. (1989). *Toward a Caring Curriculum in Nursing*. New York: NLN.

Chinn, P. L. & Watson, J. (1994). *Art and Aesthetics in Nursing*. New York: Jones & Bartlett.

Chodron, P. (2005). *No Time to Lose*. Boston: Shambhala.

Dossey, L. (1991). *Meaning and Medicine*. New York: Bantam.

Dossey, L. (1993). *Healing Words: The Power of Prayer and the Practice of Medicine*. San Francisco: Harper

Emerson, R.W. (1982). *Ralph Waldo Emerson: Selected Essays*. New York: Penguin American Library.

Green, M. (1991). Texts and margins. *Harvard Educational Review*, 61(1), 25-39.

Halldorsdottir, S. (1991). Five basic modes of being with another in D.A. Gaut and M. Leininger (eds.). *Caring: The Compassionate Healer*. New York: National League for Nursing.

Housden, R. (2005). *How Rembrandt Reveals Your Beautiful Imperfect Self*. New York: Harmony Books.

Kandinsky, W. (1977). *Concerning the spiritual in art*. New York: Dover.

Logstrup, K. (1997). *The Ethical Demand*. Notre Dame, IN: University of Notre Dame.

Quinn, J. (1992). Holding sacred space: The nurse as healing environment. *Holistic Nursing Practice*, 6(4), 26-35.

Swanson, K. (1999). What is known about caring in nursing research: A literary meta-analysis. In A.S. Hinshaw, S. Feetham & J. Shaver (eds.) *Handbook of Clinical Nursing Research*. Thousand Oaks, CA: Sage.

Watson, J. (1979). *Nursing: The Philosophy and Science of Caring*. Boston: Little, Brown. Reprinted/republished 1985. Boulder: Colorado Associated University Press.

Watson, J. (1997). The theory of human caring: A retrospective and prospective. *Nursing Science Quarterly* 10(1): 49-52.

Watson, J. & Ray, M. (1988). *The ethics of care and the ethics of cure: Synthesis of chronicity.* New York: NLN.

Watson, J. (1985). *Nursing: Human Science and Human Care: A Theory of Nursing.* Norwalk, CT: Appleton-Century Crofts. Reprinted/republished 1988 NLN. Reprinted/republished 1999. Sudbury, MA: Jones & Bartlett.

Watson, J. (1999). *Postmodern Nursing and Beyond.* Edinburgh, Scotland: Churchill-Livingstone.

Reprinted/republished 2005. New York: Elsevier.

Watson, J. (2002). *Assessing and Measuring Caring in Nursing and the Health Sciences.* New York: Springer.

Watson, J. (2005). *Caring Science as Sacred Science.* Philadelphia: F.A. Davis.

Watson, J. (2004a). Caring science web site: www.uchsc.edu/nursing.caring.

Watson, J. & Smith, M.C. (2002). Caring science and the science of unitary human beings: A transtheoretical discourse. *Journal of Advanced Nursing.* 37(5), 452-461.

QUESTIONS FOR REFLECTION

Baccalaureate

1. Select one of the 10 CPs and explain, in your own words, what it means to you.

2. You are caring for a dying patient who is "unconscious." You sit by her side quietly, imagining her peaceful transition, and gently holding her hand. What concepts from Watson's theory are evident in your caring?

3. What kind of practice have you developed or could you plan to develop that might help you to grow as a caritas nurse?

Master's

1. Advanced practice nurses may practice in settings in which their time with patients is constrained. Can transpersonal caring occur in this kind of practice? If so, how? If not, why not?

2. Select two of the 10 CPs and develop specific indicators of their presence in nursing practice with your specific population.

3. What kind of practice have you developed or could you plan to develop that might help you to grow as a caritas advanced practice nurse?

Doctoral

1. Is Watson's work a philosophy, grand theory, or middle range theory? Explain your answer.

2. How will you advance Caring Science from Watson's theoretical perspective? Describe a possible research question and sketch a design to answer it.

3. What kind of practice have you developed or could you plan to develop that might help you to grow as a caritas scholar?

IV

Seminal Research Related to Caring

ZANE ROBINSON WOLF

For decades, Dolores A. Gaut has devoted herself to the study of caring. Her dedication was evident as she promoted International Association for Human Caring (IAHC)'s caring conferences and investigations on the phenomenon of caring using human science approaches. Rather than orienting her study on caring from a philosophical perspective (Meleis, 1985), Dr. Gaut chose a philosophical method to elucidate the concept of caring. She assumed that the discipline of nursing was concerned with the caring needs of people and that caring was a value or principle for nursing action (Gaut, 1983). Through such implicit assumptions (Meleis, 1985), Gaut focused on caring nursing practice and codes of conduct for nursing.

Gaut (1983) used philosophical analysis, a form of concept analysis, to clarify the concept. She applied the elements of this qualitative, descriptive design study using techniques of semantic analysis to explain the use of the terms care/caring in ordinary language. Second-order questions or meta-questions were employed to explain the arguments and methods used by humans in speech and thought (Gaut, 1983).

Gaut (1983) conducted a search of the literature and applied semantic analysis to citations. She first examined the senses of caring derived from normal usage. Next she used "explicative analysis to refine and explain caring systematically required in the identification of a logical set of conditions necessary and sufficient to say 'S is caring for X?'" (p. 313). She then used the caring conditions to derive an action description of caring that she could justify as conceptually and theoretically adequate.

Dr. Gaut pointed out that the use of a word in scientific or scholarly literature differs from common usage. The uses of a word are comprised of a family of meanings, and literature from behavioral sciences may be vague because of behavioral scientists having to understand the meaning of the act (*of caring*) and the meaning of the interpreted action (*caring action*) (Gaut citing Kaplan, 1964).

Analysis of caring as a common word constituted the first step and revealed that caring involves a burdened state of mind and a concern for a person. Not to care indicates a lack of regard or affection. The general family of meanings for caring, cared, and cares are associated with caring in three senses as follows: (1) attention to or concern for; (2) responsibility for or providing for; and (3) regard, fondness, or attachment. These three themes structured analysis of the scholarly literature. The next step involved questions about the match of the concept of caring in scholarly versus normal usage of the word, if scholars clarified the concept of caring more precisely than common usage sense, and whether caring in nursing literature was consistently used in common and related scholarly literature (p. 315). The result was caring as giving attention to or having concern for, as responsible for or providing for; and as regard, fondness, or attachment.

Gaut (1983) next reported that caring is an action one engages in or is occupied in doing, and it is intentional in that attainment of a goal requires attention and effort (p. 318). Gaut's explicative analysis posed the conditions of caring and then refined the conditions. She collapsed five conditions (awareness, knowledge, intention, means for positive change, and the welfare-of-X criterion) into three and stated the requirements as follows:

> Any action may be described as caring, if and only if, S has identified a need for care and knows what to do for X; S chooses and implements an action intended to serve as a means for positive change in X; and the welfare-of-X criterion has been used as a nonarbitrary principle in justifying the choice and implementation of the activities as caring actions. (pp. 322–323)

The intention of the caregiver and the welfare of the other stand out as important, foundational concepts for the study and practice of nurse caring. Gaut induced an action description of caring that was conceptually and theoretically adequate.

Dr. Gaut's work has influenced that of other scholars of caring. Scholars have used the patient's need for care, action as a means for change, and the welfare of the patient as part of their orientation to the concept in nursing. In addition, the notion that nurse caring is intentional has been and continues to be debated.

Dr. Patricia J. Larson's (1984) seminal work on caring is shown through the development of the CARE-Q instrument. She framed her study in short staffing and questions about how nurse behavior has meaning for nurses. Larson's study is stellar and foundational. The study conceptualizes and operationalizes the concept of nurse caring behaviors, Larson questioned which nurse caring behaviors cancer patients' subjectively feel being cared for or were perceived as being most or least important through an instrument.

Larson (1984) framed her study in the writings of Bevis (1978), Watson (1979), Gaut (1983), and Leininger (1978). She based this study on her dissertation (Larson, 1981). She next described other measurements of caring, both nurse- and patient-oriented. Additional works cited addressed nurse behaviors denoting caring, also citing her previous development of the CARE-Q (Larson, n.d.; Larson, 1984). In this descriptive design investigation, Larson (1984) defined nurse caring behaviors as acts, conduct, and mannerisms enacted by professional nurses, which convey to the patient concern, safety, attention, and feeling cared for as a sensation of well-being and safety that is the result of enacted behaviors of another (p. 47). She assumed that the sensation of patients feeling cared for was a consequence of nurses' caring behaviors.

The CARE-Q is composed of 50 behavioral items representing six subscales as follows: accessible, explains and facilitates, comforts, anticipates, trusting relationship, and monitors and follows through. Patients sort the items. Construct validity was established by theoretical, face, and expert methods as was test–retest reliability in previous studies.

Emphasizing the intention of nurses in acting for patients and providing caring activities, Dr. Larson (1984) sampled the perceptions of hospitalized patients ($N = 57$) with cancer on caring behaviors. A Q-sort approach was used by patients as they sorted cards on 50 identified behaviors from most important to least important. Each card had a different nurse caring behavior typed on it. The Q-methodology, a technique of comparative rating, asks individuals to sort cards, called Q sorts (Burns & Grove, 2009). Patients select items printed on 3- by 5-inch cards into most important and least important categories. Patients in Larson's study were directed to sort the cards from left (most important) to right (least important) into seven pockets, with the number of cards for each pocket identified. The following were the highest ranked most important nurse caring behaviors: knows how to give shots, IVs, etc.; how to manage the equipment; and knows when to call doctor. She asserted that intended caring is not always perceived by patients as caring.

The importance of Dr. Larson's work continues to be validated by the fact that the CARE-Q items have oriented the instrument-development process of other investigators. Drs. Larson and Ferketich (1993) continued to examine the critical dimensions of nurse caring and connected caring practice and satisfaction. Larson has conscientiously studied the effect of nurses' caring on patients.

Conducting an early phenomenological study on nurse caring led Dr. Doris Johnston Rieman (1986) to address noncaring and caring in clinical settings again from the experience of patients. Dr. Rieman used phenomenological methods to enter the patients' worlds. The chapter in this section expands on findings from her dissertation, "The Essential Structure of a Caring Interaction: A Phenomenological Study" (Riemen, 1983). The method of Colaizzi (1978) directed her original study with verbal descriptions of caring and noncaring interactions with nurses provided by patients as sources of data.

Riemen (1986) compared patients' perceptions of noncaring behaviors and attitudes of nurses. As far as the elements of the noncaring interaction are concerned, the nurse's presence with the client was minimal, with the nurse physically present but emotionally distant. Significant statements were grouped as follows: being in a hurry and efficient, doing a job, being rough and belittling patients, not responding, and treating patients as objects. The nurse was just doing a job, performed using a minimal amount of energy and following rules. The client perceived the nurse who did not respond to his or her request for assistance as being noncaring (p. 34).

Rieman (1986) asserted that when asked to describe a caring and noncaring interaction with a nurse, the patients described noncaring interactions first. She explained this by speculating that patients felt humiliated, frightened, and out of control in new, strange circumstances. Patients' recollections were vivid. She noted that in clinical settings, patients perceived a lack of caring as a "lived world of noncaring interactions" (p. 31). A noncaring interaction incorporates themes of the nurse's presence, the client's response, and consequences. The noncaring interactions occur when the nurses' presence with the client is perceived as minimal with the nurse physically present but emotionally distant. The nurse is there only because it is the nurse's job and not because the client needs assistance. The nurse's response is made with a minimal amount of energy and bound by rules. The client perceives the nurse who does not respond to request for assistance as being noncaring (Riemen, 1996, p. 34). Patients are devalued and objectified as nonhuman or as children.

Riemen (1986) suggested that when a nurse is existentially *truly present* with a patient, in thought, word, and deed, the interaction would be perceived as caring by the patient and valued by both. Her work introduced the fact that sometimes patients' experiences with caring were negative and failed to value human dignity. Rather than the overwhelmingly positive literature on caring, Dr. Riemen's findings lead us to consider its antithesis. This is a serious challenge for caring scholars.

Deborah K. Mayer (1987) compared oncology nurses' and cancer patients' perceptions of nurse caring behaviors using Larson's CARE-Q in a correlational design study. She declared that investigators should relate the nurses' and patients' perceptions of nurse caring behaviors to gain insight into the foundation of the nurse–patient relationship. Furthermore, Mayer proposed that humanistic, scientific, expressive, and instrumental caring activities may comprise the construct perceptions of nurse caring.

Mayer (1987) replicated Larson's (1981) dissertation using the CARE-Q to measure the nurse caring behaviors from the most to least importance. She correlated oncology nurses' ($n = 28$) and patients' ($n = 54$) responses. Total scores on nurse rankings were related to patient rankings ($r_s = .37$, $p = < .01$), with significant agreement between the nurse and patient rankings for the following three categories of caring behaviors: explains and facilitates ($r_s = .81$, $p = .04$), trusting relationships ($r_s = .58$, $p = .01$), and monitors and follows through ($r_s = .72$, $p = .04$). The most important caring behaviors for nurses, ranked by nurses, were as follows: listens to the patients, allows the patient to express his or her feelings about his or her disease and treatment fully, and treats the information confidentially. In contrast, the patients' most important caring behaviors for nurses were as follows: knows how to give shots, IVs, and so on, and how to manage the equipment like IVs, suction machines, and so on, and is cheerful.

This study (Mayer, 1987) points out the differences between the nurse and patient perceptions regarding the caring relationship, suggesting that both involved in the caring situation or moment could perceive caring quite differently. Some of her findings supported those of Larson (1981) for nurses and patients. Mayer's investigation stands out as a replication study, early in the body of work devoted to the development of instruments that measure nurse caring.

Marilyn A. Ray (1989) has a distinguished research program. She is especially unique in her focus by virtue of her concentration on human science and the art and science of human caring in the corporate culture of the health care system. She addressed the need of executive teams to gain knowledge of the human side of nursing practice along with the business knowledge of organizations.

Dr. Ray was interested in advancing administrators' understanding of a hospital as a cultural system and clarifying the meaning of caring to hospital employees. The investigation on bureaucratic caring (Ray, 1989) was aimed at generating a theory of the dynamic structure of caring in a complex organization using a qualitative research approach. The background of the study was organized by research, culture, bureaucratic, and caring literature. Ray framed her investigation in caring as the central focus within the organizational culture. The study used ethnographic (Spradley, 1979) and grounded theory (Glaser & Strauss, 1967) research approaches to discover the meaning of caring in an acute care, urban hospital culture.

Dr. Ray (1989) interviewed informants, audio taped interviews, and used participant observation to document observations in field notes and to discern the meaning of caring to nurse and nonnurse administrators, clinical nurses, physicians, patients, and allied health personnel. Data collection was conducted in administrative and clinical phases. Rigor was established. The analysis approaches of Spradley (1979) and Glaser and Strauss (1967) were used. Themes, caring categories, definitions of clinical caring categories, and formal and substantive theories were described. The context of the hospital and the role and position of informants influenced how caring was defined and practiced in administration and on clinical units. For example, nurse executives experienced conflict between organizational goals and patient care needs (Ray, 1989, p. 35).

Political, economical, legal, technological/physiological, educational, social spiritual/religious, and ethical categories comprised the structural caring categories of clinical units. The substantive theory (Ray, 1989) induced was termed

Differential Caring; the meaning of caring was "influenced by the role and position a person had and the place within which a person worked" (p. 35) in the hospital. Ray (1989) also described a formal theory, Bureaucratic Caring, a dialectical theory built on the substantive theory. Both were present in an organizational culture. The formal theory synthesizes the thesis of caring as humanistic, social, educational, ethical, and religious/spiritual and the antithesis of caring as economic, political, legal, and technological. Bureaucratic caring is an organizational theory of caring and an important and original framework for health care organizations. It is particularly important because it is grounded in everyday hospital organizational experience. It is most likely the first formulation of such an organizational caring theory.

Agneta Cronqvist, Töres Theorell, Tom Burns, and Kim Lützén (2004) studied the experiences of moral concern in intensive care nursing using a qualitative descriptive approach. They referred to the morality of care and the increased awareness in the literature concerning complex, ethical problems in clinical practice. For example, one such problem shared by physicians and nurses in intensive care units (ICUs) is that of too much treatment. The investigators suggested that nurses may differ from physicians concerning reasoning about ethical problems, and focused on nurses' experiences of situations in ICUs that contain a moral constituent from the perspective of relational ethics or ethics of care (Cronqvist et al., 2004, p. 64). They noted that relationships are important to receivers and providers of care as well as nurses, physicians, and co-workers.

Participants worked in general, thoracic, and neonatal ICUs; ICU nurses were not satisfied with the care they provided to patients. Some of the nurses were new to the units and inexperienced. Participants provided an example of an ethical situation they experienced in the ICU; all interviews were audio taped. Qualitative content analysis proceeded through five levels of analysis. Reflections on examples of ethical situations in an ICU were organized into the following three general groups: responses that did not encompass examples of ethical situations, those that portrayed "ethics" as integrated in practice, and those that contained specific examples of the experience of ethical situations (p. 67). Two typical situations were identified, withdrawing and withholding treatment. The following five subthemes emerged: believing in a good death, knowing the course of events, feelings of distress, reasoning about physicians' "doings," and expressing moral awareness. The following main theme was formulated: caring about–caring for: moral obligations and work responsibilities in intensive care nursing.

"Caring about rests on moral grounds" and assumes that caregivers have a ". . . personal ability to know what is morally good to do in a caring situation. Caring about implies a genuine concern about the well-being of the other" (Cronqvist et al., 2004, p. 68). "Caring for is task-oriented nursing care" assigned and controlled by employers, superiors, and physicians ". . . and can be considered a moral obligation to fulfil (sic) work responsibilities." Caring for rests on organizational guidelines of practical, technical, and medical assessment (Cronqvist et al., 2004, p. 68). *Caring about* focused on genuineness, feelings, intuition, beliefs, insight, and personal values. *Caring for* focused on organization, routines, guidelines for practice, managing equipment, and environment. The investigators acknowledged the tensions nurses face in integrating caring about and caring for into nursing interventions and difficulties with balancing moral obligations and work responsibilities.

The research on nurse caring and related concepts was qualitative at the outset. However, studies began to diversify and the results generated stimulated additional scholarly work. Caring scholarship continues to use a variety of research designs and methods.

REFERENCES

Bevis, E. O. (1978). *Curriculum building in nursing.* St. Louis, MO: Mosby.

Burns, N., & Grove, S. K. (2009). *The practice of nursing research: Appraisal, synthesis, and generation of evidence* (6th ed.). St. Louis, MO: Saunders Elsevier.

Colaizzi, P. F. (1978). Psychological research as the phenomenologist views it. In R. Valle & M. King (Eds.), *Existential phenomenological alternatives for psychology.* New York, NY: Oxford University Press.

Cronqvist, A., Theorell, T., Burns, T., & Lützén, K. (2004). Caring about—caring for: Moral obligations and work responsibilities in intensive care nursing. *Nursing Ethics, 11*(1), 63–76.

Gaut, D. (1983). Development of a theoretically adequate description of caring. *Western Journal of Nursing Research, 5,* 313–324.

Glaser, G., & Strauss, A. (1967). *The discovery of grounded theory: Strategies for qualitative research.* Chicago, IL: Aldine.

Kaplan, A. (1964). *The conduct of inquiry.* San Francisco, CA: Chandler.

Larson, P. J. (1981). *Oncology patients' and professional nurses' perceptions of important nurse caring behaviors* (Master's thesis, University of California, San Francisco). Available from ProQuest Dissertations and Theses database. (AAT No. 8116511)

Larson, P. J. (1984). Important nurse caring behaviors perceived by patients with cancer. *Oncology Nursing Forum, 11*(6), 46–50.

Larson, P. J. (n.d.). *Nurse providing care to cancer patients: Perceptions of caring perceptions.* Unpublished manuscript.

Larson, P. J., & Ferketich, S. L. (1993). Patients' satisfaction with nurse caring during hospitalization. *Western Journal of Nursing Research, 15,* 690–707.

Leininger, M. M. (1978). *Transcultural nursing: Concepts, theories and practices.* New York, NY: John Wiley.

Mayer, D. K. (1987). Oncology nurses' versus cancer patients' perceptions of nurse caring behaviors: A replication study. *Oncology Nursing Forum, 14*(3), 48–52.

Meleis, A. I. (1985). *Theoretical nursing: Development & progress.* Philadelphia, PA: J. B. Lippincott.

Ray, M. A. (1989). The theory of bureaucratic caring for nursing practice in the organizational culture. *Nursing Administration Quarterly, 13*(2), 31–42.

Riemen, D. J. (1983). The essential structure of a caring interaction: A phenomenological study (Master's thesis, Texas Woman's University). Available from ProQuest Dissertations and Theses database. (AAT No. 8401214)

Riemen, D. J. (1986). Noncaring and caring in the clinical setting: Patients' descriptions. *Topics in Clinical Nursing, 8*(2), 30–36.

Spradley, J. (1979). *The ethnographic interview.* Belmont, CA: Wasworth Cengage Learning.

Watson, J. (1979). *Nursing: The philosophy and science of caring.* Boston, MA: Little, Brown.

17

Development of a Theoretically Adequate Description of Caring

DELORES A. GAUT

The concept of caring has a very special place in nursing discourse. Traditionally, nursing has been concerned with not only the caring needs of people but also with caring as a value or principle for nursing action. The interest of nurse researchers into caring phenomena has grown slowly over the last 10 years, and although there appears to be an increased use of the term *care/caring* in nursing, there has been limited interest or systematic study of the concept itself.

At a time when the nursing profession is attempting to develop a body of knowledge through research, the language used to define theoretical concepts must be precise, unambiguous, and readily communicated. This chapter discusses the beginning development of a theoretically adequate description of the concept of caring, using philosophical analysis.

Philosophical analysis is a fairly new approach to thinking about ideas and phenomena. Although the empirical researcher asks questions that require the explanation of events and causes, the philosopher asks questions that invite conceptual clarification or justification. Analysts are concerned with clarifying the arguments and methods employed by human beings in their speech and thought. Analytic strategies include the use of second-order questions (metaquestions) that require analysis of the terms themselves.

The analysis of caring reported here is the original work of the author. It began with the use of semantic analysis, which focused on the typical use of the terms care/caring in ordinary language. Using the senses of caring derived from the normal usage, the scholarly literature was surveyed to identify any extended or new senses of caring. With the senses of caring identified, the next step involved explicative analysis, wherein attempts to refine and explain caring systematically required the identification of a logical set of conditions necessary and sufficient to say, "S is caring for X."

Finally, the caring conditions were used to arrive at an action description of caring that could be justified as both conceptually and theoretically adequate. The aim of these various analytic strategies was to discover the necessary conceptual features or properties of the term *caring*.

THE USES OF CARING (EXPLICATIVE ANALYSIS)

The search for the uses of caring includes both common word usage and investigation of the literature that discusses caring in a

From Gaut, D. (1983). Development of a theoretically adequate description of caring. *Western Journal of Nursing Research*, 5, 313–324. Permission to reprint granted by Sage Publications, Inc.

scholarly or scientific manner. Common word usage is generally evaluated by nominal definitions that tell us by what combination of attributes we shall know a thing when we see it or speak of it. Once a nominal definition is established, the usage serves as a norm, and a particular utterance may be identified as a correct use or misuse of the term (Kaplan, 1964, p. 48).

However, the language of science or scholarship demands more from its terms than the usage of nominal definitions. Common language includes words that have imprecise meanings and inexactness, but in a science or a structured discipline, the technical terms must be given clear meanings if the scientific discourse is to be understood universally by members of the discipline (Feigl, 1953, p. 10).

In mapping out the uses of caring in the English language, it is important to remember the following issues:

1. Ordinary or common word usage is evaluated differently from the use of a word as a concept in scientific or scholarly literature.
2. The uses of a word do not always fit a single definition but consist of a "family of meanings." When one speaks of a family of meanings, resemblance is not a matter of some definite features common to all the members of the family, but the sharing of some features or other, enough to show the resemblance, by any two members of the family (Kaplan, 1964, p. 48).
3. In the behavioral sciences, a "fringe of vagueness" arises in the applicability of terms, and problems of clarity in language are more difficult. Such vagueness arises because data for behavioral sciences are not easily verifiable, but are actions performed in a perspective that gives them meaning or purpose. The behavioral scientist has two different things to understand—the meaning of the act itself and the meaning of the interpreted action (Kaplan, 1964, p. 23).

Keeping these issues in mind, the process was not limited to a search for any one definition that would fit all examples, but rather included a search for the many different senses the term may have acquired over time.

CARING AS A COMMON WORD

"Caring" as a word comes from the Old English and Gothic words, *carian* and *kara* or *karon*. As a noun, care derives from *kara*, meaning grief, lament, or sorrow, or bed of sickness. The earliest uses of the word (c.1000) included charging of the mind with concern, heed, or attention as in "attend to this matter with due care." With the later addition of the preposition "for," the sense of attending changed to one of "regard arising from desire or liking for."

Around 1400, care was used to indicate a sense of protection for, as prevails today in statements such as, "he is in the care of a nurse," or "I'll take her under my care." This sense of the word has become obsolete, but usage to indicate a burdened state of mind still applies.

As a verb, "cared, caring, cares" (*carian*) means having concern for, or to feel interest in; to provide for or look after; to have an inclination or liking or regard and thus be inclined or disposed to; and to have regard for in the sense of fondness or attachment for.

In the negative sense, "not to care" gives the notion of disregard, inattention, or indifference. It might even imply apathy or lack of motivation as in "He doesn't care enough to do that." In another sense, "she doesn't care for you" carries with it a lack of regard or affection.

These statements spell out some general rules regarding the correct use of care/caring as a common word in the English language. Obviously, care/caring has more than one sense, and qualifying or descriptive words must be used to clarify in what sense the speaker is using the word. "Caring for" might be used in the sense of concern or responsibility: It might also indicate a regard or fondness or attachment for a person. The statement "take care" is frequently heard and generally means to take thought of or to provide and look after, whereas "I don't care if I do" implies an inclination or disposition.

Although there is no clear-cut rule for the use of caring, the general family of meanings is all related to the notion of caring in three senses:

1. Attention to or concern for
2. Responsibility for or providing for
3. Regard, fondness, or attachment

With an understanding of the sense of caring in common usage, the next step is to examine caring in selected scholarly writings. When used as a noun, the word "care" has a number of referents. For example, care is love, care is concern, and care is understanding. When used in the grammatical form as a participle, caring denotes doing or action. The following discussion includes consideration of both care and caring.

SCHOLARLY CONCEPTIONS

The search of the scholarly literature was guided by three questions posed by this researcher:

1. Are the statements about the concept of caring in the scholarly literature contemporaneous with the normal usage of the word?
2. Have the scholars clarified and rendered the concept of caring more precise than the common usage senses?
3. Is the use of caring found in the nursing literature contemporaneous with the common word usage and the related scholarly literature?

Review of selected writings from philosophers, behavioral scientists, and nurses highlighted three points:

1. The importance of the notion of caring as evidenced by the increasing frequency of the use of the concept

2. The evolution of the concept of caring as related to some other concept or concepts
3. The discussion of activities such as feeding, touching, and talking to, which when grouped together constituted caring actions

Care as Giving Attention to or Having Concern For

May (1969) and Maslow (1975) and others spoke of care as a biological phenomenon requiring a conscious psychological awareness of caring as a fact. A human's need for care demands caring actions on the part of that person or some other person. The lack of such care is expressed by pain and illness. Caring, in the sense of feeling concern for, is the essence of a helping relationship, according to Travelbee (1966), Jourard (1971), and Rogers (1965). Concern for another person is, according to Maslow and Erikson, an essential aspect of a love relationship for another (Erikson, 1968; Maslow, 1975).

Caring as Responsible For or Providing For

Freud (1966), Gaylin (1976), and Sullivan (1953) spoke of caring as necessary for survival of the species. In pre-1960 nursing literature, caring for patients involved providing food, rest, cleanliness, and other like activities. "Giving care" was the doing of activities, or providing for needs, when patients could not provide for themselves. Caring was a one-way relationship in which the nurse provided for the needs of the patient.

Caring as Regard, Fondness, or Attachment

Discussions of caring in helping relationships by Rogers (1965), Truax (1963), and others influenced the writings of nurses such as Orlando (1961), Peplau (1963), and Travelbee (1966). Kreuter-Reiter (1957), one of the few authors discussing care/caring as a term, spoke of caring as an attitude or disposition, prompting nursing action to provide for needs. Paterson and Zderad (1976) wrote of caring as a transactional relationship for nursing, thus changing the notion of caring from a one-way relationship—nurse providing for patient—to the notion of caring as reciprocal involvement of nurse with patient.

This summarized review of the scholarly literature provides some evidence that the statements about caring in the scholarly literature appear contemporaneous with the common word usage. One exception is the work of Mayeroff (1965, 1971) wherein he expanded the notion of caring as "helping the other to grow." However, he did not concern himself with any one instance of caring or with the short-term caring relationship. Rather, he identified ingredients essential in a long-term caring relationship—devotion, permanence, patience, trust, humility, and hope. Leininger (1978) developed a taxonomic model of caring that identified 27 caring constructs including helping, touching, nurturance, protection, support, and trust.

Caring, whether used in common word usage or scholarly literature, seems to involve at least three senses: (1) disposition or feeling within the career, (2) the doing of certain activities regarded as caring activities, or (3) a combination of both attitude and action in which the caring about the other (as a value, or responsibility, or commitment) disposes the person to care for another through the doing of certain activities.

"Caring for" in the sense of providing for, or being responsible for, can be discussed apart from any sense of "caring about"; however, "caring about" the other (in the sense of a valued other) brings a quality to the relationship between the carer and the cared for. "Caring about" eliminates the apathy, indifference, obligation, withdrawal, isolation, manipulation, and possession in one-way relationships of "caring for" in the limited sense of "providing for."

As a word, or a concept, caring does not have one determinate definition and a singular meaning in all contexts of application; rather caring has a family of meanings or an indeterminate definition in which its meaning shifts across contexts. It is a word that could be considered both vague and ambiguous.

The review of nursing and other scholarly literature verified the assumption that "caring," although a frequently used term, lacks the clarity and preciseness essential to scientific endeavors. The task of the research was to arrive at a description of caring, through explication, that was both theoretically and conceptually adequate.

THEORETICAL DESCRIPTION OF CARING

A theoretically adequate description of any concept requires not only clarification of the constituents of the concept that can generate or derive any instance of the concept but also must speak of the relationship between the constituents. The description also must meet certain tests of adequacy based on nonarbitrary criteria and must include justification for accepting the description (Kerr & Soltis, 1974).

CARING COMPONENTS

Concern with the concept of caring in nursing required full attention to caring as a purposeful, human activity requiring an action description rather than a behavioral description. Thus the question, "What must be true to say that S is caring for X?" provides the framework for the logical conditions that must be met to call any action a caring action.

The necessity for consideration of caring as a practical activity relates specifically to the task of discussing caring as an activity or activities within the practice of nursing. But the discussion of "what nurses do when they care" will not be limited to discussing caring as a set of activities such as biophysical operations, movements, or events, but rather will include a discussion of caring as a set of actions that includes the perspectives of the actors, expressing certain attitudes, and expectations, thereby having a certain social and psychological significance (Kaplan, 1964).

One way to identify the conditions necessary for any caring action would be to watch someone engaged in activities recognizable as caring and then list those actions in such a way that they serve as the standards or criteria for future definitions of caring. But a stipulated list of behaviors is usually nothing more than an arbitrary set of standards that could not be justified on rational grounds.

In analyzing a practical activity like caring, the aim is not to invent some new concept or idea of caring nor even to specify what people ought to mean by caring. The objective is rather to clarify and more thoroughly understand the idea of caring that already exists in ordinary usage. The normal usage of a word then serves as one nonarbitrary criterion for the development of conditions necessary to use the word caring.

Caring as a verb denotes doing or action, but the term itself does not specify exactly what kinds of doings or actions are required to be called caring. Caring is also context dependent. Whether certain actions will count as caring is dependent on what the action is, the intention of the doer, and the context in which it is done. In one sense, we could talk about caring as an enterprise in which a person may be engaged in many activities over time. For example, "Jane is caring for Jimmy today." It is an all-day enterprise that may be broken down into many more specific activities. The word caring (as enterprise) is functioning at a general level, but if one looked at all the detailed activities of that enterprise, a variety of activities would be observed; cooking, shopping, washing, cleaning, talking, singing, and feeding. Any one of the activities may be a caring activity in a specific sense, as well as be a part of a series of activities considered

as an enterprise of caring in general. In either the specific or the general sense of enterprise, one could say that certain activities are or are not caring actions. The question of importance again becomes, how can the activity of caring be distinguished from all other activities, or "what must be true to say that S is caring for X?"

Intentional Caring

To treat caring as a verb puts the focus on its action sense and sets aside certain other senses of caring such as "care and sorrow" and to some extent caring as a virtue or quality. This analysis of caring seeks to distinguish among actions—that is, S doing something for X that may be described as caring or noncaring, rather than to distinguish among all senses of caring.

In this analysis, caring was considered as an action one engages in or is occupied in doing, and as such the action is directed toward a goal. Caring was addressed in its intentional rather than its success sense, that is, the attainment of a goal requires attention and effort, and, in the intentional sense, caring deals with the "trying to reach a goal."

CONDITIONS OF CARING (EXPLICATIVE ANALYSIS)

In answering the question, "What must be true to say that S is caring for X?," the following conditions were identified by this researcher as both necessary and sufficient to speak of S caring or not caring for X. These conditions are the result of concept explication wherein the conditions identified are put through necessary and sufficiency testing.

> First condition: S must be aware, either directly or indirectly of the need for care in X.

> Second condition: S must know that certain things could be done to improve the situation.

Third condition: S must intend to do something for X.

Fourth condition: S must choose an action intended to serve as a means for bringing about a positive change in X and then implant that action.

Fifth condition: The positive change in X must be judged on the basis of what is good for X rather than S or some other Y or Z.

To the end of refining the analysis even more the following questions were addressed:

1. In what sense must S be aware of X to care for X?
2. What must S know to care for X?
3. What is the relationship between the intended action and the need for care?
4. What could count as a positive change of direction for X?

REFINEMENT OF THE CARING CONDITIONS

In what sense must S be aware of X to care for X?

Awareness

The awareness required would seem to be in the sense of a conscious focusing of attention on a person, including self, as well as a basic recognition of what X is as something separate and distinguishable from self. Through this, S experiences the other to be cared for as an extension of self, and at the same time as something separate from self. The notion of attending to calls for the ability to concentrate, that is, focus one's senses on an object "out there." Clearly, then, the ability to attend to an object as discrete from oneself is necessary as a part of the first condition of caring. But the ability to attend to an "other" as a discrete object and attending to an "other" as similar in personhood are quite different abilities. Mayeroff called

this ability as "identity-in-difference" (Mayeroff, 1965, p. 463):

> In caring, we experience the other person as other, as apart from us, and at the same time as also one with us. . . . The word "experience" is used rather than "see" to emphasize that caring is an activity that involves the whole person and not simply a part, whether the part be mind or body, sense or reason.

For S to be able to care for X, S must be able to "attend to" or focus attention on another person. In addition, an attitude of respect must prevail as an essential condition for all rational action between persons.

Caring as Respect for Persons

In the following discussion, I will consider reasons why respect for self and others is a necessary condition for all rational action, especially caring. Although I will be speaking of regard or respect for the other, I do not mean to eliminate the possibility of attachment or affection, but rather consider the attitude of respect as a fundamental attitude necessary for caring relationships that may lead to attachment or affection.

The conceptualization of the importance of a person does not just happen in life experiences but derives from the value of "person" in a society and among individuals one seriously encounters. The concept of being a person is derivative from the value society places on individual points of view (Peters, 1961). People then think of themselves as persons, valued for their decisions and choices and determiners of their destiny. Persons grow in the conscious awareness of their agency in shaping events.

This consciousness reaches its peak in the experience of entering into and sustaining a personal relationship based on reciprocal agreement, because the relationship derives from personal appraisal and choice (Peters, 1961, p. 134).

A person is free to judge and choose, make individual assertion and actions, and as an individual, be held responsible for the consequences of those assertions or actions. At the same time, two general principles safeguard personhood: (1) not being arbitrarily interfered with in respect of the execution of our wants and decisions and (2) not having our claims and interests ignored or treated in a partial or prejudiced manner (Peters, 1965, p. 136).

The concept of respect for persons is a principle or norm for action that also must include respect for that person's actions, decisions, values, and claims. It would seem that respect is essential to the first condition of awareness when speaking of one person caring for self or another. But what is meant when we use the word respect, and how does the attitude of respect relate to the necessary condition of awareness?

Respect

The etymology of the word suggests a "looking back at or taking into account" (with respect to) as well as "to regard or treat with consideration or deference" (respect for).

The claim that all human beings have certain rights that can never be forfeited or retracted underlies the respect as consideration (*observantia*) concept.

> *Observantia:* . . . This sense of respect evolved from the very earliest notion of the powerful as deserving of respect to respectful consideration for all human beings regardless of age, sex, social status, or wealth. To see a person as having dignity, is to respect that person's moral position, to make claims against other person's conduct . . . .
>
> Certain minimal forms of consideration are due all human beings, even when they are in no position to make demands. This new attitude is the perception of an object with a legitimatized moral power over us with the ability to make demands not through force, but through claims backed up by reasons . . . .
>
> Insofar as we think of others that way, we have respect for them, and insofar as they share this image, they have self-respect. (Feinberg, 1973, p. 2)

To think of persons as having human dignity is to think of them in a position to make a claim to our services as rightfully due. To think of them as competent claimants is to respect them as persons. To respect all human beings equally, then, is to grant them the respect required for decency or practical reason. Respect or regard for another person is an attitude necessary for rational humans to be induced to act on principles, and "respect for persons" is a principle for the justification of actions of reasonable people in dealing with each other (Peters, 1961, p. 137).

The notion of "respect for persons" is crucial to the discussion of caring, for it entails an attitude necessary in the carer. Respect for other persons begins with respect for one self. Awareness of "personhood" must include not only a basic recognition of who one is but also an awareness of other human beings as persons worthy of respect in their own right.

The first condition of awareness or conscious focusing of attention on a person may not be all that is required when speaking of caring for a person. The interpretation of what one is seeing, or hearing, or feeling in relation to another person requires more than awareness.

Consider for example, the man who, after hearing of the plight of the starving people of Bangladesh, sends a cash donation to the CARE food fund established for relief aid for the country. He appears to have an awareness of persons in need (he perhaps has experienced hunger) and he respects the rights of persons to have the basic things in life and is motivated to send money to buy food. The ability to identify the needs of another involved more than just being aware that people were starving. "Need identification" also involved interpreting and then choosing actions. This brings me to the second condition of caring: S must not only be aware of X but also must know that something could be done for X to improve the situation. The question to be considered at this point is: "What exactly must S know to be caring for X?"

Knowledge

The ability of S to identify the needs of X involves more than just awareness; it also involves various kinds of knowing. To consider S caring for X requires that S not only be aware of X, and have knowledge about X to identify a need for care, but also once a need is identified, to know what to do about it. In addition, S must respect X as a person with rights, values, and choices.

An informed awareness of X as a person would involve perceiving that person, identifying a need for care (the man with two broken arms is unable to feed himself), respecting that person's desires given the reasonableness of the situation (the man would prefer to have his wife feed him), and then making a choice about what to do. S could choose to feed the man his dinner, rather than hold the food in the warmer until his wife came, in which case S is acting upon X rather than with X. In the case of S caring for a person without the element or attitude of respect, S acts upon X, just as S acts upon an object, and such actions would be questionable caring.

I would combine the first and second conditions to include awareness within the knowledge condition. To know or have knowledge of in the most general sense includes the notions of awareness, understanding, and being cognizant of. The sense of awareness required for caring includes knowing something about the object to enable S to identify a need for care. *S must have knowledge about X to identify a need for care and know that certain things could be done to improve the situation.*

Caring activity begins with the identification of a need for care. The consideration of need as something required or desired that is lacking permits me to speak in general of the needs of X whether X is an object or a person. But if one wishes to speak of X caring for X, it is not enough to say that S has identified a need for care and knows what to do, S must also choose to do something. The question then becomes, "What is the relationship between the intended action and the need for care?"

To be caring, S must not only choose an action to meet a need for care in X, but must also intend the action as a means for bringing about a positive change in X, S must implement the action chosen. It is at the stage of implementation that one might ask S, "What are you doing?" (purpose or aim of activity) and "Why are you doing that?" (justification of activity). With these considerations in mind, conditions 3 and 4 were combined into one, primarily to emphasize the relationship among the intention, action, and need constituents: *S must choose and implement an action intended to serve as a means for bringing about a positive change in X.*

But the question remains, "What could count as a positive change for X?" Could the positive change be based on what S might consider as good? Or could the positive change be based on what S knows to be good for other objects like Y and Z? To determine what might count as a positive change for X, I will first address the notion of the need for care in X, and from this discussion I will attempt to identify nonarbitrary criteria of the validation of what might count as positive change.

Positive Change Condition

The awareness/knowledge condition of caring involves identification of a need for care, that is, the identification of "a lack of something required or desired" in X. The consideration of need related to a lack entails the possibility of a change (from lack to no lack) whether it be called growth or maturation, fulfillment, movement, or any of the other terms used to designate some kind of positive alteration or progression.

When one considers change, synonyms such as variation, alteration, and modification come to mind. Change may also be considered a state in which phenomena are guided or move toward certain actualities. This usage indicates direction, and in this sense, positive change or growth indicates forward movement, while lack of movement or backward movement carries a negative connotation, the statement, "S must intend the doing as a means for bringing about a positive change in X, implies first that S must have a purpose or plan for the activity, and second that the plan be chosen to bring about a positive change in X." The planned doings will assist X in maintaining or growing in a positive direction. I do not mean to insist on a 1:1 relationship, that is, for every action considered to be caring, there must be a positive change response. However, what is required is that S intends the action chosen as a means for a positive change, or at the very least, S must not intend harmful or injurious actions.

Although the identification of a needful state in X is a necessary condition for caring, the possibility of the identification of the need for care implies that some standards or criteria exist that permit S to observe, "X needs something." The notion of change as positive or negative also suggests criteria or norms by which one might say, "that is good for X," or "what I intend to do will bring about a positive change in X" and is essential to the final discussion of nonarbitrary criteria for the judgment of positive change.

Welfare-of-X Criterion

To determine what would count as a positive change for X, one must be generally informed about criteria according to which something would be accepted as good for all X's distinguished from Y's or Z's.

One other distinction needs to be made. That is the distinction of what is good for this particular X, in this specific situation. The judgment of the intended action as a means for bringing about a positive change must be based on not only what is good for X rather than Y or Z but also what is good for X in a particular situation.

The welfare-of-X consideration then becomes a nonarbitrary criterion that serves as a norm, standard, or principle for any intended or implemented activity as "means for positive change in X." The positive change would be judged solely on the criteria identified as good for the welfare-of-X, thus excluding actions based on the whim, or wishes of S, or some other agent. With these considerations of positive change and the welfare-of-X criterion, I revised the last condition to read: *The positive change condition must be judged solely on the basis of a "welfare-of-X" criterion.*

SUMMARY

The task of this analysis has been the consideration of caring as a practical activity and the identification of conditions both necessary and sufficient for the employment of the term "caring." In an attempt to answer the question, "What must be true to say that S is caring for X?," five conditions were specified: awareness, knowledge, intention, means for positive change, and the welfare-of-X criterion. The conditions have been collapsed into three:

> Condition 1: S must have knowledge about X to identify a need for care and must know that certain things could be done to improve the situation.
>
> Condition 2: S must choose and implement an action based on that knowledge and intend the action as a means for bringing about a positive change in X.

Condition 3: The positive change condition must be judged solely on the basis of a "welfare-of-X" criterion.

To state these requirements in another way, any action may be described as caring if and only if S has identified a need for care and knows what to do for X; S chooses and implements an action intended to serve as a means for positive change in X; and the welfare-of-X criterion has been used as a nonarbitrary principles in justifying the choice and implementation of the activities as caring actions. There is a set of necessary relationships among the conditions. First, the intention or purpose of the chosen activity must be related to the need for care, and second, it must be a means for bringing about a positive change directly related to the need for care. The justification of the action is then based on the nonarbitrary criterion: welfare-of-X.

This description of caring may be justified as theoretically adequate based on the following criteria:

1. Clarification of the components of the concept is based on normal usage criteria.
2. A formal, logical approach was utilized in the consideration of the components.
3. The relationship between the components is addressed.

The usefulness of such a description of caring evolves from the necessary conceptualization process of refining abstract ideas for scientific research and specifically for nursing into caring. At a time when the nursing profession is attempting to develop its own body of knowledge as an academic and research discipline, it becomes imperative that the language used to define concepts be precise, unambiguous, readily communicated, and justifiable. If the research is ambiguous about the concepts being studied, the development of an objective, reliable method to observe or measure the phenomena is almost impossible.

In addition, this chapter attempted to show that along with empirical questions that most often receive the attention of nurse researchers, there are other kinds of questions and problems that require consideration if we are to understand the enterprise of nursing. The analysis of concepts is a coherent, logical technique, which can be applied over a wide field. Because philosophy is an analysis of language, rather than of facts, it provides a framework and purposiveness to thinking about general questions and abstract concepts.

Further development of this caring description entails utilizing the identified caring conditions as the action categories. The purpose of such activity would be the formulation of a systematic theoretical construction to which one can appeal to answer questions about how one improves research and the teaching of a practical activity such as caring.

REFERENCES

Erikson, E. (1968). *Identity, youth, and crisis.* New York, NY: W. W. Norton.

Feigl, H. (1953). The scientific outlook: Naturalism and humanism. In H. Feigl (Ed.), *Readings in the philosophy of science.* New York, NY: Appleton-Century Crofts.

Feinberg, J. (1973). Some conjectures about the concept of respect. *Journal of Social Philosophy, 4,* 1–3.

Freud, S. (1966). *Inhibitions, symptoms, anxiety.* London: Hogarth Press. (Original work published 1926.)

Gaylin, W. (1976). *Caring.* New York, NY: Knopf.

Jourard, S. (1971). *The transparent self.* New York, NY: Van Nostrand.

Kaplan, G. (1964). *The conduct of inquiry.* Pennsylvania: Chandler Co.

Kerr, D., & J. F. Soltis. (1974). Locating teacher competency: An action description of caring. *Educational Theory, 24*(1 Winter), 3–16.

Kreuter-Reiter, F. (1957). What is good nursing care? *Nursing Outlook, 5,* 302–304.

Leininger, M. (1978). The phenomena of caring. In *Caring: An essential human need.* New Jersey: C. B. Slack.

Maslow, A. (1975). Love in healthy people. In A. Montagu (Ed.), *The practice of love*. New Jersey: Prentice Hall.

May, R. (1969). *Love and will*. New York, NY: Norton.

Mayeroff, M. (1965). On caring. *International Philosophical Quarterly*, 5, 463–466.

Mayeroff, M. (1971). *Caring*. New York, NY: Harper and Row.

Orlando, J. (1961). *The dynamic nurse patient relationship*. New York, NY: G. P. Putnam and Sons.

Paterson, J., & Zderad, L. (1976). *Humanistic nursing*. New York, NY: Wiley and Sons.

Peplau, H. (1963). Interpersonal relations and the process of adaptation. *Nursing Science, 1*, 272–279.

Peters, R. S. (1961). Respect for persons and fraternity. In R. Peters (Ed.), *Ethics and education* (pp. 133–137). Palo Alto, CA: Scott and Foresman.

Peters, R. S. (1965). *Ethics and education*. London: Allen and Unwin.

Rogers, C. (1965). The therapeutic relationship: Recent theory and research. *Australian Journal of Psychology, 17*(2), 96–99.

Sullivan, H. S. (1953). *The interpersonal theory of psychiatry*. New York, NY: Norton.

Travelbee, J. (1966). *Interpersonal aspects of nursing*. Philadelphia, PA: F. A. Davis.

Truax, C. (1963). Effective ingredients in psychotherapy. *Journal of Counseling Psychology, 10*, 256–263.

QUESTIONS FOR REFLECTION

Baccalaureate

1. What does Gaut (1983) mean by the process of semantic analysis, as she began to develop the theoretical description of caring?
2. What are the *general family of meanings* about caring that Gaut (1983) described?
3. What are the differences between the common use of caring as a work and the scholarly use of caring as a word?

Master's

1. What did you learn about the process of explicative analysis? Describe the process.
2. How can you apply the component of *caring as regard, fondness, or attachment* to the care of patients in your everyday nursing work?
3. What did you like or dislike about the process Gaut (1983) used to arrive at a theoretically adequate description of caring?

Doctoral

1. How do you explain the steps of the process of philosophical analysis used by Gaut (1983)? List the steps she used to describe a theoretically adequate description of caring.
2. What would you like to learn about how Gaut's (1983) development of the theoretically adequate description of caring influenced caring theorists' work?
3. How would you explain the necessary and sufficient caring conditions to nurse colleagues at your workplace?

18

Important Nurse Caring Behaviors Perceived by Patients With Cancer

Patricia J. Larson

Caring is the essence, the very core of nursing, and is considered to be its distinguishing characteristic.[1-4] Leininger,[5] a major proponent of caring as the central focus of nursing, states, "Caring is one of the most crucial and essential ingredients for health, human development, human relatedness, well-being and survival."

Scientifically based knowledge of caring is limited, and nurses cannot be certain that their behavior consistently creates in patients a sense of "feeling cared for." From a practical perspective, the present era of short staffing, multiple tasks, and efficiency require that nurses behave in ways that have the most meaning for patients. Nurses, when asked to identify the important aspects of caring, have consistently ranked the affective aspects, such as listening, touching, and talking, as the most important ones.[6-8] We need to ask ourselves, do patients hold similar perceptions? A woman hospitalized for a second induction of therapy for leukemia was asked, "What makes you feel cared for?" She said, "Without a doubt, it is what the nurse says to me. However, the nurse must first prove to me that she knows how to manage my meds and treatments. Until then, I'm not too interested in what she has to say." It appears that a critical first step in addressing the concept of caring, as it relates to nursing, is to understand patients' perceptions of the most important nurse caring behaviors.

PURPOSE

The purpose of this study was to determine which nurse caring behaviors are perceived by patients as being most important or least important, those caring behaviors that most clearly convey to the patient a subjective feeling of being cared for, as identified by hospitalized cancer patients. Cancer patients were selected as the target population because they constitute a group of "experienced" patients, and because of their frequent contact with professional nurses, they might be better able to formulate their perceptions of the nurse behaviors that constitute caring.

BACKGROUND

Caring, a critical factor in the nurse–patient relationship, has been approached from various perspectives. Four major models for examining the phenomena of the caring process exist. Bevis' early conceptualization proposes four sequential stages (attachment, assiduity, intimacy, and confirmation) of a caring process applicable to the nurse–patient relationship. In her interpretation, Bevis notes that

From Larson, P. J. (1984). Important nurse caring behaviors perceived by patients with cancer. *Oncology Nursing Forum, 11*(6), 46–50. Permission to reprint granted by the Oncology Nursing Society.

each caring relationship is unique and the full development will require each participant, nurse, and patient to reciprocate in each activity at each stage.[1]

Watson views caring as the science of nursing derived from the integration of concepts from the humanities and the biophysical and behavioral sciences. She uses 10 factors that blend the philosophy of caring as an art into a science that can be enacted in practice.[3] For example, to implement the eighth "carative" factor (provision for a supportive, protective and/or corrective mental, physical, sociocultural, and spiritual environment), the nurse is required to assess and plan nursing care related to the internal and external variables affecting the patient's life and well-being.

In contrast, Gaut uses a philosophical analysis and proposes five essential conditions necessary for the study and subsequent practical application of the caring concept in nursing.[4] The testing of any of these conceptualizations has not been reported.

Leininger, whose work regarding care extends over many years, has identified more than 25 major caring constructs based on her transcultural and ethnoscientific study of the concept.[9] She and others have examined the constructs of support, health maintenance, and succor.[10–12]

Although these models provide an arena for a dialogue about caring, they are limited in that none define caring at the behavioral level. Leininger contends that until the professional dimensions of caring, the cognitive goals, processes, and acts are adequately researched and refined, caring will remain a nebulous term, open to various interpretations.[2]

Nursing Studies of Caring

The studies regarding caring have examined nurse behaviors that denote caring and that identify the caring behaviors most important to those who were being cared for. Ford surveyed professional nurses' descriptions of caring, nurse behaviors associated with caring, and examples of how nurses model caring. Nurses ($N = 81$) in that study defined caring primarily as having genuine concern for the well-being of another and a giving of oneself. Listening was identified as the behavior most representative of their caring and was the behavior used during role modeling of caring for others.[8]

Larson devised the Caring Assessment Instrument (CARE-Q) from two samples of professional nurses who provided care to hospitalized patients with cancer, to understand important nurse caring behaviors. The nurses in both studies ($N = 57$ and 112) identified listening, touching, allowing expression of feelings, individualizing care, talking, and including the patient in planning the care as the most important nursing behaviors that make patients feel cared for.[6,7]

Caring as a fundamental component of nursing was explored by Henry in a study of home care patients ($N = 50$). Using open-ended interview questions, she obtained patients' perceptions of what nurses do that indicates caring. Doing "extra things" (bringing flowers, getting food stamps, and finding transportation to the doctor) were the most frequent responses to the question about what the nurse does or says that made these patients feel the nurse cared. The next most frequent responses were "showing interest in the patient," "enacting skills" (taking blood pressure, giving shots), or showing patience toward the patient. Other responses were "being friendly," "listening," and "being gentle."[13]

Brown obtained hospitalized patients' ($N = 80$) perceptions of nurse behaviors that pointed toward two dimensions of care, that is, nursing tasks and effective caring. The dimension of task encompassed surveillance, availability, demonstrating professional knowledge, providing information, and supporting individuality. The affective dimension addressed the personal and professional qualities of the nurse.[14]

Perceptions of caring, based on the results of these studies, appear to be somewhat influenced by the setting in which the nurse–patient interactions occur and whether one is the enactor or the recipient of care. The professional nurses in the Ford and Larson studies perceived the affective behaviors (listening, touching, and individualizing care) as the most important dimensions of nurse caring behaviors.[6-8] Henry's home care patients perceived the nurses as caring when they did things beyond what was part of their assigned role.[13] The hospitalized patients in the Brown study saw care demonstrated by' the nurse's accessibility and professional competency.[14] These studies would indicate disagreement between professional nurses' perceptions of caring and patients' perceptions of caring and may be due to variations in sample, design, etc., or may indicate that perceptions of caring are indeed not congruent between caregiver and care recipient. Further research in this area could more fully illuminate this lack of agreement. Nonetheless, these studies indicate that a major expectation of nursing care calls for the patient "to feel cared for" as the result of nursing actions.

THE INTENT OF NURSING

Professional nursing practice incorporates the dimensions of care, cure, and coordination.[15] Caring, as conceptualized for this study, is the core of the care dimension, permeating the activities and intent of nurses even when they are engaged in the cure or coordination roles. This conceptualization is in accord with ANA *Social Policy Statement*: "Nurses are guided by a humanistic philosophy having caring coupled with understanding and purpose as its central feature."[16] The basic premise appears to be that no matter what the nurse's role, caring is an expected part of any and all nurse–patient interactions; individual patients have the right to expect that they will feel cared for.

Because of the nature of their disease and the ensuing treatments, patients with cancer have frequent contact with nurses. Nursing often becomes a major dimension in their lives, starting with the diagnostic work-up and continuing through the terminal phase of the illness. The nursing a patient with cancer experiences is generally provided by many nurses, in various settings, over a period ranging from months to years. Thus, the nursing experienced by one patient is collective in the sense that no one nurse totally represents the full care that is given to the patient over time.

In an earlier study of patients with cancer, Larson[7] found that they feel cared for as the result of nursing actions during the courses of care. Therefore, it was of interest to know which of the enacted nurse caring behaviors are seen as the most important in making patients feel cared for. The question addressed was: Which nurse caring behaviors are perceived by hospitalized patients who have cancer as being most important in making them feel cared for?

Definition of Terms and Assumption

The operational definitions of key terms used in this study were as follows: (1) nurse caring behaviors—the acts, conduct, and mannerisms enacted by professional nurses that convey to the patient concern, safety, and attention; (2) feeling cared for—the sensation of well-being and safety that is the result of enacted behaviors of another. The assumption that underlies the study was that the sensation in patients of "feeling cared for" results from nurses' caring behaviors.

METHODS

Patients and Setting

Fifty-seven adult patients with a histological diagnosis of cancer hospitalized for treatment were designated the convenience sample. All patients were informed of the purpose of the study and were assured that responses would be treated confidentially. All patients signed consent forms before participating.

The patients were chosen from three acute care hospitals in two western states; two were community hospitals and the third was a large teaching and research hospital. The patients were cared for on several nursing units, including each hospital's cancer treatment ward. Two nursing care approaches, team and primary (or modified primary), were used in the three hospitals. The settings were fairly similar: All units provided comprehensive care and treatment for hospitalized patients. Some, but not all, of these patients participated in clinical trial protocols under the auspices of three national cancer study groups.

There were also differences among the three settings. Patients hospitalized in the teaching and research hospital were primarily from large metropolitan areas. One of the community hospitals had patients who were mainly from rural areas. The patients in the third hospital were from an urban area.

Instrument

The CARE-Q, which was used to obtain the patients' perceptions of important nurse caring behavior, consists of 50 behavioral items ordered in 6 subscales of caring and ranked by importance that measures patient and nurse perceptions of nurse caring behaviors. The subscales include the following: I, accessible (6 items); II, explains and facilitates (6 items); III, comforts (9 items); IV, anticipates (5 items); V, trusting relationship (16 items); and VI, monitors and follows through (8 items).[17] The individual CARE-Q behavioral items are sorted by the patients. The scales, derived from a preliminary study with patients, provide theoretical categorizations of the CARE-Q behavioral items.

Face and content validity of the instrument were established by carefully identifying and developing the behavioral items from the perspective of both nurse and patient in two earlier studies conducted by the author. A panel of patients and a panel of nurses verified the items' representativeness of the caring behaviors of nursing. Reliability was initially tested in a small ($N = 10$) test–retest study, resulting in an r of 1.00 for one most important and one least important item. A second, recently completed test–retest study with 82 registered nurse members randomly selected from the membership roster of the Oncology Nursing Society showed the item-ranking consistency for the most important (the top 5) items to be 79.1% between Tests I and II. For the least important (the bottom 5) items, the consistency ranking was 63.4%.[7] Construct validity, due to the lack of similar instruments, has not been established.

PROCEDURES

The CARE-Q instrument examines cancer patients' perceptions of nurse caring behaviors by ranked importance. The CARE-Q format accommodates the ranking of the 50 identified behaviors from most important to least important and uses the Q methodology as designated by Stephenson.[18] The Q technique calls for individuals to sort cards, each of which contains a statement relevant to the study. The cards are called Q sorts.

The Q methodology enables identification of the most important nurse caring behavior as the measure of priority. The forced-choice distribution selected for this study required participants to select a predetermined number of items (each item printed on a 3" × 5" card) in each of the most important to the least important categories. The CARE-Q instrument follows the quasi-normal distribution in identifying one most important item and one least important item, four next most important and four next least important items, ten most important and ten less important items, and twenty behavioral items that are neither important nor unimportant. The items are placed into the designated classification by the participant.

The purpose of the Nurse Caring Behavior Study is to identify the nurse caring behaviors perceived as important in making patients feel cared for.

The Caring Assessment Report Evaluation Q-Sort (CARE-Q) packet contains seven pockets, each labeled with a number (1, 4, 10, 20, 10, 4, 1) and a deck of 50 cards, each with a different nurse caring behavior typed on it.

To identify the nurse caring behaviors perceived as most important, sort the deck of 50 cards from most important to least important by placing each card into one of the pockets—from most important to least important.

You can place one card in the pocket showing the number 1, four cards in the pocket showing 4, etc. Please count the number of cards in each pocket to make sure that the number is right.

Below is an example of how to place the pockets to aid in the sorting. They are placed from left to right.

1	4	10	20	10	4	1
Most Important	Fairly Important	Somewhat Important	Neither Important nor Unimportant	Somewhat Unimportant	Unimportant	Not Important

FIGURE 18.1

CARE-Q format and sorting directions.

The seven classifications are represented by seven appropriately labeled library cards. Figure 18.1 shows the application of the CARE-Q.

The demographic data and the CARE-Q sort of each participant were numerically coded for statistical analysis. The one most important item was coded 7. The four next most important items were coded 6, and the 10 items identified as being also important were coded 5. The 20 middle items were coded 4. The 10 items perceived as being less important were coded 3. The four items identified as being next to least important were coded 2, and the least important item was coded 1. The coded items were also categorized into the caring scale they represented.

TABLE 18.1 Background of Patients Participating in Study of Perceptions (*N* = 57)

Variable	Number	Percent
Cancer type		
Solid tumor	51	89.0
Leukemia	6	11.0
Gender		
Male	19	33.5
Female	38	66.5
Work status		
Full time	16	28.0
Part time	5	9.0
Retired	7	12.0
Unable to work	29	51.0
Place of residence		
Metropolitan area (700,000 or more)	7	12.0
City (80,000–699,000)	20	35.0
Town (10,000–20,000)	21	37.0
Ranch or farm	9	16.0

RESULTS

The 57 participating patients, all undergoing one or more treatments—radiation, surgery, or chemotherapy—ranged in age from 16 to 79 years (mean age, 48.21 years); there were 38 females and 19 males. The primary cancers of the 57 patients were solid tumors. Thirteen patients underwent the first treatment for cancer. Key demographic information is presented in Table 18.1.

The variables (hospital setting, age, gender, primary cancer site, and cancer treatment modality) were tested by the Duncan Multiple Range Test for their effect on sorting the CARE-Q.[19] The data analysis failed to demonstrate significant statistical differences among the participants; therefore, the data were treated homogeneously.

Ranking the CARE-Q Items

The means of the 50 CARE-Q items ranged from 5.04 for the most important item ("Knows how to give shots, IVs, etc., and how to manage the equipment") to 2.93 for the least important item ("Asks patients what name they prefer to be called"). Four of the 10 items ranked as most important were in the subscale, "Monitors and follows through"; three were in the subscale, "Accessible"; two in the subscale, "Comforts"; and one in the subscale, "Trusting relationship" (Table 18.2).

Five of the 10 items ranked as least important were in the "Trusting relationship" subscale, and two of the least important items were in the "Comforts" subscale. The remaining least important items were from the three subscales, "Accessible," "Explains and facilitates," and "Monitors and follows through" (Table 18.3).

Patients' Rating of CARE-Q Items

When using the forced-choice format, the patient could place only one CARE-Q item card in the pocket designated most important. There was considerable divergence in the patients' perception of what was most important in making them feel cared for. Nine patients (15.8%) agreed on, "Puts the patient first no matter what else happens," and six patients (10.5%) agreed on, "Knows how to give shots and IVs . . . and manage the equipment" as being the most important. The patients showed little agreement on the "least important" item. The item asking what name the patient prefers to be called was selected by 11 (19.29%) patients (Tables 18.2 and 18.3).

DISCUSSION

The perceptions patients with cancer have of nurse caring behaviors that make them feel cared for have thus far not been described. The patients in the study reported "being accessible" and "monitoring and following through" as most important nurse caring behaviors. These findings resemble somewhat the indicators of care surveillance and demonstration of professional knowledge identified by adult medical–surgical patients in the study by Brown.[14] The findings are also in agreement with Ford's study in which listening appeared as an important nurse caring behavior. Unlike the nurses in the Ford study, the patients in this study did not rank listening as the most important nurse caring behavior, but ranked it seventh instead.[8] In previous studies using the same CARE-Q instrument, nurse participants who interacted with patients with cancer ranked listening as "most important."[6,7]

The patients in this study did not agree with Henry's home care patients who volunteering to do little things is an important indicator of nurse caring behavior.[13] The patients ranked it fortieth (of 50) in importance.

The high ranking of nurse caring behaviors that fall within the realm of demonstrated competency on the part of the nurse indicates that for the majority of the patients in this study, demonstrated

**TABLE 18.2 Perceptions of the Most Important Nurse Caring Behaviors:
The Ten High Mean Score CARE-Q Items**

CARE-Q Subscale[a]	CARE-Q Item	X̄	SD
Monitors/follows through	Knows how to give shots, IVs, etc., and how to manage the equipment	5.04	1.34
Monitors/follows through	Knows when to call doctor	4.84	1.22
Accessible	Responds quickly to patient's call	4.61	1.15
Monitors/follows through	Gives good physical care to patient	4.60	0.98
Accessible	Gives the patient's treatments and medications on time	4.56	1.12
Trusting relationship	Puts patient first no matter what else happens	4.54	1.38
Comforts	Listens to patient	4.47	1.01
Comforts	Talks to patient	4.37	1.01
Accessible	Checks on patient frequently	4.35	1.03
Monitors/follows through	Is well organized	4.35	1.14

[a]Theoretical classifications.

**TABLE 18.3 Perceptions of the Least Important Nurse Caring Behavior:
The Ten Low Mean Score CARE-Q Items**

CARE-Q Subscale[a]	CARE-Q Item	X̄	SD
Accessible	Volunteers to do "little" things for patient	3.63	1.16
Trusting relationship	When with patient, concentrates only on that patient	3.60	1.25
Trusting relationship	Helps patient establish realistic goals	3.60	1.12
Explains/facilitates	Tells patient of available support systems	3.53	1.05
Comforts	Is patient even with difficult patients	3.46	1.12
Trusting relationship	Offers reasonable alternatives	3.46	1.15
Monitors/follows through	Is professional in appearance	3.39	1.26
	Sits down with patient time	3.39	1.33
Comforts trusting relationship	Checks out the best to talk with the patient about changes in physical condition	3.32	1.04
Trusting relationship	Asks patient what name he or she prefers to be called	2.93	1.41

[a]Theoretical classification.

competency of skills precedes the patient's need to be listened to by the nurse. Listening and talking, psychosocial skills highly valued by nurses, appeared to become important to these patients only after their basic "getting better" needs were met.

Practice Implications

The study results, because of the limitations of the Q methodology, the CARE-Q instrument, and validity and reliability concerns, preclude major recommendations regarding the practice of nursing. However, the results caution nurses who care for patients with cancer not to assume that *intended* caring is always perceived by the patient as *caring*. These patients' high ranking of nurse behaviors that demonstrate monitoring and follow through based on competency of the nurse should be heeded. We need to keep in mind that the scope of nursing practice encompasses care, cure, and coordination.[16] Caring, the major concept of the care dimension, permeates the cure and coordination dimensions as well. It may well be that these cancer patients' perceptions of caring are more closely associated with the cure dimension. Perhaps, to patients with cancer hoping for cure or palliation of symptoms, the need to put care first and have the care organized, on time, and skillfully implemented is imperative. The primary goal of patients with cancer who are undergoing active treatment for the disease is to get better, which entails receiving the proper medications and treatments at the appropriate time.[20] By being fully aware of the importance patients attach to caring behaviors, nurses can then move on to the interactions with patients nurses find meaningful—touching, being receptive to patient's needs, and providing individualized care.

Perhaps, the greatest implication of this study for practice is for nurses to validate the effect their intended caring has had on patients. By doing so, and in conjunction with further refinement of the concept of caring for nursing in studies such as this, the practical aim of making patients feel cared for can be achieved.

ACKNOWLEDGMENTS

The author wishes to acknowledge Dr. Ada M. Lindsey's assistance in the preparation of this manuscript.

REFERENCES

1. Bevis, E. O. (1978). *Curriculum building in nursing.* St. Louis, MO: Mosby.
2. Leininger, M. (1978). *Transcultural nursing: Concepts, theories and practices.* New York, NY: John Wiley.
3. Watson, J. (1979). *Nursing: The philosophy and science of caring.* Boston, MA: Little, Brown & Co.
4. Gaut, D. A. (1984). Development of a theoretically adequate description of caring. *Western Journal of Nursing Research, 5*(4), 313–324.
5. Leininger, M. (1984). Caring: A central focus of nursing and health services. In M. M. Leininger (Ed.), *Care: The essence of nursing and health* (p. 46). Thorofare, NJ: Slack.
6. Larson, P. J. Nurse providing care to cancer patients: Perceptions of caring perceptions. Unpublished manuscript.
7. Larson, P. J. (1984). Perceptions of important nurse caring behaviors. (Abstract 161A). *Proceedings of the 9th Congress of the Oncology Nursing Society, 11*(2), 90.
8. Ford, M. (1981). Nurse professionals and the caring process. (Doctoral dissertation, University of Northern Colorado). *Dissertation Abstracts International, 43,* 967B–968B (University Microfilms #81–19278).
9. Leininger, M. (1981). The phenomenon of caring: Importance, research questions and theoretical considerations. In M. M. Leininger (Ed.), *Caring: An essential human need* (pp. 3–15). Thorofare, NJ: Slack.
10. Gardner, K. G., & Wheeler, E. (1981). Patients' and staff nurses' perceptions of supportive nursing behaviors: A preliminary analysis. In M. M. Leininger (Ed.), *Caring: An essential human need* (pp. 109–113). Thorofare, NJ: Slack.
11. Uhl, J. (1981). Caring as the focus of a multidisciplinary health center for the elderly.

In M. M. Leininger (Ed.), *Caring: An essential human need* (pp. 115–125). Thorofare, NJ: Slack.

12. Leininger, M. (1984). Southern rural black and white American lifeways with focus on care and health phenomena. In M. M. Leininger (Ed.), *Care: The Essence of nursing and health* (pp. 133–135). Thorofare, NJ: Slack.

13. Henry, D. M. M. (1975). *Nurse behaviors perceived by patients as indicators of caring* (Doctoral dissertation, Catholic University, Washington D.C.). *Dissertation Abstracts International, 36*(02 652B) (University Microfilms #75–16, 229).

14. Brown, L. (1982). *Behaviors of nurses perceived by hospitalized patients as indicators of care.* (Doctoral dissertation, University of Colorado, Boulder). *Dissertation Abstracts International, 43,* 4361B (University Microfilms #DA8209803).

15. American Nurses' Association. (1965). First position on nursing education. *The American Journal of Nursing, 65*(11), 106–111.

16. American Nurses' Association. (1980). *Nursing: A social policy statement.* Kansas City, MO: American Nurses' Association.

17. Larson, P. J. (1983). *The development of an instrument focusing on nurse caring behaviors: The CARE-Q.* Paper presented at the Sixth National Caring Research Conference, Tyler, TX.

18. Stephenson, W. (1953). *The study of behavioral Q technique and its methodology.* Chicago, IL: University of Chicago Press.

19. Duncan, D. B. (1955). Multiple range and multiple-F tests. *Biometrics,* 11.

20. Weisman, A. D. (1979). *Coping with cancer.* New York, NY: McGraw-Hill.

QUESTIONS FOR REFLECTION

Baccalaureate

1. Why did Larson (1984) select oncology patients as her sample in the important nurse caring behaviors study?
2. What do you like or dislike about how the CARE-Q instrument is constructed?
3. What level of data (e.g., nominal, ordinal, interval, and ratio) does the CARE-Q instrument generate?

Master's

1. What was the construct validity process Larson (1984) described to establish the psychometric properties of the CARE-Q? Additional details are available in Larson's (1981) dissertation.
2. How do you think that patients were able to sort the cards of the CARE-Q during the data collection process of Larson's (1984) study?
3. How do the findings of Larson's study justify additional research using the CARE-Q instrument?

Doctoral

1. What information can you share about Larson's (1984) use of a *descriptive design* approach in her study on the important nurse caring behaviors study? Defend your explanation.
2. Why do you think Larson (1984) provided a ranked list of the most important and least important nurse caring behaviors?
3. If you would decide to use the CARE-Q in a future study, how would you plan the investigation? Start by describing the research question or questions.

19

Noncaring and Caring in the Clinical Setting: Patients' Descriptions

Doris Johnston Riemen

*E*verybody talks about caring. Slogans such as "caring and competent," "caring and sharing," "we care a bundle," and "to care is human" abound in nursing journals and nursing literature. But the fact is that in many clinical settings, the patients perceive a great lack of caring. The patients feel this noncaring by nurses so acutely that they can describe not only the situation but also exactly how they felt during and after the interaction. A 55-year-old former minister thus described an interaction that had taken place several years previously:

> Any contact that I had with those nurses down there, you know *it was cold* and it certainly *makes you feel very helpless* to be strapped on a bed and in such pain and when anyone speaks to you, even the *sound of their voice doesn't sound very concerned.* One nurse was washing me up, and oh, *she was so rough!* Just like she was *washing a doll and not a human being.* I remember the nurse bathing me, and just her *movements, they were so rough*, very rough physically. You know, she'd run the razor, well almost *like striking out at someone.* They *did not make me feel comfortable* or that *I was of any value to them.* And I suppose all of us like to feel that we're valuable. [Emphasis added.]

Patients have complained for years about this failure on the part of health care workers to make them feel valued as human beings. Rockefeller, writing as a consumer, states, "What the public wants is an entire health care team to give the patient the feeling that they care, that they are involved in him as a human being."[1] Chaney, writing as a former patient, states, "What I need and value most is someone concerned enough to smile, to listen . . . [they] made it very clear to me that the hospital was there to treat patients, not people."[2]

If patients perceive that nurses do not value them, what is it that nurses are doing or not doing that invites such a perception? Is it strictly physical actions that patients interpret as noncaring or is it a combination of actions, behaviors, and attitudes? And when such an interaction takes place, what are the consequences for the patient? A phenomenological approach and analysis of 10 patients' descriptions of nurse–patient interactions gives some insight into this "lived world" of noncaring interactions.

PHENOMENOLOGICAL APPROACH

The phenomenological approach is a way to look at empirical matters from the perspective of the people involved. To do this,

From Riemen, D. J. (1986). Noncaring and caring in the clinical setting: Patients' descriptions. *Topics in Clinical Nursing, 8*(2), 30–36. Permission to reprint granted by Wolters Kluwer.

it is necessary to enter the patients' world to see what is happening from their perspective. Oiler claims that the phenomenological approach is appropriate because "the nursing profession emphasizing a reverence for clients' experiences is concerned with the quality of life and the quality of the nurse–patient relationship."[3] Valle and King state that phenomenological research seeks to answer two related questions: What is the phenomenon that is experienced and lived? How does it show itself?[4]

There is not just one phenomenological method, but several different methodologies. Using Colaizzi's method, patients' descriptions of caring interactions with nurses were analyzed for significant statements, meanings were formulated, clusters of themes were identified, and finally, a description of the essential structure of the phenomenon emerged,[5] Using the 55-year-old minister's description as an example, the emphasized significant statements, when viewed through the eyes of the patient, present the following noncaring picture: a patient in a cold, rough environment hearing unconcerned voices and feeling as though he was being physically struck. He felt helpless, uncomfortable, and of no value.

Patients' Perceptions of Noncaring Behaviors and Attitudes

Consider this description of a nurse by a 21-year-old nursing student with lupus erythematosus:

> She was *always in a hurry*, she *didn't have time to talk* or even if she had time she *didn't really seem to want to talk*. Her body language let me know *she wasn't interested in what I had to say*. All she was here to do was to *perform her duty and go home*. She *stood at a distance*, she didn't even come close. She made me feel I have some kind of illness and I might rub off on her.
>
> When I was talking to her she wouldn't look at me, not directly. When I would

> ask her a question she would be snappy—even on the defensive side. She *wasn't interested in the person as a whole*. She would *cut me off short and she talked in such a rush*. She *never would say when she'd be back*. I was *not at ease*. I was *uncomfortable*. I *became depressed* by not being able to talk. I *felt I had to keep my mouth shut*. [Emphasis added.]

This description details very specific behaviors and attitudes of the nurse and the effects they had on a young patient. The specific significant statements are emphasized, and they portray the following picture: a nurse who sees nursing as a job; who is always in a hurry and doesn't take or make time to come close to, look at, or really listen to the patient; who snaps and is defensive when questioned; and who, by such attitudes and actions, makes the patient ill at ease, depressed, and convinced that the nurse didn't care about her as a whole person.

To identify more completely what it is that nurses do in the clinical setting that patients perceive as noncaring, the significant statements from other patient descriptions have been grouped under the headings "Being in a Hurry and Efficient," "Doing a Job," "Being Rough and Belittling Patients," "Not Responding," and "Treating Patients as Objects."

Being in a Hurry and Efficient

One of the views of nurses that was consistent in all 10 descriptions of noncaring interactions was that of nurses "being in a hurry and efficient." The following specific examples illustrate this perception:

- Always in a hurry
- Always in a rush
- No time to talk
- Super efficient attitude
- Acted like clockwork
- Just came in to do what had to be done
- Efficient, but no human element

Doing a Job

Patients consistently perceived nurses as just being there to "do a job," as the following examples illustrate:

- There to perform duties and then go home
- Nothing seemed to bother the nurse—it was just a job
- Acted like it (nursing) was just a hum-drum affair
- Acted like it was just an everyday job
- There just to do a job

Being Rough and Belittling Patients

The following statements are examples of patients' perceptions of the nurses being rough and treating them like children or belittling them:

- Felt as though (my) hands were being slapped
- She was mad at me
- Made me feel like a little kid
- She was really tough—no softness
- She didn't care what she said to me
- She didn't have no pity—no mercy
- She just wasn't soft
- Gave you a simple answer as though you couldn't possibly understand
- Watched you like you're a 10-year-old
- Raised and shook her finger at me
- Felt like a child being scolded
- It's insulting to be treated that way
- Talked loud and acted as though I'd lost my marbles

Not Responding

Patients perceived noncaring interactions to be even those in which there was no interaction because the nurse did not respond to their requests. Consider these examples:

- Buzz and she would not come
- Didn't pay any attention
- She would not come back to help
- Too busy talking to the other nurses to talk to me

- Did not pay any attention to what you needed
- Not come in the room
- Rang bell and would not come

Treating Patients as Objects

The following examples illustrate the patients' perceptions of noncaring nurses who wielded power and saw them as non-human objects.

- Looked at equipment and not at me
- Wasn't interested in what I had to say
- Wouldn't come close and look at me
- She did not explain
- I was not treated as a person
- It was as though I was a nobody
- Won't tell you what she's doing
- Look at you like an object
- Element of human contact lacking
- Bathed me as though she was doing a dog
- Strapped me to the bed—never talked to me, walked away
- Washed me as though I was a toy
- I was not a human being to her

Summary of Significant Statements

In all 10 descriptions not once was an ill-performed technical procedure mentioned as noncaring. It is very thought provoking to realize that a majority of perceptions fall into the two categories "being rough and belittling patients" and "treating patients as objects." It is frightening to realize that at a time when patients are so vulnerable, nurses are perceived as doing those very things that make patients even more vulnerable and helpless.

When asked to describe a caring and a noncaring interaction with a nurse, the patients consistently and immediately described the noncaring interaction first. Why do these interactions come to mind so quickly, even years after they have taken place? Part of the explanation may lie in the fact that the patients were in circumstances where everything was new and strange. But more important, as a result of the noncaring interactions, they felt humiliated, frightened, and out of control of the situation. When all of these negative and unpleasant feelings are associated with an already unfamiliar situation, it is a natural thing to be able to recall and describe the situation vividly, even years later.

Twenty-five years ago, vanKaam stated that nurses' interests in their patients had to be genuine and honest, not feigned, because "patients in their intensified sensitivity" distinguish sharply between genuine and pretended interest and care."[6] It is precisely because of this "intensified sensitivity" that patients are so acutely aware of nurses' behaviors and attitudes in the clinical setting.

Essential Structure of a Noncaring Interaction

Examples of significant statements in and of themselves do not provide the whole picture. Only when they are clustered into themes does the essential structure of a description of a noncaring interaction emerge.

After all the patients' descriptions were analyzed, three themes presented themselves: the nurse's presence, the client's response, and consequences. The nurse was present only to get the job done. For the patient, the physical presence was available briefly or not at all even when solicited. The nurse does not recognize the client's uniqueness because the nurse does not "really listen" and appears "too busy" to pay attention to the client as an individual. The client is devalued as a unique individual by actions of the nurse that are degrading and belittling. The consequence of the nurse's lack of concern for the client is that the client feels frustrated, scared, depressed, angry, and upset.[7]

These themes help develop a general picture of a noncaring interaction. The nurse's presence with the client is perceived by the client as minimal, with the nurse being physically present but emotionally distant. The nurse is viewed as being there only because it is the nurse's job and not because the client needs assistance. Any response by the nurse is made with a minimal amount of energy and is bound by the rules. The client perceives the nurse who does not respond to his or her requests for assistance as being noncaring.

Therefore, an interaction that never happened is labeled as a noncaring interaction. The nurse is too busy and hurried to spend time with the client, and, therefore, the nurse does not sit down and really listen to the client's individual concerns. The client is further devalued, seen as a child, or seemingly as a nonhuman being or object. Because of the devaluing and lack of concern, the client's needs are not sufficiently met and the client has negative feelings such as frustration, fear, depression, anger, and anxiety.[8]

IMPLICATIONS FOR CLINICAL PRACTICE

Noncaring interactions with patients are obviously not helpful or healing. Why then do nurses respond with such noncaring attitudes and behaviors? One reason is that nurses have always been praised and rewarded for efficiency, for getting the job done. Consciously or unconsciously that attitude is conveyed in nurses' actions. Another reason is that nurses themselves have not been valued or cared for as individuals but have been viewed by physicians and administrators as means to an end. Therefore, it is difficult for nurses to value caring or to care for patients as individuals. Yet another reason is that patients, on entry into the hospital, have to forfeit control of what happens to them, so it is easy for nurses to treat them as children or less than competent adults. Finally, with the tremendous increase in technology, nurses have become so attuned to monitoring the machines that the person is attached to, the machines become of secondary concern.

What is it that nurses can and must do? In order for the patients to perceive themselves as being of value, nurses must perceive nursing as more than just a job and patients as more than just objects. Noncaring behaviors must be replaced by caring behaviors that derive from caring attitudes.

Marcel, the French existential philosopher, notes one way to develop this caring attitude; he distinguishes between physically present and being truly a presence:

> It is an undeniable fact . . . there are some people who reveal themselves as "present"—that is to say, at our disposal—when we are in pain or need to confide in someone, while there are other people who do not give this feeling, however great is their goodwill. . . . The most attentive listener may give me the impression of not being present; he gives me nothing, he cannot make room for me in himself whatever the material favors he is prepared to grant me. The truth is there is a way of listening which is a way of giving, and another way which is a way of refusing. . . . Presence is something which reveals itself immediately and unmistakably in a look, a smile, an intonation, or a handshake.[9]

If nurses were such a presence, think of the difference in the patient's "lived world." Gadow advocates just such an existential philosophy for nurses, one that "unifies and enhances the experience of the individuals involved rather than devaluing and alienating."[10] Her proposal of existential advocacy as the essence of nursing points to the nurse's participation, the give-and-take, the dialogue with the patient in determining the unique meaning for the patient. For Gadow, professional involvement means directing the whole of oneself toward another's need. It is a "participation of the entire self, using every dimension of the person as a resource in the professional relation."[11]

The nurse as a presence in such a relationship would be more than just physically present and answering only the stated concerns and questions of the patient. Existential presence in a caring interaction does not have to involve extensive time. Just as Marcel stated, "Presence . . . reveals itself immediately and unmistakably."[12] Existential presence means that in each interaction, the nurse is truly present in thought, word, and deed. If the existential mode of interaction became as habitual as the hurried, brisk, efficient, objectified type of interaction, the patients would respond with the feelings of security, comfort, and relaxation. Such feelings will support healing, well-being, and a sense of value. As the patient in the first description stated, "I suppose all of us like to feel that we're valuable." In a caring interaction in which the nurse is truly present, this sense of value is felt not only by the patient but also by the nurse.

REFERENCES

1. Rockefeller, M. C. (1963). The why of citizen involvement in patient care. *Nursing Outlook, 11*(8), 580.
2. Chaney, P. (1975). Ordeal. *Nursing, 75*(6), 24, 38.
3. Oiler, C. (1982). The phenomenological approach in nursing. *Nursing Research, 31*(3), 178.
4. Valle, R., & King, M. (1978). *Existential phenomenological alternatives for psychology.* New York, NY: Oxford University Press.
5. Colaizzi, P. F. (1978). Psychological research as the phenomenologist views it. In R. Valle, & M. King (Eds.), *Existential phenomenological alternatives for psychology.* New York, NY: Oxford University Press.
6. vanKaam, A. L. (1959). The nurse in the patient's world. *American Journal of Nursing, 59*(12), 1710.
7. Riemen, D. J. (1986). The essential structure of a caring interaction: Doing phenomenology. In P. Munhall, & C. Oiler (Eds.), *Nursing research: A qualitative perspective.* Norwalk, CT: Appleton-Century-Crofts.
8. Ibid., 5–25.
9. Marcel, G. (1981). *The philosophy of existence* (pp. 25–26), In R. R. Grabon (Ed. & Trans.). Philadelphia, PA: University of Pennsylvania Press.

10. Gadow, S. (1980). Existential advocacy. In S. F. Spiker & S. Gadow (Eds.), *Nursing: Ideas and images opening dialogue with the humanities* (p. 80). New York, NY: Springer-Verlag.

11. Ibid., 90.
12. Marcel, G. *The philosophy of existence*, 26.

QUESTIONS FOR REFLECTION

Baccalaureate

1. On which original study was Riemen's (1986) article based?
2. What did you learn about patients' description of noncaring from reading the Riemen chapter?
3. How does the *forfeit of control* description by Reiman operate for adult patients on admission to hospitals, resulting in nurses' perceptions of their competency and interactions with them?

Master's

1. According to Riemen (1986), what factors may explain patients' immediate descriptions of noncaring nursing interactions before they describe caring nursing interactions?
2. Riemen's (1986) article is based on an interpretive approach. What is the research question that she posed for the investigation? How is this question consistent with the interpretive approach?
3. What is the definition of a significant statement according to Colaizzi (1978) as cited by Riemen (1986)?

Doctoral

1. What are the four elements of Colaizzi's (1978) phenomenological method as indicated by Riemen (1986)?
2. What is the essential structure of a noncaring nursing interaction as described by Riemen (1986)?
3. What follow-up studies are needed to address the problems suggested by Riemen's (1986) description of a noncaring nursing interaction along with significant statements and the main themes she identified?

20

Oncology Nurses' Versus Cancer Patients' Perceptions of Nurse Caring Behaviors: A Replication Study

Deborah K. Mayer

Caring is the central focus, the very essence of nursing, yet it is not well defined or understood. *Caring*, in its most basic definition, is "that feeling of concern, regard, and respect one human being may have for another."[1] In a professional nurse–patient relationship, caring refers to, "the direct or indirect nurturant and skillful activities, processes, and decisions related to assisting people" to achieve or maintain health.[2,3] Therefore, one may say that nurse caring is more focused and directed than caring in general.

Bevis states that "knowledge about the caring process, its purpose, organization and outcome enables nurses to understand and interact with clients more wisely and with greater caring, because they make choices based on knowledge."[4] As the technological aspects of health care have increased in complexity, so has the need to better understand and improve the caring components of nursing to provide humane health care.[5–7]

BACKGROUND

Different authors, most notably Leininger, Watson, and Gaut, have analyzed and defined the various components of caring.[2,8,9] These include the attributes of the caregiver and receiver, the caring process, and specific behaviors that convey caring. Watson and associates formulated a model of caring that includes caring interventions both *expressive* and *instrumental* in nature. Expressive activities include establishing relationships that are characterized by trust, hope, sensitivity, compassion, warmth, genuineness, and offering support, which may include nurturance, surveillance, comfort, protection, and respecting and accommodating privacy and territorial needs. Instrumental activities include physical action–oriented helping behaviors, such as assistance with gratification of human needs, administering procedures and medications, specific stress alleviation through various modalities, and maintenance of physical environment, and cognitively oriented helping behaviors, such as conducting specific teaching regimens, instructing, advising, and problem solving (p. 38).[8]

Gaut states that "because caring is a practical activity, the question of what people do when caring is appropriate (p. 32)."[9] One aspect of the caring concept that should be examined is to determine which behaviors in the context of the nurse–patient relationship, when enacted,

From Mayer, D. K. (1987). Oncology nurses' versus cancer patients' perceptions of nursery caring behaviors: A replication study. *Oncology Nurse Forum, 11*(6), 46–50. Permission to reprint granted by the Oncology Nursing Society.

make patients feel cared for. Congruence between nurses' and patients' perceptions of nurse caring behaviors is important since it may form the very foundation of the nurse–patient relationship.

Only a few nursing studies have evaluated nurse caring behaviors. Henry interviewed 50 homecare patients about their caring perceptions; responses included descriptions of what the nurse does, how the nurse does it, and how much the nurse does as the three major caring categories.[10] Brown interviewed 80 hospitalized medical–surgical patients not only to identify, describe, and classify behaviors that were indicators of care but also to examine the task and affective dimensions of these behaviors.[11] Specific categories and behaviors were identified from responses to "what the nurse does" and "what the nurse is like." Brown's data support the concept that caring is based on the attributes of the care giver as well as both expressive and instrumental behaviors. These two studies evaluated both the caring attributes and the behaviors of nurses only from the patient's perspective.

Ford surveyed 192 nurses about their definition of caring.[12] Two major categories were identified: genuine concern for the well-being of another and giving of yourself. Listening was also routinely identified as a caring behavior. This study contributed to the growing list of nurse behaviors identified as conveying caring.

Larson analyzed the perceptions of nurse caring behaviors from both the patients' and nurses' perspectives.[13] This study was unique because both nurses' and patients' perceptions were evaluated, and because of the instrument used to measure these perceptions, the Caring Assessment Report Evaluation-Q sort (CARE-Q). Utilizing the Q-sort methodology, the CARE-Q was developed to measure, by ranked importance, the differences and similarities of perceptions that nurses and patients have regarding caring behaviors. Fifty caring behaviors were classified under the following six themes: *anticipates, comforts, explains and facilitates, develops and sustains trusting relationships, monitors and follows through,* and *is accessible.* The behaviors and themes are similar to those identified by Brown and are both expressive and instrumental in nature. When administered to 57 medical–surgical nurses and 57 cancer patients, Larson found significant differences between nurses and patients (t-test, $p < .05$) in the ranked importance of 19 of the 50 caring behaviors. Patients ranked instrumental behaviors higher, whereas nurses ranked expressive behaviors as more important.

A replication of Larson's study addressed the following two questions: Is there a significant relationship between oncology nurses' and cancer patients' perceptions of nurse caring behaviors? Do the findings of this study corroborate Larson's findings?

METHOD

Sample

The convenience sample of patients consisted of 54 individuals with a variety of cancers being treated at the Biological Response Modifiers Program of the National Cancer Institute. Table 20.1 compares selected patient demographics of this study with Larson's sample. This sample included 24 men and 30 women with a mean age of 53.8 years (range 22–77 years). All patients had previously received chemotherapy, radiotherapy, or surgery, either alone or in combination for their cancer. Fifty-seven percent (31) of patients had been diagnosed within 2 years of entering this study, whereas 43% (23) were diagnosed before that time.

The convenience sample of nurses consisted of 28 female oncology nurses. Table 20.1 compares selected nurse demographics of this study with Larson's sample. The mean age was 31.1 years, and average time in nursing was 8.3 years.

TABLE 20.1 Demographics of Mayer and Larson Subjects

Demographics	Mayer	Larson
Patients (N)	54	57
Mean age, year (range)	53.8 (22–77)	42.2 (16–79)
Sex		
Male	24	19
Female	30	38
Diagnosis		
Breast	21	11
Non-Hodgkin's Lymphoma	10	6
Leukemia	7	6
Melanoma	6	0
Colon	6	4
Other	4	30
Nurses (N)	28	27
Mean age, year (range)	31.1 (22–52)	Not available
<30 yr	16	28
>30 yr	12	28
Sex		
Male	0	3
Female	28	54
Mean years in nursing (range)	8.3 (2–22)	Not available
<5	5	28
>5	23	18
Education		
AD	2	7
Diploma	10	14
BSN	13	33
MSN	3	2

Instrument

The Q-technique is a procedure for the study of interpersonal relations and is used to measure attitudes and beliefs. The Q-sort is utilized to address the correlation, or degree of similarity, between different individuals' or groups' attitudes, expectations, or opinions at a given time; and/or the degree of change in individuals' or groups' attitudes or opinions from one time to another.[14]

The CARE-Q, developed by Larson, identifies 50 nurse caring behaviors. Content and face validity were established by an expert nurse panel and psychometrician, and test–retest reliability was established by administering the CARE-Q to a random sample of 115 oncology nurses.[15]

Larson's subjects sorted the 50 caring behaviors from the most to least important into seven pockets in the CARE-Q instrument. Each behavior was given a rank number according to pocket placement. Mean rankings were then calculated for each behavior with distribution approximating a normal distribution. Theoretically, the highest possible mean ranking for a behavior was 7 and

the lowest was 1, providing that all subjects chose those particular behaviors as
the most and least important. Differences
in the mean rankings of the 50 caring
behaviors of the identified groups were
then compared. The CARE-Q was used
unmodified for this study.

Procedure

Following institutional review board
approval, informed consent was obtained
from all subjects. The patient was then
instructed in the use of the CARE-Q and
given up to 24 hours to complete it. The
majority of patients completed the test in
approximately 1 hour. At the time of testing, subjects also completed demographic
information sheets. Nurses followed the
same procedures.

The major statistical analysis of the
data was completed using descriptive statistics and Spearman's rank-order correlation
coefficients,[16,17] performing both within-
group and among-group correlations. The
Student's t-test was utilized to determine
differences between nurse and patient
rankings for each behavior. The level of statistical significance was set at $p < .05$.

RESULTS

Comparison of Nurse and Patient Responses

When evaluating all 50 behaviors, the
correlation between patients and nurses
rankings was significant ($r_s = 0.37, p < .01$).
There was also significant agreement
between nurse and patient choices for the
three of the six major categories of caring
behaviors: *explains and facilitates* ($r_s = 0.81$,
$p = .0499$), *trusting relationships* ($r_s = 0.58$,
$p = .0174$), and *monitors and follows through*
($r_s = 0.72, p = .0427$). The correlations for
the other three categories were not significant (*accessibility* $r_s = 0.26, p = .6175$; *comforts*
$r_s = 0.09, p = .8138$; and *anticipates* $r_s = 0.10$,
$p = .8729$).

The five highest and lowest ranked
nurse caring behaviors are outlined in
Tables 20.2 and 20.3, respectively. There
was no agreement in the five most important behaviors identified by the nurses and
patients. Patients chose three expressive
behaviors and two instrumental behaviors, while nurses chose four expressive
behaviors and one instrumental behavior
as most important. There was agreement

TABLE 20.2 Ranking of Top Five Most Important Caring Behaviors

Behavior	Nurse $\overline{X}$ (*N* = 28)	Patient $\overline{X}$ (*N* = 54)
Nurses' rankings		
Listens to the patient	5.61[a]	4.59
Allows the patient to express his feelings about his/her disease and treatment fully and treats the information confidentially	5.00[a]	4.41
Realizes that the patient knows himself the best and whenever possible includes the patient in planning and management of his or her care	4.82[a]	4.05
Touches the patient when he or she needs comforting	4.61[a]	4.02
Is perceptive of the patient's needs and plans and acts accordingly, e.g., gives antinausea medication when patient is receiving medication which will probably induce nausea	4.61[a]	4.11

(continued)

TABLE 20.2 Ranking of Top Five Most Important Caring Behaviors (*continued*)

Behavior	Nurse $\overline{X}$ (N = 28)	Patient $\overline{X}$ (N = 54)
Patients' rankings		
Knows how to give shots, IVs, etc. and how to manage the equipment like IVs, suction machines, etc.	4.14	5.48[b]
Is cheerful	3.28	5.42
Encourages patient to call if he or she has problems	3.86	4.92
Puts the patient first, no matter what else happens	4.28	4.90[b]
Anticipates that the "first times" are the hardest and pays special attention to the patient during the first clinic visit, first hospitalization, first treatment, etc.	4.36	4.85

[a]Also ranked top 10 by Larson's nurse sample.
[b]Also ranked top 10 by Larson's patient sample.

TABLE 20.3 Ranking of Five Least Important Caring Behaviors

Behavior	Nurse $\overline{X}$ (N = 28)	Patient $\overline{X}$ (N = 54)
Nurses' rankings		1
Is professional in appearance—wears appropriate, identifiable clothing, and identification	2.18[a]	3.24
Asks the patient what name he or she prefers to be called	2.82[a]	2.70
Suggests questions for the patient to ask her or his doctor	2.86[a]	3.26
Volunteers to do "little" things for the patient, e.g., brings a cup of coffee, paper	3.04[a]	3.33
Is cheerful	3.28[a]	5.42
Patients' rankings		
Asks the patient what name he/she prefers to be called	2.82	2.70[b]
Helps the patient establish realistic goals	4.07:	3.09[b]
Is professional in appearance— wears appropriate identifiable clothing and identification	2.18	3.24[b]
Suggests questions for the patient to ask her or his doctor	2.86	3.26
Checks out with the patient the best time to talk with the patient about changes in his or her condition	3.54	3.24[b]

[a]Also ranked top 10 by Larson's nurse sample.
[b]Also ranked top 10 by Larson's patient sample.

between the nurses and patients on three of the least important behaviors.

Although a significant degree of overall correlation exists between the nurse and patient groups, there were some obvious differences among the categories and specific behaviors. Patients ranked individual expressive activities and behaviors in the *accessible* category the highest, while nurses ranked individual instrumental activities in the *anticipates* category the highest. In five behaviors; the difference in mean rankings was one or greater. Patients ranked four of these five behaviors higher and therefore more important than the nurses (Table 20.4). However, only "is cheerful" was statistically significant ($t = 212$, $p \leq .05$), with patients ranking this behavior as more important.

Comparison With Larson's Results

Table 20.5 compares the mean scores for the six major categories of behaviors with Larson's findings. The correlation of the six mean categories between Mayer and Larson patients was $r_s = 0.87$, $p = .0248$ and between Mayer and Larson nurses was $r_s = 0.66$, $p = .1562$.

One hundred percent of the nurses' and 40% of the patients' most important caring behaviors parallel those of Larson's subjects, although the actual rankings varied somewhat. There was also agreement with Larson's data in the least important behaviors in 100% by the nurses' choices and 80% of the patients'.

TABLE 20.4 Differences Between Patient and Nurse Ranked Behaviors

Behavior	Patient X̄ (N = 28)	Nurse X̄ (N = 54)
Encourages the patient to call if he or she has problems	4.92	3.86
Is cheerful	5.42	3.28[a]
Is professional in appearance—wears appropriate identifiable clothing and identification	3.24	2.18
Knows how to give shots, IVs and how to manage the equipment like IVs, suction machines, etc.	5.48	4.14
Listens to the patients	4.59	5.61

Note. X̄ ranking difference > 1.00.

[a]$t = 2.12$, $p < .05$.

TABLE 20.5 Six Major Caring Categories—Comparison of Mayer and Larson Subjects Mean Rankings

Category	Mayer Patient (N = 54)	Larson Patient (N = 57)	Mayer Nurse (N = 28)	Larson Nurse (N = 57)
Accessible	4.39	4.18	3.80	4.07
Explains and facilitates	3.79	3.85	3.85	3.75
Comforts	4.12	3.91	4.21	4.30
Anticipates	4.11	4.12	4.22	4.08
Trusting relationships	3.83	3.85	4.04	3.98
Monitors and follows through	4.22	4.27	3.76	3.79

Most Important Behavior

The most important behavior for both samples of nurses was "listens to the patient," but both samples of patients ranked it considerably lower. Two other behaviors, "touches the patient when he or she needs comforting" and "allows the patient to express his feelings about his or her disease and treatment fully," were also identified in the top five by both nurse groups.

The most important behavior for both samples of patients was "knows how to give shots, IVs, etc. and how to manage the equipment like IVs, suction machines, etc." but nurses ranked it lower in both samples. "Puts the patient first, no matter what else happens" was also identified by both patient samples.

Least Important Behavior

Three least important behaviors in each of the nurse and patient samples of this study were also in the 10 least ranked behaviors in the Larson samples. These included: "is professional in appearance—wears appropriate identifiable clothing and identification"; "suggests questions for the patient to ask her or his doctor"; and "is cheerful" for the nurses. For the patient, these included: "asks the patient what name he or she prefers to be called"; "is professional in appearance . . ."; and "checks out with the patient the best time to talk with the patient about changes in his or her condition."

DISCUSSION

This replication study further validates the perceptions on important nurse caring behaviors reported by Larson. The overall agreement between the patients and nurses may contribute to or enhance the caring relationship, but categorical and individual differences exist. Patients appear to value the instrumental, technical caring skills more than nurses do, while nurses rank the expressive behaviors higher. Nurses may be assuming a certain level of technical competence while patients may not. Patients may not be open or receptive to the expressive caring behaviors until basic physical needs have been met through instrumental activities. For example, listening to the patient may not be perceived as caring if at the same time the nurse is not skilled in starting an intravenous injection or has not administered needed analgesics. By identifying important nurse caring behaviors as perceived by patients, nurses will be able to develop a repertoire of behaviors to convey caring.

Limitations of the Study

Benner states that caring in nursing is relational and should not be evaluated in expressive and instrumental terms. However, to have a better understanding of the whole, it may be necessary to analyze the various parts, realizing that "caring out of context will always be controversial, because caring is local, specific and individual."[18] As with any Q methodology, the least important behaviors are relative to the most important one, meaning that a particular behavior is not unimportant, only less so. Since correlational statistics summarize the degree of relationship between variables, individual differences among subjects, and specific behaviors should still be explored.

Implications for Research

The CARE-Q should be tested to establish its validity once other instruments are developed to evaluate caring behaviors. Larger samples should be obtained to conduct a factor analysis of the six major caring categories. Similar studies in different nurse and patient populations could be conducted exploring the questions that follow.

- Would the behaviors be ranked differently if the patients were homebound, in a psychiatric or surgical facility?

- Would patients' and nurses' perceptions change with repeated measure over time?
- Would primary versus team nursing alter perceptions of caring?

To further evaluate nurse caring behaviors, other questions should be asked.

- Will patients feel cared for if the five most important behaviors are consistently performed?
- If the technical aspects of patients' care are adequately performed, will they then perceive expressive activities as more important?

There is a growing body of evidence which demonstrates that the nurse–patient relationship has a significant effect on the patient's welfare.[8,19] What relationship, if any, exists between caring behaviors and health costs? Davis addresses cost containment in health care, focusing on the need for quality care to decrease hospitalization time and noting that, "renewed attention must be focused on continuity of care."[19] Research could include caring aspects in the evaluation of nursing costs (does increased caring lower costs by fostering, even if indirectly, earlier discharges?).

Implications for Practice and Education

The need to practice both humanistic and scientific caring behaviors as described by Watson is apparent.[20] Integration of both expressive and instrumental caring activities (the high tech/high touch aspects) may be more evident in the expert nurse as defined by Benner.[18]

The findings of this and other caring studies will better delineate caring behaviors that can then be taught to nurses as a central and unifying factor in nursing. The acquisition and integration of these skills should be evaluated and fostered in the student/novice nurse. Curricula should include the attributes of the caregiver/receiver, the process, and the

behaviors. These phenomena should also be initiated in the student–teacher relationship. Practice settings should also encourage and reinforce these expressive and instrumental caring behaviors. And finally, practicing nurses should validate which behaviors their patients value the most.

REFERENCES

1. Sobel, D. (1969). Human caring. *The American Journal of Nursing, 69*(12), 2612–2613.
2. Leininger, M. (Ed.). (1981). *CARING: An essential human need* (p. 9). Thorofare, NJ: C. Slack.
3. Canadian Nurses Association. (1980). *CNA: A definition of nursing practice, standards for nursing practice* (vi). Ottawa, Canada: Author.
4. Bevis, E. (1978). *Curriculum building in nursing* (p. 120). St. Louis, MO: C. V. Mosby.
5. Kelly, L. (1984). High tech/high touch—now more than ever. *Nurs Outlook, 32*(1), 15.
6. Naisbitt, J. (1982). *Megatrends.* New York, NY: Harper & Row.
7. Paulen, A. (1984). High touch in a high tech environment. *Cancer Nursing, 7*(3), 201.
8. Watson, J., Burckhardt, C., Brown, L., Bloch, D., & Hester, N. (1979). A model of caring: An alternative health care model for nursing practice and research. *American Nurses Association Publications,* (NP-59), 32–44.
9. Gaut, D. (1984). A theoretic description of caring as action. In M. Leininnger (Ed.), *Care: The essence of nursing and health* (p. 32). Thorofare, NJ: Slack.
10. Henry, O. (1975). Nurse behaviors perceived by patients as indicators of caring. *Dissertation Abstracts International, 36,* 02652B (University Microfilms No. 75–16, 229).
11. Brown, L. (1981). Behaviors of nurses perceived by hospitalized patients as indicators of care. *Dissertation Abstracts International, 43,* 4361B (University Microfilms No. DA8209803).
12. Ford, M. B. (1981). Nurse professionals and the caring process. *Dissertation Abstracts International, 43,* 967B–968B (University Microfilms No. 81–19278).
13. Larson, P. J. (1981). *Oncology patients' and professional nurses' perceptions of important nurse caring behaviors* (Unpublished doctoral dissertation). UCSF, San Francisco, CA.
14. Whitling, F. (1955). Q-Sort: A technique for evaluating perceptions of interpersonal relationships. *Nursing Research, 4*(2), 70–73.
15. Larson, P. (1984). Perceptions of important nurse caring behaviors. In *Proceedings of the Oncology Nursing Society's Ninth Annual Congress* (p. 90). Pittsburgh, PA: ONS.

16. Popham, W., & Siroinik, K. (1967). *Educational statistics: Use and interpretation.* New York, NY: Harper & Row.

17. Siegel, S. (1967). *Nonparametric statistics for the behavioral sciences.* New York, NY: McGraw-Hill.

18. Benner, P. (1984). *From novice to expert: Excellence and power in clinical nursing* (p. 209). Menlo Park, CA: Addison-Wesley.

19. Davis, C. (1983). The federal role in changing health care financing. *Nursing Economics, 1*(1), 10–17; *1*(21), 98–104, 146.

20. Watson, J. (1979). *The philosophy and science of caring.* Boston, MA: Little, Brown & Company.

21. Larson, P. (1984). Important nurse caring behaviors perceived by patients with cancer. *Oncology Nursing Forum, 11*(6), 46–50.

QUESTIONS FOR REFLECTION

Baccalaureate

1. How are replication studies the same as and different from the studies they are following?
2. What you think has happened to caring as the use of technology has increased in patient care?
3. Why is it important to study the association between patients' and nurses' perceptions of nurse caring behaviors?

Master's

1. What are the independent and dependent variables in Mayer's (1987) replication study?
2. What was the strength of the correlation and the significance level for the rankings on the CARE-Q for patients' and nurses' responses on the 50 behaviors of the CARE-Q as reported by Mayer (1987)?
3. What was the highest ranked nurse caring behavior for nurses? Did that correspond with the patients' highest ranked nurse caring behavior? Explain.

Doctoral

1. How could Mayer's results on the comparison between nurses' and patients' rankings of nurse caring behaviors be explained by one type of construct validity, convergent validity?
2. How did Mayer (1987) use the t-test in her statistical analysis of nurses' and patients' rankings of nurse caring behaviors?
3. If you decide to replicate Mayer's and Larson's studies, what would your research questions be and why? Explain.

21

The Theory of Bureaucratic Caring for Nursing Practice in the Organizational Culture

Marilyn A. Ray

Understanding and changing the emerging corporate culture of the health care system to benefit humankind is the most critical issue facing the nursing educators, administrators, and practitioners. The transformation of American and other Western health care systems to corporate enterprises emphasizing competitive management and economic gain seriously challenges nursing's humanistic philosophies and theories and administrative and clinical practices. The recent refocusing of nursing as a human science and the art and science of human caring[1-3] places nursing in a vulnerable position. When pitted against the new goal of corporate advancement in health care delivery, nursing faces a loss of self-identity and an increased risk of alienation and confusion in this competitive arena.

The need for the executive team to possess knowledge of organizations as businesses[4] while continuing to support the human side of nursing practice gives direction to new forms of theory development. Relying solely on an administrative framework designed by organizational theorists or concentrating only on nurse–patient relational theories regarding direct care jeopardizes the development of a new structure to guide practice in contemporary health care organizations. A new synthesis of blending traditional management views and the nursing perspective is necessary.[5]

The purpose of the qualitative research study on which this chapter was based was to generate a theory of the dynamic structure of caring in a complex organization. The study was conducted in the cultural system of a hospital. Two theories emerged and were discovered from a content analysis of interview responses and participant observation data concerning the meaning of caring to nurse and nonnurse administrators, clinical nurses, physicians, patients, and allied health personnel. The study was intended to advance administrative and health care professionals' understanding of the hospital as a cultural system and to clarify the meaning of caring to those who work in hospitals. The goal was to initiate new administrative caring interventions for the continual growth and development of nursing practice and organizations. To this end, a brief review of the context—research, culture, bureaucratic, and caring—through which the meaning was understood and from which the theoretical knowledge was generated will be discussed. A presentation of the data analysis, results, theory development, and implications for nursing will follow.

From Ray, M. A. (1989). The theory of bureaucratic caring for nursing practice in the organizational culture. *Nursing Administration Quarterly, 13*(2), 31–42. Permission to reprint granted by Wolters Kluwer.

CONTEXT OF THE STUDY

Research Context

Interpreting the meaning of phenomena within a context is the central aim of qualitative research. "Meaning in one form or another permeates the experience of most human beings in all societies," claimed Spradley.[6] As Mishler pointed out, "Meaning is always within context and context incorporates meaning. Both are produced by human actors through their actions."[7] Thus, ethnographic and grounded theory approaches[8–10] using the techniques of interview and observation were selected to study the meaning of caring. The cultural and bureaucratic context of the hospital facilitated the discovery of both a substantive theory (knowledge grounded in data) and a formal theory (conceptual knowledge integration) of caring in the organization.

Organizations as Cultures

The concept of culture has a long history in the discipline of anthropology and has been advanced in nursing by Leininger.[11] Only since Japanese competition made culture a real issue in North America have corporations adopted the culture concept as a metaphor for understanding how organizations work.[12–15] Culture has been defined in terms of social context or in terms of cognition.[16,17]

The most contemporary definition of culture is shared meaning systems. Geertz explained that culture is "an historically transmitted pattern of meanings embodied in symbols, a system of inherited conceptions expressed in symbolic forms by means of which men [women] communicate, perpetuate, and develop their knowledge about attitudes toward life."[18] How ideas, values, and symbols relate to or transform attitudes, feelings, and behavior is the central issue in understanding culture and organizations as cultures. As del Bueno and Vincent wrote, "Cultural norms and values are reflected in [hospital] policies and practices related to dress, personal appearance, social decorum, physical environment, communication, and status symbols" (p. 16).[19]

A framework for understanding the organizational culture can be grouped under the following properties: collective, organized, multiplex, and variable.[20] Each property helps the researcher to grasp the distinctive locus of order in culture. For example, the collective nature of culture holds that every human community functions with a group consensus about the meanings of the symbols used in the communications that constitute social life. The organized nature of culture holds that customs studied are connected and comprehensible only as parts of a large organization of beliefs, norms, values, or social action from which the meaning is derived. The multiplexity of culture relates to the integration of explicit rules and beliefs and implicit or self-evident responses or what is taken for granted. Finally, variability in culture suggests that wide variations exist in culture; however, the history of cultural diversity does not preclude the search for broad principles of order as a framework for understanding. Cultures are always in transition, and organizational cultures reflect changes in the values of the dominant culture.

Organizations as Bureaucracies

Bureaucracy plays a significant role in the meanings and symbols of organizations. Despite strong views in favor of the decentralization of decision making in formal organizations, including hospitals, much of the social life in the workplace continues to be managed and controlled by the rational-legal principles of bureaucracy outlined by the sociologist Weber.[21,22] The rational-legal principles include equal treatment of all employees; reliance on expertise, skills, and experience relative to the position; introduction of specific standards of work and output; record keeping; and rules and regulations binding on employees as well as managers. In addition, in formal organizations, power flows from official authority that is vested in hierarchical roles and principles, and the allocation and exchange of resources.[23]

Perrow remarked that criticisms of bureaucracy as inflexible, inefficient, uncreative, unresponsive, and stifling are echoes of radical left or right groups. He pointed out that less often seen in organizational literature are the charges related to bureaucracy's superiority as a social tool over other forms of organization.[24]

As bureaucratization gained greater prominence in modern social development and actually advanced as a theory of social development, Weber predicted that the future would belong to the bureaucracy, not to the working class.[25] Current sociological writings in the West have borne out Weber's predictions, pointing to the bureaucratization of enterprise that can be seen, for example, in current mergers of many industrial firms, in health care organizations evolving into large-scale systems, and in society as a whole emerging as an interdependent economic multipolarity. Thus, the concept of bureaucratization is a worldwide phenomenon. Britan and Cohen stated the following: "Like it or not, humankind is being driven to a bureaucratized world whose forms and functions, whose authority and power must be understood if they are ever to be even partially controlled" (p. 27).[26]

Caring as a Conceptual Context

Caring as nurturant behavior has been afforded little scholarly attention until quite recently, although it has been essential throughout history for the preservation of human race. Not until the human enterprise was sufficiently challenged by rapidly growing technologies did the concept of caring and interhuman knowledge reach any level of prominence. In the past decade, popularized notions of caring have evolved in the marketplace and its word usage has increased markedly,

especially in advertising on radio and television and in print. Major shifts in worldviews from positivism to postcritical philosophy and human science have contributed to the growing interest in academia in human interactive knowledge.[27]

In professional nursing from Nightingale to the present, the concept of caring has been dominant, but largely taken for granted in research activities. Many nurse scholars now recognize caring as the central focus of study in the development of nursing epistemology, but "some of the critical knowledge and methodological questions have yet to be explored by nurses."[28]

Caring was the central focus of this study within the organizational culture. Although some caring theories had been developed by nurse scholars ranging from theories and philosophies of altruistic humanism to support, oblatory love, and transcultural nursing phenomena,[29,30] all preconceived theoretical constructs of caring were held in abeyance, as data were generated to allow the substantive theory to emerge from the empirical data. A literature review of relevant information was conducted after the emergence of the substantive theory to support the discovery of the formal theory.

RESEARCH APPROACH

Ethnographic and grounded theory qualitative research was conducted in an acute care, urban hospital to address the following areas: descriptions of the meaning of caring in a hospital culture, identification of categories of caring within an organization, identification of dominant caring behaviors manifested within each clinical unit, and formulation of organizational caring theory. The principal question asked to participants was, "What is the meaning of caring to you?," and interviews evolved from a process of dialogue and exploration of caring.

DATA GENERATION

More than 200 respondents participated in the study and represented all employee groups working in the hospital. The study was divided into two phases, administrative and clinical, using purposive and convenience samples, respectively. Data generation lasted a total of 7 months—4 months for the administrative phase and 3 months for the clinical phase.

The process of data generation involved the following activities by the researcher: active involvement in the everyday activities of the hospital; documentation by field notes of experiences in administrative and clinical units; in-depth interviewing about the meaning of caring using an audiotape recorder with nurse and nonnurse administrators, nurse clinicians, physicians, patients, and allied health care personnel; participant observation of administrative and clinical caring interactions; and caregiving by the researcher to interact more closely with patients. Validity and reliability of the data were established through qualitative research principles of content, face, and concurrent validity, repeated observations, and constant comparative analysis.[31,32]

DATA ANALYSIS AND RESULTS

The analytical process of the content was adapted from Spradley[33] and Glaser and Strauss[34] and involved the following: immersing the self in the transcribed and recorded data to compare, contrast, and describe the experiences of caring phenomena; looking for categories of caring by identifying and grouping like themes of the data; developing a classification system of caring categories (previously published[35]); defining categories from the data descriptions; developing and defining clinical caring categories; watching for the emergence of a substantive theory (intensive theory) grounded in the data; analyzing the substantive theory; reviewing the relevant literature; initiating deep introspection of all relevant data to facilitate insight into the meaning of the research experience, to allow for the emergence of a formal theory or extensive, integrated theory; and engaging in another review of selected literature. The formal theory was a synthesis of caring understood as a humanistic phenomenon and influenced by competing structures and processes within the organizational culture and the society as a whole. The following subsection is a presentation of the process of the discovery of substantive and formal theories.

Discovery of Substantive Theory

Prior to the discovery of the formal theory called Bureaucratic Caring, a substantive theory called Differential Caring was discovered. The data demonstrated that caring in a hospital was grounded in a mutiplicity of meanings ranging from humanistic definitions, such as empathy, love, and concern, to political–legal definitions, such as decision making, liability, and malpractice, to ethical-religious definitions, such as trust, respect, acts of "brotherly" love, and ideals of "doing unto others," and to economic definitions, such as budget management and the economic well-being of the institution. The meaning of caring in the organization emerged as differential because no clear definition or meaning of caring was identified. The meaning of caring was markedly influenced by the role and position a person held and the place within which a person worked in the organization. Caring was defined first in humanistic terms, followed by terms related to role, and finally by terms related to one's position and place within the organization. A significant interrelationship existed between the individual personalities and the culture of the hospital.

In administration and on the clinical units, the context itself to a large extent influenced how caring was defined and practiced. Primary or dominant caring descriptors could be identified. In administration, caring was defined and played out more in relation to the competition for human and material resources to sustain the economic viability of the organization itself. Nonnurse administrators saw themselves as caring by describing empathetic dimensions, but recognized their role as maintaining the organization economically and politically so that direct care to patients could be provided. Nurse administrators generally referred to caring as a humanistic concept, and expressed the need to support both the nurse and the patient directly as well as the organization through sound political and economic decisions. Often, nurse executives were in conflict between organizational goals and patient care needs.

From the perspective of the clinical units, the meaning of caring varied. On the oncology unit, caring was described and observed as intimate and spiritual, whereas in the intensive care unit, caring was identified as technical. In the emergency department, caring was described and observed as technical, political, and legal, regulated by Medicare and Medicaid, and practiced as defensive medicine and nursing to reduce professionals' fears of malpractice suits. On the medical–surgical units, caring was described and observed more specifically as a team effort, where caring activities were divided by roles and where competition for scarce resources affected patient care; on the surgery (operating room) unit, caring was described and observed as patient advocacy, teamwork, and technical competency.

Patients primarily expressed the need for human care and had to devise strategies to get what they needed or succumb to what they claimed were injustices to their humanity. Physicians' descriptions of caring were generally within the technical sphere, but they recognized the need to convey human care to patients. Allied health personnel emphasized the

meaning of caring as support both for the organization and for staff and patients.

Development of Categories of Caring

From an analysis of the descriptions of caring values, beliefs, and behaviors, the investigator classified the data under the following structural caring categories within the organizational culture of the hospital.

Political is used to describe the following factors related to the meaning of caring: role and gender stratification in the functioning of the hospital among physicians, administrators, and nurses; team nursing (or the division of labor); decision making; patterns of communication; union activities; processes of negotiation; confrontation; external government and insurance company influences; uses of power, prestige, and privilege; and in general, competition for scarce (human and material) resources to maintain and sustain the organization.

Economic is used to describe the following factors related to the meaning of caring: money, budget, and insurance systems; and in general, allocation of scarce (human and material) resources in maintaining the economic viability of the organization.

Legal is used to describe the following factors related to the meaning of caring: accountability, responsibility, rules and principles to guide behaviors, informed consent, client and professional rights, rights to privacy, problems of malpractice, and liability leading to the practices of defensive medicine and nursing.

Technological/physiological is used to describe the following factors related to the meaning of caring: use of machinery in relation to maintaining the physiological well-being of the patient, nonhuman resources, and knowledge and skill needed to operate machinery to support the patient.

Educational is used to describe the following factors related to the meaning of caring: information, teaching, and informal and formal educational programs and use of audiovisual media to convey information.

Social is used to describe the following factors related to the meaning of caring: communication; social interaction and support; understanding interrelationships, involvement, and intimacy; knowing clients, families, and colleagues; humanistic potential for growth and development by acts of compassion and concern; and love and empathy.

Spiritual/religious is used to describe the following factors related to the meaning of caring: acts of faith and being spiritual, prayer, and acts of "brotherly" love, including "doing for the least of my brethren."

Ethical is used to describe the following factors related to the meaning of caring: "right" acting by religious, legal, and/or moral behavioral standards by respect and trust of and dedication to persons.

A total of 65 administrators participated in this study—28 non-nurses and 37 nurses. Table 21.1 represents the dominant caring descriptors and structural categories of caring of administrators in the hospital. Table 21.2 represents the dominant caring descriptors and structural categories of caring within the clinical units of the hospital.

Caring data from the in-depth interviews of administrators and nurse clinicians and from participant observation on all hospital clinical units demonstrated that the meaning of caring was distinct, yet integrally related to the culture of the organization. Thus, caring as synonymous with the organizational culture could be viewed as an organized and collective structure and represented a dynamic interplay of structural categories that were both humanistic and bureaucratic.

Theoretical sampling refined, elaborated, and exhausted conceptual categories so that an actual integration of descriptors and categories occurred forming the substantive theory itself. As a result, a major hypothesis emerged wherein the core theory was identified. Thus, the substantive theory (knowledge generated that was intensively grounded in the data) was called Differential Caring and the theoretical statement was formulated as shown in the table.

In a hospital, differential caring is a dynamic social process that emerges as a result of the various values, beliefs, and behaviors expressed about the meaning of caring. Differential caring relates to competing educational, social, humanistic, religious/spiritual, and ethical forces as well as political, economic, legal, and technological forces within the organizational culture that are influenced by the social forces within the dominant American culture.

From the discovery of the substantive (intensive) theory, the extensive or formal Theory of Bureaucratic Caring was discovered.

Discovery of the Formal Theory of Bureaucratic Caring

Social and organizational research, nursing research, substantive theory discovered in the study, and specific philosophical knowledge were the forces for generating higher level formal theory. In integrating formal theory, the design involves a progressive building up from facts (cumulative knowledge) through substantive theory to formal grounded theory,[36] and is induced primarily by

TABLE 21.1 Differential Caring in an Organizational Culture: Caring Categories of Administrators

Role	Number	Dominant Caring Descriptors	Structural Caring Categories
Non-nurse administrators	28	Empathy	Social
		Communication	Political
		Economic management	Economic
		Effective competition	Spiritual
		Responsibility/attitude	Ethical
Nurse administrators	37	Empathy	Social
		Communication	Political
		Time management	Economic
		Rapport	Spiritual
		Budget decisions	
		Spiritual concern	

Table 21.2 Differential Caring in an Organizational Culture: Caring Categories on Clinical Units

Units	Dominant Caring Descriptors	Structural Caring Categories
Admission department	Involvement	Social
	Financial involvement	Political
		Economic
		Spiritual/religious
		Ethical
Emergency department	Technical competence	Technological/physiological
	Malpractice prevention	Educational
	Government dependency	Political
		Economic
		Legal
Intensive care unit	Technical competency	Technological/physiological
	Value conflict	Ethical
Cardiac laboratories	Technical competency	Technological/physiological
	Involvement	Social
Oncology	Involvement	Educational
	Intimacy	Social
	Spiritual care	Spiritual/religious
Surgery	Advocacy	Legal
	Team interrelationships	Social
	Technical competency	Political
		Technological/physiological

(*continued*)

Table 21.2 Differential Caring in an Organizational Culture: Caring Categories on Clinical Units (*continued*)

Units	Dominant Caring Descriptors	Structural Caring Categories
Recovery room	Team interrelationships	Social
	Technical competency	Political
		Technological/physiological
Surgical	Team (intra/interhierarchical role functioning)	Social
		Political
		Economic
Medical	Involvement	Political
	Team (intra/interhierarchical role functioning)	Economic
		Social
Transitional (step down)	Involvement	Social
	Interpersonal relationships	Political
	Technical competency	Economic
		Technological/physiological
Rehabilitation (drug/alcohol, cardiac)	Involvement	Social
	Independence	Educational
	Egalitarianism	Political
Pediatrics	Safety	Legal
	Involvement	Social
	Unit maintenance	Political
Obstetrics and gynecology	Involvement	Social
	Team (intra/interhierarchical role functioning)	Political
Delivery room	Technical competency	Technological/physiological
	Teaching	Educational
	Involvement	Social

comparative analysis and insight into the whole of the experience. Bureaucratic Caring thus emerged as the formal or extensive theory represented in Figure 21.1. The discovery of the formal Theory of Bureaucratic Caring from the substantive Theory of Differential Caring within an organizational culture and the additional review of the literature on organizations as bureaucracies was a complex process. This process that led to the development and ultimate synthesis of the theory was inductive and logical. It was inductive in building on the data from the substantive theory and the literature and logical in using the philosophical argument of Hegel's dialectic[37,38] to synthesize bureaucracy and caring to a new structural form called bureaucratic caring.

DISCUSSION

The formal Theory of Bureaucratic Caring was a result of a dialectical synthesis between the thesis of caring as humanistic, social, educational, ethical, and religious/spiritual and the antithesis of caring as economic, political, legal, and technological (elements of bureaucracy). To clarify the processes

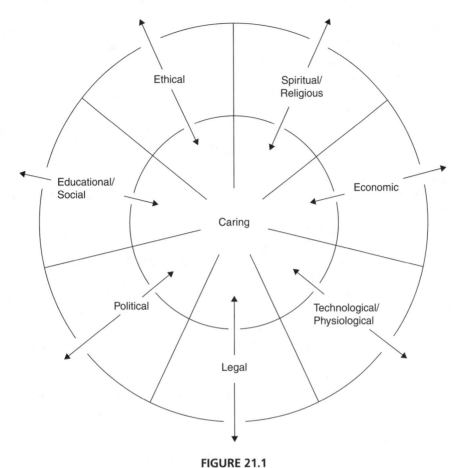

FIGURE 21.1

A bureaucratic caring structure.

involved in a dialectical theory, Moccia outlined the laws of the dialectic based on the philosophies of Hegel and Marx.

The laws of the dialectic demonstrated that the understanding of caring as a whole is merely its essential nature in contemporary organizational culture, reaching its completeness through the process of its own becoming.[39] These laws are the transformation of quantity into quality (qualitative difference), the connecting of polar opposites into a codetermining relationship (interidentification), the negation of the negation (thesis, antithesis, and synthesis), and the spiral form of development (transformation and change)[40] used to reinforce the argument in the generation of a formal Theory of Bureaucratic Caring. For nursing, the dialectic between the traditional thesis of caring as humanistic and the modern antithesis of caring as bureaucratic interidentified as a synthesis of bureaucratic caring is a superior form of caring in the contemporary world.

The logical connectedness of caring to the cosmopolitan social order demonstrates that the Theory of Bureaucratic Caring is unifying rather than alienating. It is a construct put together by analyzing the diverse changes in the nature of caring in the contemporary hospital culture. When integrated or synthesized, the concept of caring becomes coherent. Bureaucratic caring is a natural historical process for nursing. Sovie[41] wrote that nursing is experiencing the trends of a maturing profession. She identified the following concepts related to professional maturation outlined by Schein: convergence, differentiation, and bureaucratization. When these maturational concepts are applied to this study of caring in the organizational culture, significant analogies can be made. First, caring is the convergent focus of professional nursing[42,43]; second, in this research, caring is highly differential depending on its structures (ethical, religious/spiritual, social, educational, political, economical, legal, and technological/physiological); and third, caring is bureaucratic given the extent to which its meaning can be understood in relation to the rational–legal social structure of the hospital and the extent to which the concept of bureaucratization is a vital part of the whole social structure of humankind.[44,45]

Understanding the full meaning and interpretation of caring in the organization as bureaucratic caring can give clearer direction to the formulation of more purposeful caring goals within the health care organizations.

IMPLICATIONS FOR NURSING PRACTICE

The mandate for the application and implementation of nursing theory to guide nursing administration and clinical practice has been given to nurse executives.[46,47] Stevens asserted that some theories may be more effective for a given setting than another. The Theory of Bureaucratic Caring is the most effective for administrative and clinical practices because it is grounded in the everyday world of organizational experience. The Theory of Bureaucratic Caring as a synthesis of the two primary components of nursing in organizations—caring and bureaucratic components that make up the functioning of complex organizational systems—sets the stage for new organizational development.

Organizational development is an effort to democratize and humanize work; it emphasizes both executive team and staff participation.[48] People create organizational cultures and either facilitate their transformation or contribute to their disintegration. To deal with the challenges of the new corporate culture, it is helpful to view organizational development from the human side using the Theory of Bureaucratic Caring generated from the values, beliefs, and behaviors of persons within the organization. This approach can be used to develop mechanisms for creative problem solving. Thus, from this perspective, the executive team can recognize the vital nature of the bureaucratization of caring as a new structure that needs different principles for directing innovations in caring and organizational development policy.

Changes in the health care environment have raised many questions related to patient care. How are political, economical,[49] legal, and technological[50] caring decisions made? How is spiritual caring fostered? How can ethical caring be the grounds on which moral decisions are made? What new policies must be designed to enhance the human perspective in corporate policy, and how will these principles and policies guide actions? The impact of the Theory of Bureaucratic Caring on the corporate enterprise will necessitate a system shift from a narrow to a broad focus where management and caring views can exist side by side and realistically represent the transformation of health care organizations to benefit humankind.

REFERENCES

1. Leininger, M. M. (Ed.). (1981). *Caring: An essential human need*. Thorofare, NJ: Charles B. Slack.
2. Leininger, M. M. (Ed.). (1984). *Care: The essence of nursing and health*. Thorofare, NJ: Charles B. Slack.
3. Watson, J. (1979). *Nursing: The philosophy and science of caring*. Boston, MA: Little, Brown.
4. Miller, K. L. (1987). The human care perspective in nursing administration. *Journal of Nursing Administration, 17*, 10–12.
5. Jennings, B. M., & Meleis, A. I. (1988). Nursing theory and administrative practice: Agenda for the 1990s. *Advances in Nursing Science, 10*(3), 56–69.

6. Spradley, J. P. (1979). *The ethnographic interview* (p. 95). New York, NY: Holt, Rinehart & Winston.

7. Mishler, E. G. (1979). Meaning in context: Is there any other kind? *Harvard Educational Review, 49*(2), 14.

8. Hammersley, M., & Atkinson, P. (1983). *Ethnography: Principles and practices.* New York, NY: Tavistock.

9. Glaser, B., & Strauss, A. (1967). *The discovery of grounded theory: Strategies for qualitative research.* Chicago, IL: Aldine.

10. Glaser, B. (1978). *Theoretical sensitivity.* Mill Valley, CA: The Sociology Press.

11. Leininger, M. (1978). *Transcultural nursing: Concepts, theories and practices.* New York, NY: Wiley.

12. Ray, M. (1981). *A study of caring within an institutional culture* (PhD. Dissertation, University of Utah, Salt Lake City, Utah).

13. Britan, G. M., & Cohen, R. (Eds.). (1980). *Hierarchy and society: Anthropological perspectives on bureaucracy.* Philadelphia, PA: ISHI.

14. Morgan, G. (1986). *Images of organization.* Beverly Hills, CA: Sage.

15. del Bueno, D. J., & Vincent, P. M. (1986, October). Organizational culture: How important is it? *Journal of Nursing Administration, 16*, 15–20.

16. Morgan, G. (1986). *Images of organization.* Beverly Hills, CA: Sage.

17. LeVine, R. A. (1984). Properties of culture: An ethnographic view. In R. A. Shweder & R. A. LeVine (Eds.), *Culture theory: Essays on mind, self and emotion.* New York, NY: Cambridge University Press.

18. Shweder, R. A. (1984). Previews: A colloquy of culture theorists. In R. A. Shweder & R. A. LeVine (Eds.), *Culture theory: Essays on mind, self and emotion.* New York, NY: Cambridge University Press.

19. del Bueno and Vincent, "Organizational culture: How important is it?"

20. LeVine, Properties of culture: An ethnographic view.

21. Perrow, C. (1979). *Complex organizations: A critical essay* (2nd ed.). Glenview, IL: Scott, Foresman.

22. Bell, D. (1974). *The coming of post-industrial society.* New York, NY: Basic Books.

23. Blau, P. M. (1974). *On the nature of organizations.* New York, NY: Wiley.

24. Perrow. *Complex organizations: A critical essay.*

25. Bell. *The coming of post-industrial society.*

26. Britan and Cohen. *Hierarchy and society: Anthropological perspectives on bureaucracy.*

27. Bernstein, R. J. (1983). *Beyond objectivism and relativism: Science, hermeneutics and praxis.* Philadelphia, PA: University of Pennsylvania Press.

28. Watson, J. (1985). *Nursing: Human science and human care.* Norwalk, CT: Appleton-Century-Crofts.

29. Leininger. *Caring: An essential human need.*

30. Leininger. *Care: The essence of nursing and health.*

31. Brink, P., & Wood, M. (1988). *Basic steps in planning nursing research: From question to proposal.* Boston, MA: Jones and Bartlett.

32. Glaser and Strauss. *The discovery of grounded theory: Strategies for qualitative research.*

33. Spradley. *The ethnographic interview.*

34. Glaser and Strauss. *The discovery of grounded theory: Strategies for qualitative research.*

35. Ray, M. A. (1984). The development of a classification system of institutional caring. In M. M. Leininger (Ed.), *Care: The essence of nursing and health.* Thorofare, NJ: Charles B. Slack.

36. Glaser, B. (1978). *Theoretical sensitivity.* Mill Valley, CA: The Sociology Press.

37. Moccia, P. (1985, November 1–2). *The dialectics of theory development.* Paper presented at the conference, "Qualitative Research: Viable, Valuable and Visible," The University of Akron, Akron, OH.

38. Moccia, P. (Ed.). (1986). *New approaches to theory development.* New York, NY: National League for Nursing, Pub. No. 15-1992.

39. Moccia, ed. *New approaches to theory development.*

40. Moccia. "The dialectics of theory development."

41. Sovie, M. (1978). Nursing: A future to shape. In N. L. Chaska (Ed.), *The nursing profession: Views through the mist.* New York, NY: McGraw-Hill.

42. Leininger. *Caring: An essential human need.*

43. Leininger. *Care: The essence of nursing and health.*

44. Britan and Cohen. *Hierarchy and society: Anthropological perspectives on bureaucracy.*

45. Bell. *The coming of post-industrial society.*

46. Chaska, N. L. (1983). Theories of nursing and organizations: Generating integrated models for administrative practice. In N. L. Chaska (Ed.), *The nursing profession: A time to speak.* New York, NY: McGraw-Hill.

47. Stevens, B. (1983). Applying nursing theory in nursing administration. In N. L. Chaska (Ed.), *The nursing profession: A time to speak.* New York, NY: McGraw-Hill.

48. Fisher, D. (1980). A review of organizational development. *Journal of Nursing Administration, 10*, 31–36.

49. Ray, M. A. (1987). Health care economics and human caring in nursing: Why the moral conflict must be resolved. *Family and Community Health, 10*(1), 35–43.

50. Ray, M. A. (1987). Technological caring: A new model in critical care. *Dimensions of Critical Care Nursing, 6*, 166–173.

QUESTIONS FOR REFLECTION

Baccalaureate

1. Was an inductive or deductive approach used by Ray (1989) to determine the Theory of Bureaucratic Caring for nursing practice in the organizational culture?
2. How are organizations described as cultures according to Ray (1989)?
3. What were the characteristics of the respondents in Ray's study? Describe them.

Master's

1. What were the data sources identified by Ray (1989) in her study on bureaucratic caring for nursing practice in the organizational culture? Describe and list them.
2. How were the categories of caring developed? List them.
3. What were Ray's (1989) tacit and explicit assumptions as she approached the study of caring in organizational cultures?

Doctoral

1. What did you learn about the data analysis approach used by Ray (1989) to determine the results of her investigation? Explain her adaptation of Spradley's (1979) and Glaser and Strauss's (1967) methods.
2. What is the difference between the substantive Theory of Differential Caring and the formal Theory of Bureaucratic Caring? Use grounded theory sources to substantiate your answer.
3. What are the implications for clinical practice of Ray's (1989) Theory of Bureaucratic Caring for nursing practice in the organizational culture?

22

Caring About–Caring For: Moral Obligations and Work Responsibilities in Intensive Care Nursing

Agneta Cronqvist, Töres Theorell, Tom Burns, and Kim Lützén

Nursing care is claimed to be an ethical enterprise by several researchers because it is based on society's (moral) obligation to care for others[1–5] who temporarily or over a longer period of time are unable to care for themselves. Moreover, the growing amount of literature on bioethics substantiates not only a theoretical interest in understanding the morality of care but also a heightened awareness of the complexity of ethical problems in clinical practice. One such area is the intensive care unit (ICU) characterized, for example, by advanced technology, a high working tempo, and crucial end-of-life decisions for critically ill patients. These aspects of nursing raise ethical questions, particularly which situations concern nurses and what type of moral knowledge is needed to deal with ethical questions.

Sarvimäki[6] suggests that moral knowledge consists of four aspects. Briefly, these can be recognized as theoretical ethical knowledge, moral action knowledge (how to), personal moral knowledge (motivation to act), and situational moral knowledge (moral awareness). A morally integrated person exhibits these four aspects. Nurses' moral knowledge may promote a reflective, ethical attitude and thereby support them in their professional growth.[4,6]

It is well known that caring for critically ill patients in intensive care means encountering situations with an ethical constituent. Earlier studies have focused on these situations from a problematic perspective, implying that they are always prone to be problematic and conflictual in nature.[7–9] A predetermined definition of the term "ethical difficulty" was, for example, used as a focus in studies by Söderberg[7] and Sørlie.[9] In intensive care, the different ways of reasoning between nurses and physicians concerning ethical problems[10] may reflect on the different aspects of ethics. A common theme for both nurses and physicians in ICUs can be related to "too much treatment." The physicians described it from a decision-making perspective, that is, they are responsible for making decisions; the nurses described it from an executive perspective, meaning that they carry out what is ordered. In this study, we were open to the possibility that nurses could have moral concerns without viewing these as conflicts or dilemmas.

THEORETICAL PERSPECTIVE

In this study, we focus on nurses' experiences of situations in ICUs that contain a

From Cronqvist, A., Theorell, T., Burns, T., & Lützén, K. (2004). Caring about–caring for: Moral obligations and work responsibilities in intensive care nursing. *Nursing Ethics*, *11*(1), 63–76. Permission to reprint granted by Sage Publications, Inc.

moral constituent from the perspective of relational ethics, sometimes referred to as ethics of care. Within this perspective, it is understood that nursing/caring is a moral enterprise or a moral value.[1,3–5,11] Caring is a relational concept and involves caring about someone.[3,5] The way in which this relationship is described and conceptualized as a "dispositional notion of care" involves a willingness to be open for others (patients) as individuals with special needs, beliefs, desires and wants (p. 150).[5] Caring can be characterized in qualities such as compassion, competence, confidence, conscience, and commitment and can also be based on sharing and mutual respect. When a person is seen as a living being (a whole person, not fragmented into objective parts of the body), then every relationship becomes unique to both the receiver and the giver of care.[12] This type of caring relationship is not limited to the nurse–patient dyad but also comprises the relationship nurses have with other nurses, physicians, and coworkers.

To refer to the term "ethical" on a theoretical level with principles and theories and apply the term "moral" to the manifestation of what is right and wrong and good and bad in practice is an oversimplification. In the literature, there is no clear-cut difference between the two terms. In this study, they are used interchangeably, with one exception. When we formulated the interview questions, the term ethics was preferred because we understood that this is used in everyday language in Swedish health care.

AIM OF THE STUDY

The aim of this study is to analyze experiences of moral concern in intensive care nursing from the perspective of relational ethics. The main questions raised were: what situations are ICU nurses morally concerned about and how do they reason about them?

METHOD

Study Background

This study is a part of a project focusing on different aspects of intensive care nurses' experience of critical care situations and is in parts described elsewhere.[13] The participants were employed in general, thoracic, and neonatal ICUs in Sweden. High technology, a high working pace, parsimonious budgets, and frequent reorganizations of the structure of care were common characteristics of the ICU contexts. All the participants described their working situation as unsatisfactory because they could not meet the needs of the patients. All sites were filled to overcapacity at the time of the study, which meant, according to the respondents, that at times "impossible prioritization of patient care" was required. Nurses were expected, for example, to give priority to newly admitted patients. There was also a shortage of specially trained intensive care nurses. The consequence was that newly employed and inexperienced nurses were required to take full responsibility for making decisions and carrying out tasks without having sufficient experience and training.

Selection of Participants and Procedure

Ten head nurses representing the 10 ICUs in Sweden were contacted by telephone and asked to participate in the study. Contact with staff nurses who were willing to take part was made possible with the help of these head nurses. Ethical principles for conducting research were applied by giving written and oral information about the purpose of the study, obtaining informed consent from the participants, and guaranteeing confidentiality and anonymity during analysis and publication of the results. All 36 nurses who were invited agreed to participate. Their length of experience varied from 1 to 32 years; two respondents were male.

The participants were asked to give an example of an ethical situation that they had experienced in the ICU in which they worked. The interviews were conducted privately according to the participants' own choice, in a room adjacent to the ICU ($n = 32$), at a university office ($n = 2$), or in the respondents' own home ($n = 2$). The interviews were conducted either during working hours or immediately before and were all audiotaped.

Analysis of Data

A qualitative content analysis as used by Berg[14] and by Coffey and Atkinson[15] was used. The process of data analysis was also influenced by Thorne et al.'s[16] interpretive description and consisted of the following five levels.

First Level of Analysis

The interviews were listened to in order to identify the responses specifically related to the interviewer's (AC) questions about ethical situations that the participants had experienced. These parts of the interviews were transcribed. A reading of all the transcripts resulted in a general overview:

- Responses that did not encompass examples of ethical situations
- Responses that portrayed ethics as integrated in practice
- Responses that contained specific examples of ethical experiences

At the same time, relevant domains were identified for further analysis. The next step was to divide the text into meaning units, guided by the identified domains. An analysis was carried out using these text units, resulting in the designation of codes, for example, descriptions of situations, feelings, opinions, reflections (on self, physicians, patients, organization, other nurses), and beliefs.

Second Level of Analysis

The codes were compared, and the codes "examples" and "description of the situation" were subsumed and described as the examples' typical features. The remaining

codes were compared, which resulted in the formulation of five categories.

Third Level of Analysis

The categories were interpreted to uncover latent meanings and consequently to form five subthemes: believing in a good death, knowing the course of events, feelings of distress, reasoning about physicians' "doings," and expressing moral awareness.

Fourth Level of Analysis

Within each subtheme, moral tensions were identified. To raise the analysis from a descriptive level to a theoretical understanding of the findings,[16] the notion of care *about* and care *for*[17] was used. Care about is to acknowledge or pay attention to another person with his or her welfare in mind, and to care for (tend to) can be described as the task-orientated dimension of care. One can care for (tend to) someone and not care about the person and, vice versa, one can care about someone and not care for the person. Health care personnel tend (care for) others as a part of their working responsibility and may not necessarily care about these people, although they often do.

Fifth Level of Analysis

As a result of contrasting the five subthemes with the theoretical notion of care about and care for, a main theme was formulated: caring about–caring for: moral obligations and work responsibilities in intensive care nursing.

Methodological and Ethical Considerations

The first author of this chapter has extensive experience in working in ICUs, which has methodological implications. On the one hand, clinical experience can contribute to an understanding of the phenomenon studied and the context and can serve as a facilitating "bridge" between interviewer and interviewee.[16] On the other hand, the experience or preunderstanding could also bias the researcher in the process of the analysis. To counteract possible research bias, regular discussions of potential interpretations of the data were held by the research team (the authors of this chapter) and with a group of doctorally prepared nurses.

The study was reviewed by the Ethics Committee, Faculty of Medicine, Uppsala University, Sweden, which considered that a formal application was not necessary (Dnr. 99414). Confidentiality was maintained throughout the research process.

FINDINGS

General Overview of Participants' Responses

The participants' reflections on examples of ethical situations in an ICU could be divided into three general groups: responses that did not encompass examples of ethical situations, those that portrayed "ethics" as integrated in practice, and those that contained specific examples of experience of ethical situations. None of the participants referred explicitly to traditional principles or theories of ethics.

Those participants who did not give any examples of a specific ethical situation said that they had limited experience of such situations in the present unit and argued that ethical problems occur more frequently in ICUs other than in their own.

Another group of participants who did not give an example of a specific ethical situation instead claimed that the ethical dimension "was present" all the time when caring for a patient. This was expressed in "everything you do to a patient," not to expose them, not to talk about them in the third person, and also how to give adequate information to relatives. Several participants were critical of how staff members behaved and socialized in patients' rooms while carrying out nursing assignments and how they

discussed patients' medical condition with physicians.

The third group of respondents gave more detailed descriptions of ethical situations from which typical features were identified, as described below.

Typical Features of the Examples

The examples given by the participants most frequently concerned older patients who had experienced major surgery or had received advanced medical treatment, or adolescents under 12 years who had undergone organ transplantation for the first time or had received several transplants. In some examples, parents with a younger child or a newborn baby were involved. The physicians working in the unit or the anesthetist were also frequently mentioned in the participants' examples. Two typical situations dominated the examples: withdrawing and withholding treatment. These were expressed in terms of giving either too much treatment or administering meaningless treatment.

Main Theme

"Caring about–caring for: tensions between moral obligations and work responsibilities in intensive care nursing" was identified as the main theme (Figure 22.1).

The notion of caring about rests on moral grounds because moral obligation is inherent in that notion and assumes a personal ability to know what is morally good to do in a caring situation. Caring about also implies that there is a genuine concern about the well-being of the other. In this study, a genuine concern for patients in terms of feelings, beliefs, and insight into patients' vulnerability were expressed in the participants' examples of ethical situations (see Figure 22.1).

Caring for is a task-orientated nursing care that is assigned and controlled by "others" (employers, superiors, and physicians) and can be considered a moral obligation to fulfill work responsibilities. Caring for rests on what organizations provide as guidelines concerning practical,

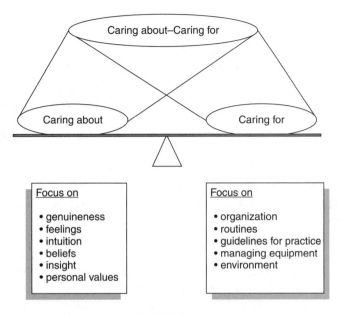

FIGURE 22.1

Caring about–caring for: Tensions between moral obligations and work responsibilities in intensive care nursing.

technical, and medical assessments (see Figure 22.1).

As the analysis shows, tensions occur when caring for and caring about a patient cannot be achieved at the same time. The four subthemes reflect this type of tension. In the fifth subtheme, the balance between caring about and caring for is in part maintained.

Subthemes

The five subthemes related to caring about and caring for were identified as: (1) believing in a good death, (2) knowing the course of events, (3) feelings of distress, (4) reasoning about physicians' "doings," and (5) expressing moral awareness. The presentation of the subthemes given below begins with a description of how they relate to the notions of caring about—caring for, followed by a presentation of the content of each subtheme. Finally, an explanation of how moral tension occurs within each subtheme is given.

Believing in a Good Death

Beliefs, or convictions of what is morally good, were found as constituents in the notion of caring about (see Figure 22.1). Beliefs were specifically expressed as values related to death and suffering. The participants believed that "to let a suffering patient die" was more morally justified than allowing him or her to suffer, for example, from painful medical interventions that would only stall the inescapable event of death. In critical care, death is a frequent reality, and the purpose of intensive care is to save lives as long as it is possible. Yet it is an inevitable fact that not all patients will survive. The participants expressed the ambiguity of these types of situations with comments such as "people have the right to die," but asking rhetorically, "why can't she [patient] be allowed to die?" Another believed that "there has to be somewhere you are allowed to die when the body has given up."

As our results showed, the participants were concerned about not allowing older patients die, as one explained: "It often happens that very old people aren't allowed to die." They also believed that patients should "die peacefully and with dignity," but "to die naturally in the ICU is not allowed." One believed that "it is a respect for life to be allowed to die" when it is time.

Some respondents attempted to explain the resistance to allowing patients to die naturally in that it could be seen as a failure and that there were no limits in what it would "cost" to keep a patient alive. As one said, "Sometimes I think this is the only ward where you eat yourself to death because they [patients] have tube feeding right to the end." What she was referring to was the routine of giving nutrition to dying patients.

The way that the participants commented on patients' death and dying, the right to die, how to die, and the possible resistance to allowing patients to die illustrates that they had an idea about what a "good death" was and that this was desirable. Moreover, they believed that caring about a "good death" is a moral and personal value. Thus, a tension seems to exist between these nurses' personal value of care, "a good death," and the wish to achieve this versus the broad purpose of intensive care, which is to save lives using all available resources.

Knowing the Course of Events

The subtheme "knowing the course of events" indicates the participants' intuitive feeling leading to an awareness of what will occur in a specific situation. In knowing the course of events, their awareness attuned to the specifics in the situation seemed to be based on their earlier experience of similar situations. Feelings and intuitions also have significance in caring about because they "tell" the individual what is at stake (see Figure 22.1). In this study, at a certain point of time during a patient's critical period, the participants

"knew" that the patient was not going to survive.

The respondents described situations in which they had been at the bedside of a patient for a long time, administering treatments and monitoring the possible effects. They also followed up patients' and families' emotional ups and downs related to arousing families' hopes at the start of new treatment and disappointment when the treatment had no effect. The participants thought that this was "an endless suffering" and believed that each new treatment effort only caused the patient more harm and was of no benefit. Feelings of meaninglessness dominated the examples, as one expressed: "They [patients] are put on a ventilator and will never come off and then you know that they will never regain consciousness."

Some respondents were convinced that all nurses in ICUs shared the same knowledge and understanding concerning the course of events. Some examples were "everybody knows about the poor prognosis," "everybody understands that this is not going to work [the patient will not survive]," and "everybody knows that he [the patient] will not make it."

This assumed that shared knowledge was identified as an attempt to justify their own knowledge of the course of events (i.e., the patient was going to die against all the odds to survive).

A tension occurs between knowing the course of events and the organizational goal to save lives via treatment. The participants were caught between their beliefs about "allowing a patient to die," as a moral "good" (caring about) and their responsibility to carry out the duties defined by the organization (caring for).

Feelings of Distress

Feelings of distress serve as a signal telling (us) that something is wrong in a situation or as a reaction to a difficult situation. That is, in certain situations, feelings of discomfort (and pleasure) arise and thereby serve to distinguish a right action from a wrong action.

These feelings can be described as a form of intuitive "knowledge" about what the participants believe is best for the patient, and, as such, be a dimension of the notion of caring about (see Figure 22.1). When the participants gave examples of moral situations, they spontaneously reflected on the situation. On behalf of themselves, they were bothered and distressed and talked about their own difficulties and limitations. Those with limited experience of nursing expressed a sort of self-reflection when discussing the care of patients who suffered from multiorgan failure and of transplant patients with complicated aftercare. One participant said, "In the beginning I had a hard time [understanding, coping] . . . I think it is very unsatisfactory, [thinks] I think it is frustrating with intensive care." The more experienced nurses also had feelings of distress when they reflected on critical situations, for example, when taking care of children: "If you are not used to care for [sick] children then it is even harder to keep a professional attitude while being terrified, [laughing] that is hard [to cope with]."

Another example of distress was when the participants came to realize that they did not agree with the physicians and said, for example,

> Sometimes you get a little frustrated when you don't feel like doing anything more or just withdraw [treatment], and then there are physicians who say "not yet" and then you are in a jam . . . [thinks] that could sometimes be very frustrating.

When the respondents expressed, for example, their own frustration in these examples, they also seemed to express their own vulnerability. A tension seems to exist between the patient's vulnerability and the nurse's vulnerability, for example, when nurses are attempting to relieve a patient's suffering while at the same time having a personal need for emotional support. Another problem is that nurses may not have the opportunity to deal with their own needs because of the time limitations of intensive care nursing.

In the high-speed ICU environment with critically ill patients demanding minute-by-minute decisions, it is distressing for nurses not to find a moment to themselves to contemplate and to obtain support.

Reasoning About Physicians' "Doings"

In the ICU, the physician is the authority governing the organization of care and has specific responsibility for the highly specialized medical treatment administered. This responsibility is upheld by an organizational structure consisting of schedules, instructions, and guidelines. These features are also characteristics of the notion caring for (see Figure 22.1). In practice, physicians are responsible for medical treatment and the guidelines that nurses must follow and execute. Collaboration between nurses and physicians is often intense, and it is necessary for them to maintain a good working relationship. Both the nurses and the physicians are expected to work together for *each* patient, although they have different responsibilities. Nurses have responsibility for fewer patients than physicians; they are at the bedside, closely monitoring the patient's condition, sometimes for many hours. Physicians have responsibility for more patients, who may be cared for on different wards. In times of heavy workload, physicians are not as available as nurses may wish. In this study, the participants reflected on or questioned the actions taken and orders given by physicians concerning withdrawing or withholding treatment. Some criticized the physicians as a group, for example:

> The physicians are more like, you know— we must try this [treatment] and this can have an effect—but in my eyes I already see a dead patient.

> The physicians do have different opinions [thinks] about what matters.

Other participants expressed criticism of physicians by describing specific situations. An example of this was when a "do-not-resuscitate-order" was made for a patient who was considered not to have any chance of survival, yet the physicians ordered dialysis and tube feeding. The participant believed that these were contradictory orders: not to resuscitate (i.e., to allow the patient to die when the heart stops) while giving dialysis so that waste products in the blood would not be toxic to the patient and lead to coma and death. The nurse thought that this was an illogical way of ordering care and the question should be asked: What type of death is acceptable when death as a consequence of severe kidney failure seems to be preferred to cardiac arrest?

Another criticism of the physicians was expressed by referring to them in the third person, as demonstrated in this example:

> when patients deteriorate on the regular ward and when they [patients] end up here [ICU] they are not allowed to die, they [physicians] push the whole battery of treatments, though you know they are not going to work [the patient will not survive].

However, other participants expressed that they acknowledge the difficulties the physicians have and felt empathy with them. An example of this is: "It is a physicians' decision to be made, perhaps in the middle of the night, and he may not be used to this ward and gets a lot of criticism from us [nurses]."

In this theme, the tension is overtly due to the participants' awareness that they disagree with what the physicians decide and do. There is disquiet between what the nurse understands as good care (caring about) and the responsibility to carry out orders as a working responsibility (caring for).

Expressing Moral Awareness

In this study, moral awareness was expressed as the ability to discuss complex caring situations from different perspectives. The feeling that "something is wrong" is an essential part of the process of becoming "aware," followed by a cognitive ability to grasp that the situations can be "looked on" from different perspectives. Caring about is characterized by the individual's ability, for example, to feel, to have insight, and to be genuine in a caring situation (see Figure 22.1). The participants expressed this dimension by the way they reflected on the situations. They also had the ability to "see" things from different angles and often referred to issues within the organizational structure, such as prioritization of patients and medical treatment (see Figure 22.1). However, they were also critical of their own beliefs and standpoints.

Most respondents gave detailed examples of situations they considered to have moral significance. Often their moral reasoning about the situation occurred without probing. When they began to analyze how and why a specific situation had originated, the participants gave various explanations of why different views among the professionals involved (e.g., on withholding treatment) were morally problematic. While deliberating about the situations they had experienced, they changed perspectives, indicating that the moral awareness of any situations concerning life or death can be contradictory in nature. An example of this type of contradiction is when one of the participants asks rhetorically, "What use is surgery on an 85-year-old person?" and then answers her own question by saying, "On the other hand we have done surgery on very old patients who have felt quite well, being grateful [thinks] then you think maybe it's worthwhile at least to try."

Another respondent claimed that nurses often have thoughts about why a treatment is not withdrawn in situations when it seems futile and there is no chance that the patient can survive. Occasionally, there is a possibility that the patient will survive against all odds, as one nurse said, "Patients that you believe do not have any chance [to survive] and then really do it."

The way in which the participants expressed their moral awareness indicates that they were also aware of the different perspectives involved in the situations. Their way of reasoning illuminated dimensions of the concepts of caring for and caring about. By expressing a moral awareness and their reflection on situations, they attempted to balance their moral obligations and work responsibilities.

DISCUSSION

The aim of this study was to explore nurses' experiences of situations that had a moral constituent in intensive care from the perspective of relational ethics. The way these intensive care nurses answered the question illuminated a most complex picture of their working situation. Shogan[17] introduced the concept of "care about–care for" as a pedagogical perspective on moral motivation (p. 7). In this study, the same interrelated concepts were found to be a relevant conceptualization for explaining intensive care nurses' experiences. As the findings imply, nurses do not seem to be able to balance moral obligations and work responsibilities that call for different actions to reduce the tension that emerges. It may be that the lack of a shared value system, different professional expectations, and different levels of knowledge and experience lead to different caring for or caring about priorities. Is this a comparison between nurses and physicians? Thus, the question becomes, how can caring about and caring for be integrated into nursing interventions without leading to tension between these two dimensions?

The results of this study seem to characterize moral dimensions of everyday practice in the context of intensive care. By feeling, knowing, and believing

(values) these nurses demonstrated a type of moral awareness, which can also be described as a personal moral knowledge.[6] A morally integrated person, according to Sarvimäki,[6] should exhibit both theoretical ethical knowledge and moral action (practical) knowledge. However, in this study, the participants did not articulate any traditional ethical principle or theory. In that sense, on applying Sarvimäki's idea, they would not have knowledge at the theoretical ethical level. Instead, they viewed ethics as a type of value system, saying that ethics is present in everything they do. Whether these nurses actually have moral action knowledge (i.e., the application of moral knowledge in practice) is a question that needs further exploration and calls for other research methods, such as participant observation.

The nurses who said that they could not give examples of any ethical situations are interesting. Whether they did not see situations as "morally" relevant or lacked the ability to reflect on moral issues, or whether they chose not to talk about them, cannot readily be answered. According to Heath,[18] nurses vary in their verbalizing skills, yet this should not be a barrier to reflection. However, if we are to believe that these nurses chose not to talk about their moral experiences, maintaining so-called moral muteness, it seems necessary to explore the reasons for this. Moreover, if reasoning abilities are indeed a central part of a caring about response[17] and if reflection is decisive for the development of clinical knowledge and ethical judgement,[4] what does this mean for a nurse who does not have these abilities?

The theme believing in a good death indicates that the process of dying, as perceived by the participants, can be viewed as good or bad. A good death is similar to the alternative concepts of a "healthy death"[19] and a "natural death."[20] Seymore[20] has identified four aspects of natural death in the ICU: (1) the process of dying is not prolonged or rushed (timing);

(2) technical death is aligned with bodily death; (3) the family has accepted the death; and (4) careful planning of withdrawal of treatment is made to enable control of the situation, so the family can witness a gradual, quiet, and dignified death. Whether these four conditions were met in the situations that the participants described is not clear. Instead, they highlighted ethical aspects of the dying process that may not be easily aligned according to Seymore's four aspects.

The nurses' mode of expressing certainty is prominent in the theme "knowing the course of events." This mode is similar to Wurzbach's[21] concept of moral certainty. When Wurzbach studied the experiences of moral certainty among acute care nurses, the basic themes identified were "speaking up," "standing up," and "refusing to participate." Several questions could be raised: Is this a way of arguing a personal trait and, if so, are nurses who exhibit such traits prone to working in acute care settings, or does the specific setting (acute care) foster the way in which nurses argue? Moral certainty could facilitate decision making, but it can also constitute a hindrance for in-depth discussion because it could lead to arbitrary decisions made by those in power.

The theme feelings of distress refers to the participants' own feelings, frustrations, and concerns in ethical situations. This state of feelings could be compared with what is considered to be moral distress.[22-24] For example, both Jameton and Wilkinson suggest that moral distress, a psychological disequilibrium or negative feeling state, refers to situations in which moral decisions are not followed through. However, the nurses in this study did not seem to express negative feelings in relation to their own decisions that were not followed. Instead, they expressed feelings, similar to distress, which had emerged in complicated caring situations. It is fair to assume that this frustration had caused feelings of stress for the nurses. In intensive

care nursing, dissonant imperatives are described as inducing stress.[13] For example, lacking the authority to act but at the same time knowing something should be done could be seen as leading to (moral) stress.

The way in which the participants reasoned about the physicians' "doings" show that nurses may approach ethical problems in different ways to physicians. Similar findings have been presented in a study from Canada[25] on end-of-life decisions, which show that physicians question themselves concerning whether they have made the right decision and nurses question the physicians' decisions. Some researchers view this divergence in collaboration as a product of power positions based on nursing existing in a highly gendered environment with strong hierarchical and patriarchal structures.[5,26,27] The tensions between the two professions continue; the boundaries between them are still somewhat diffuse and still undermined by economic constraints. Nurses attempt to handle these situations, but they are not always successful.

For the theme expressing moral awareness, the participants showed an ability to reflect but it is unclear whether this skill was applied in the situations they described. Thus, an interesting area for further research would be to explore how nurses reflect on moral concerns in concrete problematic situations and whether this reflection is put into action.

CONCLUSION

Moral concerns are inevitably inherent in intensive care. Nurses are challenged by life and death situations in which they are compelled to balance priorities. Reasoning about these situations involves believing in a good death, anticipating events, coping with feelings of distress, reasoning about physicians' "doings," and expressing moral awareness. Basic to these themes is a tension between the professional dimensions caring about—caring for and nurses' concerns about the care given. These professional dimensions are complementary but they must be kept in balance for intensive care nurses. How can these nurses be supported in maintaining this balance? Perhaps, this tension is an everyday reality for them (i.e., not all moral concerns can be solved). Therefore, there is a need to support nurses in difficult intensive care situations, for example, by mentoring focused on gaining insight into how this tension between caring about and caring for arises. This can be viewed as the first step toward developing moral action knowledge in the context of intensive care nursing.

ACKNOWLEDGMENTS

This study was supported financially by the Swedish Council for Work Life Research and the Board of Research for Health and Caring Sciences at the Karolinska Instituet (Reg. no. 3560/98 UFA and 3667/99 FFU).

REFERENCES

1. Noddings, N. (1984). *Caring—A feminine approach to ethics and moral education*. Berkeley, CA: University of California Press.
2. Bishop, A. H., & Scudder, J. R. (1991). *The practical, moral, and personal sense of nursing*. Albany, NY: State University of New York Press.
3. Tschudin, V. (1992). *Ethics in nursing: The caring relationship* (2nd ed.). Oxford, UK: Butterworth-Heinemann.
4. Benner, P., Tanner, C. A., & Chesla, C. A. (1996). *Expertise in nursing practice*. New York, NY: Springer.
5. Kuhse, H. (1996). *Caring: Nurses, women and ethics*. Oxford, UK: Blackwell.
6. Sarvimäki, A. (1995). Aspects of moral knowledge in nursing. *Scholarly Inquiry for Nursing Practice, 9*: 343–353.
7. Söderberg, A. (1999). The practical wisdom of enrolled nurses, registered nurses and physicians in situations of ethical difficulty in intensive care [Dissertation] (Umeå University Medical Dissertations, new series no. 603.). Umeå University: Umeå.
8. Bunch, E. H. (2001). Hidden and emerging drama in a Norwegian critical care unit: Ethical dilemmas in the context of ambiguity. *Nursing Ethics, 8*, 57–67.
9. Sørlie, V. (2001). Being in ethically difficult care situations. Narrative interviews with registered nurses and physicians within internal medicine, oncology and paediatrics [Dissertation] (Umeå University Medical Dissertations, new series no. 727.). Umeå University: Umeå.
10. Söderberg, A., & Norberg, A. (1993). Intensive care: Situations of ethical difficulty. *Journal of Advanced Nursing, 18*, 2008–2014.
11. Gilligan, C. (1982). *In a different voice: Psychological theory and women's development*. Cambridge, MA: Harvard University Press.
12. Bergum, V. (1994). Knowledge for ethical care. *Nursing Ethics, 1*, 71–79.
13. Cronqvist, A., Burns, T., Theorell, T., & Lützén, K. (2001). Dissonant imperatives in nursing: A conceptualisation of stress in intensive care in Sweden. *International Critical Care Nursing, 17*, 228–236.
14. Berg, B. L. (1995). *Qualitative research methods for the social sciences*. Boston, MA: Allyn and Bacon.
15. Coffey, A., & Atkinson, P. (1996). *Making sense of qualitative data*. London: SAGE.
16. Thorne, S., Kirkham, S. H., & MacDonald-Emes, J. (1997). Focus on qualitative methods. Interpretive description: A noncategorical qualitative alternative for developing nursing knowledge. *Research in Nursing & Health, 20*, 169–177.
17. Shogan, D. (1988). *Care and moral motivation*. Toronto, ON: OISE Press.
18. Heath, H. (1998). Reflection and patterns of knowing in nursing. *Journal of Advanced Nursing, 27*, 1054–1059.
19. Ornery, A. (1991). A healthy death. *Heart Lung, 20*, 310–311.
20. Seymore, J. E. (1999). Revisiting medicalisation and 'natural' death. *Social Science & Medicine, 49*: 691–704.
21. Wurzbach, M. E. (1999). Acute care nurses' experience of moral certainty. *Journal of Advanced Nursing, 30*, 287–293.
22. Jameton, A. (1984). *Nursing practice: The ethical issues*. Englewood Cliffs, NJ: Prentice-Hall.
23. Jameton, A. (1993). Dilemmas of moral distress: Moral responsibility and nursing practice. *AWHONN Clinical Issues, 4*, 542–551.
24. Wilkinson, J. M. (1988). Moral distress in nursing practice: Experience and effect.

Nursing Forum, 23(1), 16–29. (Original work published 1987)

25. Oberle, K., & Hughes, D. (2001). Doctors' and nurses' perception of ethical problems in end-of-life decisions. *Journal of Advanced Nursing, 33,* 707–715.

26. Sundin-Huard, D. (2001). Subject positions theory—its application to understanding collaboration (and confrontation) in critical care. *Journal of Advanced Nursing, 34,* 376–382.

27. Davies, K. (2001). *Disturbing gender. On the doctor–nurse relationship.* (Lund Studies of Sociology, Vol. 4.). Lund: Department of Sociology, Lund University.

QUESTIONS FOR REFLECTION

Baccalaureate

1. Why do you think that ICUs are associated with complex ethical problems of concern for nurses?
2. What is the difference between the term "ethical" and the term "moral" as explained by Cronvist et al. (2004) in the study on caring about–caring for?
3. What was the design of the study on moral obligations and work responsibilities in intensive care nursing? Explain.

Master's

1. What data were participants asked to describe during audio-taped interviews in Cronqvist et al.'s (2004) study?
2. What did you learn about Cronqvist et al.'s (2004) data analysis levels? Describe the levels used.
3. Which type of patients were often involved in the situations described by ICU nurse participants in Cronqvist et al.'s (2004) study? Why do you think that was so?

Doctoral

1. How did Cronqvist et al.'s (2004) study explain the moral obligations and work responsibilities of ICU nurses?
2. What did you learn about Cronqvist et al.'s (2004) integration of subthemes into the main theme of the investigation?
3. How would you describe Cronqvist et al.'s study to a group of ICU nurses? Do you think that the findings of Cronqvist et al.'s study would fit their experience? If so, how?

V

Research Designs and Methods for Studying Caring

ZANE ROBINSON WOLF

Research designs provide plans, structures, and strategies for investigators and help them make decisions about methods, procedures, and sources and types of data to be collected. They also assist investigators to answer research questions systematically. Many types of designs are available to scholars, for example, exploratory and descriptive and experimental and nonexperimental. In general, the design chosen is one that either values individuals' subjective experience or attempts to control variance or error. Each grouping consists of many types of designs; the ways to apply them are detailed in research texts, described in actual studies, and provided by expert methodologists in the literature.

The types of designs selected by investigators match the purposes and questions posed in studies. Qualitative investigations generate narrative, textual, or verbal data. Scholars often refer to such investigations as exploratory. Narratives portray the study results. In contrast, quantitative designs generate numerical data; measurement levels are nominal, ordinal, interval, and ratio and statistics depict findings. A variety of designs and methods have been used by researchers who study caring.

Scholars of caring produced a number of qualitative studies on nurse caring in the 1980s, and during that decade, the scholarly and research literature on caring began to proliferate. Some appeared in the books including papers presented at Caring Research Conferences, sponsored by the International Association for Human Caring (IAHC). The research designs on caring concepts began to diversify earlier than might be supposed. Some studies on caring used quantitative approaches, but these were not in the majority. Over the next three decades, more varieties of research designs were used by researchers investigating nurse caring and related phenomena.

The chapters in this part represent a variety of research designs useful to the investigators, as they pursued knowledge on the phenomenon and concept of caring in nursing. The designs represent phenomenology, methodological or instrument development, meta-synthesis, and Delphi technique approaches. They vary in relation to the data sources, for example, textual material obtained through dialogical interviews (Ray, 1991), items on an instrument elicited by a Likert-like scale (numerical) (Wolf, Giardino, Osborne, & Ambrose, 1994), studies using a variety of data collection approaches generating the textual data, (unstructured interview, participant observation, critical incidents, videotaped nurse–client interactions, and group narratives) (Sherwood, 1997), and a combination of the textual and numerical data (Wolf, Freshwater, Miller, Jones, & Sherwood, 2003). The first example in this section demonstrates a special kind and method of phenomenological research.

Dr. Marilyn D. Ray (Dee) (1991) created a distinctive qualitative method, caring inquiry as an esthetic process, for scholars of caring to use in research. Dr. Ray explored caring inquiry as a way of understanding compassion or caring and as an esthetic act. She introduced her chapter with a story about an elderly woman who suffered, communicating by speaking with her heart. Dee, the nurse in the situation, responded to the woman with her life of compassion and began ". . . the journey of sharing the pain that is nursing . . ." (Ray, 1991, p. 181). In this way, she positioned and ultimately revealed the complexity of being caring and studying caring for nurses. Dr. Ray also equated caring with love, a position shared with other scholars of caring. She later equated caring with compassion.

Dr. Ray proposed that heart and soul are synonyms and metaphorically symbolize life, living, sensitivity, reason, and integrity. Heart and soul represent a creative process. When the heart of the care provider is wounded by the suffering of the care recipient, the recipient enters the caregiver who feels compassion, communicates compassion, and is authentic and present in the experience. Ray noted that the compassionate way of being is an esthetic act. The caregiver shares in the life of the other and becomes the other.

According to Ray, the esthetic act of compassion brings forth the spiritual life within the nurse, and the meaning of this compassionate encounter is meta-physical and transcendent. Through this explanation, Dr. Ray underscored that by being compassionate and becoming one with the person cared for that, the creative process of caring was experienced. The presence of the nurse is substantial in the nursing situation. Understanding the meaning of nursing as caring goes beyond ordinary experience, and it is esthetically pleasing or appreciated artistically, not only by the nurse but by the nurse researcher studying caring/compassion.

Ray (1991) emphasized that when nurse researchers dwell with the material or text (e.g., transcribed interviews, stories, poems) provided by patients and others who share their thoughts, feelings, and perceptions, they understand the nature of caring. The text produced by patients and other individuals is communicated as shared remembrances or recollections. Furthermore, because compassion involves "we" or the caregiver and care recipient together, this research is a ". . . theological enterprise" (Ray, 1991, p. 183).

Dr. Ray envisioned that "caring inquiry as an esthetic process in research . . . [is] . . . a unique method of presence and dialogue" (Ray, 1991, p. 183). Phenomenology and phenomenological hermeneutics are used in this method of inquiry to generate interpretive human science. By means of this approach, researchers answer questions about the meaning of caring. Caring research generates descriptions and understandings of the meaning of being cared and becoming a caregiver through caring. The researcher used reflection to comprehend the nature of caring in the world of nursing. Reflection helps the investigator become transformed, deepening and expanding being; the researcher is open to creative forces within and outside of self.

The research process is an esthetic process for the researcher who is receptive and responsive to the text morally, spiritually, and psychologically. Ray (1991) acknowledged that the esthetic process of conducting the investigation incorporates methods of presence and dialogue to understand the experience of the *we* (caregiver) and the *other* (patient or client) engaged in a caring interaction. The esthetic process in caring inquiry is aimed at understanding the text more fully than previously. An example of a research question for such a study is as follows: what is the meaning of caring in your experience? By reflecting on the nature of caring in events as experienced, investigators learn about the world of nursing. The meaning of the experience of caring in nursing research is illuminated in this approach.

Ray proposed esthetic phenomenological hermeneutic inquiry as a method of answering such research questions (Van Manen, 1990). The process is a dynamic, scholarly, reflective, and a creative set of activities. The following are the elements of the process: (1) the intentionality of inner being of the researcher, (2) the process of dialogic experiencing, (3) the process of phenomenological hermeneutical reflecting and transforming, (4) the process of phenomenological hermeneutical theorizing to a theory of meaning, (5) dialoguing with written texts: examining similarities and differences, and (6) credibility and significance of the process of the phenomenology of the esthetic act (Ray, 1991, p. 184). The research process moves the investigator through reflection to a description and interpretation of the meaning of the experience of caring. Dr. Ray provided many details of the process. She explained the caring situation experienced by the nurse and patient with the nurse engaged in the creative process of caring. She also described the creative process of studying caring through phenomenological methods.

Wolf et al. (1994) used the research approach, termed methodological or instrument development design, to measure the dimensions of the process of nurse caring, a construct. At this stage of research on nurse caring, few investigators used experimental, quasi-experimental, correlational, factor analysis, and preexperimental research designs to examine the concept of caring in nursing. Some scholars had doubted the worth and feasibility of measuring nurse caring. They submitted that human experience was best explored through phenomenological and other qualitative methods. However, different research approaches began to appear in published sources.

The Caring Behaviors Inventory (CBI) was situated in the literature of Watson, Leininger, Larson, Riemen, Brown, and Mayer. The preliminary definition of the process of nurse caring was framed by Gaut, Watson, and Wolf. The CBI was built on an earlier version developed by Wolf (1981, 1986). The theoretical definition was an effort to operationalize the construct of the process of nurse caring. The principal investigator followed procedures of instrument development and applied measurement theory to further establish the qualities of the CBI. The CBI joined a few earlier examples of caring instruments. The CBI was designed for administration to hospitalized patients and nursing staff.

Wolf and colleagues collected data from patients and nursing staff using the revised, 43-item CBI using a 4-point scale to elicit responses. They established preliminary construct validity based on related literature, experts, and contrasted groups. They also established preliminary reliability using test–retest and internal consistency strategies. Nurse and patient responses differed when the test–retest procedure was used; this confirmed the findings of previous studies. Moreover, factorial validity was established by exploratory factor analysis, principal components method with varimax rotation. Consistent with the theoretical approach that caring was co-created by nursing and patients, both patient and nurse samples were combined ($N = 541$) in the factor analysis. In addition to the limitation of using a convenience sample, the investigators did not describe the directions for administration and how the scores were obtained and interpreted.

An initial six-factor solution was reduced to five by Wolf et al. (1994). One item was eliminated. The dimensions of nurse caring included respectful deference to other (courteous regard for the other), assurance of human presence (investment in the other's needs and security), positive connectedness (optimistic and constant readiness on the part of the nurse to help the other), professional knowledge and skill (nurse caring as proficient, informed, and skillful), and attentive to the other's experience (appreciation of and engrossment in the other's perspective and experience). This investigation might have been the first that used a large sample size that justified the application of factor analysis. Subsequent versions of the CBI have used a six-point scale to allow for greater variance on item responses. In addition, the investigators noted that the identified dimensions were consistent with Watson's Transpersonal Caring Theory. Different versions of the CBI are now published, and the instrument or a shorter version has been translated from English into Spanish, Tagalog, Persian, Greek, French, and Turkish. Many other instruments have been created and tested in efforts to measure the concept of nurse caring (Watson, 2009).

Dr. Gwen Sherwood is a long-standing scholar of caring. It is not surprising that as she attended successive Caring Conferences sponsored by IAHC and looked at the burgeoning literature on the concept, she could have decided to perform a study using meta-synthesis design (Sherwood, 1997). This research design summarizes qualitative studies using a systematic review, also called meta-synthesis (DiCenso, Guyatt, & Ciliska, 2005).

Sandelowski, Docherty, and Emden (1997) defined meta-synthesis as ". . . the theories, grand narratives, generalizations, or interpretive translations produced from the integration or comparison of findings from qualitative studies" (p. 366). Later, Finfgeld (2003) described the following three types of meta-synthesis: theory building, theory explication, and descriptive meta-synthesis. She also examined the methods of meta-synthesis and addressed strategies for establishing the integrity of findings.

Dr. Sherwood appreciated that many studies on caring were single, independent studies. She implemented a meta-synthesis of qualitative studies on caring and

indicated that a shift was needed toward research designs in the quantitative domain. Sherwood (1997) intended that her synthesis of findings from qualitative studies would result in generating essential patterns and themes. The findings would then help to increase caring knowledge and build caring theories; ultimately, such theories might guide nursing practice.

Sherwood (1997) developed the following inclusion criteria for study selection: qualitative studies describing nurses' caring from adult patients' perspectives. She focused on homogeneity across participant demographics. Rigor standards were applied to the studies. Dr. Sherwood (1997) reviewed different authors' methods of meta-synthesis and combined them into six phases of analysis. The textual data were collected by investigators of the selected studies using the following techniques: structured interviews, participant observation, critical incidents, videotaped nurse–client interactions, and group narratives. All of the studies reported similar data analysis techniques. The process of synthesis merged data from 16 qualitative studies published from 1973 to 1993. Key phrases and themes were identified.

Dr. Sherwood produced integrated descriptions of nurses' caring; common themes built essential patterns of caring. The meaning of the patterns was clarified by the themes, and the narrative on nurses' caring included defining attributes, attitudes, knowledge, and actions. A composite description was generated from responses across all studies; this description defined a universal therapeutic concept. The concept was translated into an operational model of caring with relational statements and propositions (Sherwood, 1997, p. 34).

The essential patterns resulted from the progressive synthesis of the studies as follows: healing interaction, nurses' knowledge, intentional response, and therapeutic outcomes. Caring was defined by its themes as nursing actions, behaviors, and interactions observable within the specific patterns (Sherwood, 1997, p. 38). Sherwood (1997) presented a narrative description of each pattern and provided a composite description framed by the context of acute care settings.

The therapeutic model specified the context (interaction pattern), the content (knowledge pattern), the process (response pattern), and the goals (therapeutic pattern) (Sherwood, 1997). The context was the interaction pattern described as the milieu or internal and external environment. Nurses' knowledge pattern incorporated their cognitive knowledge and knowledge of human behavior combined with specific attributes applied in the context of caring (the interaction pattern). The therapeutic pattern included the process or methods by which nurses act intentionally to accomplish goal-directed therapeutic outcomes. Nurses' knowledge of human behavior combined with attributes to form the content applied in the context of caring. Caring was defined as ". . . an integrative mode of human interaction (Roach, 1992) defined by goal-directed, intentioned, growth producing actions operationalized interactively with the care receiver" (Gaut, 1986) (Sherwood, 1997, p. 40).

Meta-synthesis studies may produce theories, generalizations, and interpretive translations from the integration or comparison of findings. New perspectives are achieved (Burns & Grove, 2009). Sandelowski and Barroso (2006) reported the outcomes of such studies and Sherwood (1997) achieved the following two of those outcomes in this investigation: clarification of conceptual and methodological issues pertaining to qualitative research integration and clarification and refinement of techniques for qualitative meta-synthesis. She also generated a definition of caring and a therapeutic model of caring, which other investigators might carry forward using quantitative designs. Dr. Sherwood's study most likely was the first meta-synthesis on nurse caring.

Wolf et al. (2003) used a Delphi technique to induce a standard of care for caring. They framed the rationale for the study in caregivers' search for quality health care practices and the trend of developing criteria, standards, and protocols to achieve quality outcomes. Their intent was to create a standard of performance expectations for caregivers, which would help the care recipients feel cared for. Ideally, the standard would shape caring practices or interventions. They hoped that the standard could be used as a guide to foster caring relationships among health care providers and consumers.

Delphi technique, developed for the RAND Project of the U.S. Air Force (Dalkey, 1969), is a method of systematically obtaining and combining informed opinions from a group of experts on specific questions or issues (Couper, 1984; Strauss & Ziegler, 1975, p. 253). Delphi questionnaires are composed of carefully designed and sequential questionnaires, interspersed with summarized information and opinion feedback. Both consensus and diverse opinion result. Iteration and controlled feedback structure procedures are used for data collection. A series of rounds, at least three, gradually narrow the opinions of anonymous participants (Strauss & Ziegler, 1975). First round questions elicit responses from the panel on open-ended questions, generating the textual data. These responses are analyzed and formatted into items that are next rated on Likert-type scales. Descriptive statistics are calculated at the end of the second round and brought forward to the third round. The third round item statistics are also calculated. During each round, responses from previous round are evaluated by the panel of experts (Goodman, 1987).

The Delphi study by Wolf et al. (2003) aimed at producing consensus from a group of scholars who were knowledgeable about caring, the expert panel. Collective and condensed group opinion was sought. Participants were recruited from the current membership list of IAHC and attendees of the 2000 Caring Conference. Both groups were assumed to be experts. Items in the Round I questionnaire included open-and closed-ended items. The researchers employed content analysis in each round to analyze the textual data. Respondents used a 5-point strongly agree, strongly disagree scale to identify rankings on questionnaire items and point to elements on the emerging standard to include or exclude. Descriptive statistics were calculated in Round II item responses. Round III items originated in statistics and textual data from second round responses.

Concerns about the emerging standard were expressed by respondents, including its origin in Western values and the importance of considering the cultural context of caring. The final Standard of Care for Caring included behaviors or actions clustered into four groupings. The authors suggested that the guideline might be used by caregivers to evaluate their caring behavior.

The variety of designs and methods used by the scholars of caring in this section to answer research questions show that the paths generate interesting findings that address the aspects of a complex phenomenon, nurse caring. All cited findings were invigorated by a passion to understand the concept of caring and reveal the importance of the concept in their research trajectory.

REFERENCES

Burns, N., & Grove, S. K. (2009). *The practice of nursing research: Appraisal, synthesis, and generation of evidence* (6th ed.). St. Louis, MO: Saunders Elsevier.

Couper, M. R. (1984). The Delphi technique: Characteristics and sequence model. *Advances in Nursing Science, 7,* 72–77.

Dalkey, N. C. (1969, June). *The Delphi method: An experimental study of group opinion.* Project RAND, United States Air Force.

DiCenso, A., Guyatt, G., & Ciliska, D. (2005). *Evidence-based nursing: A guide to clinical practice.* St. Louis, MO: Elsevier Mosby.

Finfgeld, D. L. (2003). Metasynthesis: The state of the art—so far. *Qualitative Health Research, 13,* 893–904.

Gaut, D. (1986). Evaluating caring competencies in practice. *Topics in Clinical Nursing, 8*(2), 77–83.

Goodman, C. M. (1987). The Delphi technique: A critique. *Journal of Advanced Nursing, 12,* 729–734.

Ray, M. A. (1991). Caring inquiry: The esthetic process in the way of compassion. In D. A. Gaut & M. M. Leininger (Eds.), *Caring: The compassionate healer* (pp. 181–189). New York, NY: National League for Nursing.

Roach, M. S. (1992). *The human act of caring: A blueprint for the health professions* (Rev. ed.). Ottawa, Ontario, Canada: Canadian Hospital association Press.

Sandelowski, M., & Barroso, J. (2006). *Handbook for synthesizing qualitative research.* New York, NY: Springer.

Sandelowski, M., Docherty, S., & Emden, C. (1997). Qualitative metasynthesis: Issues and techniques. *Research in Nursing and Health, 20,* 365–371.

Sherwood, G. D. (1997). Metasynthesis of qualitative analysis of caring. *Advanced Practice Nursing Quarterly, 3,* 32–42.

Strauss, H. J., & Ziegler, L. H. (1975). The Delphi technique and its uses in social science research. *Journal of Creative Behavior, 9,* 253–259.

Van Manen, M. (1990). *Researching lived experience.* Albany, NY: State University of New York Press.

Watson, J. (2009). *Assessing and measuring caring in nursing and health sciences* (2nd ed.). New York, NY: Springer.

Wolf, Z. R. (1981). *The concept of caring: Beginning exploration.* Candidacy paper. Philadelphia, PA: University of Pennsylvania School of Nursing.

Wolf, Z. R. (1986). The caring concept and nurse identified caring behaviors. *Topics in Clinical Nursing, 8*(2), 84–93.

Wolf, Z. R., Freshwater, D., Miller, M., Jones, R. A. P., & Sherwood, G. (2003). A standard of care for caring: A Delphi study. *International Journal for Human Caring, 7*(1), 34–42.

Wolf, Z. R., Giardino, E. R., Osborne, P. A., & Ambrose, M. S. (1994). Dimensions of nurse caring. *Image: Journal of Nursing Scholarship, 26*(2), 107–111.

23

Caring Inquiry: The Esthetic Process in the Way of Compassion

MARILYN A. RAY

Years ago, an elderly woman bedridden with a stroke looked at me with her stark, piercing blue eyes. Though I usually didn't like loud music, I turned up the radio to drown the sorrows of the sick room I was in—to drown out the sounds and, in some strange way, the sight of the suffering one before me. Unspeaking, I looked at her. She spoke with her heart. Uncomfortable in her presence, but responding to the life of compassion deep within my heart and soul, I turned off the radio. The journey of sharing the pain—that is, nursing—began.

I wrote this chapter to share ideas and an approach to the method that may capture the complexity of researching—caring. I have spent much time researching and reflecting on the nature of caring and feel intensely that it is the way of compassion, a journey of love. Caring and love are synonymous (Ray, 1981). Inquiring about caring touches the heart and translates through the soul: The "speaking together" between the one caring and the one cared for. It is an immersion into the human encounter that also reveals the human, environmental, and spiritual contexts that are nursing.

The metaphorical heart and soul are the symbols and synonyms for life, living, sensitivity, reason, and integrity. These symbols represent a creative process: The gradual or, more often, abrupt shifting of

consciousness from a focus on the "they" or "I" to a compassionate "we" (Kidd, 1990), which is also spiritual (that which deepens and moves one forward and upward) (Kandinsky, 1977). Compassion is a wounding of the heart by the other, where the "other" enters into us and makes us other. In the minutes of presence and dialogue with the other, we have the transformative powers of the esthetic—the understanding of forms of meaning within the sheer presence of the other and of dialogue or language that exercises the most penetrative authority over consciousness (Steiner, 1989).

In the compassionate way of being, the forms of "other" in consciousness communicate a depth of felt-realness or authenticity, which is intuitive (Steiner, 1989) and depends on the granting to the other to whom one communicates a share in one's being (Buber, 1965). The esthetic act in a compassionate way of being thus communicates in the understanding of forms of meaning a simultaneous immanence and transcendence—human choice to share in the life of the other, and an intuitive knowing, which, as we become "other," can be translated into a call to a deeper life, a more integrated wholeness, and a coming to understand more fully what we have understood.

From Ray, M. A. (1991). Caring inquiry: The esthetic process in the way of compassion. In D. A. Gaut & M. M. Leininger (Eds.), *Caring: The compassionate healer* (pp. 181–189). New York, NY: National League for Nursing. Permission to reprint granted by the National League for Nursing, New York, NY.

What does this mean for nursing and nursing inquiry? For nursing, real presence and dialogue as choice and intuition in compassionate forms of meaning in understanding is an act of creation. This esthetic act, this conceiving and bringing into being, is a birthing and growth of the divine or spiritual life within. Steiner has (1989) intimated that in an esthetic act, there can be no experience which does not wager on a presence of sense that is, finally, theological. He states, "So far as it [the esthetic act] wagers on meaning, an account of the act of reading in the fullest sense, of the act of the reception and internalization of significant forms within us, is a metaphysical and, in the last analysis, a theological one"; "[t]he meaning of meaning is a transcendent postulate" (1989, pp. 215–216). Transcendence in the felt-realness of the compassionate encounter is the unwritten theology. The meaning of meaning or transcendence as unwritten theology is an apprehension of the "radically inexplicable presence, facticity and perceptible substantiality of the created, it is; we are" (p. 201) because there is creation.

For nursing inquiry as the way of compassion, the esthetic (creative) act of *knowing about* the meaning of the meaning of nursing as caring, presumes creation—the conceiving of and bringing into being a knowledge of the substantiality of the created. There is transcendence that is also theological. There is a presence that, as the researcher dwells with the data to read "being anew" or to apprehend the nature of caring, "is the source of powers, of significations in the text, in the work [that is] neither consciously willed nor consciously understood . . . the unmastered 'thereness' of a secret-sharer, of a prior creation with and against which the art [esthetic] act has been effected" (Steiner, 1989, pp. 211–212). In essence, the felt-realness of compassion (caring) in nursing and nursing research, because of the focus on the compassionate "we," is a theological enterprise. As Emily Dickinson notes in one of her poems (Stone, 1990), "The soul selects her own society—Then, shuts the door—" (p. 9).

CARING INQUIRY: THE PHENOMENOLOGY OF ESTHETIC RESEARCH

Caring inquiry as an esthetic process in research is a unique method of presence and dialogue. It attends to both immanence—communion with and transcendence—and reflective intuition. When a researcher engages in caring inquiry, the compassionate "we" is enacted. Encountering the "other" to learn anew the world of caring, not the world as previously encoded by scientific analysis, is where the word and compassion (love) interact (Steiner, 1989). Both description (phenomenology) and interpretation (phenomenological hermeneutics) and esthetic knowing of the experience of caring are the means by which questions about the meaning of caring are illuminated. Phenomenology and phenomenological hermeneutics (Van Manen, 1990) are human sciences that study persons who are experiencing the lifeworld. Esthetic knowing in caring research attends to creativity, sensitivity, and the quality of presences. It is an approach of describing and understanding the meaning of being and becoming through caring. In bringing to reflective awareness the nature of caring in the events experienced in the world of nursing, the researcher (as well as possibly the research participant) is transformed, contributing to the fullness of being and the call to a deeper life—a life of integrated wholeness and openness to creative forces within and without.

Thus, what makes phenomenological hermeneutics an esthetic enterprise is an investment of one's own being in the process of the events of the research. The response to the descriptions and interpretations of the events of caring in esthetic inquiry is one of pure receptivity and responding responsibly, or being answerable to the text in the specific sense, which is at once moral, spiritual, and psychological (Steiner, 1989). The translation of data communicated as text from "shared remembrances" of participants of the meaning of caring into the general perspective of human recognition is teaching the way of the compassionate heart and soul. It illuminates a valuation of the theological or spiritual. The phenomenology of esthetic research of caring presupposes and validates an enmeshment in the metaphysical and theological. What the method is seeking is integrity—a coming to understand more fully what we have understood—where the word and love are a synthesis.

The following is a methodological process I developed based on the ideas of Husserl (Natanson, 1973), Van Manen (1990), Reeder (1984, 1988), and other philosophers of human science, art, and theology. The process is outlined as follows (Ray, work in progress):

1. The Intentionality of Inner Being of the Researcher
2. The Process of Dialogic Experiencing
3. The Process of Phenomenological–Hermeneutical Reflecting and Transforming
4. The Movement of Phenomenological–Hermeneutical Theorizing to a Theory of Meaning
5. Dialoguing with Written Texts: Examining Similarities and Differences
6. Credibility and Significance of the Process of the Phenomenology of the Esthetic Act

The general research question relates to the meaning of the experience of caring or compassion in nursing research. A specific question could be: "What is the meaning of caring in your experience?" This methodology also could be used for any other phenomenological–hermeneutical question in nursing.

THE ESTHETIC PROCESS IN CARING INQUIRY

A dynamic, disciplined, dialectical, reflective, and creative approach among the following activities forms the process of the esthetic phenomenological–hermeneutical inquiry and is outlined as follows (Ray, work in progress):

A. The Intentionality of Inner Being of the Researcher
   1. Imagining the vision of the caring in nursing—past and future within the present
   2. Listening to the "voices" within embodied consciousness, as a feeling and a form of discourse about the meaning of caring in nursing
   3. Focusing on and identifying one's presuppositions of caring in nursing
   4. Practicing bracketing to hold in abeyance one's prehistory and presuppositions about the caring in nursing
B. The Process of Dialogic Experiencing
   1. Selecting the participants for the study grounded within the imagined vision
   2. Engaging with the participants to discuss the roles of interviewer and interviewee, and securing informed consent signatures
   3. Copresencing/sensing the other by recognizing the immediate impact of each other's being on each other—the compassionate "we"
   4. Conversing with participants in tape-recorded, intensive dialogical interviews lasting approximately 1 hour, about the meaning of caring in nursing by asking the phenomenological question, "What is the meaning of caring in your experience?"
   5. Engaging in a cue-taking, talk-turning, researcher-bracketed, dialogical–dialectical interactive

process based on the participants' experience to penetrate the meaning of and experience how caring nursing is constructed for or understood by the other. The researcher at this time of dialogic interviewing holds in abeyance, or temporarily sets aside, his or her knowledge of caring that is a part of his or her embodied consciousness. There is continued controversy over the issue of bracketing in phenomenological philosophy (Stapleton, 1983). For the purpose of this research approach, bracketing of presuppositions about caring is used during the interviews by moving from the lead question of the meaning of experience of caring followed by the cue-taking, talk-turning interaction of the actual dialogue itself.

C. The Process of Phenomenological–Hermeneutical Reflecting and Transforming

The Flow of Analysis occurs through

1. Reflecting and feeling the presencing of the participants' beings in one's consciousness.

2. Transcribing the phenomenological data of the meaning of the art of nursing as texts through a computer-assisted data text and analytic system (Seidel, 1988).

3. Bracketed reflecting for a pure descriptive phenomenology or receptive knowing in consciousness while engaging in the first encounter with the transcribed data (bracketing one's interpretive tendency in relation to one's history and presuppositions about the phenomenon).

4. Attending to the speaking of language in the texts. If a transcriber, other than the researcher, transcribes the data, the researcher should listen to the tapes at the time of encountering the texts for the first time.

5. Highlighting the descriptive experiences of the art of nursing in the texts by using a highlighter pen, or device to illuminate the participants' language of experience.

6. Interpretive reflecting (hermeneutical thinking or unbracketed reflecting) to reveal the immanent themes (linguistic dimensions) emerging in the data. Unbracketed reflecting is the foundation for phenomenological–hermeneutical interpretation. Rather than bracketing one's preassumptions of caring, the history or horizon of meaning of the researcher is brought into being in the dialectic of consciousness and the text.

7. Moving back and forth in understanding the meaning of the textual data to and in consciousness (co-presencing and dialoguing with the data in consciousness).

8. Writing and transforming the themes in the transcribed text to cocreate the metathemes that are linguistic abstractions of the themes.

9. Phenomenological Reducing or Intuiting—turning to the nature of the transcendental meaning of the phenomenon by intuiting or grasping the unity of meaning as a direct, unmediated apprehension of the whole of the experience. This is an intersubjective universal—a transcendent experience of knowing wherein the researcher as knower makes a connecting leap of insight and the separateness of the phenomenon melds into a whole. The universal is reached by a "coming together" of the variations. Thus, variations or similarities of the experience are intuitively and authentically grasped and

constituted in consciousness—the primordial material of sensation out of which arises the knowing of the meaning of experience (the possibility of the phenomenological genesis or beginning, that is, what has been experienced as apart comes together as insight/new awareness, but is not put together from the different dimensions). References to the data, or themes, of experiences-as-meant of the meaning of caring in nursing from participants' experiences undergoes transformation into the researcher's intentional life, and stands out as a component of the researcher's concrete essence. A new way of experiencing, thinking, and theorizing thus is opened up for the researcher. (This experience may occur at any time in the process of reflection.) A metaphor(s) may be grasped as the unity of meaning at this time.

   10. Composing linguistic transformation of data to themes, metathemes, or metaphor (metatheme and metaphor may be the transcendent experience).

D. The Movement of Phenomenological–Hermeneutical Theorizing to a Theory of Meaning.

   1. "Putting together" a theory of meaning, which when constituted by the descriptions, themes, metathemes, and/or metaphor(s), and transcendent unity of meaning becomes the *form* or *structure* of the phenomenological meaning of caring. The theory as form may be represented as a visual model showing all the dimensions of the experience. A theory in phenomenological philosophy and method may seem contradictory given the fundamental notion of the continuous, experiencing process of the living world. However, the idea of theory in this sense is a way of

giving form to the intentional acts of the research itself—where the knower and the known are one, are integral (Reeder, 1984), and where the researcher communicates to the world the integrality of understanding the esthetic act itself. Theory in this sense aims at making explicit the universal meaning of the whole of the experience. Note the etymology of theory—theo and eros—God and love.

E. Dialoguing with Written Texts: Examining Similarities and Differences

   1. Relating the theory of meaning to literary writings in art or nursing to enhance the epistemic development of nursing theory is expressed by illustrating and illuminating similarities, and differences from the phenomenological analytic data and theory or theories previously advanced. The form or structure of the meanings, that is, the phenomenological theory, gives rise to its value in relation to the existing theories or literary works and subsequently to the implications or recommendations for nursing education, practice, administration, and research.

F. Credibility and Significance of the Process of the Phenomenology of the Esthetic Act

   1. *Recognizing, believing,* and *acknowledging* are the dynamics of credibility of the research. The phenomenological evidence of the reality-as-meant of caring is what has been lived and communicated by the participants. Reality, as expressed in experience, is not inauthentic. Meanings convince, and the meanings of the experience alter the sensibilities of those dwelling in the phenomenological written text—the researcher and other readers. Phenomenology enlarges human awareness directly

or expands the range of human perception with new ways of experiencing, rather than with new, objective, mechanistic interpretations as in traditional science. Deepening and expanding the possibilities of being—the quality of making humans more human, humane, and spiritual (the ontologic), rather than more mechanistic—is the valid experience of phenomenological esthetic inquiry.

2. *Affirming* and *confirming* the meaning of the lived experience are the dynamics of significance of the research and are expressed and understood not as agreement, conformity, or generalization, but moving toward the universal that is paradoxical. The capacity to grasp and communicate the meaning of the whole of the experience is articulated and "tested" through the reflective intuition and individuality of the researcher. The universal is deep. It is a sympathetic relationship through which the researcher is transposed into the interior lives of others. The universal is undifferentiated wholeness or caring wisdom that is ultimately both within and without—a reflective symmetry, which brings together into a unity the reflective interiority of the researcher with the possibilities and contradictions of historical–cultural horizons. The quest for meaning is a social signifier and therefore exists in the relationship between the personal–mutual, the individual–community, and the specificity–commonality of culture. The movement of phenomenological theorizing to a theory of meaning captures, through the solitude of the researcher's reflection on the meaning, the researcher's capacity to bridge participants' meaning of experience of caring and the universality of human action as esthetic. Thus, the transformations or possibilities in experiencing (the epistemologic) are open or available to all readers in the reflective symmetry or synthesis encapsulated in the theory.

CONCLUSION

This chapter focused on the sharing ideas and an approach to the method that reflects the complexity and creative power of caring inquiry as a way of compassion and an esthetic act. What I have affirmed by expressing the interiority of compassion as presence and dialogue through metaphysical and epistemological means is that caring and caring inquiry in the final analysis are spiritual and theological. The density of theological presence in nursing research has been effectively communicated by its absence in the last few decades, possibly because of the logical positivist teachings of science, or the newer dimensions of deconstructionist philosophy. It may well be that forgetting the question of the theological, in a sense forgetting to address the mystery of the hidden, yet revealed an interiority of the heart and soul that will continue to drain from nursing its creative, authentic caring potential, and the entire sphere of the esthetic—the meaning of meaning. The crisis in nursing science and practice today demonstrates an emptiness that echoes of the loss of the theological. I have communicated the loss. It could be, however, more from silence than emptiness. This chapter has given voice to this silence.

REFERENCES

Buber, M. (1965). *The knowledge of man*. New York, NY: Harper and Row.

Kandinsky, W. (1977). *Concerning the spiritual in art*. (M. T. Sadler, Trans.). New York, NY: Dover.

Kidd, S. (1990). Birthing compassion. *Weavings: A Journal of the Christian Spiritual Life, 5*(6), 18–30.

Natanson, M. (1973). *Edmund Husserl: Philosopher of infinite tasks.* Evanston, IL: North-Western University Press.

Ray, M. (1981). A philosophical analysis of caring within nursing. In M. Leininger (Ed.), *Caring: An essential human need* (pp. 25–36). Thorofare, NJ: Slack.

Ray, M. (work in progress). *Caring inquiry: The dialectic of science and art.* New York, NY: National League for Nursing.

Reeder, F. (1984). Philosophical issues in the Rogerian science of unitary human beings. *Advances in Nursing Science, 8*(1), 14–23.

Reeder, F. (1988). Hermeneutics. In B. Sarter (Ed.), *Paths to knowledge* (pp. 193–238). New York, NY: National League for Nursing.

Seidel, J. (1988). *The ethnograph.* Littleton, CO: Qualis Research Associates.

Stapleton, I. J. (1983). *Husserl and Heidegger: The question of the phenomenological beginning.* Albany, NY: State University of New York Press.

Steiner, G. (1989). *Real presence.* London, UK: Faber and Faber.

Stone, J. (1990). *In the country of hearts.* New York, NY: Delacorte Press.

Van Manen, M. (1990). *Researching lived experience.* London, Ontario: The Althouse Press.

QUESTIONS FOR REFLECTION

Baccalaureate

1. What did you observe about Ray's (1991) views on caring, love, and compassion?
2. Why is a phenomenological approach effective in investigating the esthetic process of conducting a caring inquiry?
3. How does an investigator who used phenomenological hermeneutics become enmeshed in the research process, according to Ray (1991)? Describe.

Master's

1. How is the text or material of phenomenological studies obtained by investigators?
2. What did you learn about how Ray (1991) created the methodological process to study the experience of caring or compassion in nursing research and the meaning of caring in the researcher's experience? What are the sources used in this new method?
3. What affects you about the way Ray (1991) looked at caring inquiry?

Doctoral

1. What are the steps of the methodological process outlined by Ray (1991)? Briefly summarize three steps.
2. What follow-up information do you need to expand your understanding of phenomenological reducing or intuiting?
3. What did you learn about the study of caring from a phenomenological method after reading Ray's (1991) chapter?

24

Dimensions of Nurse Caring

ZANE ROBINSON WOLF, EILEEN RIVIELLO GIARDINO, PATRICIA A. OSBORNE, AND MARGUERITE STAHLEY AMBROSE

*H*uman care is viewed as the central focus and essence of nursing (Leininger, 1986). For over a decade, nurse caring has been studied using exploratory, descriptive, phenomenological, philosophical, and model development approaches (Cronin & Harrison, 1988; Gaut, 1983; Leininger, 1981, 1983, 1984; Riemen, 1986; Valentine, 1989a, 1989b; Watson, 1979). Many nurses believe that the care they give heals, cures, and improves patients' health.

Caring is an example of a nurse's hidden work that may go unrecognized by patients and their families, except when the behaviors and attitudes that constitute caring are missed (Wolf, 1989). Riemen (1986) has noted that patients who were asked to describe caring described nursing actions that are not caring. Nurses who view caring as a key element of nursing have encouraged others to describe nurses' caring, so that the caring part of nursing will become more distinct for its practitioners (Fox, Aiken, & Messikomer, 1990; Leininger, 1980, 1984). Nurses who have analyzed caring have called for a definition of the caring process and a specification of its dimensions (Griffin, 1983; Noddings, 1981; Valentine, 1989a). The purpose of our study has been to describe the dimensions of the process of nurse caring through a factor analysis of nurses' and patients' responses to the Caring Behaviors Inventory (CBI). Nurse caring has been defined as an interactive and intersubjective process that occurs during moments of shared vulnerability between nurse and patient, and that is both self- and other-directed. Caring is directed toward the welfare of the patient and takes place when nurses respond to patients in a caring situation (Gaut, 1983; Watson, 1979; Wolf, 1981, 1986).

BACKGROUND

Watson, Burckhardt, Brown, Bloch, and Heister (1979) and Watson (1979, 1988a, 1988b, 1988c) have studied nurse caring and human caring from philosophical and ethical perspectives. Watson (1988c) has developed the transpersonal caring theory that guides this study. According to Watson, caring preserves human dignity in cure-dominated health care systems and becomes a standard by which cure is measured. Caring encompasses a metaphysical dimension and becomes a moral ideal as an "end in itself" (Watson, 1988c, p. 177). Caring–healing is communicated through the consciousness of the nurse to the one being cared for (Watson, 1988c).

From Wolf, Z. R., Giardino, E. R., Osborne, P. A., & Ambrose, M. S. (1994). Dimensions of nurse caring. *Journal of Nursing Scholarship, 26*(2), 107–111. Permission to reprint granted by John Wiley & Sons, Inc.

Caring–healing consciousness takes place during a single caring moment. There is an interconnectedness between the one cared for and the one caring.

In contrast, Leininger (1980) describes caring as human acts and processes that are concerned with helping others meet the needs of those requiring care. She asserts that the meaning and practice of nurse caring are not clear (Leininger, 1986) and she invites nurses to investigate culturally specific factors that reflect human care processes in different cultures.

Several authors have identified actions that patients view as caring. Larson (1984) has studied nurse caring behaviors using the Caring Assessment Instrument or CARE-Q. The CARE-Q has been used to measure perceptions of nurse caring behaviors, including acts, conduct, and mannerisms used by professional nurses that conveyed caring and the sensation of feeling cared for. Fifty-seven adult patients have identified their perceptions of the most important nursing caring behaviors, including knowing how to give injections and manage equipment, knowing when to phone the doctor, responding quickly to the patient's call, giving good physical care, giving the patient's treatments and medications on time, putting the patient first, listening to the patient, talking to the patient, checking on the patient frequently, and being well-organized (Larson, 1984). Fifty CARE-Q cards are administered to nurses and patients who sort items into seven packets representing a 7-point scale ranging from "Not important" to "Most important." Mangold (1991) has reported that the CARE-Q takes 45 minutes to administer.

Riemen (1986) has described caring nurse–client interactions in a phenomenological study. She has included meanings of significant statements that patients described as caring. The findings have identified the following as most significant to female patients: listening;

responding to the patient's uniqueness; being perceptive and supportive of the patient's concerns; being physically present; having attitudes and displaying behaviors that made the patient feel valued as a human being, not as an inanimate object or a thing on display; returning to the patient voluntarily without being asked; showing concern that is comforting and relaxing; using a soft, gentle voice; invoking feelings of security; and evoking patient feelings of wanting to reciprocate. The following have been important to male patients: being physically present so the patient felt concern as a valued person; returning voluntarily without being called; making the patient feel comfortable, relaxed, and secure; attending to the comfort and needs of the patient before doing tasks; and, using a kind, soft, pleasant, gentle voice and attitude (Riemen, 1986).

Brown (1986) has audiotaped critical incident reports of 50 hospitalized adult patients who described the feeling of being cared for by a nurse. Using Watson and colleagues' (1979) classification of nursing actions as instrumental and expressive actions, Brown (1986) has identified the following eight care themes: providing a reassuring presence; providing information; demonstrating professional knowledge and skill; assisting with pain; taking more time than actually needed; promoting autonomy; recognizing individual qualities and needs; and keeping the patient under watch (Brown, 1986). In addition, Mayer (1986) has described cancer patients' and families' perceptions of nurse caring behaviors as knowing how to give injections and manage equipment, being cheerful, encouraging patients to call if they have problems, putting the patient first, and anticipating that first experiences are the hardest.

Mayer (1986) has also identified family members' perceptions of the 10 most helpful nurse caring behaviors: being honest; giving clear explanations; keeping family members informed; always trying to make the patient comfortable; showing interest in answering questions; providing the necessary emergency care; assuring the patient that nursing services will be available 24 hours a day, 7 days a week; answering family members' questions honestly, openly, and willingly; allowing patients to do as much for themselves as possible; and teaching the family member how to keep the relative physically comfortable. Family members' perceptions have differed in some respects from nurse and patient views of nurse caring.

Wolf (1981) has conducted a study to identify which words and phrases registered nurses (RNs) considered as representative of nurse caring with patients. Nurses have ranked 75 items selected from the caring literature on an instrument using a 4-point Likert-like scale. This study has established content validity of the CBI by the linkage of the items to both the nursing literature and the social, psychological, and philosophical literature on caring. Subjects have ranked the following caring words and phrases among the highest: attentive listening; comforting; honesty; patience; responsibility; providing information for decision-making; touch; sensitivity; respect; calling a patient by name; and individuality. No additional validity estimates or reliability tests have been conducted during the investigation nor have been dimensions of nurse caring explored.

Larson (1987) has administered the CARE-Q to 57 oncology nurses. The following have been identified as the most important caring behaviors: listening to the patient; touching the patient when comforting is needed; allowing the patient to express feelings; getting to know the patient as an individual; talking to the patient; realizing that patients know themselves best; being perceptive of the patient's needs; giving a quick response to the patient's call; putting the patient first; and giving good physical care.

Mayer (1987) has replicated Larson's (1981) study with 28 oncology nurses and 54 cancer patients. Mayer has found that the most important caring behaviors according to the nurses were listening to the patient, allowing patients to express feelings about their disease and treatment, treating patient information confidentially, realizing that patients know themselves the best, including the patient in planning care, touching patients when they need comforting, being perceptive of the patient's needs, and planning to meet these needs. Patients have ranked the following caring behaviors the highest: knowing how to give shots, IVs, and so forth; managing equipment; being cheerful; encouraging patients to call if they have problems; putting the patient first; anticipating that first times are the hardest; and paying attention to the patient during the first clinic visit or hospitalization. Mayer's findings have been similar to Larson's. In summary, these studies show that nurses and patients viewed the process of nurse caring in a variety of ways. However, few studies have described the dimensions of nurse caring. Therefore, the purpose of our study has been to describe the dimensions of the process of nurse caring using nurse and patient responses to the CBI.

METHOD

Sample

The convenience sample has included 541 subjects: 278 nurses and 263 patients who had been hospitalized and cared for by a nurse in secondary or tertiary health-care settings. The sample subjects have been racially diverse, but the majority have been Caucasian. Table 24.1 includes the demographic characteristics of the sample. The study has been approved by institutional review boards of a hospital, a university, and a nursing

TABLE 24.1 Descriptive Statistics and Characteristics of Nursing Staff (*n* = 278) and Patients (*n* = 263) (*N* = 54)

Patients			Nursing Staff		
	n	**(%)**		*n*	**(%)**
Sex			Sex		
Female	172	**(65.4)**	Female	257	**(92.4)**
Male	82	**(31.2)**	Male	19	**(6.8)**
No response	9	**(3.4)**	No response	2	**(.7)**
Highest degree earned			Highest degree earned		
AS degree	19	**(7.2)**	AS degree	57	**(20.5)**
BS degree	8	**(3.0)**	BSN degree	75	**(27.0)**
BS other	22	**(8.3)**	BS other	23	**(8.3)**
MA/MS	11	**(4.2)**	MSN	7	**(2.5)**
MBA	1	**(4)**	MBA	2	**(.7)**
PhD	8	**(3.0)**	Master's/other	4	**(1.4)**
Other	11	**(4.2)**	Diploma	80	**(28.8)**
No response	183	**(69,6)**	No response	30	**(10.8)**
Type agency where nurse cared for patient			Nursing staffs workplace		
Teaching hospital	106	**(40.3)**	Hospital	264	**(95.0)**
Community hospital	119	**45.2)**	Home care	3	**(1.1)**
Outpatient dialysis	11	**(4.2)**	Other	6	**(2.4)**
Other	7	**(2.7)**	No response	4	**(1.4)**
No response	20	**(7.6)**			
Reason admitted to hospital			Nursing staff's position		
Surgery	103	**(39.2)**	Nursing asst.	5	**(1.8)**
Medical problem	80	**(30.4)**	LPN	22	**(7.9)**
Diagnostic study	9	**(3.4)**	Registered staff nurse	187	**(67.3)**
Emergency	15	**(5.7)**			
Childbirth	22	**(8.4)**	RN manager	16	**(5.8)**
Other	5	**(2.0)**	RN assist manager	24	**(8.6)**
No response	29	**(11.0)**	RN other	24.	**(8.6)**

research committee of a large urban hospital. Subjects have signed a consent form.

Instrument

The initial CBI developed by Wolf (1981) has included 75 items generated from the literature. The revised CBI has included 43 items, with a 4-point Likert-like scale used to elicit responses (1 = strongly disagree; 2 = disagree; 3 = agree; 4 = strongly agree). Test–retest reliability has been established ($r = .96$, $p = .000$; rho = .88, $p = .000$) on a nurse sample. The alpha coefficient has been .83. Internal consistency reliability has resulted in an alpha coefficient of .96 in the combined nurse and patient sample. Content validity has been established by a panel of four nurse experts. Construct validity of the contrasted groups type has been established comparing nursing staff ($n = 278$) and patient ($n = 263$) responses on the total scores of both groups. An unpaired t-test has revealed that the groups have been different ($t = 3.01$; $df = 539$; $p = .003$).

PROCEDURES

Nurse subject names have been obtained from computerized lists provided by a hospital and an RN-BSN program at a university. Patient names have been obtained from the database of a hospital and from diagnostic clinics, patient education groups, and personal contacts. Patients have been contacted in person or by mail. The investigators have distributed CBIs and collected completed instruments. The investigators have obtained over 10 subjects per item on the CBI.

RESULTS

An exploratory factor analysis, using principal components method with varimax rotation, has resulted in a six-factor solution on the CBI (combined nurse and patient responses) as determined by eigenvalues greater than one (Ferketich & Muller, 1990; Wilson, 1989). These six factors have explained 56.8% of the total variance. Factor loadings on the six factors that have been .4 and greater are included in Table 24.2. Item 19 has been eliminated because of factor loadings less than .4. Forty-two items have substantive loadings (>.40) on one of the remaining five dimensions. The investigators have carefully weighed the conceptual fit between the items in each factor and determined into which factor those

TABLE 24.2 Factor Analysis of Caring Behaviors Inventory Items ($N = 541$)

Item	Factor 1	Factor 2	Factor 3	Factor 4	Factor 5	Factor 6
	Varimax Rotated Factor Analysis Factor Loadings					
3. Treating patient as an individual	.73695					
8. Showing respect for patient	.66577					
1. Attentively listening to patient	.64236					
9. Supporting patient	.64073					
11. Being honest with patient	.61196					
7. Giving instructions or teaching patient	.59560					
4. Spending time with patient	.55769					
10. Calling patient by his/her preferred name	.53927					
7. Giving patient information so that he or she can make a decision	.53607					
28. Including patient in planning his or her care	.52987					.43684
15. Making patient physically or emotionally comfortable	.46791					
16. Being sensitive to patient	.46521	.43380				
19. Promoting independence or patient						

(continued)

Item	Factor 1	Factor 2	Factor 3	Factor 4	Factor 5	Factor 6
		Varimax Rotated Factor Analysis **Factor Loadings**				
36. Appreciating patient as human being		.70634				
38. Showing concern for patient		.70535				
35. Responding quickly to patient's call		.68716				
33. Encouraging patient to call if there are problems		.62831				
37. Helping to reduce patient's pain		.62538				
31. Returning to patient voluntarily		.58718				
27. Allowing patient to express feelings about his or her disease and treatment	.49306	.52998				
29. Treating patient information confidentially	.42105	.50217				
34. Meeting patient's stated and unstated needs		.49639		.46264		
32. Talking with patient		.49064		.45100		
18. Helping patient		.41415				
6. Being hopeful for patient			.64894			
24. Watching over patient			.64735			
22. Using soft, gentle voice with patient			.63156			
17. Being patient or tireless with patient			.59274			
12. Trusting patient			.55258			
26. Being cheerful with patient			.54295			
5. Touching patient to communicate caring	.40192		.53265			
14. Helping patient grow	.44133		.49594			
13. Being empathetic or identifying with patient			.46473			
20. Knowing how to give shots, IVs, etc.				.79743		
25. Making equipment skillfully				.76796		
23. Demonstrating professional knowledge and skill				.66618		
39. Giving patient's treatment and medications on time		.53024		.56902	.75692	
41. Relieving patient's symptoms						
40. Paying special attention to patient during first times, as hospitalization, treatments					.72048	

(*continued*)

TABLE 24.2 Factor Analysis of Caring Behaviors Inventory Items (*N* = 541) (*continued*)

Item	Varimax Rotated Factor Analysis Factor Loadings					
	Factor 1	Factor 2	Factor 3	Factor 4	Factor 5	Factor 6
42. Putting patient first		.44038			.66303	
43. Giving good physical care		.47284			.57856	
30. Providing reassuring presence		.45783				.57885
21. Being confident with patient				.42659		.49864
Percent of explained variance	36.5	6.0	4.5	4.2	3.2	2.4
Eigenvalue (principal component method)	15.7092	2.5775	1.94179	1.8051	1.3730	1.0268

with factor loadings in two dimensions belonged (Ferketich & Muller, 1990). The resulting five dimensions of the CBI have included respectful deference to the other; assurance of human presence; positive connectedness; professional knowledge and skill; and attentiveness to the other's experience. The investigators have named the factors based on common themes suggested by items within each factor. Table 24.3 includes the dimensions of the CBI, items in each dimension, alpha coefficient of each dimension, and correlation coefficients between dimensions. Correlation coefficients have been calculated on combined scores for each factor.

DISCUSSION

The initial factor analysis of the CBI has revealed five dimensions of the process of nurse caring. The "Respectful deference to other" factor has included 12 items

TABLE 24.3 Caring Behaviors Inventory Dimensions, Factor Items, Correlations, and Alpha Coefficients

Factor	Respectful Deference to Other	Assurance of Human Presence	Positive Connectedness	Professional Knowledge and Skill	Attentive to Other's Experience
Respectful deference to other (3, 8, 1, 9, 11, 2, 4, 10, 7, 28, 15, 29) *0.8906	1.000				
Assurance of human presence (16, 36, 38, 35, 33, 37, 31, 27, 34, 32, 18, 30) *0.9221	.7549	1.000			
Positive connectness (12, 26, 5, 14, 13, 6, 24, 22, 17) * 0.8452	.6477	.6922	1.000		
Professional knowledge and skill (20, 25, 23, 39, 21) *0.8157	.5136	.5886	.4997	1.000	
Attentive to other's experience (41, 40, 42, 43) *0.8191	.4823	.6182	.5108	.5106	1.000

*Alpha coefficients

that incorporated a courteous regard for the other. The "Assurance of human presence" factor has included 12 items that reflected an investment in the other's needs and security. "Positive connectedness" has encompassed nine items that indicated an optimistic and constant readiness on the part of the nurse to help the other, whereas the 5-item "Professional knowledge and skill" factor has indicated nurse caring as proficient, informed, and skillful. Finally, the "Attentive to other's experience" factor, with four items, has incorporated an appreciation of and engrossment in the other's perspective and experience.

A review of the five factors suggests a fit of the dimensions of nurse caring with Watson's (1988c) Transpersonal Caring Theory in that nurse caring exists in consciousness. For example, the dimensions of assurance of human presence, positive connectedness, and attentiveness to the other's experience reflect the transcendent aspects of nurse caring. These factors are consistent with the perspective that caring–healing consciousness is contained in a single caring moment, takes place between the nurse and the patient, and exists through time.

This is a preliminary study. The limitations of this study include the convenience sampling technique, because of the expense and difficulty of obtaining a large, randomized sample. Another limitation is that a combined sample of nurses and patients was used to generate the five nurse caring dimensions from the CBI regardless of the differences between both groups as reflected in t-test results. The findings of the study should be viewed cautiously because the sample cannot be replicated. Furthermore, using a 6-point Likert scale rather than the 4-point scale in future versions of the CBI would allow for greater variance on an item-by-item basis. Conducting additional factor analysis studies on the CBI, and creating factor scores, and using homogeneous nurse and patient samples may serve to reaffirm the dimensions of nurse caring identified in this study. More reliability and validity tests need to be conducted.

The findings of the study may complement findings generated from interpretive studies on nurse caring (Watson, 1988c). The five dimensions of the process of nurse caring have roots in interpretive and refutationist thinking, since CBI items have been suggested by both types of literature. It remains to be debated whether the dimensions reflect the interconnectedness and intersubjectivity of Watson's (1988c) vision of the human-caring consciousness and relationship. Respectful deference to other, assurance of human presence, positive connectedness, professional knowledge and skill, and attentiveness to the other's experience and the responses within each dimension can be explored through hermeneutical analysis. The dimensions of nurse caring can provide a framework for nurses to understand caring situations and increase their awareness of nurse and patient caring moments.

REFERENCES

Brown, L. (1986). The experience of care: Patient perspectives. *Topics in Clinical Nursing, 8*(2), 56–62.

Cronin, S. N., & Harrison, B. (1988). Importance of nurse caring behaviors as perceived by patients after myocardial infarction. *Heart & Lung, 17*(4), 374–380.

Ferketich, S., & Muller, M. (1990). Factor analysis revisited. *Nursing Research, 39*, 59–62.

Fox, R. C., Aiken, L. H., & Messikomer, C. M. (1990). The culture of caring: AIDS and the nursing profession. *Milbank Quarterly, 68*(2), 226–256.

Gaut, D. (1983). Development of a theoretically adequate description of caring. *Western Journal of Nursing Research, 5*, 313–324.

Griffin, A. P. (1983). A philosophical analysis of caring in nursing. *Journal of Advanced Nursing, 8*, 289–295.

Larson, P. J. (1981). *Oncology patients' and professional nurses' perceptions of important nurse caring behaviors.* Unpublished doctoral dissertation. San Francisco, CA: University of California–San Francisco.

Larson, P. J. (1984). Important nursing caring behaviors perceived by patients with cancer. *Oncology Nursing Forum, 11,* 46–50.

Larson, P. J. (1986). Cancer nurses' perceptions of caring. *Cancer Nursing, 9,* 86–91.

Larson, P. J. (1987). Comparison of cancer patients' and professional nurses' perceptions of important nurse caring behaviors. *Heart & Lung, 16*(2), 187–193.

Leininger, M. M. (1980). Caring: A central focus of nursing and health care services. *Nursing and Health Care, 1,* 135–143.

Leininger, M. M. (Ed.). (1981). *Caring: An essential human need.* Thorofare, NJ: Charles B. Slack.

Leininger, M. M. (Ed.). (1984). *Care: The essence of nursing and health.* Thorofare, NJ: Charles B. Slack.

Leininger, M. M. (1986). Care facilitation and resistance factors in the culture of nursing. *Topics in Clinical Nursing, 8*(2), 1–12.

Mangold, A. M. (1991). Senior nursing students' and professional nurses' perceptions of effective caring behaviors: A comparative study. *Journal of Nursing Education, 30,* 134–139.

Mayer, D. K. (1986). Cancer patient's and families' perceptions of nurse caring behaviors. *Topics in Clinical Nursing, 8*(2), 63–69.

Mayer, D. K. (1987). Oncology nurses' versus cancer patients' perceptions of nurse caring behaviors: A replication study. *Oncology Nursing Forum, 14*(3), 48–52.

Noddings, N. (1981). Caring. *Journal of Curriculum Theorizing, 3,* 139–148.

Riemen, D. J. (1986). The essential structure of a caring interaction: Doing phenomenology. In P. L. Munhall & C. J. Oiler (Eds.), *Nursing research: A qualitative perspective* (pp. 85–108). Norwalk, CT: Appleton, Century, Crofts.

Valentine, K. (1989a). Contributions to the theory of care. *Evaluation and Program Planning, 12,* 17–23.

Valentine, K. (1989b). Caring is more than kindness: Modeling its complexities. *Journal of Nursing Administration, 19*(11), 28–34.

Watson, J., Burckhardt, C., Brown, L., Bloch, D., & Heister, N. (1979a). A model of caring: An alternative health care model for nursing practice and research. In *American Nurses' Association Clinical and Scientific Sessions,* N.P. 59 (pp. 32–33), Kansas City, MO: American Nurses' Association.

Watson, J. (1979). *Nursing: The philosophy and science of caring.* Boston, MA: Little, Brown.

Watson, J. (1988a). *Nursing: Human science and human care.* New York, NY: National League for Nursing (Pub. No. 15-2236).

Watson, J. (1988b). Introduction: An ethic of caring/curing/nursing qua nursing. In J. Watson & M. A. Ray, *The ethics of care and the ethics of cure: Synthesis in chronicity* (pp. 1–3). New York, NY: National League for Nursing (Pub. No. 15-2237).

Watson, J. (1988c). New dimensions of human caring theory. *Nursing Science Quarterly, 1,* 175–181.

Wilson, H. S. (1989). *Research in nursing* (2nd ed.). Reading, MA: Addison-Wesley.

Wolf, Z. R. (1981). *The concept of caring: Beginning exploration.* Candidacy paper. Philadelphia, PA: University of Pennsylvania School of Nursing.

Wolf, Z. R. (1986). The caring concept and nurse identified caring behaviors. *Topics in Clinical Nursing, 8*(2), 84–93.

Wolf, Z. R. (1989). Uncovering the hidden work of nursing. *Nursing and Health Care, 10*(8), 462–467.

QUESTIONS FOR REFLECTION

Baccalaureate

1. What theorists were cited in the theoretical definition of nurse caring in Wolf et al.'s (1994) study?
2. What did you learn about the process of instrument development by reading Wolf et al.'s (1994) study?
3. What level of data (nominal, ordinal, interval, ratio) was generated by the items of the Caring Behaviors Inventory in Wolf et al.'s study?

Master's

1. How does this study (Wolf et al., 1994) address the need to quantify nurse caring through the development of an instrument?
2. How were nurse and patient subjects obtained?
3. What were the dimensions or subscales of nurse caring reported in this study? How would you explain them to nurse colleagues?

Doctoral

1. What additional information would you like to learn about factor analysis used in instrument development?
2. Why did Wolf et al. (1994) compare total scores of nurses and patients?
3. How do the five factors or dimensions fit with Watson's theory at the time it was conducted?

25

Meta-Synthesis of Qualitative Analyses of Caring: Defining a Therapeutic Model of Nursing

Gwen D. Sherwood

The current emphasis on intervention outcomes in health care research creates an imperative to move to new levels of caring models. The preponderance of current caring research is at beginning levels of theory development: single, independent studies that identify and describe. New research modalities are needed to move beyond qualitative designs in order to clarify the operational parameters of a caring model that can be useful in practice. Reframing the traditional ways of viewing caring can stimulate conceptualization of new models that explain, predict, prescribe, and address the needs of advanced practice nursing. Instruments can then be created to test proposed interventions leading to mid-range theoretical models of caring directly applicable in practice.

SIGNIFICANCE

Caring is postulated as the theoretical basis for specific nursing therapeutics for maintaining health, preventing illness, or confronting death (Leininger, 1991; Watson, 1988). It is a complex phenomenon that has been variously described as a concept, behavior, attitude, environment,

or process. Documenting and understanding caring are essential to explain client outcomes from nursing practice and to predict client well-being and health.

Over the past two decades, the accumulation of independent, qualitative studies defining caring from the client's perspective has created a need to synthesize the findings to continue development of nurses' caring theory and move beyond identification and description. Synthesis of client descriptions of nurses' caring, aggregated from existing qualitative studies, offers a more substantive interpretation than that available from single studies. The recovery and synthesis of the essential patterns with explanatory themes from multiple studies can refine the current state of caring knowledge, foundational for the future theory development needed to guide therapeutic nursing practice into the 21st century.

RELATED LITERATURE

Five reviews of caring literature have taken different approaches to the expanding caring knowledge base. Warren's (1988) critique and synthesis of nine caring studies have used both quantitative and qualitative research data from the perspective

This study was funded by an Intramural Grant. The University of Texas–Houston School of Nursing and the First Leininger Human Care Award.

From Sherwood, G. D. (1997). Meta-synthesis of qualitative analysis of caring. *Advanced Practice Nursing Quarterly*, 3(1), 32–42. Permission to reprint granted by WoltersKluwer Law & Business.

of nurses, clients, and the general public. Caring is found to include (a) physical care that is humane (gentle, considerate, competent, timely, and accessible) and (b) emotional care that involves concern, involvement, sharing, culturally defined touching, voluntary presence, and humor.

Using comparative analysis of conceptualizations and theories of caring, Morse, Bottorff, Neander, and Solberg (1991) have delineated and compared definitions of caring. They have arrived at five major concepts of caring: human trait, moral imperative, affect, interpersonal interaction, and intervention. A related concept examination reported by Morse, Solberg, Neander, Bottorff, and Johnson (1990) has confirmed conclusions that current views of caring are relatively undeveloped as a concept, have not been clearly explicated, and often lack relevance for nursing practice.

Boykin and Schoenhofer (1990) have used a series of ontological, anthropological, ontical, epistemological, and pedagogical questions to explicate patterns of knowing through an analysis of five caring theories. A review by Tripp-Reimer (1990) has concluded that for caring insights to be transformed into nursing interventions for improved client outcomes, continuous programs of research on caring must replace the typical single, independent study. Conclusions from these reviews reinforce the urgency of evolving research methods to advance theories of caring.

STUDY PURPOSE

The purpose of the study has been to identify the extant qualitative nursing research literature investigating caring from the perspective of clients to complete a meta-synthesis of the findings. Synthesis of the commonalities from single-study descriptions allows development of an operational model for research on care interventions. Such research can confirm the value of caring to human beings by identifying its role in enhancing recovery and promoting wellness.

STUDY DESIGN

Meta-Synthesis

Meta-synthesis is an important method of analysis. In fact, as the number of qualitative studies of basic and substantive grounded theory needed to guide nursing practice grows, its contribution increases as well (Estabrooks, Field, & Morse, 1994; Jensen & Allen, 1994).

Meta-synthesis is more than just collating research findings. Its goals are comparable to those for meta-analysis, which yields new statistical analyses of quantitative studies. Meta-synthesis integrates, synthesizes, and organizes research results into coherent patterns that can be applied more easily to clinical practice (Brown, 1991).

Findings in a single qualitative study result from a type of synthesis of participant descriptions; hence, the term "meta-synthesis" is used to communicate the additional process of synthesis of findings from aggregated qualitative studies. Just as in meta-analysis, results are limited by the quality of the original research, although rigorous selection criteria help in evaluating each study's merits for inclusion (Brown, 1991; Burns, 1989; Roberts & Burke, 1989; Sandelowski, 1986).

Steps in Meta-Synthesis

The study design involves six phases of analysis, as outlined in the box titled "Steps for Meta-Synthesis" (Estabrooks, Field, & Morse, 1994: Jensen & Allen, 1994; Noblit & Hare, 1988). A thorough search of the literature has identified studies that met the inclusion criteria of being a qualitative study that describes nurses' caring from the perspective of adult patients. Although each study had undergone peer review before publication or scientific presentation, standards for scientific rigor according to Burns (1989) and Roberts and Burke

(1989) have been applied to each study. None have been eliminated on this basis.

Steps for Meta-Synthesis

Phase I: Delineate focus of study.

Phase II: Locate studies meeting inclusion criteria.

Phase III: Read and re-read all studies.

- Rate for inclusion criteria.
- Evaluate tor scientific adequacy.

Phase IV: Determine how studies are related.

- Examine for homogeneity across studies.
- Sort according to characteristics.

Phase V: Translate studies into one another.

- Merge data from across studies into a common data pool and study for common elements.
- Collapse data into essential patterns with explanatory themes through a process of analysis and synthesis.

Phase VI: Express synthesis with a composite description narrating patterns and/or themes to explain what is taking place.

In multiple readings of the studies, comparisons have been made to determine homogeneity across respondent characteristics and to find key phrases and themes. Through a lengthy process of data synthesis, the previous findings from each individual study have been identified and organized by areas of commonality. These integrated descriptions of nurses' caring have been then further examined to yield new understandings and organizations of the data.

This process of synthesis of the merged data from all studies has rendered essential patterns of caring defined by common themes. The essential patterns relate to all aspects of what nurses do and how this activity takes place. The meaning of each identified pattern has been clarified by common themes. In the accompanying narrative, specific descriptions and quotes from respondents communicate the defining attributes, attitudes, knowledge, and actions expressing nurses' caring.

As the common themes emerge, each is related to one another and the whole. Consultation with two independent caring experts has validated and confirmed the findings. A composite description of responses from across all studies defines this universal therapeutic concept with translation into an operational model of caring. The resulting relational statements and propositions can be examined and tested in practice for theoretical confirmation.

STUDY SAMPLE

The 16 qualitative studies that met the inclusion criteria and the standards for scientific adequacy are summarized in Table 25.1. Studies are reported according to available data for gender, population, setting, and findings. The 16 studies comprising the data pool have been conducted between 1975 and 1993, with an aggregate of 353 adult respondents. Data have been collected through unstructured interviews, participant observation, critical incidents, videotaped nurse–client interactions, and group narratives. Ninety respondents are male, 190 are female, and 73 are not reported for gender. The number of respondents for each study has ranged from 8 to 50. Mean reported age has been 54.5 years, with a range of 18 to 85 years. Details of data analysis have varied, but all the studies have used similar techniques to categorize, synthesize, and validate results to derive a classification system, set of constructs, and/or exhaustive description translating nurses' caring as perceived by clients.

TABLE 25.1 Qualitative Studies Describing Caring From Patient's Perspective

Investigator	Number/ Gender	Population/Setting	Summary of Findings
Descriptive Studies			
Brown	80 24 = M 56 = F	Hospitalized patients/ hospital	1. What the nurse does: surveillance, demonstration of knowledge/skill, provision of information, assistance. 2. How the nurse does it: amount of time spent, reassuring presence, recognition of individual qualities/needs, promotion of autonomy. 3. What the nurse is like: personal qualities (friendly, cheerful, pleasant, professional).
Cronin & Harrison*	22 17 = M 5 = F	After myocardial infarction/hospital	Human needs assistance, teaching/learning, humanism/faith-hope/ sensitivity, existential/phenomenological/spiritual forces, supportive/ protective corrective environment, helping/trust, expression of positive/ negative feelings.
Dory	31 8 = M 23 = F	Recently discharged gerontological patients	Comfort, health maintenance acts, surveillance, presence, health instruction acts, protective behaviors, nurturance, health consultative acts, restorative behaviors, interest, facilitating, helping, enabling, compassion, empathy, touching, stress alleviation, sharing, tenderness, trust, and succorance.
Henry†	50 20 = M 30 = F	Home health care	1. What the nurse does: nursing skills with cognitive knowledge. 2. How the nurse does: person skills with human behavior knowledge. 3. How much the nurse does: both nursing skills and person skills with cognitive and human behavior knowledge. 4. How the patient is regarded as a person: nursing and person skills.
Knowlden	34 N/A	Home health care patients	Content: health teaching, assessment, physical care, advocacy, knowledge, supplying resources, planning for future, safety. Relationship: concern, progress, hope, listening, personal relationship, building self-esteem, touching, laughter, humor. Nurse attributes: gentle, careful, telling what the nurse found, considerate, understanding, collaborating, and counseling.
Larson*	15 N/A	Oncology patients with frequent hospitalization	Anticipates, comforts, explains/facilitates, develops and sustains trusting relationship, monitors/follows through, accessible.

(continued)

TABLE 25.1 Qualitative Studies Describing Caring From Patient's Perspective (*continued*)

Investigator	Number/ Gender	Population/Setting	Summary of Findings
		Phenomenologic Studies	
Burfitt, Greiner, Miers, Kinney, & Branyon	13 7 = M 6 = F	Formerly critically ill patients after transfer from intensive care unit	1. Vigilance: attentiveness, highly skilled, technical practices, basic care/nurturance, doing unexpected. 2. Healing: lifesaving actions, energy-freeing acts. 3. Mutuality: personal attributes of nurses, patients, family members.
Greiner & Harris	9 N/A	Psychiatric patients after transfer from critical care	1. Vigilance: constancy, tasks, time, and talk. 2. Mutuality: sensing, trust, respect, and shared humanity.
Luegenbiehl[†]	9 = F	Hospitalized labor and delivery patients	Composite: caring occurred when the nurse acted competently from a background of specific and general knowledge in a helpful, supportive, and reassuring manner.
Miller, Haber & Byrne[†]	15 N/A	Acute care/adult	Concern, connection, courteous, always there, understanding humanity, take care of you, surround with consideration, know needs to meet first. Nurse attributes: gives self, loves being there, finds satisfaction. Parallel themes: holistic understanding, connectedness, shared humanness. presence, anticipation/monitoring patient needs, beyond the mechanical.
Riemen	10 5 = M 5 = F	Previously hospitalized	Attitudinal approach of nurse (existential presence); behavioral approach of nurse (client's uniqueness): meaning generated by client (consequences).
Sherwood	10 5 = M 5 = F	Hospitalized after general surgery/ hospital	1. Assessing needs and expectations to be cared for. 2. Planning care using sound knowledge and decision-making. 3. Intervening: nursing actions, or response to need. 4. Validating nursing action and participant's condition. 5. Interactional attitude: positive, growth-producing interaction with participant.
Swanson-Kauffman[‡]	47* 2 = M 45 = F	Women who miscarried, neonatal intensive care; at-risk mothers	Knowing: avoiding assumptions, centering on one cared for, assessing thoroughly, seeking cues, engaging the self of both. Being with: being there, conveying ability, sharing feelings. Doing for: comforting, anticipating, performing competently/skillfully, protecting, preserving dignity.

(*continued*)

TABLE 25.1 Qualitative Studies Describing Caring From Patient's Perspective (*continued*)

Investigator	Number/ Gender	Population/Setting	Summary of Findings
		Phenomenologic Studies	
			Enabling: informing, explaining, supporting/ allowing, focusing, generating alternatives/thinking it through, validating/ giving feedback.
			Maintaining belief: believing in/holding in esteem, maintaining a hope-filled attitude, "going the distance."
Weaver	8 2 = M 6 = F	Hospitalized acute care/ hospital	Knowledge, nurses' presence, involvement, and commitment with subthemes: decision-making, competent clinical skills, nurses' true presence and availability, accepting, understanding, helping, and informing.

N/A = not available; M = male; F = female; N = total numbers of respondents.
*Total study has included other methods.
†Total study has included perspectives of populations other than patients.
‡Combined number of client respondents for the three studies leading to caring theory.

ELEMENTS OF CARING

Examination of the merged data pool has revealed the cross-referencing of common elements across studies. These common elements have formed the basis for subsequent synthesis into patterns and themes.

Caring is characterized within a meaning-intensive clinical context. As clients have been closer to an acute illness experience, the focus is on nurse competence (Cronin & Harrison, 1988; Henry, 1975; Larson, 1981; Riemen, 1984), lending confirmation to the importance of competence and cognitive knowledge in forming trusting relationships. Trust is built through maintaining belief that the nurses "knew what they were doing" and the constancy of their "doing what they said they would do" (Cronin & Harrison, 1998, p. 378). Nurses encourage self-care by "making you do things that help you get better even if you don't want to" (Miller, Haber, & Byrne, 1992, p. 144). Caring includes doing extra things for the client (Brown, 1981; Burfitt, Greiner, Miers, Kinney, & Branyon, 1993; Cronin & Harrison, 1988; Knowlden, 1986; Sherwood, 1988), including helping family members, providing needed personal items, and facilitating regular obligations and responsibilities.

> Caring is characterized within a meaning-intensive clinical context.

Caring has been based on knowing and being with, the meaning generated by the client (Luegenbiehl, 1986; Swanson, 1990, 1991; Swanson-Kauffman, 1986, 1988). Being existentially present or showing genuine interest in the client as a valued individual by really listening (Luegenbiehl, 1986; Riemen, 1984; Swanson, 1990, 1991; Swanson-Kauffman, 1988) has illustrated how nurses have been "interested in all of you and the environment" (Miller, Haber, & Bryne, 1992, p. 143).

Mutuality (sensing, trust, respect, and shared humanity) comes from the experience of caring (Burfitt et al., 1993; Luegenbiehl, 1986: Sherwood, 1988; Swanson-Kauffman, 1986). Constant surveillance and monitoring (Brown, 1981; Burfitt et al., 1993; Sherwood, 1988; Swanson-Kauffman, 1986, 1988) and provision for client safety help establish a supportive and protective environment (Cronin & Harrison, 1988; Henry, 1975; Knowlden, 1986; Sherwood, 1988; Swanson-Kauffman, 1986). Quoting a respondent, "The nurse is always there, and stays with you through the situation and lets you know it is okay to call, then comes quickly when you ring, and asks what you want" (Sherwood, 1988, p. 50). Nurses evaluate client responses to interventions, always helping "avoid bad outcomes" (Burfitt et al., 1993, p. 496; Swanson, 1990, p. 64).

Caring practice commands a consistent value system that recognizes each individual, giving presence, and coming together with compassionate, therapeutic care. It is not just an isolated moment—nurses' caring constitutes a way of *being* while *doing* nursing (Burfitt et al., 1993; Dory, 1989; Miller, Haber, & Byrne, 1992; Weaver, 1991). The caring paradigm is essential to prevent health care being merely a bureaucratic and technological showplace (Burfitt et al., 1993; Greiner & Harris, 1992; Miller, Haber, & Byrne, 1992; Swanson, 1991; Weaver, 1991). Teaching and informing clients about their condition indicates a caring nurse, one who "lets you know what is going on and makes sure you understand" (Sherwood, 1988, p. 65).

How nurses regard the client as a person has been conveyed instantly through interest and sensitivity, dignity, and respect: "It makes me feel someone is there if I need them" (Henry, 1975, p. 33). Caring nurses "treat you like they would want to be treated" (Miller, Haber, & Byrne, 1992, p. 144). Caring is viewed as a mode or way of being as confirmed in the parallel themes found throughout the studies: holistic understanding, connectedness/ shared humanness, presence, anticipation and monitoring of patient needs, and beyond the mechanical (Larson, 1981; Miller, Haber, & Byrne, 1992; Riemen, 1984; Sherwood, 1988; Swanson, 1990). As one patient has put it, "They were concerned about me, my progress, and helping me" (Miller, Haber, & Byrne, 1992, p. 143).

FOUR PATTERNS OF CARING

Four essential patterns of nurses' caring emerge from the progressive synthesis of the studies, each clarified by explanatory themes (Table 25.2). To define caring requires the patterns of healing interaction, nurses' knowledge, and intentional response, leading to therapeutic outcomes. One pattern cannot be present without the others. The specific themes for each pattern alternate and flow within the interactions with individual clients (Figure 25.1). Dynamic and fluid, the patterns are not

TABLE 25.2 The Essential Patterns and Explanatory Themes of Nurses' Caring

Healing Interaction	Nurses' Knowledge	Intentional Response	Therapeutic Outcomes
Created: Trust/belief	Created: Knowledgeable decision-making	Created: Helpful interventions	Created: Positive welfare
Individual uniqueness			
Availability	Knowledge of human behavior	Goal-directed actions	Healing outcomes
Personal awareness		Competent clinical skills	Resolving physical and affective needs
Vigilance/surveillance	Cognitive knowledge	Provisions for safety	
Supportive/protective environment	Personal attributes	Helping	Positive/growth enhancing relationship
Overall healing milieu		Teaching/learning process	
		Feedback	
		Advocacy	

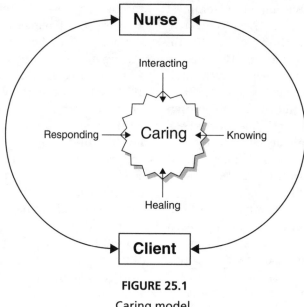

FIGURE 25.1
Caring model.

mutually exclusive categories but constantly overlap, interchanging in a multidimensional stream and each affecting the other. Therefore, represented as patterns, caring is defined by its themes as myriad nursing actions, behaviors, and interactions observable within these specific patterns. Presentation of each pattern with explanatory themes (in italics) demonstrates the synthesis of the aggregated data that have led to a composite definition.

HEALING INTERACTION PATTERN

The healing interaction pattern creates *trust and belief* between nurse and client, from the establishment of *an overall healing milieu. Recognizing the uniqueness of the individual* client, care is not rote or mechanical, but is individualized through *personal awareness* such that the affective dimensions of care are equally important as the physical acts of assistance, enabling clients' personal understanding of the health care experience. The establishment of a *supportive or protective environment* develops and

sustains the trusting relationship from the nurses' reassuring presence, availability, and accessibility. In *making the self available* with physical and mental presence, nurses display involvement and commitment, respecting the client as an individual of value. The constant *vigilance and surveillance* ensures that nurses are available quickly when called.

Concern and commitment are communicated through actions: smiling; looking into the patient's eyes when talking; asking how the client felt, if the medication helped, or if the client needed anything; being courteous in interactions; addressing clients by name; stopping by to sit and listen; and using humor and touch appropriately. Nurses show concern with physical and mental needs through empathy evidenced by supporting, anticipating, helping, nurturing, and succoring (assisting in distress). Making comfortable, preserving dignity, and surrounding with consideration are expressed by waking the client gently, showing care for needles in the arms, being compassionate about physical care, and offering back rubs.

NURSES' KNOWLEDGE PATTERN

The nurses' knowledge pattern is defined by themes of *nurses' personal attributes, knowledge of human behavior, and cognitive knowledge,* creating knowledgeable decision-making. Caring nurses use their knowledge of human behavior to develop person skills, the ability to convey personal attributes. Interactions are thus characterized as gentle, careful, informative, considerate, understanding, collaborative, client friendly, cheerful, pleasant, solicitous, and personally interested. Nurses' personal attributes are determinants in the way a nurse does things with, to, or for a client. The nurses approach their work with a readiness to give of themselves, a love of being there, satisfaction, and a sense of purpose. Their interest and concern in the welfare of another confirm the worth of each client.

Caring requires cognitive knowledge for health consultative acts. By observing, anticipating, and monitoring client needs, knowledge is applied in the assessment of physical and affective needs to determine the plan for managing care. Sound decision making to prioritize needs demonstrates competence and leads to an organized schedule, planning for the future, and acquiring resources to secure therapeutic outcomes.

INTENTIONAL RESPONSE PATTERN

Nurses knowledgeably choose nursing actions in response to identified needs or problems, creating *helpful interventions.* The intentional response pattern requires application of a nurse's knowledge in performing *competent clinical skills,* which helps maintain trust and belief in the nurse. Getting to know the client and identifying the nursing actions needed are not enough; actually, following through with *goal-directed actions* utilizing a nurse's cadre of attributes and knowledge patterns is essential to direct therapeutic outcomes. *Provisions for client safety* add to feelings of security and confidence of "being taken care of" (Miller, Haber, & Byrne, 1992).

> Task and affective dimensions of care are not separable.

Helping clients with human needs assistance, health maintenance acts, lifesaving actions, and restorative behaviors arise from the client's need to have others do tasks during a time of duress. Nurses do what clients would normally have done for themselves if the necessary knowledge, physical energy, or emotional strength were available. These energy-freeing acts are a bridge for ill clients until they are able to return to self-care, inspiring client autonomy.

Task and affective dimensions of care are not separable. Assisting with pain management, doing extra things, offering to help, alleviating stress, and spending time with a friendly small talk overlap with the interaction pattern in creating trust and belief in the nurses' caring response. Specific nursing care knowledge is applied to handling equipment, decisions to call the physician, basic nursing practices, and highly skilled, technical interventions.

Assessing clients' intellectual needs, the *teaching/learning process* provides details of the illness as well as health information. Health instruction acts include explaining progress, telling what to expect, teaching about the specifics of nursing care, sharing health information, and answering questions in a clear and understandable way. Serving as *client advocates,* nurses activate other care resources extending to innovative, collaborative, multidisciplinary interventions. Critical thinking of assessed needs, use of knowledge and skills, and the overall interaction pattern are evaluated for effectiveness in resolution of patient needs. *Giving feedback* on managing responsibilities for interventions allows nurses to generate alternative approaches.

THERAPEUTIC OUTCOMES/HEALING PATTERNS

Respondents have indicated that caring interactions made them feel better, creating *positive welfare*. Healing patterns enable clients to achieve the maximum level or state of wellness possible. *Healing outcomes*, the goals of caring, are accomplished by *resolving the client's physical and affective needs*, resulting in feelings of self-care, autonomy, comfort, security, peace, and relaxation.

Caring leads to a *positive, growth-enhancing interrelationship* with the client, characterized by mutuality between the caregiver and the receiver of care. Interactions evolve out of the behavioral and attitudinal approach of the nurses, the mutual process driven by the personal attributes of both nurse and client. Being with the client goes beyond knowing to actually feeling with: a connection happens between nurse and client through interpersonal communication based on personal and professional interest.

There is sensitivity to how the person is coming to terms with an illness experience. To be able to maintain hope, clients need to have others believe in their capacity to get through the experience and to find a point of comfort, enabling a way of dealing with the effects of the illness. The interaction of caring facilitates the capacity to grieve and get through a loss, to heal, to reach the highest level of wellness, or achieve peaceful death.

COMPOSITE DESCRIPTION

Caring is defined by a model of interaction defined by essential patterns and themes fulfilled by nurses' knowledge leading to healing outcomes. The nurses' concerned, interactive presence forms the foundation for a healing environment. Vigilance and surveillance to anticipate the unique physical and mental needs of each client creates trust that nurses are "right on top of things" (Miller, Haber, & Byrne, 1992). Based on knowing and being with, nurses' belief in the client leads to a hope-filled attitude, enabling the client's personal understanding of the health-care experience.

Both nursing and personal skills are the required content of caring. The nurses' attributes and human behavior knowledge are essential; without the person skills, nursing skills are mere technical, physical acts—a robot performance emphasizing cure instead of wellness and healing. The process of caring requires intentional response and intervening for the clients' positive welfare. Knowing that they would not be left alone, clients see caring nurses as "going the distance" (Swanson, 1991) to help achieve therapeutic outcomes.

DEVELOPING A THERAPEUTIC MODEL

An inductively derived therapeutic model demonstrates the overlay and dynamic nature of the essential patterns with explanatory themes and descriptions (Figure 25.2). Caring is viewed within the basic building blocks of theoretical model development, context, content, and process, within a goal-directed framework (Barnum, 1994). *Context* forms the background, the environment, on which theory plays out. Here, environment includes the entire milieu, the internal and the external environment, where nursing care takes place and is defined as the interaction pattern. *Content* includes the subject matter and forms the main building blocks that interact on the background. As shown in the model, the nurses' knowledge pattern represents the nurses' cognitive knowledge and knowledge of human behavior combined with specific attributes to form the content applied in the context of caring. *Process*, the methods by which nurses act, is the movement or action, where intention is acted out to accomplish goal-directed, therapeutic outcomes. In theory

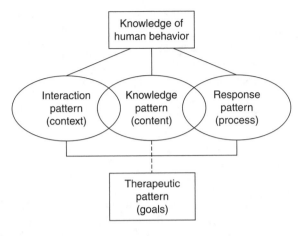

FIGURE 25.2

Building an operational, therapeutic model of caring.

building, *goals* are the intentions that set the operational direction for the context, content, and process of the model.

The operational definition creates a typology of caring needed to clarify and isolate phenomena influencing human responses related to nursing practice (Eisenhauer, 1994). The congruency of findings in these 16 studies is significant to be able to predict subsequent client responses (Sherwood, 1993).

IMPROVING PRACTICE OUTCOMES BY ADVANCING HUMAN CARING THEORY

Through meta-synthesis, a state-of-the-science definition of caring can lead to the design of nursing approaches to ensure client well-being and healing. Explicating clients' expectations of caring by nurses will enable delivery of personalized, culturally congruent care (Leininger, 1991). Understanding caring will allow new predictions of therapeutic interventions for the well-being and health of individuals, families, and groups for movement along the wellness continuum.

Caring is often cited as what the nurse does, how the nurse does it, and how much the nurse does (Henry, 1975); the

being and doing by the nurse (Sherwood, 1988); the instrumental and expressive actions of the nurse (Brown, 1986); and the technology versus the human touch of nurses (Barnum, 1994). The composite of the 16 studies shows that caring cannot be split into such formal parts. Caring is an *integrative* mode of human interaction (Roach, 1992) defined by goal-directed, intentioned, growth-producing actions operationalized interactively with the care receiver (Gaut, 1986).

The correlation between behaviors of caregivers and receivers of care in producing therapeutic client care outcomes must be defined. People respond as approached; knowing how consumers perceive nursing care delivery will provide approaches to produce desired results. More than just feeling and acting, caring requires an informed awareness of the recipient of care; knowing the client creates the integral link between the technologic and behavioral sciences with patient outcomes (Jenny & Logan, 1992; Tanner, Benner, Chesla, & Gordon, 1993). Care that matches a client's unique set of needs and realities impels nurses to document, know, predict, and explain systematically what is nurses' caring, overcoming the current impersonal health care delivery (Sherwood,

1995; Swanson, 1993). The mutuality of the caring process renews and energizes the nurse, aiding renewal and retention of staff (Marck, 1990; Sherwood, 1992). Study of other environmental factors could determine the healing impact of a spiritual atmosphere where staff and clients experience growth. The caring patterns and themes derived in this meta-synthesis provide the structure to define the therapeutics of caring operationally, propelling nursing to the forefront of health care delivery.

REFERENCES

Barnum. B. (1994). *Nursing theory: Analysis, application, evaluation.* Philadelphia, PA: J. B. Lippincott Co.

Boykin, A., & Schoenhofer, S. (1990). Caring in nursing: Analysis of extant theory. *Nursing Science Quarterly, 4,* 149–155.

Brown, L. (1981). Behaviors of nurses perceived by hospitalized patients as indicators or care. *Dissertation Abstracts International, 42*(11), 4361B. (University Microfilms No. DA 82–09, 803)

Brown, L. (1986). The experience of care: Patient perspectives. *Topics in Clinical Nursing, 8*(2), 56–62.

Brown, S. (1991). Measurement of quality of primary studies for meta-analysis. *Nursing Research, 40*(6), 352–355.

Burfitt, S., Greiner, D., Miers, L., Kinney, M., & Branyon, M. (1993). Professional nurse caring as perceived by critically ill patients: A phenomenological study. *American Journal of Critical Care, 2,* 489–499.

Burns, N. (1989). Standards for qualitative research. *Nursing Science Quarterly, 2*(1), 44–52.

Cronin, S., & Harrison, B. (1988). Importance of nurse caring behaviors as perceived by patients after myocardial infarction. *Heart and Lung, 27,* 374–380.

Dory, V. B. (1989). Nursing behaviors perceived as caring by gerontological patients (master's thesis, University of Florida, 1987). *Master's Abstracts International, 27,* 93.

Eisenhauer, L. (1994). A typology of nursing therapeutics. *Image: The Journal of Nursing Scholarship, 26*(4), 261–265.

Estabrooks, C. A., Field, P. A., & Morse, J. M. (1994). Aggregating qualitative findings: An approach to theory development. *Qualitative Health Research, 4*(4), 503–511.

Gaut, D. (1986). Evaluating caring competencies in practice. *Topics in Clinical Nursing, 8*(2), 77–83.

Greiner, D. S., & Harris, D. (1992). *Professional nursing caring as perceived by critically ill psychiatric patients: A phenomenologic study.* Unpublished study. University of Alabama School of Nursing, University of Alabama at Birmingham, Birmingham, Alabama.

Henry, O. M. (1975). Nurse behaviors perceived by patients as indicators of caring. *Dissertation Abstracts International, 36*(02), 652B. (University Microfilms No. AAC7516229).

Jenny, J., & Logan, J. (1992). Knowing the patient: One aspect of clinical knowledge. *Image: The Journal of Nursing Scholarship, 24*(4), 254–258.

Jensen, L., & Allen, M. (1994). A synthesis of qualitative research on wellness-illness. *Qualitative Health Research, 4*(4), 349–369.

Knowlden, V. (1986). The meaning of caring in the nursing role. *Dissertation Abstracts International, 46,* 2574A.

Larson, P. (1981). Oncology patients' and professional nurses' perceptions of important nurse caring behaviors. *Dissertation Abstracts International, 42*(2), 568B. (University Microfilms No. AAD 81165111).

Leininger, M. M. (1991). *Cultural care diversity and universality: A theory of nursing.* New York, NY: National League for Nursing.

Luegenbiehl, D. L. (1986). The essence of nurse caring during labor and delivery. *Dissertation Abstracts International, 47*(06), 237B.

Marck, P. (1990). Therapeutic reciprocity: A caring phenomenon. *Advances in Nursing Science, 13*(1), 49–59.

Miller, B. K., Haber, J., & Byrne, M. (1992). The experience of caring in the acute care setting: Patient and nurse perspectives. In D. Gaut (Ed.), *The presence of caring in nursing* (pp. 137–156). New York, NY: National League for Nursing.

Morse, J. M., Bottorff, I., Neander, W., & Solberg, S. (1991). Comparative analysis of conceptualizations and theories of caring. *Image: The Journal of Nursing Scholarship, 23,* 119–126.

Morse, J. M., Solberg, S. M., Neander, W. L., Bottorff, J. L., & Johnson, J. L. (1990). Concept of caring and caring as a concept. *Advances in Nursing Science, 13*(1), 1–14.

Noblit, G., & Hare, R. D. (1988). *Meta-ethnography: Synthesizing qualitative studies.* Newbury Park, CA: Sage Publications.

Riemen, D. (1984). The essential structure of a caring interaction: A phenomenological study. *Dissertation Abstracts International, 44,* 3041B. (University Microfilms No. ADG8816567)

Roach, M. S. (1992). *The human act of caring: A blueprint for the health professions* (rev. ed.). Ottawa, ON: The Canadian Hospital Association Press.

Roberts, C. A., & Burke, S. O. (1989). *Nursing research: A quantitative and qualitative approach.* Boston, MA: Jones & Bartlett.

Sandelowski, M. (1986). The problem of rigor in qualitative research. *Advances in Nursing Science, 8*(3), 27–37.

Sherwood, G. (1992). The caregiver's response to the experience of suffering. In P. Starck & J. McGovern (Eds.), *Human suffering: An invisible dimension of illness.* New York, NY: National League for Nursing.

Sherwood, G. (1993). A qualitative analysis of patient responses to caring: Basis for a caring practice. In D. Gaut (Ed.), *Caring: A global agenda.* New York, NY: National League for Nursing.

Sherwood, G. (1995). The chemistry of nurses' caring: A model for humane health care. *Humane Medicine: A Journal of the Art and Science of Medicine, 11*(2), 62–65.

Sherwood, G. D. (1988). Nurses' caring as perceived by post-operative patients: A phenomenological study. *Dissertation Abstracts International, 49*(06), 2133B. (University Microfilms No. ADG8816567)

Swanson, K. M. (1990). Providing care in the NICU: Sometimes an act of love. *Advances in Nursing Science, 13*(1), 60–73.

Swanson, K. M. (1991). Empirical development of a middle range theory of caring. *Nursing Research, 40*(3), 161–166.

Swanson, K. M. (1993). Nursing as informed caring for the well-being of others. *Image: The Journal of Nursing Scholarship, 25*(4), 352–357.

Swanson-Kauffman, K. M. (1986). Caring in the instance of unexpected early pregnancy loss. *Topics in Clinical Nursing, 8*(2), 37–46.

Swanson-Kauffman, K. M. (1988). Caring needs of women who mis-carried. In M. Leininger (Ed.), *Caring discovery and uses in clinical and community nursing.* Detroit, MI: Wayne State University Press.

Tanner, C., Benner, P., Chesla, C., & Gordon, D. (1993). The phenomenology of knowing the patient. *Image: The Journal of Nursing Scholarship, 25*(4), 273–280.

Tripp-Reimer, T. (1990). Qualitative approaches to care: A critical review. In J. Stevenson & T. Tripp-Reimer (Eds.), *Knowledge about care and caring.* Kansas City, MO: American Academy of Nursing.

Warren, L. (1988). Review and synthesis of nine nursing studies on care and caring. *Journal of the New York State Nurses Association, 19*(4), 10–16.

Watson, J. (1988). *Nursing: Human science and human care—A theory of nursing.* New York, NY: National League for Nursing.

Weaver, R.A. (1991). A phenomenological study of caring in the nurse-patient relationship: The patient's perspective. *Master's Abstracts International, 29,* 269. (University Microfilms No. AAC1342329).

QUESTIONS FOR REFLECTION

Baccalaureate

1. What did you learn about meta-synthesis studies by reading Sherwood's (1997) investigation?
2. How did Sherwood (1997) explain the need in caring literature to conduct a study using meta-synthesis design?
3. How did Sherwood go about selecting studies to analyze in her meta-synthesis on caring from the perspective qualitative studies on nurses' caring conducted with adult patients?

Master's

1. How did Sherwood (1997) explain the elements of nurses' caring regarding the clinical context?
2. What did you learn about how Sherwood (1997) arrived at specifying the *essential patterns* and *explanatory themes* of nurses' caring?
3. How would you explain the nurses' knowledge pattern to other nurses with whom you work?

Doctoral

1. Why is the pattern, therapeutic outcomes/healing patterns, particularly important in health care settings?
2. What did you learn about the development of an operational, therapeutic model of caring that you could share with nurse administrators?
3. How does this study benefit current scholars who investigate the concept and process of nurse's caring?

26

A Standard of Care for Caring: A Delphi Study

ZANE ROBINSON WOLF, MARGARET MILLER, DAWN FRESHWATER,
REBECCA A. PATRONIS JONES, AND GWEN D. SHERWOOD

The literature of professional nursing is replete with references to caring. Schoenhofer and Boykin (1993) provide one example; they propose that when nurses offer their service to people, "that offer is an offer to care" (p. 84). For many years, caring has been declared an essential element, and a central and unifying focus of nursing (Leininger, 1977). Some suggest that caring is the quintessence of the profession (Fox, Aiken, & Messikomer, 1990). Furthermore, caring helps to keep the person as a central focus of the health-care system (Callahan, 1990) and is considered by patients and families to be the hallmark of good nurses (Joiner, 1996).

However, nurses' ability to provide compassionate care is undermined daily by the forces of specialization, science, technology, cost containment, and the interference of organizational priorities (Knowlden, 1998). Large patient assignments, caseloads, and brief office visits leave little time to expand interventions during interactions between care receiver and provider (Forrest, 1989; Green-Hemandez, 1997). The constraints of the health care delivery system affect nurses' ability to provide an optimum level of quality care and negatively influence patient satisfaction, an indicator of quality nursing care (Moore, Lynn, McMillen, & Evans, 1999; Williams, 1998).

The emphasis on measuring the quality of health care practices and on the development of criteria, standards, and protocols has challenged clinicians and administrators in the last two decades. Health care practices have been evaluated, and patient outcomes have been targeted across health care agencies (McLaughlin & Kaluzny, 1997) in the pursuit of quality services. Guidelines and standards have been developed to improve quality care and monitor health care outcomes. Professional standards of care, as authoritative bases, set expectations of practitioners and patients at a high level. Standards are generally accepted, objective measurements, such as rules or guidelines, supported through findings from expert consensus, based on specific research and/or documentation in scientific literature against which an individual's or organization's level of performance can be compared (Joint Commission on Accreditation of Health care Organizations, 1996, p. GL25). An absolute or normative standard, developed by consensus from experts in the field, may reflect an ideal practice of healthcare practitioners to achieve the best possible outcomes (McLaughlin & Kaluzny, 1997). Standards help to ensure a level of

From Wolf, Z. R., Freshwater, D., Miller, M., Jones, R. A. P., & Sherwood, G. (2003). A standard of care for caring: A Delphi study. *International Journal for Human Caring, 7*(1), 34–42. Permission to reprint granted by the International Association for Human Caring.

care for patients and families (Reese & Reese, 1994) and foster interdisciplinary and interinstitutional consensus building (Dozier, 1998). Furthermore, they are often used to help institutions assess quality performance (McLaughlin & Kaluzny, 1997) and link the accountability areas of professional practice, including care, quality, and competence (Dozier, 1998). Standards and guidelines form the foundation for improvement efforts (Joiner, 1996).

The concept of quality continues to generate some confusion, and the growing number of concepts linked to quality further compounds this. The concepts of structure, process, and outcome are often used to distinguish among criteria against which a specific service is compared (Clinton & Nelson, 1998; Donabedian, 1980). The term "standard" is central to the development of quality assurance systems. Standards have been used in reference to both the quality and effectiveness of care. While the notions of quality and standards increasingly have become the concern of health care organizations, quality cannot be considered in isolation from the management of health care systems, the practitioners working within them, and, more importantly, patients and their families. A standard of care for caring can help clinicians consistently provide caring interventions across health care agencies and communities, and serve as a precursor to quality. It can legitimize the caring component in the activities of health care professionals. A standard can serve as a starting point for debate among clinicians who are challenged by cost containment initiatives and the effects of the nursing shortage.

The purpose of this study has been to create an international standard of care for caring useful by nurses, and other health-care providers, in health care agencies and communities. A Delphi method has been used. In the first round, the standard has been created from the highest ranked elements and textual responses have been identified by members of the International Association for Human Caring (IAHC), and attendees of the research conference held in Boca Raton, Florida (USA), in 2000. During the second and third rounds, the current members of IAHC have been asked to judge the standard as it emerged, and to comment and suggest revisions in a narrative style.

A standard of care for caring is defined as a performance requirement that describes strategies to ensure that patients, family members, and communities feel cared for consistently during care episodes. The standard of care for caring is not framed in a perspective that sees caring as a uniquely nursing phenomenon that is necessarily conceptualized across cultures (Smith, 1999), nor as an end in itself. Furthermore, such a standard should not be viewed as an all-encompassing one. It may offer nurses a starting point to incorporate a caring standard into nursing care delivery models in their own institution with matching performance standards to evaluate quality of care.

Nurse investigators do not agree on the nature of care and caring; this lack of agreement justifies the current study (Andrews, Daniels, & Hall, 1996; Sherwood, 1997). The confusion about what constitutes caring in practice and the operationalization of a seemingly nebulous and abstract concept presents a contemporary challenge to nurses and health care professionals alike, never more so than in the era of evidence-based practice. It is timely to articulate caring practices, that is, to make private knowledge public, since the professional and academic credibility of the science of nursing continues to emerge. Additionally, nurses and other health care providers, who give direct care services, may benefit from conforming to such a standard (Smith, 2000). Providing a standard of care for caring may provide "a new path through the maze of tradition, convention, and dogmas" (Watson, 1987, p. 15). The standard may serve as a yardstick against which nurses and other health care providers can compare their performance of caring practices, strengthening human caring in the workplace (Ray, 1997), and thus improve quality of care. The standard may serve as a guide to foster caring relationships among healthcare providers and consumers. Conversely, it may stimulate debate among nurses of diverse cultures. Nonconformance to such a standard or failure to create one carries a high price; it sacrifices caring at the bedside, devalues professional services, and negatively influences patients' perceptions of health care organizations (Williams, 1998) and care providers.

LITERATURE REVIEW

According to Williams (1998), patients perceive quality nursing care as caring, interpersonal interactions. Caring is personal; patients want to be treated as unique individuals by caregivers who are careful, gentle, kind, friendly, respectful, attentive, and considerate. Williams' three investigations on the dimensions of nurse caring, using the holistic caring inventory, contribute information about patients' perceptions of quality and nurse caring behaviors, and the holistic, humanistic caring element of provider–patient interaction. Williams conclude that patients value care that recognizes their uniqueness, their need to share feelings with providers, and their need to be accepted and listened to. Patients perceive physical caring (e.g., sharing information about physiological needs, being sensitive to assisting patients to meet needs) and sensitive caring (e.g., listening, sharing concerns) more than other dimensions of caring.

Joiner (1996) has described the efforts of the Nursing Quality Management and Research Council of Akron General Medical Center to improve survey results regarding patient satisfaction. Council members have examined policies and other printed materials for evidence of themes of caring and empathy in nursing

practice. Staff nurses and council members have created a document that represented empathy: caring, respect, encouragement, and "going the extra mile" (Joiner, 1996, p. 39). Standards of caring have been developed and implemented through presentations to nursing staff, have been incorporated into orientation classes, and have been used in nursing staff performance evaluations. They include effective communication, courtesy, respect, attentiveness, and promotion of a sense of protection and rest. The standards focus not only on nurses, patients, and families but also on diffusing caring to other departments and services of the hospital.

Reactions to the standards vary. New nurses welcome the caring standards since they have not been emphasized in their education. Unexpectedly, seasoned nursing staff consider the standards so intrinsic to nursing care that they are insulted to have them explicitly stated.

Joiner (1996) and colleagues have continued to disseminate the standards for a year, to focus on service excellence and to monitor patient satisfaction. Subsequently, other departments have wanted service standards, resulting in organization-wide standards that have been based on the original four standards of caring. Overall, the service excellence initiative has influenced the larger health care community and has resulted in improved results on patient satisfaction surveys.

Popovich (1998) has affirmed that standards reflect the values and priorities of health care providers and institutions. She has presented a multidimensional measurement model that organized the evaluation of performance by classifying primary sources of standards: regulatory, professional, and institution- or system-specific. Once a standard of care for caring is created and implemented, assessment sources may help nurses and other health care providers to determine its institution-wide impact.

Caregivers are more able to care for patients and are more effective when they feel supported (Down, 2002). Care interventions are intensified when caregivers feel cared for by families and friends, as well as colleagues (Freshwater, 2000; Green-Hemandez, 1996; Sheridan, Abruzzese, O'Grady, & Green-Hemandez, 1996). Staff support fosters high-quality patient care (Beeston & Jesson, 1999). Therefore, application of a standard of care for caring to include nurse colleagues and employees from other departments and services in a work setting can benefit nurses and patients. Reflective practice through clinical supervision builds an environment that fosters caring for staff, as well as local ownership of the caring standards for development and debate (Johns & Freshwater, 1998).

To examine the impact of shortened stays on ambulatory surgery patient outcomes, Swan (1998) has studied the relationship of postoperative patient-perceived nurse caring behaviors to symptom distress and functional status in ambulatory surgical patients at 24 hours, 4 days, and 7 days postsurgery. Subjects with a higher rating of postoperative patient-perceived nurse caring behaviors have experienced less symptom distress and higher levels of functional status. Swan's and other's (Duffy, 1990; Wolf et al., 1994) investigations have emphasized the association of nurse caring with positive patient outcomes. If a standard of care for caring is developed and adopted by clinicians across a health care institution, researchers could document the effect of such a standard on patient outcomes.

Morse, Bottorff, Neander, and Solberg (1991) have compared theories and conceptualizations of caring by analyzing nursing literature on caring. They have also considered the implications of caring for nursing. Five conceptualizations have been specified: caring as human trait, as moral imperative, as affect, as interpersonal interaction, and as therapeutic intervention. Three outcomes of caring have been identified: (a) patient's subjective experience, (b) patient's physical response, and (c) nurse's subjective experience. Morse et al. have pointed out the lack of definitions and clarity in descriptions on caring. The authors have invited investigators and theorists to delineate caring strategies for families and small groups, therefore expanding beyond the focus on individual patients. Finally, Morse and colleagues have called for research that strengthens the link between caring and patient outcomes. A standard of care for caring, once implemented, may provide that link.

Gaut (1983) has conducted a philosophical analysis of caring in order to develop a theoretically adequate description of caring. She has identified the necessary and sufficient conditions for the practical activity of caring and specified three conditions for any action described as caring: (a) the caregiver identifies a need for care and knows what to do for the care recipient, (b) the caregiver chooses and implements action intended as a means for positive change, and (c) the welfare of the cared for is used as a nonarbitrary principle, justifying the choice and implementation of the caring actions (Gaut, 1983). By adopting a standard of care to improve the outcomes of patients, families, and groups, nurses and other employees satisfy Gaut's condition of intention.

Watson's caring theory (1990) provides a framework for this study. Caring is posited as a moral ideal and an end in and of itself. Transpersonal caring–healing helps nurses, who are intimately involved with patients, preserve human dignity and humanity in the rapidly changing, highly technological health care system. Watson (1979) has positioned caring in "universal human values—kindness, concern, and love of self and others" (p. 10). Carative factors are emphasized as a philosophical basis for the science of caring, for example, the formation of a humanistic-altruistic value system, instillation of faith-hope, and cultivation of sensitivity to self and others (pp. 10–19). Consistent with

Watson's (1988a, 1988b, 1988c) theory, caring preserves human dignity in cure-dominated health care systems and becomes a standard by which cure is measured. Caring is therefore linked with patient outcomes. Watson's theory illustrates the transcendent, the intersubjective, and the in-the-moment nature of human care, and caring as nurses and others share environments and caring experiences.

METHOD

The investigators have employed a Delphi technique, using a panel of experts and iteration with controlled feedback (Dalkey, 1969), to elicit elements of a standard of care for caring. This approach uses sequential rounds of questionnaires to obtain consensus (Dennis, Howes, & Zelauskas, 1989). The technique has been used to feed information back from a first-round, open-end, and close-end item questionnaire to participants in second and third rounds after responses have been condensed and revised. Through this technique, collective group opinion is obtained in the next two iterative rounds. Condensed group opinion (Waltz, Strickland, & Lenz, 1984) is sought and incorporated into the last two versions of the questionnaire. The second round enables participants to add responses that have been incorporated into the third-round instrument (Goodman, 1987). Responses to the Round III questionnaire are incorporated into a draft of the final version of the standard.

Sample and Setting
Study Rounds I, II, and III have enlisted a respondent group from all of the current membership on a list provided by IAHC ($n = 354$), and for Round I alone, attendees ($n = 125$) at lAHC's Boca Raton conference in 2000. IAHC members, in attendance at the Boca Raton conference, have been asked to complete the

Round I questionnaire only once. The members of IAHC have been assumed to be experts, well versed in the practice, education, research, and literature of human care and caring. The demographic characteristics of Round I ($n = 98$) subjects are included in Table 26.1. Round II has surveyed IAHC members solely ($N = 354$); 72 respondents have completed the Round II instrument with a response rate of 20.3%. Round II results have been reviewed by several nurse managers or administrators ($n = 5$) who suggested revisions. Round III surveys have been sent to IAHC members ($N = 354$). Seventy respondents have completed the round; the response rate has been 21.1% ($n = 75$).

Ethical Considerations
An institutional review board of a university has approved the study for human subjects' considerations. Responses have been maintained in confidence, since no data have been linked to individual respondents. Demographic data have been aggregated. Completion of surveys has implied consent during the three rounds of the study.

Instrumentation and Procedures for Data Collection
The Round I questionnaire has included open- and closed-ended items to elicit words and phrases that describe elements of a standard of care for caring, an invitation to add themes or elements to be included in the standard, and an open-ended question to specify elements to exclude. Close-ended items have been ranked using the following Likert scale: 1 = Strongly Disagree; 2 = Disagree; 3 = Uncertain; 4 = Agree; 5 = Strongly Agree. The initial-round questionnaire, including instructions, has been pilot tested with five graduate-prepared registered nurses. It has been subsequently revised. Average time to complete the questionnaire has been 10 to 20 minutes.

Next, the Round II instrument has been constructed by content analysis and descriptive statistical analysis from Round I responses. Tentative elements of a standard of care for caring have been incorporated into this version of the tool. Items have been added based on Round I content analysis results. The Round II instrument has been reviewed by the coauthors and revised based on suggestions and questions. To encourage responses, potential elements of the standard have been listed along with the same Likert scale. Also, a comment/revision section has been provided to encourage subjects' textual responses.

The Round III instrument has been based on Round II statistical (i.e., clustering of four dimensions through factor analysis) and thematic results. As with Rounds I and II questionnaires,

TABLE 26.1 Demographic Characteristics of Round I Respondents (*N* = 98)

Age		
	Mean	51.34
	SD	8.56
	Range	28–72
Sex, *n* (%)		
	Female	88 (89.8)
	Male	3 (3.1)
	No response	7 (7.1)
Marital Status, *n* (%)		
	Married	65 (66.3)
	Single	14 (14.3)
	Divorced	11 (11.2)
	Widowed	2 (2.0)
	Partner	1 (1.0)
	No response	5 (5.1)
Country of Residence, *n* (%)		
	USA	71
	Canada	12
	Indonesia	2 (2.0)
	Denmark	2 (2.0)
	New Zealand	6 (6.1)
	England, Slovenia, Austria, Wales, Finland (1 each)	
	No response	4 (4.1)
Highest Degree Earned, *n* (%)		
	Doctoral	51 (51.1)
	Master's	32 (32.6)
	Bachelor's	5 (5.1)
	No response	10 (10.2)
IAHC Member, *n* (%)		
	Yes	84 (85.7)
	No	8 (8.2)
	No response	6 (6.1)

the Round III version of the standard of care for caring has provided directions (Couper, 1984) and the same Likert scale. Standard dimension items, comments, and suggested revision sections have been included. Based on Round III results, the investigators have revised the standard.

The items used on the Round I questionnaire have originated in caring literature and have established content validity of the questionnaire. Reliability of the responses has been supported by consistent themes across the sample for each round. The investigators have reviewed responses, and have recorded changes based on subject responses and consensus.

The first-round surveys have been conducted by mail or distributed at IAHC's 2000 research conference in Boca Raton. Rounds II and III have been mailed. Potential respondents have been asked to

participate in the study through a letter included with the instrument. Respondents have been asked to complete a demographic profile for Round I of the investigation. Addressed, stamped envelopes have been inserted in the mailings to increase the response rates. Three rounds have been considered adequate to elicit consensus regarding a standard of care for caring.

RESULTS

Descriptive statistics have been computed on the demographic characteristics of respondents (Table 26.1) and the Likert-scaled items on Round I (Table 26.2), and Round II (Table 26.3) surveys using Statistical Package for the Social Sciences for Windows. Items in Table 26.2 and Table 26.3 are arranged from highest to lowest

TABLE 26.2 Element of a Standard of Care for Caring Prioritized in Delphi Study (*N* = 98)

Rank Element	Round I		Rank Element	Round I	
	Mean	SD		Mean	SD
Showing respect	4.91	0.27	Being gentle	4.30	0.83
Listening	4.90	0.41	Supporting independence	4.30	0.75
Establishing trust	4.82	0.41	Teaching	4.30	0.92
Being present	4.81	0.48	Spending time	4.30	0.79
Being competent	4.80	0.44	Giving information for decision-making	4.29	1.00
Seeing person as a unique individual	4.78	0.54	Explaining	4.29	0.76
Being with	4.72	0.67	Helping	4.24	0.84
Being attentive	4.69	0.54	Giving feedback	4.24	0.92
Being clinically competent	4.69	0.56	Putting the person first	4.23	0.95
Giving emotional support	4.66	0.55	Helping the person grow	4.23	0.80
Ensuring confidentiality	4.65	0.67	Being hopeful for the future	4.17	0.80
Staying during difficult time	4.63	0.67	Feeling with and for	4.15	0.89
Advocating	4.62	0.56	Knowing the person	4.15	1.10
Being nonjudgmental	4.60	0.67	Teaching	4.13	0.86
Answering questions honestly	4.59	0.60	Anticipating needs	4.10	0.71
Providing safety	4.57	0.70	Keeping watch over	4.09	0.90
Encouraging to express positive and negative feelings	4.53	0.72	Building self-esteem	4.06	1.89

(*continued*)

TABLE 26.2 Element of a Standard of Care for Caring Prioritized in Delphi Study (N = 98)
(continued)

Rank Element	Round I Mean	SD	Rank Element	Round I Mean	SD
Encouraging to ask questions	4.53	0.64	Being hopeful	4.04	0.93
Following through	4.53	0.59	Providing reassurance	4.01	0.90
Picking up cues	4.52	0.74	Monitoring	3.96	0.99
Acting to decrease pain	4.51	0.66	Giving physical care	3.93	0.99
Supporting spiritual growth	4.50	0.73	Telling what is found	3.81	0.92
Protecting from injury	4.48	0.81	Touching	3.76	1.02
Ensuring privacy	4.46	0.67	Giving medications and treatments	3.74	1.07
Showing concern	4.40	0.74	Being humorous	3.61	0.85
Providing a safe place	4.40	0.77	Overcoming problems	3.53	0.99
Being accessible	4.39	0.77	Serving	3.50	1.04
Being involved	4.35	0.81	Being close	3.48	1.03
Comforting	4.34	0.81	Meshing or fitting with the person	3.46	0.95
Explaining procedures, treatments, and medications	4.34	0.79	Holding	3.41	1.02
Intending to care	4.34	0.96	Being consoled	3.41	1.11
Including in planning	4.33	0.87	Being engrossed in the person's experience	3.37	1.13
Responding quickly to a request for help	4.32	0.78	Being firm	3.17	1.16
			Being available by phone	3.04	0.90

TABLE 26.3 Round II Potential Elements of Standards (N = 72)

	Mean	SD
Nurses and other caregivers will . . .		
Listen and be responsive to the patient	4.73	.68
Give information for decision making	4.71	.72
Provide privacy for the patient and keep patient information in confidence	4.68	.73
Include the patient in planning and follow through with plans	4.68	.73
Explain procedures, treatments, and medications	4.66	.73
Approach the patient (family, group, community) reflecting the intention of improving his or her welfare/situation by caring about and for the patient.	4.64	.77
Be courteous and respectful	4.64	.73
Provide a safe place and protect the patient from injury	4.64	.74
Encourage the patient to ask questions and honestly answer the patient's questions	4.64	.77
Act to decrease the patient's pain and suffering	4.64	.74
Demonstrate clinical competence and self-confidence in their performance	4.60	.78
Will monitor the patient and keep watch over the patient	4.57	.83
Advocate for the patient and support the patient's independence	4.55	.81

(continued)

TABLE 26.3 Round II Potential Elements of Standards (*N* = 72) (*continued*)

	Mean	SD
Pay attention to the patient's cues and respond to them	4.55	.89
Be present/available for the patient	4.55	.81
Be accessible and attentive to the patient	4.51	.78
Be gentle, compassionate, and concerned	4.51	.84
Encourage the patient to express positive and negative feelings	4.48	.78
Support the patient	4.48	.89
Attempt to earn the patient's trust	4.44	.96
Connect with the patient and create an authentic relationship with the patient	4.44	.86
Be nonjudgmental	4.42	.96
Teach the patient	4.42	.86
Respond quickly to a patient's request for help	4.42	.83
Anticipate the patient's needs	4.37	.80
Be attuned to the patient's story	4.33	.82
Give the patient feedback	4.33	.85
Mobilize resources for the patient	4.33	.85
Give physical care, medications, and treatments	4.31	.84
Support the patient's spiritual growth	4.17	.91
Reassure and console the patient	4.11	.91
Encourage the patient's development of self-esteem	4.08	.82
Use humor appropriately	4.08	.79
Witness what the patient is experiencing	3.82	.98
Show hope for the patient's immediate and long-term future	3.80	1.01
Be engrossed with the patient's experience	3.40	.93

means. An exploratory factor analysis procedure has been used to cluster Round II results into standard dimensions or factors. Content analysis has been used to analyze textual data elicited as comments for Round I, II, and III surveys.

Respondents have noted some concerns about the Round II standard. One has written that reducing caring "to a list seems to diminish the process." While expressing positive reactions to the standard, another has pointed out its grounding in Western values.

The problem remains, however, how can we teach "caring." Heidegger speaks of caring as the core value as we have moved into communal life. Caring, however, is one of those omni-directional words, since completely opposite actions can be carried out in its name whose caring values, or perceived values, dominate? Can we as nurses accept all values, even "destructive" ones as we understand them? The rhetoric of "caring" assumes, for example, Western caring values that are associated with liberty, truth, justice, and rights. All are rhetorical terms of sophistic splendor.

A respondent has voiced strong opposition to the standard, considering caring and care influenced by cultural context and that context "greatly influences outcome." Care, according to the respondent, is "meaningless and dangerous unless known and understood within cultural context, values, beliefs, and lifeways." The respondent has warned that the standard was not necessarily culture bound or appropriate for different generations. She has emphasized the importance of the cultural context for patients, families, and communities.

Another respondent, who questioned whether nurses have autonomy, has expressed a concern about the professional status of nursing. That respondent has asserted that, in most cases, nurses do not have autonomy. Still, another has suggested that taking responsibility for errors and asking to correct them should be added to the standard. One respondent has pointed out that the standard seemed more of a fit with acute care settings.

In contrast, 20 respondents from Round III have noted that the standard was very good to excellent. Several ($n = 4$) have indicated that the standard required no revisions. One has written that it was very complete.

TABLE 26.4 Standard of Care for Caring

A standard of care for caring may be useful to nurses and other caregivers. The standard serves as a behavioral guideline for those interested in comparing themselves to a caring "yardstick." It assumes that nurses and other caregivers have the capacity to care and recognize the vulnerability of clients. They do not exploit these vulnerabilities for gain or self-interest. The standard also assumes client and nurse autonomy over their own actions, caring as a way of being in relationship, variations in the competencies of nurses and other caregivers, and caring as a moral imperative and virtuous activity.

The standard has been developed with the understanding that clients, families, and communities are culture bound. Thus, the standard is of use only when nurses and other caregivers are sensitive to the cultural context of those cared for.

Standard Dimension

1. Nurses and other caregivers . . .

1.1	Approach the client (family, group, community) with the intention of enhancing his or her welfare/situation by caring about, for, and with the client
1.2	Are courteous, respectful, and unbiased
1.3	Are compassionate, gentle, and empathetic
1.4	Seek to discover the client's values, beliefs, and desires and advocate for them in a culturally sensitive manner
1.5	Safeguard the client's rights and respect his or her dignity
1.6	Support the client's culturally based practices
1.7	Provide privacy for the client and keep client information in confidence
1.8	Establish a trusting relationship with the client
1.9	Encourage the client to ask questions and provide honest answers
1.10	Verify that the client understands the information provided
1.11	Support the client's independent decision making
1.12	Assist the client in decision-making and planning, and follow through with the prioritized plan of care
1.13	Teach the client and explain procedures, treatments, treatment alternatives, and medications
1.14	Encourage self-care
1.15	Anticipate the client's needs and concerns and help the client mobilize necessary resources
1.16	Address the client's priority needs and concerns
1.17	Perform knowledgeably, skillfully, confidently, and competently, consistent with role and responsibility
1.18	Develop their knowledge and skills
1.19	Competently provide physical care, medications, and treatments

(continued)

TABLE 26.4 Standard of Care for Caring (*continued*)

Standard Dimension

2. Nurses and other caregivers . . .

2.1	Monitor and vigilantly watch over the client
2.2	Make themselves available to the client
2.3	Provide a safe environment and protect the client from injury
2.4	Address issues in the health care system that infringe on client rights or that may cause harm to the client
2.5	Facilitate seamless care and foster collaboration among caregivers by communicating and planning with caregivers and the client
2.6	Respond in a timely manner to the client's request for help or indications of deterioration
2.7	Follow up with the client as promised
2.8	Act promptly to decrease the client's discomfort, distressing symptoms, and suffering

3. Nurses and other caregivers . . .

3.1	Learn the client's story, situation, and context
3.2	Act in a genuine manner to create a therapeutic relationship with the client
3.3	Engage in the client's experience
3.4	Pay attention to the client's cues and respond to them
3.5	Give feedback to and receive feedback from the client
3.6	Promote the client's self-esteem
3.7	Support the client's spiritual, emotional, mental, physical, and social needs
3.8	Pay attention to the client's healing

4. Nurses and other caregivers . . .

4.1	Encourage the client to express his/her feelings, beliefs, concerns, and positive and negative feelings
4.2	Listen to and support the client
4.3	Accept the client's silence
4.4	Respond to, reassure, empathize with, and console the client
4.5	Support decisions regarding the client's immediate and long-term future
4.6	Respect the client's expressed wishes regarding end-of-life care
4.7	Support the client and family through the dying and grieving process

The standard of care for caring is included in Table 26.4. Four groupings of dimensions are presented along with introductory comments.

DISCUSSION

The results of the study should be viewed with caution, and the standard of care for caring has been used carefully and strategically. Response rates have been low. The standard of care for caring has been generated from the responses of IAHC members and attendees of the Boca Raton conference—the panel of experts. Because of their countries of residence, members of IAHC are strongly influenced by Western cultural ways. Another limitation is that feedback from each round serves to focus respondents' opinions (Bums & Grove, 2001), thus possibly limiting the content of answers. Additionally, a nurse administrator has noted that the standards could be used as guidelines, and that health care providers, other than nurses, should review and evaluate the standards.

The standard of care for caring may serve as a starting point for discussion and debate. It can also guide the development of a nursing practice model. Nurses must confirm the importance of their contributions to health care. Lang and Krejci (1991) have considered standards necessary to reflect nursing's holistic contributions, and have called for the measurement of the outcomes of subjective experiences, such as caring, on health. Consumers and providers recognize the value and effect of subjective experiences on health and quality of life. The creation and dissemination of a standard, as one for caring, and measurement of associated outcomes respond to Lang and Krejci's request. The standard, based on this study, can help to provide evidence caring for patients and providers, and change health care in the process.

AUTHOR NOTE

The authors would like to thank Sharon Beck, DNSc, RN, and Carol Uccelletti, BSN, RN, for their support during this study. Correspondence concerning this chapter should be addressed to Zane Robinson Wolf, La Salle University School of Nursing, 1900 West Olney Avenue, Philadelphia, PA, 19141 USA. Electronic mail may be sent via Internet to wolf@lasalle.edu. Other authors may be reached via electronic mail: Dawn Freshwater, dawn.freshwater@btintemet.com; Margaret Miller, margaret.a.miller@widener.edu; Rebecca Jones, wsjonesra@wscn.edu; and Gwen Sherwood, gwen.sherwood@uth.tmc.edu.

REFERENCES

Andrews, L. W., Daniels, P., & Hall, A. G. (1996). Nurse caring behaviors: Comparing five tools to define perceptions. *Ostomy/Wound Management, 42*(5), 28–37.

Beeston, H., & Jesson, A. (1999). Caring for staff: Setting quality standards. *Nursing Standard, 13*(16), 43–45.

Burns, N., & Grove, S. K. (2001). *The practice of nursing research: Conduct, critique, & utilization* (4th ed.). Philadelphia, PA: W. B. Saunders Company.

Callahan, D. (1990). The primacy of caring. *Commonweal, 117*(4), 107–112.

Clinton, M., & Nelson, S. (1998). Quality discourse and nursing as therapy. In R. McMahon & A. Pearson (Eds.), *Nursing as therapy* (2nd ed.). Cheltenham, UK: Stanley Thornes.

Couper, M. R. (1984). The Delphi technique: Characteristics and sequence. *Advances in Nursing Science, 7*(1), 72–77.

Dalkey, N. C. (1969). *The Delphi Method: An experimental study of group opinion*. Santa Monica, CA: United States Air Forces, Project Rand.

Dennis, K. E., Howes, D. G., & Zelauskas, B. (1989). Identifying nursing research priorities: A first step in program development. *Applied Nursing Research, 2*(3), 108–113.

Donabedian, A. (1980). Criteria, norms and standards of quality: What do they mean? *American Journal of Public Health, 71*(4), 409–412.

Down, J. (2002). Therapeutic nursing and technology: Clinical supervision and reflective practice in a critical care setting. In D. Freshwater (Ed.), *Therapeutic nursing*. London, UK: Sage.

Dozier, A. M. (1998). Professional standards: Linking care, competence, and quality. *Journal of Nursing Care Quality, 12*(4), 22–29.

Duffy, J. R. (1990). An analysis of the relationship among nurse caring behaviors and selected outcomes of care in hospitalized medical and/or surgical patients. Ann Arbor, MI: Catholic University of America. University Microfilms, 119137361.

Forrest, D. (1989). The experience of caring. *Journal of Advanced Nursing, 14*, 815–823.

Fox, R. C., Aiken, L. H., & Messikomer, C. M. (1990). The culture of caring: AIDS and the nursing profession. *Milbank Quarterly, 68*(2), 226–256.

Freshwater, D. (2000). Cross currents: Against cultural narration. *Journal of Advanced Nursing, 32*(2), 481–484.

Gaut, D. (1983). Development of a theoretically adequate description of caring. *Western Journal of Nursing Research, 5*(4), 313–324.

Goodman, C. M. (1987). The Delphi technique: A critique. *Journal of Advanced Nursing, 12*, 729–734.

Green-Hemandez, C. (1996). Engendering collegial caring: A mandate for staff development. *Nursing Staff Development Insider, 5*(1), 5–8.

Green-Hemandez, C. (1997). Application of caring theory in primary care: A challenge for advanced practice. *Nursing Administration Quarterly, 21*(4), 77–82.

Johns, C., & Freshwater, D. (Eds.). (1998). *Transforming nursing through reflective practice*. Oxford, UK: Blackwell.

Joiner, G. A. (1996). Caring in action: The key to nursing service excellence. *Journal of Nursing Care Quality, 11*(1), 38–43.

Joint Commission on Accreditation of Health care Organizations (1996). *Comprehensive accreditation manual for hospitals*. Oakbrook Terrace, IL: Author. (May 2000 Update, p. GL9 Glossary 25).

Knowlden, V. (1998). *The communication of caring in nursing*. Indianapolis, IN: Center Nursing Press.

Lang, N. M., & Krejci, J. W. (1991). Standards and holism: A reframing. *Holistic Nursing Practice, 5*(3), 14–21.

Leininger, M. (1977). Caring: The essence and central focus of nursing. *Nursing Research Reports, 12*(2), 2, 14.

McLaughlin, C. P., & Kaluzny, A. D. (1997). Total quality management issues in managed care. *Journal of Health Care Finance, 24*(1), 10–16.

Moore, K., Lynn, M. R., McMillen, B. J., & Evans, S. (1999). Implementation of the ANA Report Card. *JONA, 29*(6), 48–54.

Morse, J. M., Bottorff, J., Neander, W., & Solberg, S. (1991). Comparative analysis of conceptualizations and theories of caring. *Image: Journal of Nursing Scholarship, 23*(2), 119–126.

Popovich, J. M. (1998). Multidimensional performance measurement. *Journal of Nursing Care Quality, 12*(4), 14–21.

Ray, M. A. (1997). The ethical theory of existential authenticity: The lived experience of the art of caring in nursing administration. *Canadian Journal of Nursing Research, 29*(1), 111–126.

Reese, R., & Reese, C. (1994). Guidelines for developing a new standard in hospice care. *Caring, 13*(9), 8–9, 69–70, 72.

Schoenhofer, S. O., & Boykin, A. (1993). Nursing as caring: An emerging general theory of nursing. In M. E. Parker (Ed.), *Patterns of nursing theories in practice* (pp. 83–93). New York, NY: National League for Nursing.

Sheridan, D. R., Abruzzese, R. S., O'Grady, T., & Green-Hernandez, C. G. (1996). Nursing staff development in the 1990s. In R. S. Abruzzese (Ed.), *Nursing staff development* (2nd ed., pp. 16–29). St. Louis, MO: Mosby-Year Book.

Sherwood, G. D. (1997). Meta-synthesis of qualitative analyses of caring: Defining a therapeutic model of nursing. *Advanced Practice Nursing Quarterly, 3*(1), 32–42.

Smith, M. (2000). The standard of caring. *Emergency Medical Services, 21*(1), 32, 83.

Smith, M. C. (1999). Caring and the science of unitary human beings. *Advances in Nursing Science, 21*(4), 14–28.

Swan, B. (1998). Postoperative nursing care contributions to symptom distress and functional status after ambulatory surgery. *MEDSURG Nursing, 7*(3), 148–158.

Waltz, C. F., Strickland, O. L., & Lenz, E. R. (1984). *Measurement in nursing research*. Philadelphia, PA: F. A. Davis.

Watson, J. (1979). *Nursing: The philosophy and science of caring*. Boston, MA: Little, Brown & Company.

Watson, J. (1987). Nursing on the caring edge: Metaphorical vignettes. *Advances in Nursing Science, 10*(1), 10–18.

Watson, J. (1988a). *Nursing: Human science and human care*. New York, NY: National League for Nursing (Pub. No. 15-2236).

Watson, J. (1988b). Introduction: An ethic of caring/curing/nursing qua nursing. In J. Watson & M. A. Ray (Eds.), *The ethics of care and the ethics of cure: Synthesis in chronicity* (pp. 1–3). New York, NY: National League for Nursing (Pub. No. 15-2237).

Watson, J. (1988c). New dimensions of human caring theory. *Nursing Science Quarterly, 1*(4), 175–181.

Watson, M. J. (1990). Transpersonal caring: A transcendent view of person, health and healing. In M. E. Parker (Ed.), *Nursing theories in practice* (pp. 277–288). New York, NY: National League for Nursing.

Williams, S. A. (1998). Quality and care: Patients' perceptions. *Journal of Nursing Care Quality, 12*(6), 18–25.

Wolf, Z. R., Colahan, M., Costello, A., Warwick, F., Ambrose, M. S., & Giardino, E. R. (1994). Relationship between nurse caring and patient satisfaction. *MEDSURG Nursing, 7*(2), 99–105.

QUESTIONS FOR REFLECTION

Baccalaureate

1. What did you learn about the Delphi technique by reading Wolf et al.'s (2003) study?
2. Why do you think it is important or unimportant to describe a standard of care for caring?
3. How were the nurse participants established as experts for the rounds of the Delphi study on the standard of care for caring?

Master's

1. What did you learn about the methods of the Delphi technique? Describe the steps.
2. How did the Delphi study on the standard of care for caring combine qualitative and quantitative analysis techniques?
3. How could the standard of care for caring be implemented with your nurse colleagues?

Doctoral

1. What do you like or dislike about the standard of care for caring?
2. What challenges would you confront if you decided to implement the standard of care for caring at your workplace?
3. What follow-up steps would be needed to implement the standard of care for caring at your workplace?

VI

Caring-Based Nursing Practice Models

MARIAN C. TURKEL

Nursing is a discipline of knowledge and professional practice wherein nursing theories and conceptual models, essential to the discipline, guide what is to be studied for the practice of nursing. Theories describe and explain the phenomena of interest about the nature, goals, and practice of nursing in diverse nursing situations. Conceptual models have varied definitions and actions ranging from abstract ideas or systems, to sets of values and beliefs, to methods of procedures for guiding research and practice (Parker, 2001). Theory-guided practice advances both the discipline and the profession of nursing. Theories are part of the knowledge structure of any discipline (Parker & Smith, 2010). According to Parker and Smith (2010), the major reason for structuring and advancing nursing knowledge through nursing theory is to develop, understand, and transform nursing practice.

Professional nursing practice models have been studied in the nursing literature since the 1970s and have traditionally focused on methods of patient care delivery and organization of care. The models included primary care, modified primary care, team nursing, and care or case management. Focus of these models was on the work and role of the registered nurse; they were not grounded in the tenets of a specific nursing theory.

The American Nurses Credentialing Center (ANCC) Magnet Recognition Program® (Magnet) recognizes excellence in professional nursing practice. This emphasis on professional nursing practice has resulted in organizations integrating nursing research and professional models of care delivery using nursing theory into the practice setting. Nursing theory has moved from its central place in academia and research to practice (Davidson, Ray, & Turkel, 2011).

The majority of Magnet hospitals have implemented a theoretical framework grounded in caring science. Through the lens of caring science, contemporary nursing practice focuses on creating caring–healing professional practice models for nurses, patients, and families within today's complex health care organizations. The philosophy and Theory of Human Caring has become a theory of choice as direct care registered nurses return to caring values. Watson's Theory of Human Caring is being used to inform nursing practice at both the national and international levels. According to J. Watson (personal communication, October 7, 2010), approximately 500 hospitals are using the theory to guide, inform, and transform professional nursing practice.

Caring-based professional practice models illuminate the meaning and value of caring and clarify how caring is portrayed in diverse practice situations to improve the quality of nursing care. These professional practice models make explicit the caring relationship, values, beliefs, and philosophies that guide advanced nursing practice (Watson, 2008). Professional practice models generated from caring theories continue to emerge, and original models have been advanced. A few of the sentinel works are represented in this section.

Duffy and Hoskins (2003) provided an evidence-based practice framework to demonstrate the value of professional nursing practice in terms of quality health outcomes and translated the invisible work of nursing into objective terms linked to quantifiable outcomes through the Quality-Caring Model©. The Quality-Caring Model© reaffirmed the nature of nursing's work as relationship-centered, focused on the two dominant relationships of independent relationships (patient or family–nurse) and collaborative relationships (Health Care Team–Nurse). The unique feature of the model is the explicit association between caring relationships and positive outcomes for patient or families, health care providers, and health care systems. In addition to the presentation of the model, the authors exposed the hidden work of nursing, described the conceptual–theoretical–empirical linkages between quality of care and human caring, and proposed approaches for testing the accuracy of the model (Duffy & Hoskins, 2003).

The authors presented an overview of research supporting a linkage among professional nursing care, nurse caring, and patient outcomes. Although the linkages exist, what specifically accounts for this is unknown (Duffy & Hoskins, 2003). As part of the section related to nursing's work, they reviewed that the work of nursing theorists focused on the nurse–patient relationship. The authors acknowledged the concept of nurses' activities being separate from the work of medicine and the essence of nursing (caring) as separate

but complementary to medicine (curing) (Watson, 1985) as foundational to caring based professional models of care. They identified various definitions of caring from the perspectives of various scholars. Boykin and Schoenhofer (1993, p. 27) described nursing as a unique "form of caring," while Gordon (2002) stated that the caring in nursing practice, although often silent, is "educated caring." This view is consistent with the thinking of Mayeroff (1971) and Benner (1984) who believed that knowledge is required for caring to be part of nursing practice.

Duffy and Hoskins (2003) presented an analysis of Watson's Theory of Human Care (1985) and the original carative factors, which evolved into Clinical Caring Processes (Watson, 1999). Watson described transpersonal relationships as having a benefit to both patients and nurses and theorized that outcomes from such relationships include preservation of human dignity, protection from harm, and inner harmony. The authors acknowledged that this postmodern view of nursing is not supported in the traditional biomedical institutional model of tasks, technology, and procedures. According to the authors, relationships with patients and family remain the primary focus of nurses' work, although relationships with other members of the health care team have been linked to specific patient outcomes.

The authors identified that the Quality-Caring Model© integrated the works of Donabedian (1992) and Watson (1985) and was influenced by contributions from King (1981), Mitchell, Ferkeitch, and Jennings (1998), and Irvine, Sidani, & Hall (1998). The major components of the model are structure, process, and outcomes. Structure involves the participants of providers, patient or family, and system. Factors that influence outcomes are identified under each category. For example, the attitudes and behavior of providers, patient comorbidities or age, and system staffing patterns may directly or indirectly influence outcomes of care. Process, the second major component of the model, is the focus of the model and includes the concept of caring relationships. They defined caring relationships as human interactions grounded in clinical caring processes (p. 82). The authors described the two types of relationships as independent and collaborative. Independent relationships include patient or family–nurse interactions, which nurses implement autonomously and hold sole accountability for. The specific intervention performed by the nurses, such as pain management, is measured in terms of nurse–sensitive patient outcomes. Medication titration is a nursing activity and responsibility shared by other members of the health care team and is an example of a collaborative relationship. Relationship-centered professional encounters represent the majority of nursing's work, and it is during these encounters that nurses form caring relationships with patients and families independently and in collaboration with other members of the health care team. The relationships are grounded in the clinical caring processes, essential to quality care, and result in positive outcomes for the patient, provider, and the health system. Outcomes related to patient or family, provider, and system constitute the third component of the model and are defined as intermediate and terminal outcomes. Examples include increased quality of life and satisfaction with care.

The purpose of the model is to provide evidence that nurse caring does positively affect patient outcomes. The authors affirmed that additional research involving independent nursing interventions grounded in the clinical caring processes on patient outcomes and correlational studies of the nurse–patient relationship to patient outcomes will provide needed empirical evidence linking caring nursing practices to quality health care in terms of nurse–sensitive indicators and patient outcomes. Nursing practice often occurs in a traditional medical industrial model governed by tasks. The Quality-Caring Model© originated by Duffy and Hoskins recognized and valued relationship-centered professional encounters as a way to guide professional nursing practice and provide evidence on the value of nursing caring practices.

Turkel and Ray (2004) viewed the soul of nursing "as seeking the good of self and others through compassionate caring" (p. 249) and introduced the concepts of healing and caring for oneself as being integral to having the energy to compassionately care for others. They feel that nursing leaders have a moral responsibility to integrate, role model, and value self-care, practice renewal, and healing within organizational cultures to foster caring and trusting relationships. This allows nurses to provide holistic nursing practices grounded in caring values and caring science as part of the professional practice model. At the time this manuscript was published, nurses in the practice setting were beginning to intently implement caring theory–guided practice intently. The authors referenced Watson (1985) in terms of the idea of the nurse being holistic body–mind and spirit. For nurses to practice authentic presence and create harmony within the caring moment, self-caring is integral.

The authors recognized the writings of Tzu (Wing, 1986) in relation to the universality of compassionate caring. Compassion involves looking inward and outward, being insightful to the forces of spirit and nature to reveal a path of personal excellence. Turkel and Ray were also informed by the concept of "lead with the soul" (Bohman & Deal, 2001) and the recognition that healing and caring for oneself is critical to successful relationships and organizations (Kahn, 1994) and enforces how self and others are interconnected (Chappell, 1993).

Turkel and Ray (2004) examined the definitions of caring as proposed by various caring scholars (Leininger, 1981; Leninger & McFarland, 2003; Ray, 1981, 1989; Roach, 1992, 2002; Turkel & Ray, 2000, 2001; Watson, 1979, 1985, 2001). These illuminate caring as transcultural, a human trait, a way of being, and moral ideal, grounded in organizational contexts including economics and a complex dynamic. Although caring was expressed differently by theorists, it centers on caring as a way of being and encompasses a body of knowledge grounded in human science and spirituality.

The authors reflected on the meaning of caring within organizations and espoused the view that "when organizations are infused with compassionate caring values, they reflect a human face, which is necessary for the continued existence of humanity" (p. 251). The role of nursing leaders is recognizing the power of caring for self to awaken the creative caring sprit and to create a caring workforce environment. The authors cited the work of Schuster (1997) who was one of the first caring scholars to make explicit the value of self-care and self renewal to co-create communities of caring. Schuster stated that "our creative selves need consistent acknowledgment, respect and nurturing" (p. 251). Turkel and Ray also referenced Sister Simone Roach's (1992/2002) definition of competence, which includes having the needed energy required for technical proficiency. They provided specific examples of how nurse leaders can integrate caring for self activities into the practice setting. One example was to include a healing modality such as meditation, massage, or aromatherapy into yearly competency education for nursing staff. Innovative for the time, this approach is now being implemented in many hospitals that use Watson's Theory of Human Caring to guide the professional practice model of care delivery.

They reaffirmed that in order for self-care to be fully valued and integrated within a culture, organizational culture needs to be recreated. Specific strategies for recreating organizational culture were presented. The strategy of creating a "healing room" for nurses to meditate, rest, and reflect is emerging in many hospitals that are using Watson's Theory of Human Caring and outcomes are being recognized in terms of increased registered nurse satisfaction and feelings of self-renewal. Another strategy of having nurses develop a plan for self-care as part of their annual evaluation is becoming part of the professional practice model within several organizations.

The authors honored the work of Florence Nightingale (1969) as the first nursing scholar to discuss the role of the physical environment to allow for healing. Examples of health care organizations developing healing gardens, using Feng Shui for design, and creating labyrinths were presented. Turkel and Ray (2004) ended by restating the belief that caring nurse leaders need to have the vision, wisdom, and knowledge to advance opportunities for self-care to create caring compassionate organizations. This in turn allows registered nurses to find new meaning in work and integrate caring–healing practices into the professional practice model.

Watson and Foster (2003) developed the Attending Nurse Caring Model® (ANCM) as a way to integrate caring–healing practices into acute care hospital settings where nursing practice has been influenced by the medical paradigm and focused on technology, diagnosis, and treatment of acute illness and product line management. The authors identified that nurses are torn between the human caring values of the profession and the biomedical model, that is, the practice reality where they spend the majority of their time. The authors referenced Swanson (1999), who identified that nurses become hardened, oblivious, and robot-like when they are not able to practice within a caring environment. The Attending Nurse Caring Model® is an exemplar for advancing the discipline and transforming nursing practice within a reflective, philosophical, theoretical context informed by caring science (Watson & Foster, 2003). In this model, nursing practice moves away from the routine, industrial, task-oriented approach to a "focused intentionality towards caring and healing relationships with a shift towards the spiritualizing of health" (p. 361).

The authors reviewed the traditional physician practice hospitalist model and the nurse hospitalist model (Mustard, 2002). The nurse hospitalist model consists of advanced practice registered nurses who report to the chief nurse executive and are responsible to oversee other nurses. Focused education for the nursing staff and improvement of competency through critical thinking and interpersonal skills as ways to improve nurse performance are emphasized. The hospitalist nurse coordinated care, informed the patient, respected the patients' values, and involved the patient and family in decision making. Caring theory did not serve as the foundation for the model. This model reflected a professional practice model of care delivery rather than a caring-based professional nursing practice model.

The Attending Nurse Caring Model® incorporated and extended Mustard's (2002) work to incorporate caring theory as foundational with a focus on the integration of "heart-felt" caring–healing practices. Nurses practicing within this model develop and oversee a plan of caring theory–guided care for patients and families. The attending caring nurse (ACN) is responsible for overseeing this plan of caring–healing 24 hours a day. Specific responsibilities of the ACN were identified. These included establishing and sustaining a continuous caring relationship

with patients and families and developing a comprehensive assessment of caring needs and concerns using caring theory as a guide. The knowledge, values, philosophy, and practices are grounded in caring theory and have resulted in a new pattern for the delivery of professional nursing care.

The authors presented an overview of the pilot project on a 37-bed surgical unit at the Children's Hospital in Denver, Colorado. The model was used to guide a comprehensive program of pain management for hospitalized children. Specific caring–healing modalities related to pain management were incorporated into the plan of care to complement physicians' orders for analgesics to create a caring healing environment for patients. Nurses involved in this pilot project participated in educational sessions related to Watson's theory and the 10 Carative Factors (Watson, 1979), identified caring–healing practices for self-care, and engaged in reflective practice activities of recording caring moments and focus group discussions.

MOVING FORWARD

Caring-based nursing practice models have been developed by other scholars interested in theory-guided practice. Bent et al. (2005) used action research to guide the implementation of Watson's Theory of Human Science and Human Care (1985) within the Veterans Administration Eastern Colorado Health Care System. Nightingale units were created and tangible expressions of human caring were integrated into daily nursing practice. A registered nurse with expertise in translating caring theory into practice was present on the units 1 or 2 days per week. She assisted staff in advancing caring–healing modalities such as aromatherapy and reflexology and emphasized the relational aspect of caring for patients. A change of shift report that engaged patients and supported their healing was developed, and the staff break room was painted to serve as a retreat for the staff. Other innovations included dimming the lights, playing soft music, and initiating a computerized documentation system with the carative factors to encourage staff to think about their care in terms of the theory. Caring–healing-guided practices include focusing on relationships and connectedness, authentic presence, patient–family-centered care, holistic assessment of patient needs, and holistic therapeutic interventions.

Boykin, Schoenhofer, Smith, St. Jean, and Aleman (2003) shared their experience of how the theory Nursing as Caring (Boykin & Schoenhofer, 1993) was actualized in practice on an 18-bed telemetry unit. The values and assumptions of the theory guided the value statements, intended project outcomes for patients/families, nursing staff, and system, and project implementation. Dialogues were held where all members of the nursing staff were invited to share stories that portrayed caring and then asked to reflect on caring, and what made this a caring experience. Themes emerged from the dialogue and nursing practice was redesigned to embrace the values of the staff. Changes in practice included giving each new patient a greeting card with information on how to reach members of the nursing staff, inviting patients and families to share what mattered most to them at that time, and then using this information to guide daily nursing practice. In addition, staff intently focused on coming to know each other and how they each expressed caring. Staff created new ways of being within the organization, respecting and honoring the unique gifts each brings to practice. All patient satisfaction questions related to nursing care on the Press Ganey survey increased significantly and nurses verbalized that their practice of nursing was transformed through sharing stories of focusing on what matters most to patients.

The Theory of Nursing as Caring informed the transformation of the practice of nursing in the emergency department of a community hospital (Boykin, Bulfin, Baldwin, & Southern, 2004; Boykin, Bulfin, Schoenhofer, Baldwin, & McCarthy, 2005). The team focused on introducing the concept of caring to the staff, so they came to understand that technical expertise, diagnostic skills, compassion, commitment, and respect for person are all part of caring. To transform care from object-centered to patient-centered involved staff knowing self and other as caring person. Staff including nursing leaders reflected on What does it mean to live caring in everyday life? and How do I express caring in practice? Through dialogue and reflection, they began to see caring as something real and committed to intentionally focusing on creating a caring-based value system for practice. Examples of practice changes included focusing on hearing what mattered most and then supporting and sustaining this for patient and family, giving Thank-You cards to all patients discharged from the hospital, and leaders sending hand-written notes to the staff honoring and celebrating their caring practices with patients and families.

Brown et al. (2005) described how Watson's Theory of Human Science and Human Care (1985) and the carative factors served as the framework for creation of the patient care facilitator (PCF) role at the Baptist Hospital of Miami. In 2001, this hospital was one of the first to adopt Watson's theory to guide nursing practice. Caring was identified as one of the primary needs of the patients, yet nurses had less time to spend with patients, additional responsibilities, and patients saw many different caregivers during their stay. The authors felt that caring is essential for continuity of care, while continuity of care reinforces caring. In this caring-based professional practice model, the patients' needs are at the center of the delivery system and the

PCF acts as the CEO for a small group of patients, usually 12 in total. The PCF is an experienced registered nurse who demonstrates expertise at bedside caring and clinical expertise who provides leadership for a team of nurses assigned to 12 to 16 patients, and the primary role of the PCF is to know each patient in this area, serving as their advocate during the hospital stay. The PCF turns caring for patients into a way to fully exemplify caring by the nurses (p. 52). The authors identified that the PCFs feel a strong sense of connection with patient and family, and the nurses in role this feel that the role brings out their passion for being a nurse and that "the soul of the PCF role is caring" (p. 55).

Duffy (2010) continued to advance the original Quality-Caring Model©. In the revised model, the link between caring relationships and quality care is made more explicit and the revised model is considered a middle range theory. The four main concepts include humans in relationship, relationship-centered professional encounters, feeling cared for, and self-caring. Duffy stated "the overall role of the nurse in this model is to engage in caring relationships with self and others to engender feeling 'cared for'" (p. 405). The author acknowledged that quality nursing care is based on the use of best evidence from caring research. The model is currently being used by registered nurses by direct care registered nurses in at least 10 hospitals as a way to practice nursing centered on caring relationships and to guide specific nursing interventions.

Touhy, Strews, and Brown (2005) used the theory of Nursing as Caring to create a caring-based professional practice model within a 60-bed skilled nursing facility. All staff, residents, and families were invited to participate in interviews. They were asked to share thoughts about what is most important to you when caring for someone or being cared for and to share a story that best represents those aspects of care. Practice changes identified by the authors included posters with pictures of staff, residents, and families in caring interactions; creating and exchanging special occasion cards made by residents and staff; celebration of diverse cultural holidays, heart-shaped pens for staff, creating unit-based caring themes such as "staff care from the heart"; caring awards; including nursing assistants in the planning of care and development of a " Coming to Know" booklet describing the unique calls for caring of each resident. The authors used the Caring Behaviors Inventory (Wolf, 1994; Wolf et al., 1998; Wolf, Giardino, Osborne, & Ambrose, 1994) for post-project evaluation. Results indicated an increase in scores related to listening, treating the person as an individual, spending time, touching to communicate caring, and being hopeful.

ONGOING REFLECTION

Having nursing practice grounded explicitly in caring theories supports caring being the essence of nursing, a unifying focus of the discipline, and allows for research linking caring practices to traditional and nontraditional outcomes. The publications in this section represent sentinel work of caring scholars, integrating the concepts of caring theory into the practice setting as a way to advance the discipline and inform and transform the practice of nursing. The way the theory was translated into practice models varied based on the nursing situation and practice setting, but the intentional focus on developing caring–healing relationships was central to all. It is through this person-centered approach to care grounded in caring values that nursing is able to humanize the health care system with tangible outcomes for patient/family, nurse, and system.

The creation of the Watson Caring Science Institute (WCSI) and the resulting educational opportunities for registered nurses interested in translating caring theory into practice has resulted in registered nurses creating new professional practice models within their respective systems. The unifying focus of these practice models is in the tangible expression of the 10 Caritas Processes™ (Watson, 2008) within specific practice settings and the intentional focus on the integration of self-care into practice. Outcomes include registered nurses having a renewed sense of passion in nursing, practicing loving kindness to self and others, reframing the language of nursing in terms of documentation, changing the culture from a focus on tasks to the integration of caring–healing modalities including aromatherapy, singing bowls, healing touch, and healing rooms for employees. The development of the Watson Caritas Patient Score (Watson, Brewer, & D'Alfonso, 2010) allows for research to empirically validate the outcomes of caring practice, further advancing the science of caring scholarship and the value of caring-based nursing professional practice models. As a discipline with a social mandate, the profession needs to take responsibility for the transformation of patient care delivery based on caring-based professional practice models.

REFERENCES

Benner, P. (1984). *From novice to expert: Excellence and power in clinical nursing practice.* San Francisco, CA: Addison-Wesley.

Bent, K., Burke, J., Eckman, A., Hottman, T., McCabe, J., & Williams, R. (2005). Being and creating caring change in a health care system. *International Journal for Human Caring, 9*(3), 20–25.

Bohman, L., & Deal, T. (2001). *Leading with soul.* San Francisco, CA: Jossey-Bass.

Boykin, A., & Schoenhofer, S. (1993). *Nursing as caring: A model of transforming practice.* New York, NY: National League for Nursing.

Boykin, A., Schoenhofer S., Smith, N., St. Jean J., Aleman, D. (2003). *Nursing Administration Quarterly, 27*(3), 223–230.

Boykin, A., Bulfin, S., Baldwin, J., & Southern, S. (2004). Transforming care in the emergency department. *Topics in Emergency Medicine, 26*(4), 331–336.

Boykin, A., Schoenhofer, S., Bulfin, S., Baldwin, J., & McCarthy, D. (2005). Living caring in practice: The transformative power of the theory of Nursing as Caring. *International Journal for Human Caring, 9*(3), 15–19.

Brown, C. L., Holcomb, L., Maloney, J., Naranjo, J., Gibson, C., & Russell, P. (2005). Caring in action: The patient care facilitator role. *International Journal for Human Caring, 9*(3), 51–58.

Chappell, T. (1993). *The soul of business: Managing for profit and the common good.* New York, NY: Bantam Books.

Davidson, A. W., Ray, M. A., & Turkel, M. C. (2011). *Nursing, caring, and complexity science: For human-environment well-being.* New York, NY: Springer Publishing Company.

Donabedian, A. (1992). The role of outcomes in quality assessment and assurance. *Quality Review Bulletin, 8,* 356–360.

Duffy, J. R., & Hoskins, L.M. (2003). The Quality-Caring Model© blending dual paradigms. *Advances in Nursing Science, 26*(1), 77–88.

Duffy, J. (2010). Joanne Duffy's quality caring model. In M. E. Parker & M. C. Smith, (Eds.). *Nursing theories and nursing practices* (3rd ed.). (pp. 402–416). Philadelphia, PA: F. A. Davis Company.

Gordon, M. (2002). *Keynote address, National Teaching Training Institute.* Atlanta, GA: American Association of Critical Care Nurses.

Irvine, D., Sidani, S., & Hall, L. M. (1998). Linking outcomes to nurses' roles in health care. *Nursing Economics, 16*(2), 58–64.

King, I. M. (1981). *A theory for nursing: System, concepts, process.* New York, NY: Wiley.

Leininger, M. (1981). *Caring: An essential human need.* Thorofare, NJ: Charles B. Slack Inc.

Leininger, M., & McFarland, M. (2003). *Transcultural nursing.* (3rd ed.). New York, NY: McGraw-Hill.

Mayerhoff, M. (1971). *On caring.* New York, NY: Harper & Row.

Mitchell, P., Ferketich, S., & Jennings, B. (1998). Quality health outcomes model. *Image: Journal of Nursing Scholarship, 30*(1), 43–46.

Mustard, L. (2002). Caring and competency. *JONA's Health care, Law, Ethics, and Regulation, 4*(2), 36–43.

Nightingale, F. (1969). *Notes on nursing: What it is and what it is not.* Philadelphia, PA: Lippincott. (Original work published in 1859.).

Parker, M. (2001). *Nursing theories and nursing practice.* Philadelphia, PA: F. A. Davis Company.

Parker, M., & Smith, M. (2010). *Nursing theories and nursing practice* (3rd ed.). Philadelphia, PA: F. A. Davis Company.

Ray, M. (1981). *A study of caring within an institutional culture.* Unpublished doctoral dissertation. University of Utah, Salt Lake City, UT.

Ray, M. (1989). The theory of bureaucratic caring for nursing practice in the organizational culture. *Journal of Nursing Administration, 13*(2), 31–42.

Roach, M. (1992/2002). *The human act of caring.* Ottawa, Ontario: The Canadian Hospital Association.

Schuster, E. A. (1997). *Caring for self.* Boca Raton, FL: Christin E. Lynn College of Nursing Curriculum, Florida Atlantic University.

Swanson, K. (1999). What is known about caring in nursing science. In A. S. Hinshaw, S. L. Feetham, & J. L. F. Shaver (Eds.). *Handbook of clinical nursing research* (pp. 31–60). Thousand Oaks, CA: Sage.

Touhy, T. A., Strews, W., & Brown, C. (2005). Expressions of caring as lived by nursing home staff, residents, and families. *International Journal for Human Caring, 9*(3), 31–37.

Turkel, M. C., & Ray, M. (2000). Relational complexity: A theory of the nurse-patient relationship within an economic context. *Nursing Science Quarterly, 13*(4), 307–313.

Turkel, M. C., & Ray, M. (2001). Relational complexity: From grounded theory to instrument development and theoretical testing. *Nursing Science Quarterly, 14*(4), 281–287.

Turkel, M. & Ray, M. (2004). Creating a caring practice environment through self-renewal. *Nursing Administration Quarterly, 28*(4), 249–254.

Watson, J. (1979). *Nursing: The philosophy and science of caring.* Boston, MA: Little, Brown.

Watson, J. (1985). *Nursing: Human science and human care.* Norwalk, CT: Appleton-Century-Crofts.

Watson, J. (1999). *Postmodern nursing and beyond.* Edinburgh, Scotland, UK: Churchill Livingstone.

Watson, J. (2001). *Post-modern nursing.* London: Churchill-Livingston.

Watson, J., & Foster, R. (2003). The Attending Nursing Caring Model®: Integrating theory, evidence and advanced caring-healing therapeutics for transforming professional practice. *Journal of Clinical Nursing, 12*, 360–365.

Watson, J. (2008). *Nursing: The philosophy and science of caring* (2nd Rev. ed.). Boulder, CO: University Press of Colorado.

Watson, J., Brewer, B. B., & D'Alfonso, J. (2010, September). Caritas: A theory guided scale to measure human caring. Poster presented at the 2010 State of Science Congress on Nursing Research. Washington, DC.

Wing, R. L. (1986). *The Tao of power (Lao Tzu's classic guide to leadership, influence, and excellence).* New York, NY: Doubleday & Co Inc.

Wolf, Z. R. (1994). *Caring behaviors inventory.* (Available from 27 Haverford Road, Ardmore, PA 19003.)

Wolf, Z. R., Giardino, E. R., Osborne, P. A., & Ambrose, M. S. (1994). Dimensions of nursing caring. *Image: Journal of Nursing Scholarship 26*(2), 107–111.

Wolf, Z. R., Colahan, M., Costello, A., Warwich, F., Ambrose, M., & Giardino, E. (1998). Relationship between nurse caring and patient satisfaction. *MED-SURG Nursing, 12*(2), 99–110.

27

The Quality-Caring Model©: Blending Dual Paradigms

JOANNE R. DUFFY AND LOIS M. HOSKINS

The rapidly changing health care system, together with recent advances in outcomes research, is stimulating the nursing profession to examine the quality of its services in an empirical, systematic manner. Providing quality health care is a professional responsibility and a patient expectation. It has traditionally been defined in terms of the structure–process–outcomes health model developed by Donabedian.[1] The structural component focuses on characteristics of patients, providers, and the health care environment that may influence the processes and outcomes of care. Processes of care are those specific interventions or care practices that health professionals provide. Outcomes are the endpoints or results of the health care process; they have recently assumed the highest priority among insurers, health care institutions, accreditors, and providers. Nursing-sensitive outcomes reflect "an established or theoretical link to the availability and quality of professional . . . nursing services,"[2(p. 9)] and may include variables such as health status, patient safety, patient satisfaction, comfort, increased knowledge, and quality of life.

Increasingly, objective evidence is supporting that linkages exist between nursing care and patient outcomes. Most impressive is the beginning evidence of associations between the amount of professional nursing care and positive health outcomes. Nurse staffing levels and selected patient outcomes have now been linked in several studies.[3–5] Recently, in a retrospective study of 700 hospitals in 11 states, Needleman et al.[6] reported that increased amounts of registered nurse (RN) care were associated with better quality in hospitalized patients. Interestingly, no relationships were found between increased amounts of care provided by licensed practical nurses (LPNs) or nursing assistants (NAs). The findings remained even after differences in patient characteristics, including age, comorbidities, and other pertinent variables, were controlled. These staffing studies suggest that lower numbers of RNs are related to higher adverse outcomes in the acute care population.

Preliminary investigations have also suggested that the features or characteristics of nursing interactions with patients lead to improved health care outcomes. In a study of 86 acute care medical–surgical patients, Duffy[7] demonstrated a link between nurse caring and patient satisfaction. An RN telephonic case management intervention recently demonstrated lower hospital readmission rates and costs and higher patient satisfaction levels in heart failure patients.[8] Advanced practice nursing studies have also reported similar results.[9–12]

It is clear that linkages exist between professional nursing and patient outcomes; yet, what specifically accounts for those linkages is unknown. According to Lang,[13] the behaviors and decisions that nurses carry out remain invisible. Nursing services are provided around the clock, across many settings, and throughout the health care continuum. They are accountable for the majority of health-related activities observed in hospitals, clinics, and nursing homes as well as in private homes, schools, work settings, and even faith communities. Professional nursing services are known to contribute to specific outcomes that benefit patients and their families. Yet, the work of nursing remains unexposed and little has been documented that demonstrates the value of these services. Based on preliminary evidence, the caring, relationship-centered nature of nursing may be connected to positive health outcomes. The primary purpose of this chapter is to present a blended Quality-Caring Model© for professional evaluation and analysis. The three secondary purposes are to (1) reaffirm and expose the hidden work of nursing, (2) describe the conceptual–theoretical–empirical linkages between quality of care and human caring, and (3) propose approaches for testing the accuracy of the model.

NURSING'S WORK

From the beginnings of professional history, the activities nurses performed were considered distinct from medicine.[14] Henderson[15] believed that nurses performed independently from physicians, but acknowledged that the health care team was also important. Watson[16] spoke about the essence of nursing (caring) as separate, but complementary to medicine (curing). As the knowledge base has matured, the work of nursing is more frequently described in relational terms. In fact many nursing theorists speak to the nurse–patient relationship. For example, Johnson,[17] Travelbee,[18] Peplau,[19] Patterson and Zerad,[20] Leininger,[21] Benner and Wrubel,[22] King,[23] and Watson[16] all view establishing meaningful relationships with patients and families as a predominant aspect of nursing work. Chinn and Kramer[24] describe human interaction as the primary focus of nursing that distinguishes it from other health care disciplines. Moreover, they view the technical and medical aspects of nursing work as supportive to the primary focus, human interaction.

Although not intending to be quantifiable and testable, Watson[16] took the step of specifying the attributes or properties necessary for adequate relationships with patients and families and labeled them *Carative Factors*. Watson[16] described the essence or core of nursing as caring, and in the last few decades, caring has emerged as a central paradigm in nursing.[25] It has been studied extensively both qualitatively and quantitatively. Recently, the original carative factors have evolved and are now known as Clinical Caring Processes.[26] Caring processes are considered transformative and dynamic both for the carer and the one being cared for.

While caring exists in a generic sense in all cultures[21] and between relatives and friends, the caring that exists in nursing practice is embedded or integrated in the daily work of nursing and has as its aim health and healing. Boykin and Schoenhofer recently described nursing as a "unique lived form of caring,"[27(p. 23)] while Gordon[28] stated that the caring embedded in nursing practice remains silent and labeled it "educated caring." These views are consistent with those of Mayerhoff,[29] who believed that knowledge is required for caring to occur, and with Benner's[30] expert practice work.

Caring is the predominant adjective used by nursing students and nurses to characterize nursing practice[31] and remains a major component of nursing curricula. The American Nurses Association recently described nursing as the "pivotal health care profession, highly valued for its specialized knowledge, skill, and caring in improving the health status of the public."[32(p. 7)] The Theory of Human Care[16] espouses that through transpersonal caring relationships, both providers and patients benefit. Although unconfirmed, outcomes from caring relationships, such as preservation of human dignity, protection from harm, self-knowledge, health, and inner harmony, have not only been theorized but are necessary for quality health care. While theorized to be central to nursing, most nurses would agree that traditional, institutionalized nursing does not support this postmodern approach to care. The focus on biomedical tasks, productivity, control, and individual autonomy does not encourage mutual interaction or relating, openness, body–mind–spirit approaches and alternative possibilities. Yet, in today's uncertain world of fast-changing technology, violence and terrorism, diverse cultures, rampant chronic disease, and the worst nursing shortage in history, it is clear that caring relationships may be relevant to quality health care, perhaps more so than ever before. Caring relationships with nurses are an expectation of patients and families that when unfulfilled cause unnecessary angst.[7] Understandably, nurses are longing for the time and energy[33] to do the work for which they were educated, that is to have caring relationships with patients and families.

Relationships with patients and families are the primary focus of nurses' work; however, evidence exists that relationships with other health care providers have become a factor in quality health care. For example, cooperation and coordination among members of the health care team have been demonstrated to impact patient outcomes in certain patient populations.[34-36] The multidisciplinary nature of modern health care requires that providers work together for the benefit of patients and families. Nurses typically are the supportive glue that holds the health care team together for the benefit of the patient and family.

The work of nursing, then, is relationship centered. Time spent initiating, cultivating, and sustaining caring relationships is an often overlooked and undervalued aspect of professional nursing services that runs counter to the traditional scientific nature of health care. Blending the societal need for measurable outcomes with the unique relationship-centered processes imbedded in daily nursing practice presents a postmodern approach that may benefit patients/families, members of the health care team, and nurses themselves.

QUALITY HEALTH CARE AND HUMAN CARING: A BLENDED MODEL

An environment that is constantly searching for "evidence" to quantify outcomes of health care is understandably data driven. Using the structure–process–outcomes[1] framework, health care organizations spend enormous resources on mandated data collection such as ORYX[37] (acute care), the Outcomes Assessment Information Set[38] (OASIS, home health care), the Minimum Data Set[39] (MDS, long-term care), and associated external benchmarking activities. Emphasis is placed on searching for ways to demonstrate clinical effectiveness, improve timeliness, maintain safety, and decrease costs of health care. Although the Joint Commission on Accreditation of Health care Organizations lists respect and caring as dimensions of quality,[40] little has been done to demonstrate the value of these relational processes of health care to the patient, provider, or the health care system. The caring processes that are imbedded in nursing practice may in fact be a key independent factor in improving health care outcomes.

The Quality-Caring Model© reflects the trend toward evidence-based practice while simultaneously representing nursing's unique contribution to quality health care. The model integrates biomedical and psychosociospiritual factors associated with quality health care. Under girding the model is the philosophical belief that persons are multicontextual beings who are connected to the larger pluralistic world. Persons are viewed *in relation to* and thus are interdependent with others. Nurses, patients and families, and other health care providers work in partnership to effect positive changes in health. Inherent in the model is the continuous search for evidence that care provided does in fact benefit patients and families. This evidence is viewed dynamically with endless possibilities for improvement. The model is grounded in the works of Donabedian[1] and Watson[16] and influenced by contributions from King,[23] Mitchell et al.,[41] and Irvine et al.[42] The overriding structure–process–outcomes components[1] are blended with major constructs in the Human Caring Model[16] and provide the central components of the model (see Figure 27.1).

The first major component, *structure*, of the Quality-Caring Model© is blended with the construct, causal past, and includes the concept, participants. This central component refers to important factors that are present prior to the delivery of health care. Such factors are present in the participants of the model, namely, the patient/family, various health care providers, and the health care system. Within each of the participants, unique attributes and characteristics that comprise their

causal pasts are apparent. For example, the subconcepts life experiences, descriptors such as demographics, various physiological, psychosociocultural, and spiritual factors are properties exclusive to providers and patients. In addition, the subconcept phenomenal field, a unique frame of reference or context known only to that person,[16] is also included. Regarding the health care system, factors such as the staffing patterns, organizational culture, available resources, and others that are unique to the setting are included. Since systems function within unique contexts, phenomenal field is integrated into this subconcept as well. Concepts and subconcepts included in the structure component influence the process of care and may directly or indirectly influence outcomes of care. For example, a patient with multiple comorbidities who lives alone may have different outcomes than one who has no comorbidities and lives with a supportive spouse, regardless of the process of care.

The second major component, *process*, involves interventions or practices that health care providers offer and is the focus of this model. Donabedian refers to process as "what is done for patients"[1(p. 357)] and suggests that it is composed of two broad categories of activities: technical and interpersonal. Watson[16] spoke to caring occasions where nurses utilized the carative factors[16] with patients and families. Nursing practice, however, is complex and multidimensional. King[23] viewed interpersonal systems formed by any number of human beings as complex relationships influenced by values, perceptions, communication, transactions, roles, and stress. King's focus on interpersonal systems supports that the process aspect of the model is in relation to others and is goal oriented. Irvine et al.[42] observed nursing as a discipline with three roles: independent, dependent, and interdependent. She believed the appropriate enactment

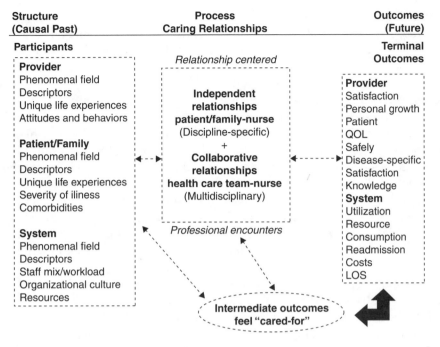

FIGURE 27.1

The Quality-Caring Model©.

of these roles affected the outcomes of patient care. Mitchell et al.,[41] on the other hand, proposed that clinical processes are direct and indirect. They view dynamic, reciprocal relationships among structure, process, and outcomes constructs, with a need to consider teams of health care providers in interaction with patients and families.

In the Quality-Caring Model©, caring relationships dominate the process and establish the groundwork for the two relationships that are the predominant focus of nursing. Nurses function primarily in relationship with patients and families, but also in relationship with members of the larger health care team. Although many of the concepts of the Quality-Caring Model© have been previously defined, four new concepts within the process component require definition. *Caring relationships* are human interactions grounded in clinical caring processes. They incorporate physical work (doing), interaction (being with), and relationship (knowing).

Two predominant relationships comprise nursing's work: independent relationships (discipline specific) as well as collaborative relationships (multidisciplinary). *Independent relationships* include those patient/family–nurse interactions that nurses implement autonomously and are solely held accountable for. This relationship is primary and includes values, attitudes, and behaviors that nurses carry out in partnership with patients and families. Independent relationships facilitate discipline-specific interventions such as managing pain and lead to nursing-sensitive patient outcomes. They may affect other outcomes of care as well. (See example of how the patient/family–nurse independent relationship might be applied in a clinical situation in Figure 27.2.) *Collaborative relationships* include those activities and responsibilities that nurses share with other members of the health care team. Interventions such as titrating medications, group counseling, and coordinating home oxygen equipment represent many health care disciplines working together in collaborative relationships that ultimately lead to shared outcomes of care. Taken together, independent and collaborative relationships constitute *relationship-centered professional encounters*, the greater part of nursing's work. During professional encounters, nurses initiate, cultivate, and sustain caring relationships independently (discipline specific) with patients and families and collaboratively with a designated health care team (multidisciplinary). Professional encounters are thus three dimensional with caring relationships existing among patients, nurses, and other health professionals. Because nurses work both independently and collaboratively with many members of the health

care team, their contributions to patient outcomes are simultaneously unique and shared. Relationships grounded in the clinical caring processes[26] are key to this balance.

Clinical caring processes are uniting; they provide the glue that holds relationships together. Relationships that are based on mutual respect, faith, hope, trust, and sensitivity to needs create the necessary foundation for human connection. Watson[16] calls such connection transpersonal because a new relationship forms that is more inclusive than that of the individuals alone. This new relationship is a genuine, authentic one that engenders feelings of being "cared for" in the recipients. When one feels "cared for," a sense of security develops that makes it easier to learn new things, change behaviors, take risks, and follow guidelines.

While independent relationships with patients/families are primary, collaborative relationships are essential to quality care. Appropriately balancing these

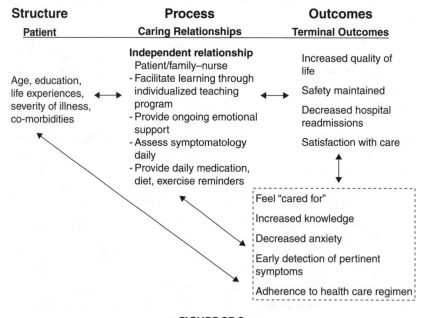

FIGURE 27.2

Application of the Quality-Caring Model©, patient/family–nurse independent relationship.

complementary professional relationships while keeping patient/family needs a central focus is a function of the nurse, one that expert nurses know well. Professional encounters that are relationship centered are outcomes-enhancing for the patient, the provider, and the health care system. The *role of the nurse* is to be the link between the patient, the health care team, and the unseen possibilities known as outcomes.

The third major component of the Quality-Caring Model©, *outcomes*, corresponds to the future construct of the Human Caring Model[16] and refers to the end results of health care. Two forms of outcomes are apparent. Intermediate outcomes represent "a change in the patient/family's behavior, emotions, or knowledge that can influence the end-result outcomes."[43(pp. 2–7)] Intermediate outcomes frequently include the goals on care plans and clinical pathways, but can also include feelings about the health care process. Terminal outcomes are those major end-result concepts that affect the future, such as quality of life, costs, disease-specific variables, and satisfaction with care. The subconcepts associated with outcomes are the same participants that comprise the structural component of the model. Both forms of outcomes can be affected in the patient/family, provider, and system at different times and sequences. Furthermore, there are reciprocal interactions between intermediate outcomes and terminal outcomes (Figure 27.2). System outcomes are important to consider because these reflect the current stability and future capability of a health care institution to prosper in a competitive market. Outcomes are dynamic and can be continually improved. Success in outcomes realization is heavily dependent on the dynamic and balanced independent and collaborative relationships that comprise professional encounters.

Assumptions of the Quality-Caring Model© are as follows: (1) caring must be done in relationship, (2) caring is submerged in the daily work of nursing, (3) caring

relationships are tangible concepts that can be measured, (4) knowledge of caring relationships is a significant issue for nursing and health care, (5) increased use and study of nurse caring will determine nursing's contribution to health care. The major *proposition* of the model is that relationships characterized by caring contribute to positive outcomes for patients/families, health care providers, and health care systems.

An important tenet of the Quality-Caring Model© is the understanding that the structure–process–outcomes components are a function of time and circumstances and are not simply a linear chain of events. The nature of human beings and human interaction implies variation in characteristics, ongoing feedback, and resultant alterations. The Quality-Caring Model© depicts an unlimited number of interrelated factors that influence all three central components in a dynamic cycle of possibility, consistent with a continuous search for excellence. Such ideas are postmodern by definition because they are ambiguous and unpredictable and suggest multiple interpretations. Although a source of instability and perceived loss of control for some, use of the model in practice and research may be uplifting and liberating for many health care providers.

CONCEPTUAL–THEORETICAL– EMPIRICAL LINKAGES BETWEEN QUALITY OF CARE AND HUMAN CARING

Although quality health care and human caring are different phenomena, there are multiple similarities. Both are concerned with human beings, health, and environmental variables that affect the delivery of health care. Most importantly, both models are concerned with providing the highest quality of care. Concepts and subconcepts within the Quality Health Model[1] and the Theory of Human Care[16] have been identified and defined. Linkages have been established via propositional statements. There are similarities in the models in terms of constructs, concepts, and relational statements. The models are future oriented and dynamic in nature with antecedents and consequences. In spite of this, the cornerstone component of importance to nursing, process, remains elusive especially in the Quality Health Model.[1]

In the last two decades, however, theory has evolved to a point that the process component of quality as it relates to nursing has become more explicit. The clinical caring processes unique to nursing[16,26] and evident in expert nurses[22] have been defined and are oftentimes the basis for standards of performance, curricula, and research. Throughout the 1990s, various measures of nurse caring have been developed, albeit with differing conceptual foundations and in specialized populations. Many of the existing instruments are now consolidated in a recent publication.[44] Measures of caring among teams of health care professionals have not been studied.

In light of nursing's contribution to improving the quality of health care, conceptual–theoretical–empirical linkages between the models exist. The major quality constructs of structure, process, and outcomes can be equated with the human caring constructs of causal past, clinical caring processes, and the future. Four levels of concepts and subconcepts can be identified and tied to empirical indicators such as demographics, degree of nurse caring, and specific patient outcomes (see Figure 27.3). Higher levels of measurement now exist allowing for more sophisticated analytical techniques. This fit between the components of Health Care Quality[1] and the Theory of Human Care,[16] together with the ability to operationalize theoretical concepts, provides the logical consistency necessary for empirical validation.

ACCURACY OF THE QUALITY-CARING MODEL©

While the Clinical Caring Processes[26] and the Theory of Human Care[16] have provided the foundation for caring knowledge, a model of the multidimensional relational aspects of human caring blended with the quality components may help us more

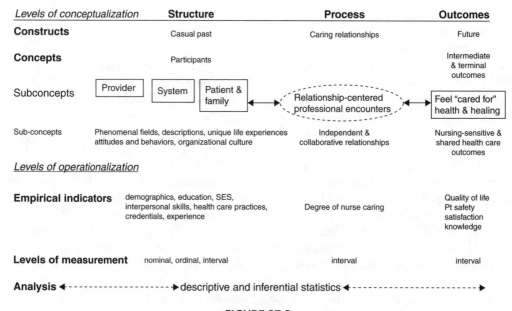

FIGURE 27.3

Conceptual–theoretical–empirical linkages between quality of care and human caring.

efficiently provide evidence that nurse caring does indeed positively affect patient outcomes. Use of this blended model in practice and research will help continue the knowledge development begun in caring science by exposing the hidden work of nursing, demonstrating its value, validating and refining theory, and providing evidence of nursings' contribution to quality health care.

In the postmodern view of knowledge development, there are no rigid laws or linear patterns governing inquiry; rather a longitudinal, dynamic, interactive process of study can provide multiple ways of understanding phenomena. To understand the inherent accuracy of the Quality-Caring Model©, however, it is important to examine the relationships between the concepts and the subconcepts of the model. Since high-quality empirical indicators already exist, correlational studies using LISREL might be designed to test relationships between the degree of nurse caring and intermediate and terminal outcomes in various patient populations. Independent nursing interventions grounded in the clinical caring processes can be tested for their effects on selected patient outcomes using experimental designs and comparative inferential statistics. Results generated from such studies would provide evidence of the success or failure of the model in specific patient populations. Simultaneously, continued qualitative inquiries may help health care professionals understand in more depth the nature of relationship-centered professional encounters.

As evidence for caring nursing practice becomes tied to positive patient outcomes, it becomes essential for nurse educators to better understand how to teach and measure caring behaviors in nursing students. Measuring end-of-program competency in nurse caring and improving knowledge of what teaching–learning strategies best develop nursing students' caring behaviors will provide nursing educators with priceless information about how to more thoroughly educate nursing students for relationship-centered practice.

Finally, nursing administrators have the foremost challenge of creating caring practice environments with limited resources, both financial and human. Studies that measure the degree of nurse caring in proportion to staff mix and RN hours per patient day, the relationship between a caring practice environment and nurse retention, and cost–benefit analyses of caring practice environments will provide the evidence required to sustain needed change in nursing work environments.

CONCLUSION

Existing theory and beginning science are crucial not only to improved patient outcomes but also to the advancement of the profession. The important link between nursing and health care outcomes has already been established. A blended approach incorporating nursing's unique relationship-centered practice may provide the impetus for advanced study and application. The Quality-Caring Model© represents a way of safeguarding and preserving the essence of nursing while simultaneously demonstrating its value. The scope of the model is broad and is applicable to individual patients and families as well as specialized patient populations. Several subconcepts for which operational definitions exist lend the model to empirical testing. The Quality-Caring Model© can be used as a guide for practice and research as well as the basis for nursing interventions.

Health care and nursing is in a period of transition between what was and what will be. Today, there is a genuine need for a pragmatic, effective, inclusive model that provides a simple and direct foundation for practice and research. Nursing continues to be driven by the task-oriented biomedical model; yet, the business of nursing is relationship centered. Cultivating independent relationships with patients and families and helping to build mutually cooperative collaborative relationships with members of the health care team is nursing's work. Unfortunately, in the fast, impersonal, technological context of modern health care, the centrality of relationships is often lost and considered "soft." The Quality-Caring Model© helps to translate such perceptions into more objective language that can be tested and applied. The clinical caring processes that are buried in everyday nursing practice and are the basis for effective relationship-centered professional encounters can now be tied more effectively and efficiently to improved health care outcomes. Relationships characterized by caring not only alleviate suffering for patients and families and facilitate teamwork among health care providers but also support and uphold professional nursing.

Nursing's Agenda for the Future: A Call to the Nation[32] contains 10 major objectives. First, the Quality-Caring Model© directly relates to seven and peripherally to two of these objectives. Foremost is the design of "integrated models of health care delivery that are interdisciplinary . . . and that advance evidence-based practice."[32(p. 11)] Second, the Quality-Caring Model© is tied to the public relations objective that nursing becomes valued for its unique knowledge and expertise. Application of the model will undoubtedly demonstrate that nursing "makes a difference in peoples' lives"[32(p. 14)] by demonstrating quality, cost-effective health care outcomes. Third, as the model is used to guide research and quality improvement activities, reliable evidence will be generated that will support health policy formulation. Finally, the model will help nursing become viewed as a "strategic, critical, health care asset,"[32(p. 15)] helping nurses

to achieve external professional recognition and perhaps positively influencing the recruitment and retention of a diverse workforce. In fact, by practicing caring, nurses are caring for themselves since that is what they were meant to do.

Nursing must let go of the old ways and begin to work both independently and collaboratively toward providing evidence that demonstrates how its real work contributes to health care quality. Scientifically demonstrating its worth will provide nursing with a rich understanding of its inherent value and offer much needed evidence to the health care system. This evidence linking nurse caring to both nursing-sensitive and shared patient outcomes is essential for the survival of the nursing profession, especially in the current health care market. The Quality-Caring Model© provides a framework of possibilities for healing the profession. Evidence that emerges from the model may protect and transform the nursing profession from the inside out, leading to a more mature profession secure in its own identity!

REFERENCES

1. Donabedian, A. (1992). The role of outcomes in quality assessment and assurance. *Quality Review Bulletin, 8,* 356–360.
2. American Nurses Association. (1995). *Nursing care report card for acute care.* Washington, DC: American Nurses Association.
3. Aiken, L. H., Smith, H. L., & Lake, E. T. (1994). Lower mortality among a set of hospitals known for good nursing care. *Medical Care, 32,* 771–787.
4. Blegen, M. A., & Vaughn, T. (1998). A multisite study of nurse staffing and patient occurrences. *Nursing Economics, 16*(4), 196–203.
5. Kovner, C. T., & Gergen. P. J. (1998). Nurse staffing levels and adverse events following surgery in U.S. hospitals. *Image—The Journal of Nursing Scholarship, 30,* 315–321.
6. Needleman, J., Buerhaus, P., Mattke, S., Stewart, M., & Zelevinsky, K. (2002). Nursing staffing levels and the quality of care in

hospitals. *Netherlands Journal of Medicine, 346*(22), 1715–1720.

7. Duffy, J. (1992). The impact of nurse caring on patient outcomes. In D. Gaut (Ed.), *The presence of caring in nursing.* New York, NY: NLN Press.

8. Reigle, B., Carison, B., Kopp, A., LePetrie, B., Glaser, D., & Unger A. (2002). Effect of a standardized nurse case-management telephone intervention on resource use in patients with chronic heart failure. *Archives of Internal Medicine, 162,* 705–712.

9. Mundinger, M. O., Kane, R. L., Lenz, E. R., Totten, A. M., Tsai, W. Y., Cleary, P. D. . . . Shelanski, M. L. (2000). Primary care outcomes in patients treated by nurse practitioners or physicians: A randomized trial. *Journal of the American Medical Association, 283*(l), 59–68.

10. Naylor, M. D. (2000). A decade of transitional care research with vulnerable elders. *Journal of Cardiovascular Nursing, 14*(3), 1–14.

11. Wheeler, E. C. (2000). The CNS's impact on process and outcome of patients with total knee replacement. *Clinical Nurse Specialist, 14*(4), 159–172.

12. Reeve, K., Calabro, K., & Adams-McNeill, J. (2000). Tobacco cessation intervention in a nurse practitioner managed clinic. *Journal of the American Academy of Nurse Practitioners, 12*(5), 163–169.

13. Lang, N. (1999). Discipline-based approaches to evidence-based practice: A view from nursing. *Journal on Quality Improvement, 25*(10), 539–543.

14. Nightingale, F., (1992). *Notes on nursing* (Com. Ed). Philadelphia, PA: Lippincott.

15. Henderson, V. (1996). *The nature of nursing.* New York, NY: Macmillan.

16. Watson, J. (1985). *Nursing: Human science and human care.* Norwalk, CT: Appleton-Century-Crofts.

17. Johnson, D. E. (1980). The behavioral system model for nursing. In J. P. Riehi & C. Roy (Eds.), *Conceptual models for nursing practice.* New York: Appleton-Century-Crofts.

18. Travelbee, J. (1966). *Interpersonal aspects of nursing.* Philadelphia, PA: FA Davis Co.

19. Peplau, H. E. (1988). *Interpersonal relations in nursing.* New York, NY: Springer.

20. Patterson, J. G., & Zerad, L. T. (1976). *Humanistic nursing.* New York: Wiley.

21. Leininger, M. M. (1988). Leininger's theory of nursing: Culture care diversity and universality. *Nursing Science Quarterly, 1,* 152–160.

22. Benner, P., & Wrubel, J. (1989). *The primacy of caring: Stress and coping in health and illness.* Menlo Park, CA: Addison-Wesley.

23. King, I. M. (1981). *A theory for nursing: System, concepts, process.* New York: Wiley.

24. Chinn, P. L., & Kramer, M. K. (1999). *Theory and nursing: Integrated knowledge development.* St. Louis, MO: Mosby.

25. Saewyc, E. M. (2000). Nursing theories of caring. A paradigm for adolescent nursing practice. *Journal of Holistic Nursing, 18*(2), 114–128.

26. Watson, J. (1999). *Postmodern nursing and beyond.* Edinburgh, Scotland, UK: Churchill Livingstone.

27. Boykin, A., & Schoenhofer, S. (1993). *Nursing as caring: A model for transforming practice.* New York, NY: National League for Nursing Press.

28. Gordon, M. (2002). *Keynote address, National Teaching Training Institute.* Atlanta, GA: American Association of Critical Care Nurses.

29. Mayerhoff, M. (1971). *On caring.* New York, NY: Harper & Row.

30. Benner, P. (1984). *From novice to expert: Excellence and power in clinical nursing practice.* San Francisco, CA: Addison-Wesley.

31. Duffy, J. The influence of professional values on nursing career choice. *Nurse Education Peers.* In press.

32. American Nurses Association. (2002). *Nursing's agenda for the future: A call to the nation.* Washington, DC: American Nurse Publishing.

33. Chinn, E. (2001). From the editor—Making a difference in health care. *Advances in Nursing Science, 24.*

34. Knaus, W. A., Wagner, D. P., & Zimmerman, J. E. (1986). An evaluation of outcomes from intensive care and major medical centers. *Annals of Internal Medicine, 104,* 410–418.

35. Rich, M. W., Beckham, Y., Wittenberg, C., Levin, C. L., Freedland, K. E., & Carney, R. (1955). A multidisciplinary intervention to prevent the readmission of elderly patients with congestive heart failure. *Netherlands Journal of Medicine, 333*(18), 1190–1195.

36. Stewart, S., Marley, J. E., & Horowitz, J. D. (1999). Effects of a multidisciplinary, home-based intervention on unplanned readmissions and survival among patients with chronic congestive heart failure: a randomized controlled study. *Lancet, 354,* 1077–1083.

37. www.jcaho.org/pms/core+measures/cr_hos_cm.htm. Accessed June 25, 2002.

38. Crisler, K. S., Campbell, B. M., & Shaugnessy, P. W. (1997). *OASIS Basic: Beginning to use the outcomes and assessment information set.* Denver, CO: Center for Health Services and Policy Research.

39. Won, A., Morris, J. N., Nonemaker, S., & Lipsltz, L. A. (1999). A foundation for excellence in long-term care: The Minimum Data Set. *Annals of Long Term Care, 7*(3), 92–97.

40. Joint Commission on Accreditation of Health care Organizations. (1997). *National library of health care indicators.* Oakbrook Terrace, IL: Joint Commission on Accreditation of Health care Organizations.

41. Mitchell, P., Ferketich, S., & Jennings, B. (1998). Quality health outcomes model. *Image—The Journal of Nursing Scholarship, 30*(1), 43–46.

42. Irvine, D., Sidani, S., & Hall, L. M. (1998). Linking outcomes to nurses' roles in health care. *Nursing Economics, 16*(2), 58–64.

43. Huethner, C. (1998). *Toward a safer 21st century: Aviation safety research baseline and future challenges.* Washington, DC: National Aeronautics and Space Administration.

44. Watson, J. (2002). *Instruments for assessing and measuring caring in nursing and health sciences.* New York, NY: Springer.

45. Sitzman, K. L. (2002). Interbeing and mindfulness: A bridge to understanding Jean Watson's theory of human caring. *Journal of Nursing Education, 23,* 376–383.

QUESTIONS FOR REFLECTION

Baccalaureate

1. What professional practice model is in place where you are currently working or doing a student rotation? How could you integrate components of the Quality-Caring Model© into this setting?

2. What nurse-sensitive outcomes are being collected where you are currently working or doing a student rotation? Does the organization link these findings to the professional practice model?

3. Provide examples of caring relationships, independent relationships, and collaborative relationships that you observe or participate in where you are currently working or doing a student rotation.

Master's

1. How has Watson's Theory of Human Caring influenced the Quality-Caring Model©?

2. Can you link empirical outcomes to caring in the organization where you are currently practicing? Why or why not? What changes would you initiate to allow for this information to be collected?

3. What evidence-based nursing practices are in place in the organization where you are currently working or doing a student rotation? Can caring be integrated into these practices?

Doctoral

1. How has the connection between human caring and patient or system outcomes been advanced since Duffy's original work in 2002?

2. Is Donabedian's work of structure, process, and outcome still relevant within the quality initiatives of contemporary nursing practice? Why or why not? Does this approach allow for the integration of caring theory? Why or why not?

3. What research question can you identify to link caring practices to empirical outcomes? What research design would you use to carry out this research? What key articles would be included within the review of the literature?

28

Creating a Caring Practice Environment Through Self-Renewal

Marian C. Turkel and Marilyn A. Ray

"Leaders whose position will endure are those who are the most compassionate"[1(p. 67)] The words of the ancient philosopher Lao Tzu in the *Tao of Power* speak to the universality of compassionate caring for those in positions of power and leadership, namely nurses. Compassion is looking inward and outward—insightfulness to relational caring forces of spirit and nature, and integrity that can reveal the path to personal excellence and outstanding social influence. The individual contains the whole universe, as Lao Tzu remarked.[1] Nurses are aware of the whole, the self, patients, organizations, and communities. They can exercise the power of caring. The recent Institute of Medicine study[2] exposed the dilemmas confronting the professions of nursing, medicine, and health care administrations in the safety and protection of patients. Trust, a central aspect of the organizational caring relationship, was emphasized.

Loss of trust has occurred because of stressors regarding economic concerns and managed care, insurance and legal issues, and disrespect for the profession of nursing. The shortage of nurses and the crisis in health care have resulted.[3] The inability to "lead with the soul"[4] underscores all these problems. The soul of nursing is seeking the good of self and others through compassionate caring. Healing and caring for oneself is critical to successful relationships and organizations[5] and enforces how the self and others are interconnected.[6] People as well as corporations are shaped by others' minds and spirits. Values and corporate identities are not mere reflections of organizations but are a metacommentary on the health of a society.[7] As such, there is a call for change from the society at large and change from nursing within the culture of health care organizations. The change speaks to the need to revise the value of compassionate caring, promote creativity in worklife, preserve autonomy, create feelings of interconnectedness, manage the business of corporations within the ideal of seeking the good, and respond to community. The first step is to facilitate the creation of caring in complex health care organizations. The purpose of this chapter is to discuss caring in nursing, self-care and healing, and caring in complex organizations. Strategies for self-care, renewal, and healing in the organizational culture will follow.

From Turkel, M. C., & Ray, M. (2004). Creating a caring practice environment through self-renewal. *Nursing Administration Quarterly, 28*, 249–254. Permission to reprint granted by Wolters Kluwer.

CARING IN NURSING

In the last three decades, caring has been described as the essence of nursing by many scholars, such as Leininger,[8] Leininger and McFarland[9] Ray,[10–12] Roach,[13] Watson,[14–16] Turkel and Ray,[17,18] and Morse et al.[19] Theories illuminate caring as transcultural, a human trait, a way of being, a moral ideal grounded in organizational contexts, and a holographic, complex dynamic. Newman and colleagues.[20] claimed that caring in the human health experience and the unitive transformative paradigm are the foci of the discipline. A paradigm signifies a cluster of basic assumptions that form a worldview, a way of screening knowledge and experience to bring forth a new way of understanding the world.[12] Some scholars would agree that caring is what unites and transforms the discipline and profession; others do not. Reflect on, for example, the current focus of evidence-based practice, which, for the most part, is guided by the logical positivist worldview of objective, scientific knowledge.[21] Administrators and practitioners who engage with physicians and management personnel see evidence-based practice as a logical and business-minded approach, whereas scholars in the field of caring science see it as limited and not within the framework of holism or what can be referred to as the soul of nursing. Although caring has been expressed differently by theorists, it centers on caring as a way of being and encompasses a body of knowledge that is grounded in the intersubjective and interpretive human science and spirituality. How can nursing unite with seemingly uncommon values about the nature of its discipline? Although coming to terms with a common philosophy of nursing may be difficult, one ideal value that does unite is the notion of seeking the good and committing to the health and well-being of self and others within diverse institutional and community practice environments.

Self-care highlights the greatest asset of all—the individual.[4] Self-care is critical to health and healing. The idea of the nurse as holistic—body, mind, and spirit—was illuminated by Watson[15] in her theory of caring. A nurse who is holistic and self-caring can create harmony with others through authentic presence in the caring moment. If one does not appreciate the self as a caring person or if the nurse does not care for self, it is impossible for her to compassionately care for others. This notion can also refer to nurse administrators who often abandon caring for self and others for the sake of the "bottom line" in health care organizations. The inability to care for self frequently shows up as violence at the workplace.[22] One particularly alarming area of practice that has been discovered is horizontal violence—where, nurses, who do not care for themselves and feel that they are not cared for by administrators, develop destructive behaviors toward self and other nurses, especially, younger, idealist nurses who are beginning their professional journey. Self-esteem is often damaged for good in terms of professional nursing practice. When nurses do not have a strong sense of self and caring, they do not provide total patient care.[10] The ability to self-organize is a part of caring for self. In the philosophy of Lao Tzu,[1] the character for organization relates to a strong individual. Strength emerges from struggle, which is necessary for growth, development, and healing. As nurses struggle in their wounded state,[13] compassionate caring holds the key to the meaning of suffering within selves and others. Healing self is a way of "walking the talk."[5]

THE MEANING OF CARING ORGANIZATIONS

What does caring mean in organizations? How do nurses and other administrators create caring organizations? Ray's research[10,11] showed that caring in the organization is complex, dynamic, and a part of the bureaucracy. "The formal theory of Bureaucratic Caring symbolized a dynamic structure of caring which was synthesized from a dialectic between the thesis of caring as humanistic, social, educational, ethical, and religious/spiritual (elements of humanism), and the antithesis of caring as economic, political, legal, and technological (elements of bureaucracy."[12(p. 425)] Thus, the meaning of caring was not only expressed as human, social, ethical, and spiritual but also expressed in relation to the structure of the organization. Caring interactions and symbolic systems of meaning are formed and reproduced from the constructions or dominant values held within the culture of an organization. In subsequent research, Ray et al.[3] discovered from grounded theory research that losing trust was the central response not only of nurses but also of administrators. The study showed that hospitals were driven by the need to economically survive, resulting in nurses experiencing disillusionment with nursing practice and decreased loyalty toward organizations. However, nurses did communicate what was needed to transform hospitals into caring organizations. A model of relational caring self-organization emerged, highlighting transformational elements of respecting, communicating, maintaining visibility, and participating in decision making. The path toward relational caring self-organization and ultimately, the soul of business[4,6] is choice, or more specifically, moral choice. Respect for individuals and communities of caregivers, including organizational structures, is choosing the path of right action for the common good. Health care systems exist for the common good as well as managing business. When organizations are infused with compassionate caring values, they reflect a human face, which is necessary for the continued existence of all humanity.

A new meaning of work will emerge as nurses direct their own professional practice. "Caring is not always agreeable; it is sometimes frustrating and rarely easy."[23(p. 52)] Nurse administrators and staff nurses do have voices and they need to exercise them through compassionate caring leadership. Caring nursing leaders recognize that nurses find themselves by finding their place in nursing and health care organizations. Nurses find their place in nursing by engaging others who need their caring and, in turn, are cared for by them. A description of how to help nurses find a place in the world of health care, create caring organizations through self-care, and caring organizational strategies will follow.

VALUE OF SELF-RENEWAL

To awaken the creative, caring spirit within each of us, it is essential to acknowledge the power of caring for self as being essential to creating a caring, harmonious work force environment. With all the challenges nurse leaders and nurses face on a daily basis, they rarely have time or energy for themselves. Failure to care for self leads to burnout or compassion fatigue.[24] However, discovering or rediscovering the caring self is an important source of nourishment for the emergence of creative, caring energy. From this unshakable foundation, we nourish our inner strength and beauty as we reach out to others from our authentic caring selves. The following value statements reaffirm the importance of awakening the creative, caring self to cocreate communities of caring[25]:

- Our lives are grounded in our creative, caring selves.
- Our creative selves need consistent honest acknowledgment, respect, and nurturing.
- When we relinquish attention to our creative foundation, imbalance occurs

and we are unhappy at our deepest levels ("dis-ease").

- Any choice we make either supports or diminishes our creative selves.
- The creative self is always there; we cannot lose it but we can ignore or abandon it, to our peril as whole persons.
- There are no shortcuts.
- There are no "excused absences"; we can either do the work or not. We have the choice.
- Paradoxically, our creative selves respond only to light, playful, loving attention and not to a taskmaster "have to" approach.
- When we are a life artist, we bring that artistry to ail our roles and we create new roles to accommodate our artistry.
- The life artist blends and balances the roles of teacher, healer, leader, and visionary.
- Our technologies, which we respect, come from without—"how to do"; our artist comes from within—"how to be."
- Our lifeline is in paying attention to our doing and our being; the artistry is in maintaining the balance.

As self is renewed, personal and professional commitments become balanced and inner energy is replenished. Sister Roach[13] describes competence as "having the needed skills, judgment and energy required for technical proficiency." However, how many nurse leaders focus on the energy aspect of competence? Are caring for self strategies part of management or staff orientation? Is caring for self valued by administration? Within traditional health care organizations, there is an intense focus on managerial skills related to performance improvement, financial analysis, conflict resolution, and productivity measures. Considering that most health care environments are intense, high-stress environments, it is essential for nurse leaders to value and respect the concept of caring for self. Following are examples of how nurse leaders can

integrate caring for self activities into the practice setting[26]:

- Model caring for self by striving for wellbeing and maintaining a balance between the demands of work and time for self-renewal.
- Start the workday with a centering or relaxation experience and encourage managers to do this in every nursing unit.
- Allow for nurses to have mini-relaxation experiences during the course of a 12-hour shift.
- Invite a holistic nurse practitioner to monthly management, staff, or educational meetings.
- Incorporate caring for self activities into the orientation programs for both managers and nursing staff.
- Honor the request from managers or members of the nursing staff to take off for personal renewal or reflection.
- Include a healing modality (meditation, aromatherapy, massage) into yearly competency education for nursing staff.
- Sponsor a daylong retreat for nurses where they can experience healing activities and come together to reflect on practice.

RECREATING ORGANIZATIONAL CULTURE

By transforming the perspective on tasks and productivity, nurse leaders can create a culture that will help nurses to rediscover their values, their mission, their creativity, and even their productivity. Caring for nurses results in nurses transmitting their own caring values to both the patient and the patient's family.[27] Strategies for recreating organizational culture include the following[26]:

- As a hospital organization, dedicate a regular time each month for nurses to contemplate and communicate their visions and goals for the organization.

- Provide a public and private sharing forum and then as a leader, follow up on the ideas.
- Begin executive and board meetings with a story where a nurse's caring made a difference in his or her patient's care.
- Posters, charts, and photographs used during organizational meetings should celebrate the human spirit instead of focusing solely on the bottom line.
- Create a "healing room" for nurses where they can meditate, rest, or simply reflect on their thoughts. In time, you will begin to see them creatively solving more challenges on their own without intervention from nursing leadership.
- Set aside time each day for creative/reflective thinking activities and discussions. Post these times in plain sight and encourage all nurses to attend.
- Assist nurses in having a work/life balance by not expecting overtime or frequent shift rotation. Offer flexible scheduling and on-site classes, such as yoga, journaling, or art therapy, which focus on self-healing.
- Have nurses develop a plan for self-care as part of their annual evaluation and respect the implementation of their plan.

CREATING A HEALING ENVIRONMENT

Florence Nightingale[28] contended that the role of the nurse was to monitor the environment and make improvements as needed so that nature could act to cure the patient. The nurse leader can expand on this concept and create physical environments designed to destress the nursing staff and provide a healthy healing environment. An example of this type of innovation would be to integrate Feng Shui theory into the design and construction of a hospital building or nursing unit. Feng Shui is an ancient Chinese art of building design and furniture placement that helps ensure a balanced, healthy environment by creating positive energy.

Another example is the creation of a labyrinth walk outside the hospital for both nurses and visitors. Labyrinth walks are reflective of life itself, for life does not run in a straight line. The winding path, its right and left turns, is known to calm the mind and settle the emotions.

Healing gardens within a hospital environment provide an opportunity for nurses to view and be in proximity with nature. Research has shown that healing gardens provide a stress-reduction benefit to those who choose to experience them. A beautiful example of this in practice is the Healing Garden at Banner Good Samaritan Medical Center in Arizona.[29] The Healing Garden is used by patients, visitors, and nurses, and fosters a sense of serenity and healing.

RELEVANCE TO PRACTICE

Most nurses feel they are missing something in their professional lives and this results in compassion fatigue.[24] Allowing nurses the time to heal through self-care will enhance their sense of meaning, passion, and purpose at work. The role of the nurse leader is to support nurses on their personal journey of reflection and renewal. The nurse, in turn, needs to be receptive and responsive to the beauty of renewal and not view this creative approach to practice as "something I must do." Once a nurse has completed his or her personal journey, he/she will have reached his/her full potential and become reengaged within the work environment. As more nurses experience self-renewal, they are creating a community of caring for self, colleagues, patients, and visitors and establishing deep personal connections with each other. Work is now viewed as a place of renewal and friendship, and a sense of family begins to form. As nurses are less vulnerable to exhaustion, stress, and frustration, they will be freer to let their creative, caring spirit emerge.

CONCLUSION

Nursing has entered a new era in its history, one in which political power, technological change, and business principles including legal issues have dominant consequences for the profession and for patient care. In the struggle for wisdom and knowledge of self-care and the creation of caring organizations, nurse leaders can develop a new vision or recapture their traditional vision of compassionate caring to direct the process toward mutual fulfillment for nurses, administrators, and patients in the work environment. By intelligent and knowledgeable caring, nurse leaders can advance their range of possibilities toward a new meaning of work. Only spiritual, ethical caring leaders will be able to overcome the polarities of economics, technologies, legalities, and politics in health care. Caring nurse leaders will recognize that caring and the characteristics of the organizational context must be viewed as necessary poles of the same existence by advancing notions such as economic spiritual–ethical caring, political spiritual–ethical caring, technological spiritual–ethical caring and so forth.[10–12] Transformation toward relational caring self-organization cannot only be the goal but also the process toward self-fulfillment and the meaning of work.

REFERENCES

1. Wing, R. L. (1986). *The Tao of Power (Lao Tzu's classic guide to leadership, influence, and excellence)*. New York, NY: Doubleday & Co Inc.
2. Page, A. (Ed.). (2004). *Keeping patients safe: Transforming the work environment of nurses*. Washington, DC: The National Academies Press.
3. Ray, M., Turkel, M., & Marino, E. (2002). The transformative process for nursing in workforce redevelopment. *Journal of Nursing Administration, 25*(1), 1–14.
4. Bohman, L., & Deal, T. (2001). *Leading with soul*. San Francisco, CA: Jossey-Bass.
5. Kahn, S., & Saulo, M. (1994). *Healing yourself: A nurse's guide to self care and renewal*. Albany, NY: Delmar Publishers, Inc.
6. Chappell, T. (1993). *The soul of business: Managing for profit and the common good*. New York, NY: Bantam Books.
7. Turner, V., & Bruner, E. (Eds.) (1986). *The anthropology of experience*. Chicago, IL: The University of Illinois Press.
8. Leininger, M. (Ed.) (1981). *Caring: An essential human need*. Thorofare, NJ: Charles B. Slade, Inc.
9. Leininger, M., & McFarland, M. (Eds.) (2003). *Transcultural nursing* (3rd ed.). New York, NY: McGraw-Hill.
10. Ray, M. (1981). *A study of caring within an institutional culture* [doctoral dissertation]. Salt Lake City, UT: University of Utah.
11. Ray, M. (1989). The theory of bureaucratic caring for nursing practice in the organizational culture. *Journal of Nursing Administration, 13*(2), 31–42.
12. Ray, M. (2001). The theory of bureaucratic caring. In M. Parker (Ed.), *Nursing theories and nursing practice* (pp. 421–431). Philadelphia, PA: FA Davis Co.
13. Roach, M. (1992/2002). *The human act of caring*. Ottawa, Canada: The Canadian Hospital Association.
14. Watson, J. (1979). *The philosophy and science of caring*. Boston, MA: Little Brown & Co.
15. Watson, J. (1985). *Nursing: Human science and human care*. Norwalk, CT, Appleton-Century-Croft.
16. Watson, J. (2001). *Postmodern nursing*. London, Churchill-Livingstone.
17. Turkel, M., & Ray, M. (2000). Relational complexity: A theory of the nurse-patient relationship within an economic context. *Nursing Science Quarterly, 13*(4), 307–313.
18. Turkel, M., & Ray, M. (2001). Relational complexity: From grounded theory to instrument development and theoretical testing. *Nursing Science Quarterly, 14*(4), 281–287.
19. Morse, J., Solberg, S., Neander, S., Bottorff, J., & Johnson, J. (1990). Concepts of caring and caring as a concept. *Advances in Nursing Science, 13*, 1–14.
20. Newman, M., Sime, A., & Corcoran-Perry, S. (1991). The focus of the discipline of nursing. *Advances in Nursing Science, 14*(1), 1–6.
21. Dawes, M., Davies, P., Gray, A., Mant, J., Seers, K., & Snowball, R. (1999).

Evidence-based practice. London: Churchill Livingstone.

22. McKenna, B., Smith, N., Poole, S., & Coverdale, J. (2003). Horizontal violence: Experiences of registered nurses in their first year of practice. *Journal of Advanced Nursing, 42,* 1332–1342.

23. Mayeroff, M. (1971). *On caring.* New York, NY: Harper & Row.

24. Henry, J., & Henry, L. (2004). The soul of the caring nurse. Stories and resources for revitalizing professional passion. Washington, DC: American Nurses Publishing.

25. Schuster, E. (1997). *Caring for self.* Boca Raton, FL: Christin E. Lynn College of Nursing Curriculum, Florida Atlantic University.

26. Turkel, M. (2001). Challenging contemporary practices in critical care settings. In N. Locsin (Ed.), *Advancing Technology, Caring and Nursing.* Westport, CT: Auburn House.

27. Turkel, M. (2003). A journey into caring as experienced by nurse managers. *International Journal Human Caring, 7*(1), 20–26.

28. Nightingale, F. (1969). *Notes on nursing: What it is and what it is not.* Philadelphia, PA: Lippincott, original work published in 1859.

29. Geary, M. (2003). Facilitating an organizational culture of healing in an urban medical center. *Nursing Administration Quarterly, 27*(3), 231–239.

QUESTIONS FOR REFLECTION

Baccalaureate

1. What self-care practice are you currently engaged in? How does this impact your personal sense of balance and inner peace? If you are not currently engaged in a self-care practice, what can you begin doing? After 2 months, reflect on how this has made a difference for you.

2. Are registered nurses where you are currently working or doing a student rotation encouraged to practice self-care? What small ritual or practice can you do at work to promote self-care?

3. Does the organization where you are currently working have any initiatives in place to create a healing environment for employees? If yes, please describe. If no, what can be initiated on the nursing unit where you work or do a student rotation to create a healing environment?

Master's

1. Develop a personal plan for self-care and a self-care contract that will be part of your student evaluation or performance evaluation where you are working.

2. How has the work of Nightingale influenced the concept of nursing and the environment? How would you introduce the value of creating a healing environment to nursing leaders within the organization where you are currently working or doing a student rotation?

3. How does the organization where you are currently working or doing a student rotation promote self-care and caring within the organizational culture?

Doctoral

1. Identify key findings or themes from three research studies published within the last 5 years related to the value of self-care. Do they support the ideas of Turkel and Ray?

2. How does this sentinel work contribute to the scholarship of caring science?

3. What research questions would you identify related to the personal and professional value of self-care?

29

The Attending Nurse Caring Model®: Integrating Theory, Evidence, and Advanced Caring–Healing Therapeutics for Transforming Professional Practice

JEAN WATSON AND ROXIE FOSTER

BACKGROUND

Numerous studies in the United States continue to document publicly that patient deaths are tied to lack of nurses (*New York Times*, August 8, 2002: A14). Recent crises related to safety concerns have brought new attention to nursing and physician practices and models for how to address the shortage and crisis of care in acute care hospitals (Mustard, 2002).

These system dilemmas are compounded by the fast-paced health care delivery system of the 21st century, which has brought a nursing profession's struggle for identity and survival to a new level of public attention. Nurses are torn between the human caring model of nursing that attracted them to the profession and the task-orientated biomedical model and institutional demands that consumes their practice time. Nurses who are not able to practice within a caring context are reported to be hardened, oblivious, robot-like, frightened, and worn down (Swanson, 1999). In the context of a nationwide nursing shortage in the United States, if not in other Western countries worldwide, the viability of the profession is as much at stake as is the viability of care practices throughout acute care inpatient institutions.

Proposed solutions for recruitment and retention, like better compensation packages and increased numbers of undereducated nurses or even less-prepared assistants, comprise superficial and short-term approaches to a deeper, philosophical value-based issue prevalent throughout the profession. Ultimately, the ability to resolve conflicts between what nursing is (e.g., the theories, philosophies, ethics, and knowledge that guides their practices), and *what nurses do*, may be the cutting-edge difference, which dictates the discipline and profession's existence and survival into this new millennium.

From a social–political lens, nursing remains invisible and externally controlled, in spite of the scientific facts and evidence that nursing care and caring are crucial variables that make a positive difference in patients' (and nurses') outcomes of health and well-being (Swanson, 1999). Meanwhile, many mainstream systems are struggling to comprehend, conform to, or catch up with the past era of hospital-centric, cure-centric approaches, which are already dissolved (Watson, 2001, p. 78).

From Watson, J., & Foster, R. (2003). The attending nurse caring model®: Integrating theory, evidence, and advanced caring–healing therapeutics for transforming professional practice. *Journal of Clinical Nursing, 12,* 360–365. Permission to reprint granted by John Wiley & Sons, Inc.

Resolution of this philosophical professional value–system–culture conflict requires renewal of the profession and the system from inside out, allowing nursing to reconnect with the foundations of professional nursing and its theoretical, knowledgeable, ethical, and philosophical principles to revision nursing practice. However, to resolve practice dilemmas, abstract conceptualizations of what nursing is, must translate to the concrete realm of what nursing does and must guide integrative professional clinical judgment for those actions within the context of a system and culture in crises and conflict.

As institutions grope for new ways to solve the care and safety and institutional cultural dilemmas, which seem to be accelerating in Western medical institutions, new integration models of advancing caring–healing practices for inpatient acute care systems are becoming a growing trend. This movement is occurring both in nursing and medicine, as well as in hospitals themselves.

REORIENTATIONS FOR HOSPITAL CARE DELIVERY MODELS AND PATTERNS

There are dramatic shifts required within established patterns of care delivery that now warrant an orientation, away from traditional hospital structures and their routinized, industrial practices. The traditional hospital treatment delivery model was characterized by a care delivery system driven by technology, diagnosis and treatment of acute illness, and product line management. The shifting trend is toward managed care environments, integrated with a caring–healing emphasis; this trend holds promises for transforming both practices and settings (Miller & Apker, 2002; Watson, 1999).

The new caring–healing practice environment is increasingly dependent on partnerships, negotiation, coordination, new forms of communication pattern, and authentic relationships. The new emphasis is on a change of consciousness, a focused intentionality toward caring and healing relationships and modalities, a shift toward a spiritualizing of health vs. a limited medicalized view. Thus, new standards, principles, guidelines, and models for advancing and sustaining professional nursing caring practice are required (Miller & Apker, 2002; Tressolini & Pew-Fetzer Task Force, 1994; Watson, 2002).

It can be argued that these complex and somewhat chaotic changes create not only uncertainty for medicine and nursing, but also new opportunities for leadership. However, one interprets these complexities, and it is clear that the responsibilities, activities, and practice models of professional nursing are under fire and nursing is mandated, along with others, to rethink conventional industrial models of care delivery. It is also clear that responsibilities of nursing will continue to be substantially transformed (Miller & Apker, 2002) whether we agree with the changes or not.

The dynamics of relational, human-to-human caring practices and comprehensive therapeutic modalities for caring–healing seem to be eclipsed by the daily routines, mechanics, and demands of economic, management, physical, and technological aspects of care. The heart of the necessary changes needed for renewal and transformation seem to be dependent on human dimensions and skills that result in transforming patterns and depths of communication, relationships, and healing modalities. These human caring–healing dimensions transcend profession, system, and institutional structures.

Miller and Apker (2002) have identified some of the key pattern shifts in communication and in the roles of nursing that move us beyond conventional systems. While the nurse has traditionally served as caregiver, educator, and emotional support for patients, families and so on, the new demands and responsibilities extend into new dynamics and relational aspects of care delivery. They identify several key new areas for new relationships and communication expectations. They include, for example (Miller & Apker, 2002, p. 155, authors' parentheses):

- More interaction with nursing assistants (and technicians)
- Increased (change in nature and patterns of) communication with physicians, medical residents, and other professional health practitioners (e.g., PharmDs)
- Liaison with increasing numbers of hospital-specific personnel (chaplains, massage therapists, complementary practitioners) which are an increasing discipline
- Interaction (and cooperation) with insurance companies and outside agencies charged with coordinating care across the care continuum

They characterized these new communication patterns within managed care hospitals as the four Cs of nurse communication. The four Cs include:

- Collaboration with wide range of hospital personnel
- Conflict resolution around costs and care issues
- Change management leadership roles and communication experts
- Construction of new nursing identity, personally and professionally

These changing communication and relationship patterns and expectations have generated new visions of nursing and medicine. Likewise, efforts to revision leadership initiatives to address the shifting patterns in hospital structures are beginning to emerge. Growing public scrutiny around issues of safety and mortality rates in hospital systems is also contributing to the call for dramatic changes in professional nursing and physician practice models.

PHYSICIAN *HOSPITALIST* MODEL

A growing physician practice model, termed the *hospitalist* movement in the United States, has been underway for the past 5 years or so. The *hospitalist* is structured as a daily on-site practitioner (usually a physician) who is an inpatient generalist (or specialist on cardiac intensive care units) who is employed by the hospital to oversee direct care protocols and care regimes for hospitalized patients (Cram, 2002). The physician hospitalist mediates treatment programs and clinical care issues between and among the interdisciplinary treatment team. The goal is to facilitate total quality improvement prospectively, rather than retrospectively. The hospitalists are generally accountable to the hospital administration and tend to see themselves as practitioners "who run hospitals and have an ethical and moral obligation to make sure that when people come into our (systems) we treat them as guests who come into our home" (Cram, 2002).

NURSE HOSPITALIST AS EMERGING MODEL?

The recent work of Mustard (2002) has connected issues of caring and competency to address current attention and concerns with patient safety and day-to-day examples of substandard patient care. He proposes a new model of the *nurse hospitalist*, as a daily teacher and facilitator for hospital nurses based on living examples of substandard care that have been documented within the institution. He envisions the inpatient generalist advanced practice hospitalist nurse as one who is employed by the hospital, but who reports to the chief nurse executive. This role of hospitalist nurse, proposed by Mustard, would be "devoted entirely to collaborating with nurse leaders, educators, charge nurses, and floor nurses in advancing the competency of nursing" (Mustard, 2002, p. 36).

Mustard's model requires no structural change in the institution, but introduces an educational agenda with the nursing staff, with nursing and hospital administration, to assist in creating a new learning environment, thus changing the culture of care practices, helping to increase oversight, decrease injury, accidents, deaths, and improve overall safety standards. In Mustard's model, the nurse hospitalist becomes an expert in both caring and competency as a means to improve the performance of the acute care nurse. In this model, there is more emphasis on critical thinking and interpersonal skill, rather than just clinical and technical skill. The attributes required for the hospitalist nurse, in Mustard's model, are related to attributes of our humanness and stress the humanities of nursing practice (Mustard, 2002, p. 38). He reports some of the necessary attributes that have been identified for such a nurse, for example:

- Coordinating care among different disciplines of the clinical team
- Informing the patient on the level of detail of care being rendered, including prognosis based upon the patient's preference or desire to know
- Respecting the patient's values, privacy, and dignity, especially in decision making; making the patient comfortable in the hospital environment
- Providing emotional support and reducing fears and anxieties
- Involving family and friends in patient support and decision making
- Addressing the patient's anxieties in discharge planning and providing support for successful recovery after discharge

While we agree that all these attributes are congruent with professional nursing care, there is no theory or overarching disciplinary foundation for Mustard's hospitalist nurse model. The hospitalist nurse model is not responsible for direct patient care, nor advanced practice approaches that are explicitly guided by theory, but rather is designed more as a staff educator role.

While the hospitalist nurse model is posited as a proactive and prospective model for improving nursing performance in a facilitative manner, in contrast with the retrospective model of quality control, it can be enhanced if created more explicitly within a professional collegial cooperative model, that is discipline specific, while simultaneously transcending any disciplinary myopia. If nursing is to be renewed for mature caring practices, any model must be grounded both in time-honored values of caring and be guided by an explicit disciplinary perspective. It is true that proactive, prospective approaches and solutions to competency and caring issues are preferred, and we concur that true total quality improvement, practiced retroactively, is ineffective. However, acknowledging, and building upon, the intellectual, theoretical, and moral grounding of the model, along with an implementation approach that endorses and facilitates nurses advancing in their caring practices (informed by congruent theories, values, and knowledge/evidence), will significantly improve the hospitalist nurse concept. Offering new structures, patterns, and possibilities for nurses' unity and self-renewal from within hold promise for nurses actively to cocreate the very caring–healing models they envision for their patients, the public, and their profession.

EXTENDING *HOSPITALIST* NURSE: TURN TOWARD CARING THEORY-GUIDED, EVIDENCE-BASED PRACTICE MODEL

The proposed nurse hospitalist model, its general premises and directions, are consistent, to a large extent, with a proposed advanced professional nursing caring model. A process termed "theory-guided, evidence-based, reflective practice" offers a promising approach to this hospitalist concept, but frames it within a new professional practice model that is grounded in a disciplinary foundation. Therefore, offering hope to improve and advance nursing's time-honored caring–healing practices in both inpatient and community settings (Fawcett, Watson, Neuman, Walker, & Fitzpatrick, 2001).

ATTENDING NURSE CARING MODEL® (OPERATIONALIZING THEORY-GUIDED, EVIDENCE-BASED REFLECTIVE PRACTICE)

The Attending Nurse Caring Model® (ANCM) can incorporate some, if not most, of Mustard's hospitalist notions, while extending it, allowing more actualization of nursing as a mature caring and healing profession.

The ANCM, in some ways, parallels, but expands, Mustard's nurse hospitalist model. For example, the ANCM is designed to deliver and oversee a program of collaborative, comprehensive, continuous caring–healing nursing therapeutic practices for a group of identified patients/families, all within the context of relationship-centered care (Tressolini & Pew-Fetzer Task Force, 1994). In the hospitalist nurse model, the advanced nurse oversees other nurses, rather than having the direct opportunity for developing, practicing, and overseeing a comprehensive plan of theory-guided care for patients/families.

The ANCM incorporates a caring theory as a philosophical–ethical base that grounds nurses in a shared world view and culture. It allows the emergence of a collective vision, whereby shared knowledge, values, goals, and advanced caring therapeutics can extend practices. This process, in turn, can generate a new pattern and structure for care delivery. A culture of shared knowledge and values guide heart-felt caring practices that are grounded in both theory and evidence. This approach helps to translate theory and evidence into advanced nursing therapeutic practices. Thus, the ANCM extends and advances professional caring practices and patterns while expanding, supporting, and simultaneously sustaining independent and interdependent care goals. The ANCM is both discipline specific and transdisciplinary.

DEFINING THE ATTENDING CARING NURSE (ACN)

The Attending Caring Nurse (ACN) within the ANCM is responsible for:

- Establishing and sustaining a continuous, caring relationship with patients/families; this relationship may begin before hospital admission or on hospital admission and continue after discharge with follow-up
- Comprehensive assessment of caring needs and concerns, from patient's frame of reference, using caring theory as a guide for caring needs
- Assessing meaning of the subjective as well as objective concerns
- Cocreating with the patient/family a plan for comprehensive caring and healing that intersects with and is coordinated with the medical plan of care
- Overseeing and assuring comprehensive care planning and in some instances directly carrying out the therapeutic regime plan related to the caring–healing modalities of nursing
- Creating plans for direct communication with other nurses, physicians, and team members to assure continuity

Moreover, the ACN is responsible for writing comprehensive nursing directions for continuous care. This plan includes assuring caring theory-guided, evidence-based caring and healing therapeutic modalities. The ACN is responsible for oversight of this comprehensive plan of caring and healing, 24 hours a day. The ANC practitioner is considered an independent-interdependent professional nurse, who works collaboratively in full partnership with other nurses, physicians, and other health disciplines within the hospital and community.

The ANCM parallels an Attending Physician Model, except the ACN is "attending to" comprehensive nursing care–healing practices and therapeutics, and their integration with medical treatments. The ACN is informed and guided by an ethic and theory of caring, a caring relationship and evidence. In summary, the ANCM seeks to make explicit the caring relationship, the knowledge, values, philosophy, theory, and therapeutics that guide advanced professional caring–healing practices, Finally, the ACN creates a new pattern and structure for delivery of professional nursing that transforms conventional approaches while activating and renewing nursing caring paradigm.

PILOT PROJECT: THE ANCM: INTEGRATING THEORY AND EVIDENCE TO TRANSFORM PRACTICE

The ANCM is currently underway as a pilot project on one unit at The Children's Hospital in Denver, Colorado. It is constructed as a Nursing-Caring Science, theory-guided, evidence-based, collaborative practice model by applying it to the conduct and oversight of pain management on a 37-bed, postsurgical unit. The ANCM is designed to operationalize a disciplinary focus for advancing nursing practice in collaboration with physicians and other members of the team. This caring science initiative is informed by values, theory, and knowledgeable caring practices. It becomes both nursing specific and transdisciplinary, in that the ANCM model guides a comprehensive, continuous caring–healing program and pain management for children/parents.

CARING THEORY AND PAIN

The construct of pain is particularly well suited to this approach because effective pain management has historically been constrained by lack of a common theoretical/philosophical perspective (biological vs. a comprehensive unitary, whole person approach) and by limitations in accessibility and utility of the sizeable literature on assessment and management. The urgency to define effective practice models in the United States has recently been heightened by the need to implement the Joint Commission on Accreditation of Health care Organizations (JCAHO) standards for pain management. Caring theory and pain theory are congruent in their contemporary focus on the subjective human experience, the inner life processes, and meaning of the experience. Pain theory describes the pain experience as a dynamic interaction among biological, physiological, psychosocial, cultural, and spiritual influences. The human caring process requires knowledge of human behavior including the unity of mind, body, and spirit; one's strengths and limitations, and responses; and knowledge of how to comfort, offer compassion and empathy within the context of a caring relationship (Watson, 1985, p. 227).

ANCM: PROPOSED THEORY-GUIDED EVIDENCE PROGRAM

In the pilot project, nurses who self-select to apply and participate in the ANCM are being introduced to a series of educational sessions of caring theory, including the 10 carative factors (Watson, 1979) to understand the structure of the caring process. More recent work related to caring theory incorporates notions of caring consciousness, intentionality, and caring–healing modalities that are being incorporated into "caring moments" in direct care situations. In addition to manifesting caring into practice, the model of care simultaneously assists professionals with their own caring–healing practices for self-care. Another aspect of knowledge is that available through clinical evidence and clinical judgments. Sackett, Richardson, Rosenberg, and Haynes (1997, p. 2) defined evidence-based practice as "the conscientious, explicit and judicious use of current best evidence in making decisions about the care of individual patients." Evidence encompasses not only the empirical and theoretical literature but also clinical expertise and feedback from patients and families. In the ANCM pilot project, participants are initiating the search for evidence, as they define clinical problems in pain management. The nurses participating in the project are learning how the ANCM can increase their caring consciousness and intentionality to use knowledge and evidence, as well as to help increase autonomy, enhance interdisciplinary teamwork, and reduce suffering in children. Reflective activities, such as focus group discussions and individual recordings of caring moments help participants integrate the theoretical knowledge into their day-to-day practices with children in pain. Nurses are also writing nursing directions on the order sheet in the medical record for use of caring–healing modalities and nursing therapeutics for comfort measures, pain control, creating a sense of well-being, relaxation, and so on. These nursing modalities complement the physician's orders for analgesics. To date, collaborative practices among interdisciplinary participants are changing, with enhanced patterns of communication and dialogue between nurses and physicians and other members of the team.

Finally, the ANCM elevates contemporary nursing caring values, relationships, therapeutics, and responsibilities to a higher/deeper order of caring science and professionalism, intersecting with other professions while sustaining the finest of its heritage and traditions of healing. In summary, the proposed ANCM offers new options for addressing the dissonance between nursing theory and practice; between nursing caring philosophy, knowledge and values, and system constraints. The ANCM seeks to transcend conventional problematic practice patterns, generating new possibilities for self-renewal of time-honored values of nursing, combined with the most contemporary knowledge and advanced modalities of nursing. As such, it offers hope for transforming both nurse self and system while working within the context of the most contemporary crises and challenges facing today's health care structures, systems, and society, at this point in human history.

REFERENCES

Cram, P. (2002). Physicians critical of fast food at nation's top hospitals. *Hospitalist & Inpatient Management Report, 4*(7), 108.

Fawcett, J., Watson, J., Neuman, B., Walker, P. H., & Fitzpatrick, J. J. (2001). On nursing theories and evidence. *Journal of Nursing Scholarship, 32*(2), 115–119.

Miller, K. I. & Apker, J. (2002). On the front lines of managed care: Professional changes and communicative dilemmas of hospital nurses. *Nursing Outlook, 50*, 154–159.

Mustard, L. (2002). Caring and competency. *JONA's Health care, Law, Ethics, and Regulation, 4*(2), 36–43.

Sackett, D. L., Richardson, W. S., Rosenberg, W., & Haynes, R. B. (1997). *Evidence-based medicine.* New York, NY: Churchill Livingstone.

Swanson, K. (1999). What is known about caring in nursing science. In A. S. Hinshaw, S. L. Feet-ham, & J. L. F. Shaver (Eds.),

Handbook of clinical nursing research (pp. 31–60). Thousand Oaks, CA: Sage.

Tressolini, C. P., & the Pew-Fetzer Task Force. (1994). *Health professions education and relationship-centered care. Report of Pew-Fetzer Task Force.* San Francisco, CA: Pew-Fetzer Task Group, Pew Health Commission.

Watson, J. (1979). *Nursing. The philosophy and science of caring.* Boston, MA: Little, Brown.

Watson, J. (1985). *Nursing. Human science and human care* (p. 227). New York, NY: NLN.

Watson, J. (1999). *Postmodern nursing and beyond.* New York, NY: Harcourt–Brace.

Watson, J. (2001). Post-hospital nursing: shortage, shifts, and scripts. *Nursing Administrative Quarterly, 25*(3), 77–82.

Watson, J. (2002). Intentionality and caring-healing consciousness: A practice of transpersonal nursing. *Holistic Nursing Practice, 16*(4), 12–19.

QUESTIONS FOR REFLECTION

Baccalaureate

1. Identify two concepts that Watson and Foster identify as the responsibility of the Attending Caring Nurse.
2. What caring–healing modalities/practices have you observed in the clinical setting where you work or are doing a student rotation?
3. How do you involve families in patient support and decision making?

Master's

1. What two concepts that Watson and Foster identify as the responsibility of the Attending Caring Nurse could you implement in the practice setting where you work or are doing a student rotation?
2. Discuss the similarities and differences among the nurse hospitalist, physician hospitalist, and Attending Nurse Caring Model®?
3. Watson and Foster discussed the importance of a focused intentionality toward caring and healing relationships and modalities. What does this mean to you as a nurse? How do you integrate this into your practice of nursing?

Doctoral

1. Watson and Foster discuss that complex and chaotic changes create uncertainty for nursing but also new opportunities for leadership. Provide two examples from recent (within the past 5 years) nursing literature where this has been identified.
2. What evidence-based caring–healing modalities have been advanced to treat pain for patients in acute care settings since 2003? What outcomes are associated with these modalities?
3. What type of research study would you design to show the economic and human caring value of implementing the Attending Nurse Caring Model®?

VII

Caring, Health Policy, and the Community

MARIAN C. TURKEL

This part includes several classic articles related to caring within a community context. In this section, the traditional context of community has been expanded to include the environment.

Historically, nurses have responded to the needs of persons in communities. However, the majority of extant nursing literature related to caring theory guided practice, and caring-based nursing practice models emphasized the integration of the models into the acute care setting within hospitals. As discussed in the previous section, the advancement of caring theory guided practice was influenced by the American Nurses Credentialing Center (ANCC) Magnet Recognition Program® recognizing excellence in professional nursing practice. Nursing theory moved from its central place in academia and research to practice (Davidson, Ray, & Turkel, 2011). Since formal inception in 1997, the focus of the Magnet Recognition Program® was acute care hospitals. Currently, no criteria are available for community settings to obtain this designation. However, the concept of expanding beyond the traditional acute care systems is being reviewed by the leaders of the program.

Nursing practice is always evolving and changing in response to the needs of those we serve and is guided by the substantive knowledge that has been a part of the heritage of the discipline. Florence Nightingale (1859/1969) did not develop a theory of nursing; however, she could be considered the "first theorist for community health" in terms of the integration of the environment into her writings, beliefs, and practices. Her work during the war exemplified caring within and for the community. Nightingale's commitment to the environment influenced the delivery of care during the Crimean War. As a result, infection and mortality rates fell (Nightingale, 1859/1969). Her ideas and practices related to the environment, and the intent focus on keeping populations healthy and free from diseases remain relevant to contemporary nursing practice within the community and global health issues. Nightingale (1859/1969, 1992) is recognized as the "mother" of professional nursing. She laid the foundation for caring as central to nursing and was deeply concerned about others' suffering. Her vision of nursing was seeing nursing caring actions as improving health within the human–environment relationship. Many of Nightingale's ideas parallel the thought and action present in nursing today. Nightingale demonstrated the importance of nursing as nature and nurture in caring and health (Davidson et al., 2011).

The metaparadigm of nursing is part of the domain of the discipline (Fawcett, 1984). The four concepts within the metaparadigm include persons, environment, health, and nursing. In this section, sentinel articles related to caring and community are reviewed and synthesized. In all the articles, the concept of environment is stated either explicitly or implicitly by the authors and is integral to the relationship between nursing and the community served.

Rafael (2000) used Watson's philosophy, science, and Theory of Human Caring as a conceptual framework for guiding community health nursing practice. The author recognized the congruency between Watson's theory and the contemporary global approaches to community health and health promotion. This classic article was one of the first to apply the theory, developed for individuals, to the practice of community health nursing.

Rafael (2000) discussed that public health nurses use theories from other disciplines to inform practice as most nursing theories do not seem relevant. Two specific reasons included the focus of nursing theories on the individual and the development for practice within the context of hospitalization and disease. Public health nurses did not see the applicability to the community population-focused care of health promotion. Rafael (2000) maintained that Watson's (1985, 1988b) Theory of Human Caring was philosophically congruent for community health nursing. This belief was grounded in Watson's focus on nonmedical determinants of health, the author's personal experience of using the theory as a practicing public health nurse, and working with nursing students to frame practice based on the theory.

Rafael (2000) presented an overview of Watson's theory and the evolution of the theory over the last 20 years. Watson's (1988a, 1990, 1999) work was influenced by consciousness theory, noetic sciences, and quantum physics; she envisioned a future where the caring–healing practices of nurses moved from the margins to the center of societal health. Rafael (2000) identified three reasons that the theory is unique among nursing theories. First, the caring moment reflects the lived experience of both the client and the nurse.

Second is the mindbodyspirit dimension of the theory, and third is the explicit inclusion of multiple ways of knowing, including empirical, aesthetic, ethical, and personal.

The author discussed underpinnings and beliefs that are central to the theory. Specific beliefs include individual's potential for self-healing, striving for self-actualization of the spiritual self as a basic human need, value of the transpersonal relationship for healing, and the 10 carative factors. Rafael (2000) presented a detailed overview of the 10 carative factors, including the relevance of specific carative factors to the preparation of the nurse to enter into a transpersonal caring relationship with another, the transpersonal caring relationship, and the caring processes. It is through the caring processes that client health and healing is promoted, and the patient and nurse together decide on the caring processes to be used. Watson's (1985) conceptualization of the environment in facilitating healing was informed by Nightingale. Watson expanded this work in terms of relevance to contemporary and futuristic nursing practice and included the notion of the spiritual and sociocultural environment.

Rafael (2000) detailed the relevancy of Watson's theory to the practice of community health nursing, global approaches to health, health promotion, and models of community development and empowerment. The holistic nature of the theory supports a focus on the community as a whole while still honoring and valuing the uniqueness of individuals and families who are part of the community. Watson's definition of health as "unity and harmony within body–mind–spirit and with the world" (p. 41) resonates with community health nurses; disease or other community problems such as homelessness and crime are more likely to occur when the community is in disharmony. Rafael (2000) acknowledged that Watson's view of health is consistent with that of the World

Health Organization, Canadian Public Health Association, Health and Welfare Canada (1986) and the view of health promotion is consistent with the definition within the Ottawa Charter (1986) and Jakarta Declaration (1997). Watson's (1985) focus on the environment guides public health nurses to assess and address the social, political, economical, and environmental determinates of health.

The relevance of the carative factors to specific aspects of community health nursing practice was highlighted by Rafael (2000). Practicing loving kindness to self and others includes clarifying values and authentic presence that are important in caring for communities. Community caring evolves when a helping–trusting relationship is developed between the nurse and the members of community and when the caring involves protecting and enhancing the dignity of others. Creative problem solving focuses on the health goals established by the community and involves active participation and mutability between the nurse and the community when working toward these goals. Health education in the community is guided by transpersonal teaching–learning. The nurse explores the meaning of the situations and allows for empowerment through the development of skills and education for individuals to have greater control over their health. Community health nurses attend to the basic needs of communities in partnership with members to allow for achievement of health goals. The carative factor of allowing for existential phenomenological forces is lived out in practice when a community health nurse helps a community find meaning in the face of disaster.

Rafael's (2000) writing reaffirmed that Watson's philosophical beliefs and tenets of the theory are congruent and relevant to the contemporary practice of community and public health nursing. As nurses use the theory to guide practice, they are actually returning to

a practice that is in harmony with the original values and practices of the founders of public health nursing (Rafael, 1999). The author continues to advance this sentinel work. Baccalaureate students and public health nurses have integrated Watson's Theory of Human Caring into practice and have shared their experiences with Rafael (2005). Rafael (2005) expanded her thinking related to Watson's theory, caring science, and empowered caring and developed a theory of critical caring that integrated critical feminist theories as a guide for public health nursing practice.

Schuster (1990) was a true avant garde caring scholar who the authors of *Caring Classics* had the pleasure of knowing on a personal and professional basis. Dr. Schuster was "green" before it was cool or trendy to be green, and her philosophical beliefs were actualized in all ways of her being, knowing, and doing. At the time her article was published, the faculty at the Christine E. Lynn College of Nursing at Florida Atlantic University had created a nursing curriculum grounded in the tenets of caring science and the Theory of Nursing as Caring. The focus was on integrating caring into the educational foundation, using caring to guide the practice of nursing students, and having the theory guide research. Dr. Schuster recognized the need to care for self and to extend the concept of caring beyond persons. The courses developed and taught by Dr. Schuster related to caring for self and the specific course titled Women, Witches, and Healing were very popular and always received high ratings from students.

This sentinel article that explored the interrelationship among environment, nursing, and caring, was written to challenge the readers and to have us expand our definition of caring to include Mother Earth (Schuster, 1990). Schuster (1990) reminded us that as nurses, we have a moral obligation to honor earth caring values not only for our own quality of life and survival but for the well-being of the planet. Current environmental issues were presented and the 10 key values of the Greens' social commitment outlined. The limited number of scholarly publications linking nursing to the environment were reviewed and presented. The few that were published focused on radiation, smoking policies, water pollution, chemical hazard identification, and working in toxic environments (Schuster, 1990).

Schuster (1990) acknowledged that the nurses most interested in the environment at this time were the members of the American Holistic Nurses Association (AHNA, 1989). In the handbook for holistic nursing practice, authors Dossey, Keegan, and Guzzeta (1989) expanded the definition of environment beyond the physical and stated,

> environment is everything that surrounds an individual or group of people; may be physical, social, psychological, cultural or spiritual; includes external and internal, animate and inanimate objects, seen and unseen vibrations and frequencies, climate and not yet understood energy patterns. (p. 27)

Schuster (1990) applauded the professional statement released by AHNA (1989) outlining the responsibilities of nurses to be a role model and educate others on relevant environmental issues to preserve our home Mother Earth.

Schuster (1990) reviewed the nursing theories of Rogers (1980) and Watson (1988b). Although not explicitly stated, the philosophical tenets of both theories are congruent with expanded definitions of the environment in terms of the higher energy fields. Without providing specific statements or examples, Schuster (1990) strongly espoused the idea that Leininger's (1981) current definition of caring as the essence of nursing and unifying focus of the discipline be expanded to include the needs of the environment.

Schuster's (1990) thinking was philosophical in nature versus directive. Her vision was for caring scholars to reflect on caring as engagement for the environment from an ontological and epistemological perspective. Dr. Schuster (1990) questioned the first goal of the International Association for Human Caring to "identify major philosophical, epistemological and profession dimensions of care and caring to advance the body of *knowledge* that constitutes nursing and to help other disciplines use care and caring in *human* relationships" (p. 29). Caring scholars used the term human caring, and Schuster felt that the use of the word human did not "readily allow for the nonhuman interchange of care or caring" (p. 29). This article was Schuster's (1990) opportunity to share somewhat provocative for the time, views, and reflections about the earth and caring for the purpose of stimulating thinking and disclosure within the discipline so that we all would grow and thrive. Schuster ended the article with a poetic reflection from a Native American tribe (Allen, 1986).

Other authors have written about the relationship between the environment and nursing. Schuster's (1990) work remains unique with the metaparadigm perspective focus on the relationship among caring, nursing, and environment. Schuster (1990) felt that as nurses our commitment to caring for Mother Earth should be grounded in philosophical tenets and as intentional as our caring for persons.

Zerwekh (2000) conducted a phenomenological study with seven community health nurses to understand the lived experience of caring for disenfranchised patients and the meaning of caring for individuals "on the ragged edge of society." According to Zerwekh (2000), nurse informants revealed that the practice of caring for disenfranchised and outcast patients involved fearless caring. Prior to this publication, Zerwekh (2000) had a research trajectory related to public health/community health nursing practice; however, this classic article was explicitly grounded in a caring science framework.

Zerwekh performed a review of the literature from the perspective of caring theory. The beliefs of Boykin and Schoenhofer (1990, 1993), Parse (1993), Rafael (1996, 1998), Rogers (1980), Smith (1986, 1989), and Swanson (1993) were synthesized and served as the theoretical foundation for understanding the findings of this research study. The specific research method for the study was Ray's (1991) phenomenological approach. In accordance with this method, the author's beliefs and assumptions were bracketed, and the author identified seven nurses who had developed compassionate relationships while serving the disenfranchised patient population. Three questions guided the interview process. They included: "What is it like to care for persons whom mainstream often does not care?"; "Would you tell me one or two experiences of caring for marginalized people that have special meaning for you?"; and "What is the meaning of caring for the patient population you serve?" (p. 49).

Zerwekh (2000) characterized significant findings as metaphors, themes, and meta-themes. All included direct quotes, stories, and vivid descriptions reflecting the lived experiences of the participants' nursing practices. The metaphor of Going around the Wall illustrated the work of nurses caring on the ragged edge. Clients are separated from family and the community by the wall of fear; the community pulls away, builds barriers, and the wall is developed (Zerwekh, 2000). Nurses go around the wall and client circumstances, seeing them as humans, and providing the needed resources. Ten themes were clustered into three meta-themes. The meta-themes include The Human Connection, the Community Connection, and Making Self-Care Possible.

Human Connection described the nurses' beliefs of sharing a common humanity with those individuals who are referred to as the disenfranchised. Nursing practices included "honoring the clients' humanity, knowing the clients' humanity, and sharing one's own humanity" (p. 54). A direct quote from one of the participants reveals this dimension of practice. "I see their worth as people rather than treating them like a disease or symptom" (p. 54). Community Connection illustrated the practices of "connecting the disconnected, haunting the case and mediating to provide clients on one side of the wall with needed community services and resources on the other side" (p. 55). The final meta-theme of Making Self-Care Possible referred to ways the nurses strengthen clients' self-care. The approaches included "getting clients through emotionally, teaching them to understand themselves, helping them take control, and confronting fear at the community level" (p. 57).

Zerwekh (2000) identified caring on the edge as the emergent theoretical theme of the research. Caring on the edge is "caring that courageously nurtures possibility in the face of separation and fear; nurses go around the wall" (p. 59.) However, rather than developing another nursing theory, Zerwekh (2000) expanded Swanson's (1993) theory of Caring for the Well-Being of Others as the framework to illustrate caring for disenfranchised people. Zerwekh (2000) described how the five caring processes identified by Swanson (1993) are applicable when caring on the edge.

Maintaining belief (Swanson, 1993) refers to nurses having faith for those living outside the wall, believing in their clients' possibilities, and growing themselves through the experience. Knowing and being with (Swanson, 1993) is congruent with Zerwekh's (2000) theme of honoring humanity, knowing humanity, and sharing humanity. Doing for (Swanson, 1993) is practiced by nurses caring on the edge through connecting, haunting, and mediating. Swanson's (1993) caring process of enabling relates to Zerwekh's (2000) theme of Making Self-Care Possible where the registered nurses help clients get through, teach them to understand, help them take control, and work with them to confront fear at the community level.

Zerwekh (2000) remains concerned philosophically and politically about the care of those who are marginalized. She encouraged nurses to advocate at a personal and professional level for those living at the edge and to see possibilities and hope for this group. Zerwekh (2000) asserted her personal belief that through concern and caring, self-love and self-regard increase.

MOVING FORWARD

Barry and Gordon (2005) illustrated how the theory of Nursing as Caring was used to create a model for the practice of school nursing. The Community Nursing Practice Model was developed to guide the practice of caring for students and families within the school setting. Nursing practice within this model was centered on the values of respect for person, caring, and wholeness (Barry & Gordon, 2005). A nursing situation provided an exemplar of how a school nurse used the values to be authentically present and listen to the concerns of a student and his or her family. Through this intentional caring, the nurse made a difference by meeting social and health care needs. Within this model, the concept of environment has been expanded to include the relationships between social and health issues that influence one's life. Drawing upon the ideas of Schuster (1992), the authors acknowledged the importance of considering the interconnectedness of all animate and inanimate environmental elements when coming to understand the context of how one lives. This model is used in the Florida Atlantic school-based wellness centers where access to care is provided for students, staff, and community members living in underserved areas. The work continues to be advanced and has been expanded from underserved communities in southeast Florida to a school-based community wellness center in Uganda (Barry, Gordon, & Lange, 2007). As in the United States, the intent was to focus on collaboration and partnership and one of the first questions the nurses asked members of the community in Uganda, was "How can I be helpful to you?" (p. 176).

Bent (1999) explored the concepts of caring, community, health in community, and community interventions and presented a model of eco-caring as a philosophical foundation reflective of community health nursing praxis or the integration of being, knowing, and doing. This approach differed from the work of Barry and Gordon who offered a tangible model of how caring is lived and expressed by nurses and members of the community being served. Bent felt that in community nursing nurses needed to understand the philosophical foundations of: "What does it mean to be in relation or to be in community?," "What does it mean to be in a caring community?," and "What does it mean to care for community and interconnectedness?" (pp. 30–31). Bent (1999) presented on overview of the literature related to the ethics and ontology of caring, definition of communities, health in communities, and caring community partnerships. In the model developed by Bent (1999), eco-caring reflects the process of community relatedness with a focus on changing individual behaviors rather than holding individuals responsible for changing the health of the community as a whole. She further acknowledged that caring in the community is interactive and includes the connection among economics, politics, policy, and law. According to Bent (1999), the actual process of engaging in community caring through the lens of critical thinking results in change and positive health outcomes.

Schuster (1992) continued to advance thinking related to environmental ethics and how value systems guide decision making that is not always earth friendly. The writing is prolific and meant to bring into question how one chooses to practice global responsibility as a way of being in the world. She provided no clear-cut directions or strategies but acknowledged the need of understanding self in relation to how we choose to be in and relate to the world. Schuster (1992) believed that as humans we make deliberate choices of how to be in the world including the decision to pollute in one way or another. She invited humans to see ourselves as "Earth Dwellers," to honor the sacredness and mystery of the earth and to preserve and care for world's creation by being environmentally responsible. Throughout the article, Schuster (1992) acknowledged that world creation is not limited exclusively to humans and the need to reaffirm the human connectedness to all things. She firmly believes that for these changes to occur nursing theory, nursing practice, and nursing research needed to expand the concept of environment beyond the physical environment of the patient, family, and nurses. Schuster (1992) identified that when nurses value the relationship of self to the earth practice changes will occur as nurses voice concern over how supplies are procured and disposed of within the work environment.

ONGOING REFLECTIONS

Initially, many of the caring nursing theories focused upon the individual (patient) or family within a specific setting. Caring within the community continues to be advanced by caring scholars who view the role of nursing practice outside of the hospital as relevant to meeting the health care needs of specific populations, society, and the world at large. Common themes across the various community settings is nursing practice grounded in caring science and caring values. The work of these scholars allows for the creation of caring, healthy communities at the national and international levels. At the societal level, health care outcomes for communities are improved through the absence of disease, illness, and injury. At the human level, nursing practice grounded in values of caring and compassion for vulnerable communities allows for health and healing to occur. This holistic approach to the community facilitates health promotion by meeting the basic needs of the body, mind, and spirit.

REFERENCES

Allen, P. G. (1986). *The sacred hoop: Recovering the feminine in American Indian traditions*. Boston, MA: Beacon Press.

American Holistic Nurses Association political position statement in support of a healthy environment. (1989). *Beginnings: The official newsletter of the American Holistic Nurses' Association, 10*(8), 7.

Barry, C., & Gordon, S. (2005). Caring for students in school using a community practice model. *International Journal for Human Caring, 9*(3), 38–42.

Barry, C., Gordon, S., & Lange, B. (2007). The usefulness of the community nursing practice model in grounding practice and research: Narratives from the United States and Africa. *Research and Theory for Nursing Practice: An International Journal, 21*(2), 174–184.

Bent, K. N. (1999). The ecologies of community caring. *Advances in Nursing Science, 21*(4), 29–36.

Boykin, A., & Schoenhofer, S. (1990). Caring in nursing: Analysis of extant theory. *Nursing Science Quarterly, 4*, 149–155.

Boykin, A., & Schoenhofer, S. (1993). *Nursing as caring: A model for transforming practice*. New York, NY: National League for Nursing.

Davidson, A. W., Ray, M. A., & Turkel, M. C. (2011). *Nursing, caring, and complexity science: For human-environment well-being*. New York, NY: Springer Publishing Company.

Dossey, B. M., Keegan, L., & Guzzetta, C. E. (1989). Environment: Protecting our personal and planetary home. In *Holistic nursing: A handbook for practice*. Rockville, MD: Aspen Publisher.

Fawcett, J. (1984). *Analysis and evaluation of contemporary nursing knowledge*. Philadelphia, PA: F.A. Davis.

Jakarta declaration on health promotion into the 21st century. (1997). *Health Promotion International, 12*, 261–264.

Leininger, M. M. (1981). *Caring: An essential human need*. Thorofare, NJ: Charles B. Slack.

Mitchell, G. J. (1993). The view of freedom within the human becoming theory. In R. R. Parse (Ed.), *Illuminations: The human becoming theory in practice and research*. New York, NY: National League for Nursing.

Nightingale, F. (1969). *Notes on nursing: What it is and what it is not*. New York, NY: Dover. (Original work published 1859)

Nightingale, F. (1992). *Notes on nursing: What it is and what it is not*. Philadelphia, PA: J. B. Lippincott.

Rafael, A. R. F. (1998). Nurses who run with the wolves: The power and caring dialectic revisited. *Advance Nursing Science, 21*(1), 29–42.

Rafael, A. R. F. (1999). The politics of health promotion: Influences on public health promoting nursing practice in Ontario, Canada, from Nightingale to the nineties. *Advances in Nursing Science, 22*(1), 23–39.

Rafael, A. R. F. (2000). Watson's philosophy, science, and theory of human caring as a conceptual framework for guiding community health nursing practice. *Advances in Nursing Science, 23*(2), 34–49.

Rafael, A. R. F. (2005). Advancing nursing theory through theory-guided practice: The emergence of a critical caring perspective. *Advances in Nursing Science, 28*(1), 38–49.

Ray, M. (1991). Caring inquiry: The esthetic process in the way of compassion. In D. Gaut & M. Leininger (Eds.), *Caring: The compassionate healer*. New York, NY: National League for Nursing.

Rogers, M. E. (1980). Nursing: A science of unitary man. In J. P. Reihl & C. Roy (Eds.), *Conceptual models for nursing practice* (2nd ed.). New York, NY: Appleton-Century-Crofts.

Schuster, E. A. (1990). Earth caring. *Advances in Nursing Science, 13*(1), 25–30.

Schuster, E. A. (1992). Earth dwelling. *Holistic Nursing Practice, 6*(4), 1–9.

Smith, M. (1999). Caring and the science of unitary human being. *Advances in Nursing Science, 21*(4), 14–28.

Smith, M. J. (1986). Human environment process: A test of Rogers' principle of integrality. *Advances in Nursing Science, 9*(1), 21–28.

Swanson, K. (1993). Nursing as informed caring for the well being of others. *Image, 25*(4), 352–257.

Watson, J. (1985). *Nursing: The philosophy and science of caring*. Boulder, CO: Colorado Associated Press.

Watson, J. (1988a). New dimensions in human caring theory. *Nursing Science Quarterly, 1*(4), 175–181.

Watson, J. (1988b). *Nursing: Human science and human care: A theory of nursing*. New York, NY: National League for Nursing.

Watson, J. (1990). The moral failure of the patriarchy. *Nursing Outlook, 38*(2), 62–66.

Watson, J. (1999). *Postmodern nursing and beyond*. New York, NY: Churchill Livingstone.

World Health Organization, Canadian Public Health Association, Health and Welfare Canada. (1986, November 17–21). *Ottawa charter for health promotions*. Presented at the First International Conference on Health Promotions, Ottawa, Ontario, Canada.

Zerwekh, J. V. (2000). Caring on the ragged edge: Nursing persons who are disenfranchised. *Advances in Nursing Science, 22*(4), 47–61.

30

Watson's Philosophy, Science, and Theory of Human Caring as a Conceptual Framework for Guiding Community Health Nursing Practice

Adeline R. Falk Rafael

Commonly, public/community health nursing scholars lament the paucity of nursing conceptual frameworks that are useful in guiding community health nursing practice. Their concern is frequently echoed by public health nursing practitioners who, not uncommonly, dismiss nursing theories as irrelevant to their work. Yet, at the same time, either knowingly or unknowingly, public health nurses inform their practice with theories from other disciplines as diverse as medicine, sociology, psychology, and even business.[1] Because many of those theories emanate from paradigms incongruent with a nursing philosophy, it seems logical to assume that they contribute to the increasing loss of identity and invisibility that has been reported among public health nurses.[2-5] Although the reasons that nursing theories frequently are not perceived as useful to community health nurses and, at the same time, those from other disciplines are enthusiastically embraced are many and complex, the limitations of existing nursing theories for community health nursing practice are an important factor and bear further consideration.

Two major criticisms of existing nursing theories are that they focus on individuals, and they have been developed primarily for practice within the context of infirmity and disease. They are, thus, inadequate for a population-focused health promotion approach in which the focus of nursing attention moves beyond the individual to the community, population, or group. Although considerable work has been done to extrapolate Neuman's theory to the community,[6] and Helvie[7] recently developed a systems-based theory for community health nursing practice, a conceptual framework that recognizes the primacy of relationship in community health nursing work and informs an empowering approach to the health promotion of communities is lacking.

This chapter proposes that Watson's philosophy/science/theory of human caring, although also developed with individuals in mind, has the potential to be such a framework because of its philosophic congruence with community health nursing. That congruence was evident in the first publication of Watson's theory in 1979 when, remarkably for the time, she offered a critique of the medical domination of health care and devoted a whole chapter to nonmedical determinants of health.[8] Watson's position at the time was

From Falk Raphael, A. (2000). Watson's philosophy, science, and theory of human caring as a conceptual framework for guiding community health nursing practice. *Advances in Nursing Science*, 23(2), 34–49. Permission to reprint granted by Wolters Kluwer.

in keeping with those of others that began to surface internationally at approximately the same time and formed the basis for contemporary global approaches to health and the health promotion of communities.[1] Watson's critique, however, is grounded as much in Florence Nightingale's legacy and vision of nursing as it is influenced by health care critics such as Illich. As such, it offers the hope of returning community health nursing practice to a nursing center and restoring the strong nursing identity and vision of early community health nursing leaders such as Nightingale and Wald.

My explication of the relevance of Watson's work to community health nursing practice is grounded in my own experiences with using Watson's theory as a practicing public health nurse, examining public health nursing practice through research, and facilitating the learning of students who use Watson's work to guide their community health nursing experiences. Before examining Watson's theory as a conceptual framework for community health nursing practice, however, a brief overview of the theory itself is instructive.

OVERVIEW OF WATSON'S THEORY OF HUMAN CARING

Watson's[8,9] Theory of Human Caring has evolved over the past 20 years. First published in 1979 as a basic nursing text for baccalaureate students, Watson later expanded her ideas to "elucidate the process of human caring [and to] preserve the concept of the person in our science."[8(pix)] In her latest book,[10] Watson continues her visionary quest to move nursing's caring–healing practices from the margins to the center of societal health and healing practices. This work strongly reflects the influences of consciousness theory, noetic sciences, quantum physics, transpersonal psychology, Jungian psychology, and feminist theories, among others, that have gained prominence in her work over the past decade.[11–15]

At least three factors make Watson's theory unique among nursing theories. First, it stresses the importance of the lived experience not only of the client but also of the nurse. Both come together in a caring moment that becomes part of the life history of each person. Second, the theory acknowledges the unique dimensions of mind/body/spirit without compromising the wholeness of the person. Although some critics insist that acknowledging dimensions of a whole is tantamount to reducing it to parts, Watson's approach may be viewed as similar to appreciating the unique contribution of each color of a rainbow to the beauty of the whole or each musical note to the grandeur of a symphony. Her assertion of acknowledging parts without compromising the whole is based on the holographic paradigm that suggests the whole is in the parts.[12] Third, Watson's theory of nursing values and explicitly acknowledges multiple ways of knowing, including empirical, aesthetic, ethical, and personal knowing.

Watson's humanistic, existential, and metaphysical conceptualization of human beings underpins her view of both the transpersonal caring relationship that is central to her theory and her conceptualization of health–illness. She views human beings as beings-in-the-world with dimensions of mind/body/soul that, in health, exist in harmony.[9] Conversely, illness results from conscious or subconscious disharmony and may lead to disease. Inherent in Watson's conceptualization of human beings is the metaphysical potential for self-healing and transcendence to higher levels of consciousness. From her perspective, the patient/client is the agent of change and is primarily responsible for allowing healing to occur with or without external coparticipant agents of change (of which the nurse may be one).

Watson describes her concept of soul as "spirit, or higher sense of self"[9(p. 45)] and notes that it most closely resembles the psychologic concept of self-actualization.

Unlike Maslow's theory, however, in which the need for self-actualization is only activated after all other needs are met, striving for actualization of one's spiritual self is for Watson the most basic human need to which all other needs are subservient. Spirit is "greater than the physical, mental, and emotional existence of a person at any given point in time" and is tied to a "higher degree of consciousness, an inner strength, and a power that can expand human capacities … and cultivate a fuller access to the intuitive and even sometimes allow uncanny, mystical, or miraculous experiences."[9(pp. 45–46)]

The human potential for self-healing and transcendence to higher levels of consciousness informs Watson's vision for nursing, which is "to help persons gain a higher degree of harmony"[9(p. 49)] through a transpersonal caring relationship. She characterizes this relationship as one of mutuality in which the whole nurse engages with the whole client, each bringing her or his own experience and meaning to an actual caring occasion. The transpersonal caring relationship at once recognizes the value and importance of both the client's and the nurse's subjectivity. As a result, a number of the carative factors identified in Watson's theory focus on preparation of the nurse before interaction with the patient/client.

The Carative Factors in Watson's theory are not linear "steps" to human caring but represent the *core* of nursing (in contrast to the *trim*).[15] Watson described the carative factors further as "those aspects of nursing that actually potentiate therapeutic healing processes and relationships; they affect the one caring and the one-being-cared-for."[15(p. 50)] Although the carative factors are the attributes of caring that characterize the transpersonal caring relationship,[9] some more clearly focus primarily on the nurse, the relationship, or the processes of caring. Important to note is that the 10 Carative Factors are based on a knowledge base, clinical competence, and healing intention.[8]

Preparation of the Nurse

Watson values and attaches importance to both the nurse and the client in the transpersonal caring relationship. Caring–healing within her caring framework begins with the preparation of the nurse as indicated in the first three carative factors: a humanistic–altruistic system of values, faith-hope, and sensitivity of self and others.

Human caring, according to Watson, is based on human values such as "kindness, concern, and love of self and others."[8(p. 10)] She differentiates altruism from self-sacrifice and describes it as a fullness of being that allows the nurse to be authentically present with clients.[16] Watson states that a humanistic–altruistic value system begins early in life but continues to be influenced through interactions with parents, family, friends, and others, including nurse educators. Furthermore, she asserts that such values can be developed through consciousness raising and introspection. Watson believes that the carative factor she labels as "faith-hope" interacts with the first to enhance caring–healing.[8] From the perspective of the nurse's belief and value systems, this involves gaining knowledge of mind-bodyspirit integration and valuing the therapeutic effects of faith-hope.

Influenced by the work of Carl Rogers, Watson asserts that a balanced sensitivity to one's self is foundational to empathy.[8] Sensitivity to self includes reflection on one's own thoughts, feelings, and experiences in the clinical setting and development of one's own potential. It allows the nurse to be fully present to the client, not hidden behind professional detachment. Developing sensitivity to self involves values clarification regarding personal and cultural beliefs and behaviors such as racism, classism, sexism, ageism, and homophobia, among others, that might pose barriers to transpersonal caring. Finally, sensitivity to self includes an awareness of the interconnectedness of all things and beings and of the social, historical, and political context that shapes nursing practice and nurses' vision of what is possible.[10]

The Transpersonal Caring Relationship

Four of Watson's carative factors focus on the transpersonal caring relationship.[9] Two, which have been discussed from the perspective of the nurse, are also important to the client–patient relationship. Faith-hope extends beyond the nurse's understanding of the integration of mindbodyspirit and also involves fostering faith and hope in clients, based on the client's, and not the nurse's, belief systems.[16] Whereas sensitivity to self is clearly important in the preparation of the nurse to care, sensitivity to others refers to a way of being in relation to clients and is critical to the caring relationship. It allows for the nurse to be changed through the caring relationship and is fundamental to facilitating authentic communication.

Two carative factors relate to interpersonal communication as the basis for the therapeutic relationship. Establishing a helping–trusting, human care relationship is pivotal to Watson's theory and is informed by the first three carative factors.[16] Watson states that the development of a helping-trusting relationship involves intentionality and a consciousness directed at preserving the integrity of the person. As noted, she credits much of her thinking on therapeutic relationships and communication to the work of Carl Rogers and identifies congruency, empathy, and warmth as foundational to a caring relationship that facilitates the client's expression of emotions. Congruency refers to authenticity and genuineness, empathy reflects understanding of both the content and the emotion the client is communicating, and warmth is the degree to which the nurse conveys caring to the client.[17] Gazda, Childers, and Walters[17] note that warmth reflects respect and acceptance and is communicated extensively by nonverbal behaviors.

Caring Processses

The remaining five carative factors address those aspects of caring that primarily involve assessing client health priorities and needs, planning to address those priorities, contributing to meeting client health goals, and evaluating the effectiveness of the caring processes in promoting client health and healing. These carative factors, as do the others, occur within a context of mutuality in which both patient and nurse together decide not only what caring processes will be used but also the role each will assume.[18]

Watson identifies the creative, reflective use of problem solving as a carative factor.[16] However, she stresses that this is not a linear, cause-and-effect approach to problem solving, but it is a creative process that allows interaction of multiple factors and requires not only scientific knowledge but also personal or intuitive, aesthetic, and ethical knowledge. In addition, the whole process is reflective, suggesting that evaluation is constantly occurring and influencing the assessment, caring process, and caring relationship. Watson prefers the term "caring process" to "intervention," because she notes the latter has a mechanistic connotation that is inconsistent with her ideas.[9]

Each carative factor interrelates with the creative, reflective use of the problem-solving (nursing) process and guides the process and content of assessment and evaluation, the nature of planning, and the direction of nursing actions. The last three carative factors are particularly helpful in guiding content and organizing assessment of clients and are discussed in more detail later. Watson rejects the connotations of power conveyed by diagnostic language as well as the diagnostic process in which nurses assess and judge other human beings.[10] Instead, the nurse and client mutually determine conclusions about client strengths, goals, and needs. This requires that the nurse create an opportunity for active participation of the client in the caring process to the extent that the client is able/willing. In this process, in contrast to a consumeristic approach, nurses actively facilitate clients' authentic self-determination, including making their knowledge, expertise, and professional judgment available to clients for use in making health decisions.[19] Nurses help clients express realistic health goals, facilitating clients' empowerment to assume as much of the responsibility for health work as they are willing or able.

One of the nursing activities that the client and nurse may decide will be helpful for the client in achieving health goals is the carative factor related to transpersonal teaching–learning. Although an understanding that the nurse and client both teach and learn from each other is implicit in the label for this carative factor, teaching–learning is concerned with enhancing a client's response to health concerns.[8] It is not the didactic giving of information, but it includes an exploration of the meaning of the situation for the client.[16] Teaching–learning is based on the tenets of teaching–learning theory and involves the acquisition of knowledge and skills that are important in the development of self-efficacy. It often contributes to clients' empowerment by enabling them to gain or regain some control over their health.

Action contributing to a supportive, protective, or corrective mental, physical, sociocultural, and spiritual environment is the carative factor that has perhaps undergone the most dramatic change in emphasis over the past 20 years. Although environment was broadly conceptualized in Watson's earliest work to include mental, physical, social, and spiritual environments, her early emphasis was much narrower than her more recent work. Discussion of internal and external environments focused on stress, comfort,

privacy, safety, and clean esthetic surroundings.[8] In broadening the focus of the immediate environment, Watson revisited Nightingale's model and reframed her discussion from the perspective of Nightingale's wisdom regarding the importance of the environment in facilitating healing. Watson has brought each of the tenets of Nightingale's 19th-century model into the 21st century by illustrating them with contemporary and futuristic nursing actions to create healing environments.[10]

In her most recent works, Watson also developed further the notion of spiritual environment. Drawing on sources as diverse as Eastern philosophy, 12th-century mystic Hildegard von Bingen, and 20th-century artist Alex Grey, Watson situates body within spirit within a field of consciousness that is connected and integral to all consciousness.[10] Within this conceptualization, the nurse moves beyond creating healing environments to becoming a healing environment through the intentional use of consciousness.[20] Watson believes consciousness can be shared, creating new energy fields with healing potential in the process.[10] The implications she draws from the interconnectedness of all things do not stop with human interactions but extend to issues that are critical to the health, healing, and survival of the earth and all life on it, revealing an ecologic aspect to her theory.

The sociocultural environment of the patient/client is the least developed aspect of this carative factor. Although issues traditionally associated with sociocultural concerns, for example, economic status, ethnicity, cultural values, norms, and healing practices, are not explicitly discussed, Watson's emphasis on interconnectedness, mutuality, and the nurse's goal to facilitate client self-determination implies their consideration. Aspects of the social, cultural, and political environments that are discussed at length relate to a postmodern analysis of the place and value of caring, healing, and women's voice in a patriarchal society.[10,13] Clearly, this discussion, although focused largely on the implications for nurses and nursing, also has significance for clients.

To frame her discussion of human needs assistance, Watson initially drew on the work of Maslow. She described this carative factor as being a systematic way of attending to an individual's comfort and well-being, including symptom management.[16] Depending on the role that the nurse and client negotiate, the nurse may advocate for the client with other health professionals and health care agencies and may assist the client in advocating for himself or herself. In her earlier work, Watson categorized human needs in terms of biophysical needs such as food and fluids, elimination, and ventilation; psychophysical needs such as activity, rest, and sexuality; psychosocial needs such as achievement and affiliation; and intrapersonal-interpersonal needs such as self-actualization.[8] This framework for human needs, along with a systematic review of internal and external environments and consideration of existential–phenomenological–spiritual forces, provides a useful schema for organizing an assessment.

The allowance for existential–phenomenological–spiritual forces is perhaps the most difficult of all carative factors to understand. Watson notes that this factor is closely related to self-actualization, but whereas self-actualization is concerned primarily with the pursuit of life goals, this factor focuses on a person's search for meaning in experience and purpose in life. Carative processes related to this carative factor center around being fully present with clients and helping them explore the meaning of an experience, the means by which they transcend life's predicaments, the meaning of life and death, and belief systems through which they find a sense of purpose.

A brief overview cannot possibly reflect the intricacies of Watson's philosophy, theory, and science of caring. It can, however, serve as a basis for extrapolating key concepts into a framework that may be used to guide community health nursing practice.

WATSON'S THEORY OF HUMAN CARING AS A CONCEPTUAL FRAMEWORK FOR COMMUNITY HEALTH NURSING

Resistance to using Watson's work to guide community health nursing practice is usually related to the centrality of the transpersonal relationship to her theory and the question of how it can translate into nursing practice in which communities are the focus of attention. Gadow, who significantly influenced Watson's conceptualization of the nurse–patient caring relationship, believes the philosophy underpinning a person-to-person relationship extends to a person-to-community relationship (personal communication, July, 1993). Her work with Schroeder[21] explicated that relationship in a reconceptualized notion of community as partner, in which the goal of the nurse is to enhance community self-determination. That idea of partnership is congruent with the concept of mutuality that is central to a transpersonal caring relationship. It is equally congruent with global approaches to health articulated in the tenets of primary health care,[22–24] the principles of health promotion,[25,26] and models of community development and empowerment.[27–29]

The centrality of relationship to effective public health nursing practice also has been documented in recent community health nursing research.[2,30] These studies not only show the integral connection of the nurse with the community, but they also provide evidence that effective public health nursing practice cannot dichotomize the community from the individuals within it. Although such a statement may seem self-evident to community health nurses, external pressures on community health nursing practice have in some instances shifted nurses' practice away from communities to individuals[5] and in others from individuals and families to communities and populations.[1]

A holistic approach that recognizes the interconnectedness of a community's health with that of its constituent members would not be congruent with a view of holism that denied attention to parts. Watson's theory, which recognizes the whole in the parts, supports a focus on the wholeness of a community, aggregate, or population, while still attending to the individuals and families within it. In extrapolating ideas such as mindbodyspirit to community, it is not difficult to see how "body" of a community may refer to physical attributes of the environment, the services it offers, and the demographics of a community. "Mind" might well refer to a community's cultural norms, laws, and political structures. Community spirit may be exemplified in the community's value systems. Yet, each of these dimensions of a community are not parts that can be summed to represent the whole community any more than the sum of mind, body, and spirit represent a whole person. Rather, consistent with the holographic model, individual parts provide information about the whole that in themselves produce a less-detailed and coherent projection of the whole than they do together.[31]

Health, according to Watson, is unity and harmony within bodymindspirit and with the world. Likewise, harmony within the various aspects of the community described earlier, as well as its relationship to the outside world (other jurisdictions and the environment), reflects health, while disharmony is indicative of illness. Disease is qualitatively different from illness but is more likely to occur in a state of disharmony. A community example might be that an outbreak of disease is less likely to occur when a community is in harmony, that is, when services such as immunization are in place to prevent anticipated diseases. "Disease" in the community extends beyond biologic epidemics. Community problems also may be thought of as a form of community disease. Homelessness and crime are more likely to occur in communities that do not have an established social safety net or what might be considered harmony of the various dimensions of a community. Watson's conceptualizing of health is consistent with the World Health Organization (WHO) definition of health as "a positive concept emphasizing social and personal resources, as well as physical capacities."[25]

The qualitative differentiation of health and disease in Watson's theory marks a significant departure from the dominant biomedical model. An example of the latter, the Leavell and Clark model, is been continuously used widely in public health and situates health promotion as a prepathogenic strategy.[32] One study revealed that this model had been used widely to support the elimination of public health nursing services that were not considered to be primary prevention because disease (such as mental illness or heart disease) was already present and therefore health promotion was deemed not possible.[1] Nurses in that study expressed the ethical dilemmas they faced because of administrative directives that, in the opinions of several, amounted to patient abandonment. Most nurses, however, did not recognize that the basis for the directives was a medical model, and the reason for their discomfort was, at least in part, related to the incongruence of that model with their own nursing paradigm. Consciously informing practice with a nursing theory in which health promotion can occur whether or not disease is present may strengthen nurses' voice to advocate for services that meet expressed community health needs and enable them to resist external pressures to eliminate those services.

Not surprising, given that Watson's conceptualization of health is consistent with WHO's definition, health-promoting nursing practice guided by her framework is also consistent with the definition of health promotion articulated in the Ottawa Charter[25] and affirmed most recently in the Jakarta Declaration,[26] which is "the process of enabling people to increase control over, and to improve, their health." The centrality of empowerment to health promotion is as clear in the WHO definition as it is in Watson's strikingly similar assertion that caring involves "helping a person gain more self-knowledge, self-control, and readiness for self-healing."[9(p. 35)] Health-promoting actions identified in the Ottawa Charter, such as strengthening community actions, are consistent with this aspect of caring. Another of the Charter's five health promotion actions, the development of personal skills, is demonstrated in Watson's carative factor related to transpersonal teaching-learning. The other three—creating supportive environments, building healthy public policy, and reorienting health services toward a health promotion approach—are encompassed by the carative factor that attends to the support, protection, or correction of sociopolitical environments.

Health promotion practices that flow logically from Watson's theory and her early attention to nonmedical determinants of health are also supported by nursing literature. One aspect of health according to Watson[9] is harmony with the world or environment. It is easy to see how her theory guides the community health nurse to examine and address social, economic, political, and other environmental determinants of health. In fact, the carative factor relating to nursing activities that support, protect, or correct mental, physical, sociocultural, and spiritual environments in community health nursing encompasses the social or political activism that has been advocated in nursing literature for some time.[33-36] Broadening a nursing focus from individual determinants of health to include sociopolitical determinants also addresses the challenges issued in nursing literature over the past decade to reconceptualize both the environment[37,38] and the health promotion to be consistent with nursing's legacy and paradigm.[39-43]

Expanding community health nursing practice to include broad determinants of health is also congruent with contemporary global approaches to health. The Ottawa Charter identified nine prerequisites to health: peace, shelter, education, food, income, a stable ecosystem, sustainable resources, social justice, and equity.[25] More recently, the Jakarta Declaration added social security, social relations, the empowerment of women, and respect for human rights to the initial nine, acknowledging poverty as the single greatest threat to health.[26] Identifying such sociopolitical issues as prerequisites to health recognizes that although they may greatly affect the health of individuals and communities, the supportive, corrective, or protective measures to address them must be directed beyond the individual to societal social and political structures.

Many of Watson's other carative factors are helpful for community health nurses working within her framework. Several factors focus on the nurse's part of the caring relationship in clarifying values and being authentically present to clients. Understanding one's self and being sensitive to others is as important in caring for communities as individuals. Community caring occurs within a helping-trusting relationship and is directed toward protecting and enhancing the dignity of others.

The reflective and creative use of the problem-solving process is consistent with contemporary ideas of health promotion because, according to the theory, it occurs within the context of a relationship of mutuality where the community's health goals are paramount, and there is at least an opportunity for the community's active and equal participation in the process. Watson's theory informs not only the process of assessment but also its scope and focus. A community assessment tool reflects Watson's emphasis on strengthening the client's resources or capacities, as well as mutuality, in planning, taking, and evaluating health actions. As with individual clients, the nurse and the client together decide on the role each will play in working toward health goals. (It should be noted that this assessment tool was recently developed to assist students to assess communities holistically and to make the abstract notion of broad determinants of health more concrete. At this point, it is an untested tool.)

Transpersonal teaching-learning is an important part of the health education in which community health nurses frequently engage. As with individuals, this refers not to the didactic giving of information but to an exploration of the meaning of the situation for the community and the provision of information and development of skills that client and nurse identify as necessary to enable the client to gain greater control over health. Health education is an important health promotion activity in facilitating the development of personal skills. It is important that it be guided by the same empowering approach that characterizes other caring/ health-promoting actions.

Human needs assistance is described by Watson as a systematic way of attending to a client's needs and, again, can be applied to communities. The promotion of self-responsibility and the development of personal skills are an integral part of this carative factor and are consistent with similar principles in the Ottawa Charter.[25] A community's salient health needs may or may not initially be expressed explicitly. Farley noted that the involvement of others outside the community is sometimes necessary "for citizens to recognize and meet the needs of

their community ... because the citizens may have become insensitive to the great need in their own backyard, or may feel helpless in the face of apparently overwhelming need."[22(p. 247)]

It is quite possible that even initially, explicit expressions of need later will be augmented as the nurse, in partnership with the community, systematically assesses the community. The role of the nurse in facilitating authentic community self-determination, as with individuals, involves making professional knowledge, expertise, and judgment available to the community, thereby enabling it to express and achieve health goals and facilitating its empowerment to assume as much responsibility for health as it deems appropriate.[21]

Allowance for existential–phenomenological–spiritual forces in community health promotion acknowledges the wholeness of the community. One way this carative factor may become part of community health nursing practice is in helping a community find meaning in the face of disaster. Although community health nurses are often involved in responding to crises such as storms and disease outbreaks, they also frequently participate in debriefing sessions in which they can help strengthen the community's capacity to respond to future crises as well as help the community make sense of the events.

Watson's theory of human caring is philosophically congruent with contemporary empowering approaches to community health. The primacy of caring, holism, and ecology to her theory is clear and mirrored in the Ottawa Charter, which asserts that they are "essential concepts in health promotion."[25] Concepts related to caring for individuals can be readily extrapolated to communities in a manner consistent with nursing literature and community health nursing practice. Using Watson's theory to guide community health nursing practice may assist community health nurses to withstand the pressures to shift their practice to reflect every passing theoretical fad and political trend[4] and return their practice to a nursing center, that is, to a practice that is consistent with the philosophy and practices of the founders of public health nursing.[1]

APPENDIX COMMUNITY ASSESSMENT GUIDED BY WATSON'S THEORY

Community Identity

1. Who makes up the community (population, age distribution, ethnicity, and family types)?
2. What makes this a community (e.g., shared geography, common characteristic, shared problem, and relationship of community members with one another)?
3. What is this community's history? If this is a temporary community (e.g., a group), how long have members been together, and how long are they likely to stay together? Is the community membership stable or does membership change frequently?
4. What are the community's sources of pride? What does it believe it does well?
5. What barriers to health does the community identify?
6. What is the community's self-image?
7. What vision does this community have for its future?

Community Spirit

1. What values are evident?
2. What is the community spirit and how is it evident?
3. What belief systems are most prevalent, including presence of worship centers and organized religions?
4. What are common community explanations for events, such as natural disasters, that are beyond human control?

Internal and External Environments

1. Describe the physical setting in which this community is located. (In a geographical setting, use information from a "windshield" survey. What do you see as you drive through this community: parkland, terrain, dense housing, industry, pollution, climate, and so on. For communities confined to a single location, look at facilities and resources, for example, in a classroom you might look at size, layout, light, noise, temperature, and adequacy and state of repair of desks.)
2. What is the economic status of the community?

   - What are income levels, unemployment rates, industry, and sources of employment?
   - How equitably is income distributed across the community?
   - What is the relative wealth of this community in comparison with national, state/provincial, or regional levels of wealth?
   - What are the major sources of revenue (e.g., taxes, exportable resources, and tourism), and how sustainable are they?
   - What proportion of children live below the poverty level?

3. What is the political structure of the community (or power dynamics of a group)? How are leaders/representatives chosen? What is the community's perception of how well this political/power structure represents and advocates for its members outside of the immediate community?

Community Capacity to Meet Basic Needs of Members

1. What housing types predominate (e.g., high density and single dwelling)?

   - How affordable is housing?
   - To what extent is homelessness a problem, and how is it addressed?

2. How does the community address nutritional needs?

   - To what extent is food homemade or purchased?
   - How do community members purchase groceries (e.g., small specialty stores, superstores, and comer stores)?
   - How accessible and affordable are groceries?
   - What labeling regarding nutritional content, additives, and genetic engineering is required?
   - What mechanisms govern the safety of food?
   - What food supplemental services exist (e.g., breakfast programs and food banks)?

3. How does the community meet needs for clean air and water?

   - What are the adequacy, safety, and sustainability of water supplies?
   - How are biologic and industrial wastes disposed?
   - What is the air quality: are advisories frequently issued, what are sources of pollution, and what mechanisms are there for dealing with polluters?

4. To what extent do community health services (promotive, preventive, curative, rehabilitative, and emergency) meet the health needs of community members?

   - How affordable and accessible are health services to community members?
   - How acceptable are health services to community members, that is, to what extent have they emerged from the community's involvement in identifying needs and planning to meet those needs?

5. What public policies or programs promote and support health?

   - How well do laws protect public safety (e.g., seatbelt laws,

nonsmoking areas, and access for physically challenged members)?

   - To what extent is health promoted in public places (e.g., breastfeeding friendly workplaces, restaurants, and shopping malls; identification of healthy food choices on restaurant menus)?
   - How are families supported in promoting the healthy growth and development of their children?
   - To what extent is health promoted in schools (e.g., comprehensive school health programs and school-based clinics)?
   - What sectors besides health are involved in promoting health and how?

6. How does the community ensure the safety of its members (e.g., police, fire, and rescue services)?

7. What crises services does this community have in place depending on nature of the community (e.g., disaster plan, tornado warning system, fire drills, and sprinkler systems)?

Community Capacity to Care for Its Most Vulnerable Members

1. What social services are provided to community members through tax dollars (e.g., day care, income assistance, welfare, and pensions)? What additional user-paid services are available?

2. How are the needs of older residents met?

   - To what extent do families care for elderly family members at home?
   - Are there sufficient and appropriate living environments that promote maximum independence while providing adequate supports to meet older adults' health and safety needs?

3. How are needs of diverse community members met (e.g., culturally sensitive

services, translators, support for integration into the educational system, and English as a second language courses)?

- How does the community integrate new members?
- To what extent is diversity welcomed and supported?
- To what extent are some community members advantaged or disadvantaged by virtue of race, ethnicity, gender, class, or sexual orientation?

Community Capacity to Meet Social Needs of Members

1. How do community members communicate with each other and outsiders (e.g., newspapers, newsletters, media, person to person, posters, and key informants)?
2. What social programs and activities exist within the community, and what facilities exist to promote them (e.g., community centers and churches)?
3. What is the major mode of transportation within the community and to other communities?

- To what extent are services accessible to all members of the community (e.g., how disadvantaged is someone who does not have a car)?
- Is public transportation adequate and accessible?

Community Capacity to Promote Growth and Development of Its Members

1. How does the community promote the growth of its members?
   - What educational programs are provided, for example, preschool, prekindergarten, kindergarten through 12th grade, and postsecondary education?
   - To what extent are these educational opportunities accessible to all community members (e.g., public versus private funding)?

- What continuing education opportunities are provided?
2. What supports exist in the community for recreational activities?

- Playgrounds with equipment;
- Organized sports/fitness activities across the life span;
- Hobby groups/classes, card clubs, and so on; and
- Facilities (e.g., swimming pools, hockey rinks, tracks, and tennis courts).

3. To what extent are recreational supports accessible to all community members?
4. To what extent are the arts and culture promoted in the community, and how accessible are such events to community members?

Summary

- Nurse/community perceptions of community strengths
- Nurse/community perceptions of challenges to community health
- Community health goals
- Nurse/community plan for achievement of health goals

REFERENCES

1. Rafael, A. R. F. (1999). The politics of health promotion: Influences on public health promoting nursing practice in Ontario, Canada, from Nightingale to the Nineties. *Advances in Nursing Science, 22*(1), 23–39.
2. Rafael, A. R. F. (1999). From rhetoric to reality: The changing face of public health nursing in Southern Ontario. *Public Health Nursing, 16*(1), 50–59.
3. Zerwekh, J. (1992). Community health nurses—A population at risk. *Public Health Nursing, 9*(1), 1.
4. Laffrey, S., & Page, G. (1989). Primary health care in public health nursing. *Journal of Advanced Nursing, 13,* 1044–1050.
5. Salmon, M. E. (1993). Public health nursing—The opportunity of a century. *American Journal of Public Health, 83*(12), 1674–1675. Editorial.

6. Neuman, B. (1997). *The Neuman systems model.* Norwalk, CT: Appleton and Lange.

7. Helvie, C. O. (1997). *Advanced practice nursing in the community.* Thousand Oaks, CA: Sage.

8. Watson, J. (1985). *Nursing: The philosophy and science of caring.* Boulder, CO: Colorado Associated Press.

9. Watson, J. (1988). *Nursing: Human science and human care: A theory of nursing.* New York, NY: National League for Nursing.

10. Watson, J. (1999). *Postmodern nursing and beyond.* New York, NY: Churchill Livingstone.

11. Watson, J. (1995). Advanced nursing practice … and what might be. *Journal of Nursing & Health Care, 16*(2), 78–83.

12. Watson, J. (1988). New dimensions in human caring theory. *Nursing Science Quarterly, 1*(4), 175–181.

13. Watson, J. (1990). The moral failure of the patriarchy. *Nursing Outlook, 38*(2), 62–66.

14. Watson, J. (1995). Postmodernism and knowledge development in nursing. *Nursing Science Quarterly, 8*(2), 60–64.

15. Watson, J. (1997). The theory of human caring: Retrospective and prospective. *Nursing Science Quarterly, 10*(1):49–52.

16. Watson, J. (1994). *Applying the art and science of human caring* (Video). New York, NY: National League for Nursing.

17. Gazda, G. M., Childers, W. C., & Walters, R. P. (1982). *Interpersonal communication: A handbook for health professionals.* Gaithersburg, MD: Aspen Publishers.

18. Rafael, A. R. F. (1995). Advocacy and empowerment: Dichotomous or synchronous concepts? *Advances in Nursing Science, 18*(2), 25–32.

19. Gadow, S. (1990.). Existential advocacy: Philosophical foundations of nursing. In T. Pence & J. Cantrall (Eds.), *Ethics in nursing: An anthology.* New York, NY: National League for Nursing.

20. Quinn, J. F. (1992). Holding sacred space: The nurse as healing environment. *Holistic Nursing Practice, 6*(4), 26–36.

21. Gadow, S., & Schroeder, C. A. (1994). Ethics and community health: An advocacy approach. In E. Anderson & J. McFarlane (Eds.), *Community as partner: Theory and practice in nursing.* Philadelphia, PA: JB Lippincott.

22. Farley, S. (1993). The community as partner in primary health care. *Nursing Health Care, 14*(5), 244–249.

23. World Health Organization. (1993). Declaration of Alma-Ata. In J. M. Swanson & M. Allbrecht (Eds.), *Community health nursing: Promoting the health of aggregates.* Philadelphia, PA: WB Saunders.

24. Hildebrandt, E. (1996). Building community participation in health care: A model and example from South Africa. *Image: Journal of Nursing Scholarship, 28*(2), 155–159.

25. World Health Organization, Canadian Public Health Association, Health and Welfare Canada. (1986). *Ottawa charter for health promotion.* Presented at the First International Conference on Health Promotion November 17–21, Ottawa, ON.

26. The Jakarta declaration on health promotion into the 21st century. (1997). *Health Promotion International, 12,* 261–264.

27. Eng, E., Salmon, M. E., & Mullan, F. (1992). Community empowerment: The critical base for primary health care. *Family & Community Health, 15*(1), 1–12.

28. Petersen, A. R. (1994). Community development in health promotion: Empowerment or regulation? *Australian Journal of Public Health, 18*(2), 213–217.

29. Robertson, A., & Minkler, M. (1994). New health promotion movement: A critical examination. *Health Education Quarterly, 21*(3), 295–312.

30. Diekemper, M., SmithBattle, L., & Drake, M. A. (1999). Bringing the population into focus: A natural development in community health nursing practice, part I. *Public Health Nursing, 16*(1), 3–10.

31. Weber, R. (1985). The enfolding-unfolding universe: A conversation with David Bohm. In K. Wilbur (Ed.), *The holographic paradigm and other paradoxes: Exploring the leading edge of science.* Boston, MA: Shambhala.

32. Leavell, H. R., & Clark, E. G. (1979). *Preventive medicine for the doctor in his community: An epidemiologic approach.* Huntington, NY: Robert E. Krieger.

33. Backer, B. A. (1993). Lillian Wald: Connecting caring with activism. *Nursing & Health Care, 14*(3), 122–129.

34. Bent, K. N. (1999). The ecologies of community caring. *Advances in Nursing Science, 21*(4), 29–36.

35. Moccia, P. (1988). At the faultline: Social activism and caring. *Nursing Outlook, 36*(1), 30–33.

36. Kendall, J. (1992). Fighting back: Promoting emancipatory nursing actions. *Advances in Nursing Science, 15*(2), 1–15.

37. Kleffel, D. (1991). Rethinking the environment as a domain of nursing knowledge. *Advances in Nursing Science, 14*(1), 40–51.

38. Chopoorian, T. (1986). Reconceptualizing the environment. In P. Moccia (Ed.), *New approaches to theory development.* New York, NY: National League for Nursing.

39. Butterfield, P.G. (1990). Thinking upstream: Nurturing a conceptual understanding of the societal context of health behavior. *Advances in Nursing Science, 12*(2), 1–8.

40. Gott, M., & O' Brien, M. X. (1990). The role of the nurse in health promotion. *Health Promotion International, 5*(2), 137–143.

41. Lowenberg, J. S. (1995). Health promotion and the "ideology of choice." *Public Health Nursing, 12*(5), 319–323.

42. Maben, J., & Clark, J. M. (1995). Health promotion: A concept analysis. *Journal of Advanced Nursing, 22*(6), 1158–1165.

43. Williams, D. M. (1989). Political theory and individualistic health promotion. *Advances in Nursing Science, 12*(1), 14–25.

QUESTIONS FOR REFLECTION

Baccalaureate

1. Identify the three factors that Falk Rafael described as making Watson's theory unique among nursing theories.
2. How does Watson describe the Carative Factors that are part of her theory?
3. How is Watson's theory congruent with the concept of health promotion?

Master's

1. Watson's theory values multiple ways of knowing (empirical, esthetic, ethical, and personal). How are these ways of knowing integrated into the practice of community health nursing?
2. Describe a transpersonal caring relationship that you have experienced with a patient within the acute care setting. How would this relationship be different if you were practicing within the community setting?
3. What are the main health promotion concerns within the community that you live in? How would you use Watson's Theory of Human Caring to address these concerns?

Doctoral

1. In addition to the discussion by Rafael how has the work of Nightingale and Eastern philosophy informed the writings of Watson?
2. Is Watson's theory still relevant to the current practice of community health nursing? Please support your response with cited literature.
3. Would having a caring theory to guide community health nursing practice make a difference in your community? Why or why not? What different outcomes would emerge if Watson's theory guided the nursing practice?

31

Earth Caring

Eleanor A. Schuster

Helped are those who love the earth, their mother, and who willingly suffer that she may not die; in their grief over her pain they will weep rivers of blood, and in their joy in her lively response to love, they will converse with trees.[1(p. 288)]

As we enter the decade of the 1990s, in what ways do we expect to honor our earth connections and relate this wisdom to our way of being on this planet as planetary citizens who have chosen to enact our being as nurses? Is it possible through the economic model of our work world, where profit is the driving force, to successfully reconcile Earth-caring values with those of the marketplace?

I suggest and am convinced that these are the primary and most salient questions of our time and for the foreseeable future. Indeed, the way we choose to acknowledge, to specify, and to work out these relationships through our personal and professional lives is linked directly to our survival, the quality of our lives, and the well-being of the planet. As a current environmental slogan asserts, "We are crew members, not passengers."

NEW ENVIRONMENTALISM

Recent polls put environmental issues at the top of Americans' social concerns, along with crime, drugs, and acquired immunodeficiency syndrome (AIDS), and ahead of the economy, nuclear war, and communism.[2] There is a proliferation of new periodic journals representing a range of environmental issues from the microcosm of our own backyards (*Garbage: Practical Journal for the Environment*) to global and international considerations (*Colorado Journal of International Environmental Law and Policy*).

The new environmentalism is broad based and local, a grassroots movement in the making that could become a universal and potent political theme for the 1990s. Many are not so much protecting the environment as protecting their families, homes, and communities. Others, such as the "Greens,"[3] the "deep ecologists,"[4] and the ecofeminists,[5] acknowledge and champion a deep interconnection of all life with social processes, claiming that neither environmental nor social problems can be solved in isolation from one another. The Greens' social commitment and broad vision for a transformed society are outlined in their 10 key values[6]: (1) ecologic wisdom, (2) grassroots democracy, (3) personal and social responsibility, (4) nonviolence, (5) decentralization, (6) community-based economics, (7) postpatriarchal values, (8) respect for diversity, (9) global responsibility, and (10) sustainability/future focus.

From Schuster, E. (1990). Earth caring. *Advances in Nursing Science*, 13(1), 25–30. Permission to reprint granted by Wolters Kluwer.

GROWING ENVIRONMENTAL INTEREST

Environmental groups have been proliferating in the past 10 years.[7] National, mainline organizations such as the Sierra Club and the National Audubon Society report doubled and tripled memberships. The fastest growth, however, has been outside these groups. For example, the Clean Water Action Project has little name recognition but has 500,000 members. The Citizens' Clearinghouse for Hazardous Waste has grown to 9,000 and increases by 100% yearly. Greenpeace USA is reported to gain 60,000 adherents monthly. Even so, the average citizen is increasingly estranged from environmental affairs. For many organization members, there is little to be done other than send in annual dues and additional donations when canvassed for special needs. These monies usually support lobbying and legislative efforts. A vast number of Americans express concern about the environment but do not know how to turn their concern into action, to act personally as well as politically. Denis Hayes, a California attorney, hoped to change this through Earth Day 1990. As a student in 1970, he organized the first Earth Day, a national day for education, ecology fairs, and serious discussion that ultimately propelled political forces and resulted in congressional enactment of the Clean Air Act and the establishment of the Environmental Protection Agency.[7]

NURSING AND ENVIRONMENT

Is it important, or to what extent and for what reasons is it important for nursing to demonstrate or to claim linkage with contemporary or future environmental issues? The nursing literature to date is sparse in that regard. We know from a historical perspective, of course, that nursing can appropriately claim many social reformers, such as Florence Nightingale, Lillian Wald, Margaret Sanger, and Wilma Scott Heide, whose work was closely related to environmental concerns.

A literature search of the categories *caring* and *nursing* in relation to *environment* resulted in 20 citations from the past 10 years. Of these, five were from nursing journals: radiation effects,[8] developing corporate smoking policies,[9] giardiasis water pollution,[10] chemical hazard identification,[11] and working in toxic environments.[12] The remaining English and foreign journals were from the fields of epidemiology, public health, anesthesia, and medicine. One[13] examined the relationship between fetal loss and occupational exposure of nurses to antineoplastic drugs and reported a significant risk for fetal loss in the first trimester. If this is an adequate representation of nurses' systematic reporting of their environment-specific work, we may want to rethink or redirect our efforts as caring responses in these ecologically troubled times.

HOLISTIC NURSING PERSPECTIVES

A recent handbook[14] for holistic practice addresses the subject of the environment from a nursing perspective. An illustration in the chapter enumerates the physical manifestations of environmental hazards and reflects the themes identified from the literature review: noise pollution, air pollution, radiation, chemicals, water pollution, and land pollution. The definition of environment in the chapter is notable because it goes beyond physical parameters. The definition is as follows: "Environment is everything that surrounds an individual or group of people; may be physical, social, psychological, cultural or spiritual; includes external and internal, animate and inanimate objects, seen and unseen vibrations and frequencies, climate and not yet understood energy patterns."[14(p. 182)]

A nurses' handbook[15] on wellness devotes a chapter to wellness in the immediate environment, which includes a discussion of the impact of sound, light, and color in relation to wellness. The internal as well as the external environment is considered. Variables other than physical are discussed.

A statement in support of a healthful environment was approved by the American Holistic Nurses Association (AHNA) at their annual meeting during the summer of 1989.

> The environment involves both our immediate and our global surroundings. Many of us are aware of a need to expand our consciousness regarding environmental issues and believe that this can have an effect on our own personal and community well-being. Our concerns come from a reverence for the beauty of the earth, which sustains us and is our home, our Mother Earth. Relevant environmental issues including preserving the integrity of the air, soil, and water as well as issues such as global warming, acid rain, and other equally challenging situations [sic]. We believe as holistic nurses, we have the responsibility for increasing responsibility in others regarding these issues through role modeling and educating within our communities. The AHNA encourages self-responsible behavior as well as participation in socially responsible environmental groups, to protect and support improvement of the health of our environment.[16(p. 7)]

Based on the foregoing information, nurses involved in wellness work and those claiming holistic practice are currently the most obvious in the environment–nursing relationship, at least in public pronouncements having to do with environment.

Another relational aspect is reported in the literature, although it is not highly visible at this time: nurse researchers are testing theory based specifically on Rogers' science of unitary human beings.[17] As one example, Smith[18] reports that the integrity of the mutual human-environment field process was strengthened through her work with an environment of varied harmonic sounds. In this quasiexperimental study, participants perceived themselves as rested following exposure to harmonic auditory input, "supporting the notion that human-environmental field process integration is strengthened when auditory input for those confined to bed is patterned."[18(p. 27)]

From another theory base, that of human care and caring, Watson[19] proposes expanded dimensions of human caring wherein human caring and healing become transpersonal and intersubjective, opening up a higher energy-field consciousness that has metaphysical, transcendent potentialities.

Smith[18] and Watson[19] and those of similar thought believe that we as humans inhabit, are integral to, and are in exchange with a universe pulsating with life, vigor, zest, and birthing. Our spoken language, as we know it now, falls far short of representing these realities. That is why some nurses, and others, speak more accurately and eloquently in metaphor, which gives rise to varied and perhaps new investigational methods.

HUMAN CARE AND CARING

Environmental concerns and issues elicit human caring in one form or another, be it self-interest or other directed. It seems that theory development in nursing on human care and caring might reveal specific connections with environmental concerns. So far, that relationship is elusive.

The basic philosophy of nursing's human caring efforts asserts that care and caring are the essence of nursing and the unique and unifying focus of the profession.[20] This direction, begun by Leininger[21] and others with similar vision and commitment, is gaining momentum, as can be noted in the nursing theory literature and by other indices, such as clinical research, schools of nursing philosophy, and service agencies whose activities are directed through a human caring model.

I propose, for reader consideration, five speculations about the paucity of obvious linkages of human caring theory and praxis with the needs and claims of the environment. It seems reasonable to assume that the stated goals[20] of the International Association of Human Caring (IAHC) provide insight into human care and caring as conceptualized by the founders and the membership (with the caveat that goals can change as understanding evolves and as experiencing may direct over time). The first goal of the IAHC states, "Identify major philosophical, epistemological and professional dimensions of care and caring to advance the body of *knowledge* that constitutes nursing and to help other disciplines use care and caring in *human* relationships"[20] [emphasis added].

SPECULATIONS

The major points I propose for consideration are as follows:

1. Developmental stage: Human care and caring as theory in and of nursing is new, perhaps 15 years into its evolution. So far, focus has been on human-human interrelationships, which is hardly surprising given the conventions and legal parameters of practice. So lack of obvious engagement with environment as such could be a function of developmental process.
2. Expecting more than a given theory or construct can or should deliver: Perhaps, it is unrealistic or illogical from an ontologic perspective for the caring model to accommodate environmental exigencies.
3. Anthropocentrism: The notion of *human* caring does not readily allow for nonhuman interchange of care or caring. Is it desirable, or even expedient, to particularize care and caring to humankind? If we do, what are the ramifications? Anthropocentrism is that world view that posits the

human (usually stated "man") as the ultimate aim of the universe. Subjugation of nonhuman species, compromise of the quality of the physical world, and various other forms of oppression and domination result from most forms of anthropocentrism.
4. Primacy of the intellect: Caring *knowledge* in human relationships may be at the expense of *experiencing* caring; this can limit caring to "knowing about," without living as a "carer" or "caree." Intellectualization often means assigning recognition and rewards to left-brain activities while ignoring or trivializing right-brain intuitive or synthesizing functions.
5. Nurse "ownership" of human care and caring ("help other disciplines use care and caring knowledge in human relationships"[20]): Might we not learn about the nature of care and caring from many sources, including other disciplines? This statement can be construed as unilateral and elitist by inference if not by intent.

The intention behind these reflections and observations is to share in public forum my concerns, about environment, about the earth, and about caring, and to respectfully present these concerns for dialogue and, perhaps, for friendly argument, so that we all may grow and thrive.

Allen, a scholar from the Native American tradition, reminds us that all creation is dynamic, responsive, "for relationships among all the beings of the universe must be fulfilled; in this way each individual life may also be fulfilled."[22(p. 56)] This old song from the Keres tribe expresses that belief:

I add my breath to your breath
That our days may be long on the earth
That the days of our people may be long

That we may be one person
That we may finish our roads together
May our mother bless you with life
May our life paths be fulfilled.[22(p. 56)]

REFERENCES

1. Walker, A. (1989). *The temple of my familiar.* Orlando, FL: Harcourt Brace Jovanovich.
2. Erlich, E. (1989, September 25). The new American. *Business Week, 154,* 155.
3. Tokar, B. (1987). *The green alternative: Creating an ecological future.* San Pedro, CA: R & E Miles.
4. Devall, B., & Sessions, G. (1985). *Deep ecology.* Layton, UT: Gibbs M. Smith.
5. Plant, J. (1989). *Healing the wounds: The promise of ecofeminism.* Philadelphia, PA: New Society Publishers.
6. *Building a Green Environment.* (Pamphlet). Kansas City, MO: National Clearinghouse Green Committees of Correspondence.
7. Steinhart, P. (1990). Bridging the gap: Can earth day 1990 bring together greens and mainline conservatives? *Audubon, 92*(1), 21–23.
8. Halstead, M. A. (1987). Caring for the radiation accident victim. *AORN Journal, 46*(1), 68–72.
9. Gaughan, S. E. (1988). Developing corporate smoking policies. *AAOHN Journal, 36*(9), 358–360.
10. Loken, S. (1986). Giardiasis: Diagnosis and treatment. *The American Journal of Primary Health Care, 11*(20), 20–26.
11. Raniere, T. M. (1978). Chemical hazard identification—Our need to work together. *Occupational Health Nursing, 26*(9), 19–21.
12. Mackinick, C. G., & Mackinick, J. W. (1987). Toxic new world: What nurses can do to cope with a polluted environment. *International Nursing Review, 34*(2/272), 40–42.
13. Seleven, S. S., Lindbohm, M. L., Homung, R. W., & Hemminki, K. (1985). Relationship between fetal loss and occupational exposure to antineoplastic drugs in nurses. *The New England Journal of Medicine, 313*(19), 173–178.
14. Dossey, B. M., Keegan, L., Guzzetua, C. E., & Kolkmeier, L. G. (1989). Environment: Protecting our personal and planetary home. In *Holistic nursing: A handbook for practice.* Rockville, MD: Aspen Publishers.
15. Swinford, P. A., & Webster, J. A. (1989). *Promoting wellness: A nurse's handbook.* Rockville, MD: Aspen Publishers.
16. American Holistic Nurses Association. (1989). AHNA political position statement in support of a healthy environment Beginnings. *The Official Newsletter, 10*(8), 7. AHNA is a nonprofit national organization, headquartered in Raleigh, North Carolina, whose membership is open to nurses and others interested in holistically oriented health care.
17. Rogers, M. E. (1980). Nursing: A science of unitary man. In J. P. Reihl & C. Roy (Eds.), *Conceptual models for nursing practice* (2nd ed.). New York, NY: Appleton-Centuiy-Crofts.
18. Smith, M. J. (1986). Human environment process: A test of Rogers principle of integrality. *Advances in Nursing Science, 9*(1), 21–28.
19. Watson, J. (1988). New dimensions in human caring theory. *Nursing Science Quarterly, 1*(4), 175–181.
20. International Association for Human Caring. Brochure for membership.
21. Leininger, M. M. (Ed.). (1981). *Caring: An essential human need.* Thorofare, NJ: Charles B. Slack.
22. Allen, P. G. (1986). *The sacred hoop: Recovering the feminine in American Indian traditions.* Boston, MA: Beacon Press.

QUESTIONS FOR REFLECTION

Baccalaureate

1. According to Schuster the Greens have 10 key values. Identify three and how they are relevant to your community.
2. Does your community have an Earth Day? Would you attend? Why or why not?
3. According to Schuster what nurses are most involved in the environment–nursing relationship? Do you agree with this? Why or why not?

Master's

1. Does the hospital organization where you work or do a practice rotation have any "Green eco-friendly" initiatives in place? If yes please describe. If no, what could you implement?
2. How does Watson's theory integrate the concepts of nursing and environment as described in Schuster's' reflections?
3. Perform a literature search on caring, nursing, and the environment. What topics are discussed within nursing journals? Which journals have the most articles?

Doctoral

1. How has the interrelationship among environment, nursing, and caring been advanced from a theoretical perspective since Schuster's work in 1990? Cite references to support your response.
2. Review the website for the International Association of Human Caring (www.humancaring.org). Re-write the goals to be inclusive of Schuster's philosophical tenets.
3. Schuster referred to the American Holistic Nurses Association (1989) statement in support of a healthful environment. Has this idea been advanced? Support your response with cited references and examples.

32

Caring on the Ragged Edge: Nursing Persons Who Are Disenfranchised

Joyce V. Zerwekh

All of us at some level have a fear of the disenfranchised, whether it's because we could be in that place or because there may be potential harm to us. But I seek to break that fear and see someone as a human. The more I work with her, the more I see her as human.

The above words are from a nurse informant who has contributed to my search to understand the nature and meaning of caring on the ragged edge of society. What is it like to care for people when mainstream society often does not care? This study applies a hermeneutic phenomenological approach to bring to reflective awareness the unique nature of caring for disenfranchised and often outcast patients. To be disenfranchised is to be deprived of the rights and privileges of society. It is to be outcast, thrust beyond the walls of community. As nurse informants reveal, this practice involves fearless caring with clients who are separated and fearful. Often, they are blamed for their own problems. Such caring involves belief in the possibilities of marginalized people and taking a stance with them in difficult circumstances. Courage makes such hopefulness possible and hope makes courage possible.[1]

FOUNDATIONS FROM THE LITERATURE

Selected concepts form a foundation for exploring the results of this inquiry. Caring theory affirms the intrinsic value of all persons and identifies caring as a reciprocal process of learning from one another.[2,3] By entering into the life world of the other, new possibilities for growth are recognized. Parse[4] asserts the ever-present possibility of choice despite the estrangement, deprivation, and struggle of disenfranchised clients. People are inherently free to choose how they will live; possibility is ever-present in even the most desperate circumstances. Rafael[5,6] has developed the concept of empowered caring, in which both nurse and client are active participants. Nurses practicing empowered caring have a heightened sense of interrelatedness and a strong sense of responsibility for engagement, in contrast to the long-standing nursing practice of avoidance and distancing.[7] Empowered caring creates possibilities for choice and control. Smith[8] synthesizes caring theory and Rogers' Science of Unitary

From Zerwekh, J. V. (2000). Caring on the ragged edge: Nursing persons who are disenfranchised. *Advances in Nursing Science*, 22(4), 47–61. Permission to reprint granted by Wolters Kluwer.

Human Beings to describe the following five constitutive meanings:

1. Manifesting intentions that affirm human possibilities
2. Appreciating the pattern of wholeness in another person
3. Attuning to the rhythms of another
4. Experiencing the infinite in the connection and sacredness of another
5. Inviting creative emergence of the possibilities for another's well-being

In a qualitative study of public health, nurse family caregiving competencies, Zerwekh[9] identified the central focus to be developing family capability to take charge of their own lives and make their own choices. Expert nurses working with vulnerable mothers believe in client capacity for choice. The groundwork for doing this is building trusting relationships and developing the capacity for self-help. In summary, caring nurtures possibility.

Swanson[10] proclaims that nursing is informed caring for the well-being of others. This chapter concludes with an expansion of her five caring processes to incorporate dimensions vital to nurture human possibilities when caring on the ragged edge. Swanson emphasizes client capacity for choice while acknowledging that the range of possibilities is not equal for all persons.

METHOD

This inquiry was inspired by Ray's phenomenological approach to study the lived experience of caring.[11] The purpose is to learn anew the world of caring, not that previously encoded. First, the author's presuppositions from practice, reflection, and study, as well as prior qualitative studies of expert nursing, were bracketed, setting them aside for the moment. Nursing leaders identified seven nurses who maintain compassionate and effective relationships with disenfranchised patient populations. These exemplary seven persisted in celebrating the wholeness and humanity of those on the ragged edge. They sustained interconnection with people from whom our society and most caregivers withdraw. Informed consent for interviews was obtained through a process approved by the university's Institutional Review Board. Interviews were recorded by extensive handwritten notes and concurrently recorded by audiotape. Three questions guided the interview as follows:

1. What is it like to care for persons for whom mainstream often does not care?
2. Would you tell me about one or two experiences of caring for marginalized people that have special meaning for you?
3. What is the meaning of caring for the patient population you serve?

Following Ray's strategy, interview dialogues proceeded using a clue- and cue-taking process after the initial question. Detailed descriptions were sought from the informants.

Answers were transcribed into text, and both the typed and the handwritten notes were reviewed over and over to bring to awareness the nature of caring for disenfranchised people. Conscious dialogue with the text revealed themes, meta-themes, and metaphors that capture the essence of caring on the ragged edge. In this chapter, selected qualities of the nurses and their clients are captured and summarized. Then the nature of the client experience is explored. Finally, the meaning and essences of caring on the edge are presented.

THE SEVEN NURSES

Nurses' ages ranged from 39 to 63 years. They averaged 21 years of active practice as registered nurses; this ranged from 11 years of practice to 35 years. Three held associate degrees in nursing, two had bachelor's degrees in nursing, and two had master's degrees.

The nurse narrators describe their practice in community health, school nursing, critical care, mental health, health promotion, and oncology. Some of their clients live and die with devastating illnesses, including cancer and AIDS. Many are legal and illegal immigrants. Several are mentally ill and/or abusing drugs. Most are poor. All seven nurses speak vividly with profound conviction about their work. One views her clients as part of her extended family; her advocacy for them often gets her into "hot water." Another describes her work building community among fearful psychiatric patients. A nurse who has practiced with the mentally ill and those living with AIDS proclaims the necessity of making authentic connections with clients. He faces his antithesis, "You who scare me." The oncology nurse describes herself as a specialist with those who are angry and afraid. Another nurse informant describes her practice with people who have "been shut out of the human family" and considers all of us at risk of becoming marginalized because of illness. And finally, a nurse

describing her work with impoverished Caribbean and Latin American immigrants explains her practice as "Going around the Wall," which is a vivid metaphor for the work of caring on the ragged edge. The words of these nurses colorfully illustrate the following descriptions of their clients, the meaning of their practice, and the essential dimensions of their practice.

SEPARATION: CLIENTS BEHIND THE WALL

In the 25 nursing situations described in interviews, clients are characterized as separated from human community and as people who are afraid and bring about personal fear in others. What we fear, we back away from. Separation and fear are pervasive themes describing the disenfranchised. A nurse explains, "They have been pushed out of the human family." The client and the community, separated by a wall of fear, are illustrated in Figure 32.1. In another metaphor, Hilfiker[12] imagines his homeless clients on an island separated

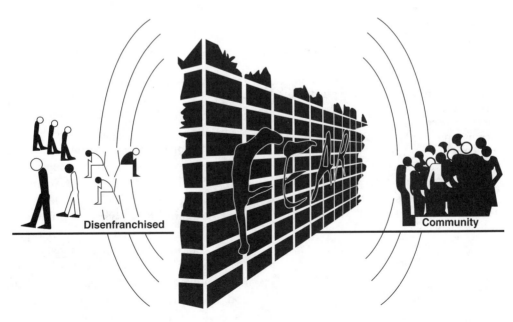

FIGURE 32.1

The wall.

from the mainland by deep waters; he practices what he terms "poverty medicine." His narrative poignantly describes his clients' despair. Not only are they abandoned by society, but they also have internalized their abandonment and now see themselves as unlovable and unable to influence the course of their lives. The wall separating them from the mainstream has devastating human consequences. An interviewed nurse uses yet another metaphor, that of a locked door, "The door is shut and you can't get back in." That all of us have the potential for being disenfranchised is vividly illustrated by the tragedy of two nurse clients described by two different nurse informants.

> She was a nurse who worked with us, born and raised in the local community, a single mother. She was diagnosed with lupus and unable to work. She could no longer be kept on the payroll and had no income to afford insurance. No one came to visit her from her family. Eventually, we had her in a geriatric chair, restrained, and incoherent. It was the nursing staff who brought her laundry home, fed her, and plaited her hair. Hospital administration seemed unable to acknowledge that this was happening to one of our nurses. We put her in the nurse's station and she would let us know the phone was ringing because she would yell out. But one of the doctors happened to arrive on the floor and went crazy. Even though he had worked with this woman side by side, he wanted nothing to do with her. He didn't want to see her. That experience with her as a coworker, as a woman, and as a potential patient myself made me realize what really happens. Her illness moved her further and further away from everyone. We all have the potential to be disenfranchised literally over night. The door is shut and you can't get back in. Who will open the door?

> He was a lieutenant commander, in the service for about 18 years. That's all he knew. He was well respected as a nurse educator. It was 1986 and every 6 months we had what was called a command sweep. Everybody got tested for HIV. When you popped up positive, you were immediately withdrawn. You were

shunned from community. When he came up positive, Naval Investigative Services set up a witch hunt. This was my colleague. He had given up certain aspects of his life to strive for his career. The embarrassment and humiliation in that man's face is one thing that I will never forget. At a certain point, he would break down with the fear of dying, dying alone, and the fear of having nothing: no insurance, no pension, no friends. His whole world was turned upside down. And I thought, "You are just one. How many?"

Many are the causes for such separation from human community. Certainly, there is stigmatizing disease as has been described: physical and emotional illness. Perhaps, they have had repeated alcoholic or drug-related relapses. Perhaps, they are immigrants or without homes. Perhaps, they are persistently poor with no sense of personal choice. Some proclaim defiantly to those who would help them, "You don't know where I have walked." Perhaps, they are dirty and disheveled and talking to themselves. Perhaps, they hear "voices tell them all day long that they are no good, ugly." Whatever their clients' circumstances, these nurses see themselves as fellow humans, vulnerable also.

PERVASIVE FEAR

Disenfranchised people are defined by their own fear and by the avoidance of others because they are afraid of their behavior or afraid of encountering their intense level of hardship and suffering. They make us weary; we develop "compassion fatigue." The Wall develops as the community pulls away and builds barriers. One nurse explains that "what is unfamiliar makes us uncomfortable." Another proclaims that unruly people are most afraid, "As soon as a person doesn't follow the rules, nobody wants to take care of him and those are the people who need the most care because they are really the most afraid." She gives an example of a 5-year-old rural Mexican child refusing to follow the protocols needed for a bone marrow transplant. He could not get out of bed or leave the room. He threw things and would not do any of the traumatic treatments. Her response to his fear and agitation was to take him into her arms in a rocking chair and watch *The Little Mermaid* and rock and rock while administering his treatments.

Psychiatric patients may try to be frightening because they are afraid of other people as they perceive them.

> They may act violent or be disturbing because they fear you. If they act up and talk loud, most people will back up. If you don't feed into their behavior and act afraid, they see that doesn't work. Then you reach them personally and draw them out, "What's really bothering you?" A patient told me she was sometimes irritable because when she looks at my face it would change. It becomes colors and then the shape of it changes. That must be horrific to try to trust people, take medicine from people, and their face is going from one kind of a face to another kind of face.

Adolescents practicing dangerous drug use and sexual behavior frighten us; they take undue risks for immediate gratification because they have no hope for their future.

> The poverty brings the hopelessness and the hopelessness causes these individuals to take undue risk for immediate gratification. They're so poor and the men will come along and say, "I am going to show you a better life, for the next 6 months move in with me and be my girlfriend and I am going to support you with all these material goods." I say, "Five years from now you finish high school, you go to the vocational school, and you'll be able to buy as many pairs of shoes as you want once you're working." But there is no way they can envision 5 years from now. It's poverty and hopelessness causing all these risks: pregnancy and AIDS.

Sometimes the consequences of risk behavior and the dehumanized medical response can be terrifying.

If they think the holocaust is over, it's here. In critical care, I had people that dreamed of coming to this country and there they were dying in the United States of America. Incontinent of urine and feces, orange sputum dribbling out of their endotracheal tubes, and there wasn't a person in the place who could at least ask them in Creole, "How are you?" They were Haitian refugees dying of AIDS. If there was any group we would want to say was disenfranchised, I've often thought of them. Living their American dream, dying in America.

Another nurse described his work with the first U.S. AIDS patients and with one man in particular whose behavior was especially challenging and frightening.

> They were the ones coming down with it first; they were the ones who did all the wrong things and made no apologies for it. Angelo had lived his life very joyously. People loved him. That was part of his ingratiating character. If you stripped him down and took away the defenses, there was nothing more than a shallow human being who hadn't received a lot of nurturing or brain exercise. He was my antithesis. I thought, "You are just too cool." We had a wellness program with exercise that made him more healthy and then he went back to the same situations that made him unhealthy: drugs, indiscriminate sex, and unprotected partners. No duty. Nonexistent sense of ethics. Angelo would respond, "Yeah, there's rules but they don't affect me." So releasing my judgment was the hardest thing I had to do with this population.

THE MEANING OF NURSING THOSE WHO FRIGHTEN US OR WHO ARE AFRAID

Interpretation of the nurses' stories reveals four dimensions of meaning. Nurses caring on the ragged edge perceived the work as rewarding because of the challenges overcome, as a calling, as a family legacy, and as an experience of common humanity.

Meaning as Challenges Overcome

This practice is described as gratifying, rewarding, rejuvenating, invigorating, and challenging. The nurses describe many ways that they are nourished by the kind of challenges involved. One nurse likens her efforts to an athletic competition, "Fighting for a way to help keeps me going. I won't stop until I can get whatever they need." The very reality that other people do not care is the challenge that keeps the nurses doing the work. Somebody has to "look out for the people." A nurse concludes, "I am putting an end to letting them fall through the cracks." Fearless caring is evident, "facing that fear with you, you who scared me because you are different." After working with HIV patients practicing sex destructive of themselves and others, a nurse explains his reflections about working with the patients' fears, "I am able to be a better human being as a result of facing my own prejudices and preconceived notions." Challenges lead to personal growth.

Meaning as Calling

Nurses used religious and nonreligious language to describe their internal conviction that "these are the people I am meant to help." The most religious stance was from a nurse who proclaimed, "I have to answer to God. You never know who God is in disguise." Another nurse described the work as "my sense of mission" and asks people of faith to view those infected with HIV as Jesus would view them. He would hope that at the end of his life he would be seen as "somebody who heard the call." Says another highly experienced nurse, "I persist because, number one, I have a deep religious faith, and when I need strength I can go back and draw from my religion." Another asserts that her work with the poor is "a call for my life—the driving force." One nurse feels that she is a perfect match with her work, "I am a round peg in a round hole." These nurses feel unique in the trusting relationships they develop

and the strong effort they make on behalf of clients.

Meaning as Family Legacy

Four of the nurses spoke about their work with the disenfranchised as connected to their family histories. One had a brother who was terminally ill during her childhood and associates that legacy with her current calling. Another nurse explained her relationship with the poor who are mentally ill as "I come from my family." She has a brother who is alcoholic and had an aunt who lived for many years in their extended family. The aunt used to scream out the windows and run up and down the stairs calling for the police. But she belonged to the neighborhood and therefore was accepted. Another nurse has a son who is schizophrenic, which has given her powerful insight into the suffering of her patients' families. She recognizes the look on parents' faces and talks to them about what to expect, "There will be good times and bad times. We have to reset what is realistic."

Struggling to help the underdog is another family legacy.

> I grew up in a poor family and my father always found a way to provide for us. My whole practice is a model from the way I was brought up. My parents were unbelievable people who were always for the underdog. They would give you the shirt off their back. They would do without everything so that we as children could have it. But also in the community, my parents were right there when people needed help.

Meaning as an Experience of Common Humanity

All nurses interviewed held strong convictions about common humanity with those that they were helping, and that every person has a right to sustenance and respect. Disenfranchised people are seen as fellow human beings, and the nurses assert that it is important that nurse and client see each other's authentic humanity. In one nurse's words, "This could be me. I value life. Every person deserves every opportunity" "We are all the same. Pain and anger fuel me. We need to be there." Nursing presence represents humanity, perhaps as "the only caring person in hell." Another nurse proclaims, "I've been on the other side of this bedpan." Another colorful explanation is that authentic caring relationships only happen when "I open my raincoat to reveal my true self." The underlying purpose of the work is proclaimed, "This work means life. To preserve a life and dignity. Dignity living." Two nurses describe patients as family and, indeed, have members of their own family living with mental illness.

Several nurses commented on the reciprocal experience of giving and receiving help and learning from clients, "They are giving back more than you're giving."

CARING FOR THOSE WHO FRIGHTEN US OR WHO ARE AFRAID

Reflection on the nurses' narratives reveals that fearless caring with separated and often frightened clients has 10 themes that can be organized into three meta-themes: the Human Connection, the Community Connection, and Making Self-care Possible (Figure 32.2). The nurse goes around the separating wall of fear. The power of fearless caring is illustrated in the nurses' own words.

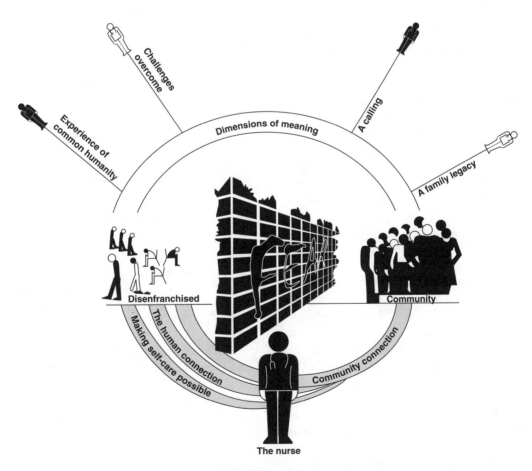

FIGURE 32.2

Caring on the ragged edge.

The Human Connection

This caring meta-theme is grounded in the nurses' strongly held conviction that they share a common humanity with disenfranchised people. The Human Connection is characterized by actions that involve honoring their humanity, knowing the people, and sharing one's own humanity.

Honoring Their Humanity

The nurses believe that they are consulted and trusted by clients because they treat them with respect. "I see their worth as people rather than treating them like a disease or symptom." All the stories emphasize high regard for shared humanity. One nurse recalls honoring the humanity of a just-deceased penniless Mexican migrant worker who had no family. She agreed to not immediately call to arrange a county burial. After a few hours, his friends arrived with their finest cowboy boots and hats and pulled out rolls of bills to pay for a small service at a local funeral home. She was able to intercede with county officials. Although she could not do much for him when he was in critical condition, she could after his death. She proclaims, "It was a perfect ending for me. I think they saw that I was another human being that really cared about a respectful honorable way to acknowledge their friend's death. This was the final act of caring."

Knowing Their Humanity

Expert nurses practicing with marginalized people are able to discover what is going on in their clients' lives. They know their past, they are familiar with their patterns, and they know how to ask questions to draw out their stories. A psychiatric nurse explains her insight into one woman's refusal to take a shower, "I have found you have to sit down and ask them why, which was because she saw snakes in that shower."

Another psychiatric nurse knows her patients' patterns of drug abuse. She interceded when a patient, denying the seriousness of her problems, was not going to be admitted. "I know that when she overdoses on prescription pain pills, her mind starts to play tricks on her, and she hallucinates and is delusional. She would go home, take more pills, and maybe really kill herself because her mother said that she was putting a knife to her chest."

Sharing One's Own Humanity

Nurses caring expertly for disenfranchised people do not hesitate to share their own worlds with clients and imagine themselves in the client's position. "With this kind of population, like a new mother who has a drug-addicted child or a psychiatric patient or a homeless patient or an HIV patient, they have to perceive me as real. Is the interaction real?" The following words affirm that conviction.

> Do what is natural to you without worrying about what anybody else is going to think. Cry with the patients. Allow yourself to express yourself. You can't stay disconnected. The patients stay disconnected because they are embarrassed. They feel like totally nothing because they have to allow someone to help them with toileting. Let them know that, yeah, I've had experiences like this, too. It makes them feel more human.

The Community Connection

This meta-theme involves the overlapping dimensions of connecting the disconnected, haunting the case, and mediating. The nurse links clients on one side of the wall with each other and with community services on the other side of the wall.

Connecting the Disconnected

Going around the wall of fear, the nurses strengthen community among the disconnected as well as pulling in community resources on behalf of their clients. Caring requires going around the walls between estranged individuals and between estranged individuals and community. The following is a powerful anecdote about building community among hospitalized indigent psychiatric patients.

> I tell them, "I expect you to help one another. I expect you to take care of one another." They begin to realize that they are special, that they all need help. They kind of align and start doing positive things that they should be doing instead of a lot of negative bickering and fighting. I tell them that I expect more of them because they know what it's like to hear things, to be afraid, to be alone, to be alienated, and for your family not to trust you. And I say, "Well, you know when you came in you were very manic too." So you find one patient tagging behind another and telling us, "They are manic and give them something to do. They need something to do." They need to reach out to one another.

All the nurses relate their aggressive efforts to get community services going on behalf of their clients. Examples range from mobilizing the fire department when housing is unsafe, to working with a grandmother to secure child custody when her daughter is abusing drugs, to accessing dentistry and affordable medications. One nurse describes a nursing role of "single handedly opening the door" to community services. Another colorfully describes her aggressive efforts to find help from the mainstream community for her disenfranchised clients.

> We've been able to pull in all our resources. For one family, we now have Family Builders, we have Medicaid for the children, and we got them food stamps. I visualize a giant wall and if I can tunnel through at any point, I just have to find a weak spot in that wall. I'm a little rat. Then behind the wall, there is a maze with roadblocks.

At the same time, this nurse is intensely conscious of the importance of not making people dependent on all the resources she wants to mobilize for them. She describes a fiercely independent Appalachian woman who was "really adamant about wanting to be able to

provide for her children in her own way. She wanted to be independent and was fighting to be responsible and not have all these people coming in and doing for her family that she's worked so hard to hold together." Pulling in resources must be expertly balanced with fostering personal power and self-sufficiency as the ultimate goal.

Haunting the Case

Even when clients are connected to resource people and agencies, they may remain unheard and not get needed attention. One nurse describes herself as "haunting the case" in her unrelenting effort to get the mental health team to respond to client needs. Indeed, all the practice experts saw themselves as unique in persisting to advocate for disenfranchised individuals and families. They are proud of their assertion when others give up.

Mediating With the Bureaucracy and Making Exceptions

The nurses speak to team members and administrators on behalf of clients. One nurse describes herself as getting into "hot water" as she advocates for clients with viewpoints that counter those of administration or physicians or social services. Another advocate for the disenfranchised describes his primary role as mediator.

> My place is to mediate. To do that, you've got to have people identify something about you. You're the messenger. So if they see me as anywhere left or right of center, immediately their value judgment comes. So I try to stay very much in the center, very conservative. Stay within the system, yet clearly articulate the injustice.

Other nurses deal with the bureaucracy by quietly making exceptions to usual practice. When clients need "somebody to really close the door and sit down and look at them and talk to them," one nurse informant promises to come at the end of the shift. She stays as late as patients need to talk. Another nurse visiting in the home describes making exceptions like giving people $5 for food or extra clothing if they are cold in winter.

Making Self-Care Possible

This meta-theme describes strengthening self-care by getting clients through emotionally, teaching them to understand themselves, helping them take control, and confronting fear at the community level.

Getting Them Through Emotionally

These nurses specialize in working with people who are living in intense emotional turmoil, often alternating between anger and fear, A nurse explains her listening and consulting with a grandmother caring for four grandchildren with one daughter deceased and another diagnosed with chemical dependency.

> The new mother was a cocaine addict and the newborn was with Grandma. Grandma had two sons, both incarcerated, and three daughters. One daughter had just died of AIDS and left her three little children. When the daughter was dying at Grandma's house, HIV counselors had come in and talked down to the daughter and belittled the family. So the morning I first went she was at first very guarded about outsiders. But then she sat me down and she ranted and raved for maybe a full hour and a half, and then she broke down and wept. I validated her feelings as she went along, and this was my entry to her family.

Another describes her work with angry cancer patients in treatment as "getting them through the rough spots." She describes one patient in particular.

> She came to us with metastatic breast cancer, already throughout her back and hips. From what I can ascertain, she was a very angry person to start with. She didn't trust anybody and didn't want to do anything. If you sent her to another doctor, she would throw things and curse and have fits. Everybody would react by telling her, "If you don't want to do the treatment, don't do it." I sat many, many hours with her to discover what it is she needed to know. And I finally realized that she needed everything explained, verbally and written down, and then re-explained. She had a very hard time understanding. If she didn't understand, it angered her. Repeated explanations were hard on everyone working with her. She learned to bargain with me. I agreed to answer her questions as many times as she needed as long as she gave me a little leeway and time. Angry people have to have one center person to trust.

Teaching Them to Understand Themselves

The nurses teach people to understand their own bodies and feelings to maximize their own health. They teach them to understand their disease and its management. One nurse says to clients, "You should know more about the illness than I do because you have to walk it, wash it, live it, breathe it." If clients are not motivated by respect for others and their own body, an expert declares that he uses "selfishness and conceit" to motivate behavior change on their own behalf. The nurses teach clients to pay attention to their own condition.

Helping Them Take Control

These nurses practice empowered caring by strengthening clients so that they can take charge, "always, always let them know they are in control." Discovering what kind of control people need is essential, "Find out what they need to control and work out a plan." The psychiatric nurses encourage clients to reject stereotypes, get back self-esteem, and look for a "niche in life." One explains how to guide them to separate from the fearful hallucinatory voices and recognize their own capability.

> Talk to them about the voices and let them know that the voices are part of the illness. Try to help them separate from the voices, which are not real, and get back to reality. And though all during the day the voices say you are bad, that's just not real. But I see a good person. You help another person. I know what you can do.

The nurses help clients develop resilience to the stereotyping and rejection that can prevent a person from taking charge of his or her life. This involved "developing calluses" in the ostracized Navy nursing educator. The nurse sought to raise the educator's sense of self-esteem and help him develop defenses when people were talking all around him about his being gay and having AIDS. The goal was to bring out his strengths and sense of control.

Confronting Fear at the Community Level

Three of the nurses reflected on the need to break down the wall altogether so that caring becomes possible. One nurse was interviewed during a period when the United States was bombing Yugoslavia, intending to stop Serbian aggression against Kosovar Albanians. She fantasized about how she could demonstrate the profound suffering of her immigrant families on the national news, just as the suffering people of Yugoslavia had been portrayed on TV. She proclaims that "It's like a war for them, comparable. If I could videotape it, ask somebody to walk with me for a day, and show that on the 8 o'clock news."

Another nurse had different fantasies, of an intensely supportive "cradle through high school" program. At-risk children would have "positive role models who could say there is a life beyond what they see at home. Let them be exposed 10, 12 hours a day to hope." One nurse had actually taken action at the "big picture" or community level by developing an HIV educational program for the Roman Catholic diocese.

> I speak to all the archdiocese schools. I speak to their PTAs. I speak to their principals and I speak with the message of compassion and understanding, using biblical references and papal encyclicals, I tell them, "I want you all to view HIV as Jesus viewed the Lepers, as he viewed Mary Magdalene, as he viewed anybody else who was cast out. He could do it and

> stand up for them in a time that was so frightening. I am asking you to let somebody else find fault, not you. Don't judge."

AN ELABORATION OF CARING FOR THE WELL-BEING OF OTHERS

Caring on the Edge is caring that courageously nurtures possibility in the face of separation and fear; nurses go around the wall of fear. Rather than developing yet one more theory, it is useful to consider how Swanson's Caring for the Well-Being of Others can be expanded beyond perinatal context to capture the unique dimensions of caring for disenfranchised people. Her caring definition is reaffirmed, "a nurturing way of relating to a valued other toward whom one feels a personal sense of commitment and responsibility."[10(p. 354)] To elaborate, Caring for the Well-Being of Disenfranchised Others emphasizes valuing those others whom society frequently does not value and taking responsibility for people whom American society frequently abandons. Swanson's midrange theory describes five caring processes that have unique dimensions when caring on the edge.[10]

Maintaining Belief

Swanson[10] asserts that caring is founded on a commitment to people and their capacity for change and growth. Many who live securely within the walls of social convention do not have any faith in those who are outside the walls, but it is affirmed by nurses who practice fearless caring. The meaning of Caring on the Edge includes the experience of being challenged through nurses' engagement in caring when others see the same clients as overwhelming and frightening. The strong sense of purpose is sometimes connected to family history. Nurses caring on the edge are willing to acknowledge common vulnerability, "This could be me." They grow and are empowered by their belief in clients' possibilities.

Knowing and Being With

Swanson describes "knowing" as striving to understand the reality of another person and "being with" as authentic presence that conveys "availability and the ability to endure with the other."[10(p. 355)] The Human Connection through Caring on the Edge is consistent with this caring process through *honoring humanity, knowing humanity, and sharing humanity.* These provide illustration and vivid detail regarding practice with clients whom this unique group of nurses chooses to be with and know.

Doing For

Swanson describes psychomotor nursing activities as well as interpersonal skills that include setting up programs or systems, "doing for the other what they would do for themselves if it were at all possible."[10(p. 356)] The Community Connection through Caring on the Edge significantly expands understanding of this caring process with extensive description of *connecting, haunting*, and *mediating.* Because the most fundamental underlying problem is estrangement for those on the edge, it is not surprising that a vital nursing activity is going around the wall of fear.

Enabling

This caring process fosters clients' practice of self-care; the purpose is "to facilitate the other's passage through difficult events and life transitions."[10(p. 357)] According to Swanson, enabling is practiced through coaching, informing, supporting, assisting the other to focus, helping the client to identify alternative choices, guiding him or her to think through issues, providing feedback, and affirming reality. Making self-care possible through Caring on the Edge expands understanding of how this is done with marginalized clients by *getting them through, teaching them to understand themselves, helping them take control, and confronting fear at the community level.*

CONCLUSION

Questioning readers may assert that these nursing actions appear too individualized. They may say that nursing the disenfranchised is not "good enough" unless it focuses upstream and builds community capacity to challenge existing power structures. They might believe that those who "truly" care for the oppressed must guide them as a group to struggle against the sources of their oppression. Certainly, this is the stance of critical theorists, whose position I have been advocating philosophically and politically for nearly 30 years.

However, we must honestly face the true circumstances of our own lives, those of our mainstream clients, and those of our marginalized clients. "More than a century after Marx, 80 years after women gained the vote in the United States, 35 years after the landmark Civil Rights Acts, and 30 years after the Stonewall rebellion for gay rights, no greater enigma exists in the social sciences than the participation of people in the very sociopolitical and cultural systems that oppress them."[13(p. 45)] Fear and silencing keep us from "rising up" at all levels of organization and community; truth is rarely spoken who oppress them, that certainly should not stop wise nurses from understanding the nature of power structures that deprive human beings from sustenance, rights, and dignity. As nurses, I believe we must challenge those oppressive structures through civic involvement at every personal and professional level. Likewise, by strengthening individual clients, we enhance the possibility of their acting as empowered communities.

We have much to learn from nurse colleagues courageously practicing on the ragged edge. We can validate, explain, teach, and replicate fearless caring with clients subject to innumerable societal injustices and fears. As the gap between rich and poor widens,[14] a unique group of outstanding nurse colleagues persistently struggle to affirm humanity and build individual capacity of the most disadvantaged. They go around walls where others fear to tread to stand beside the fearful and the feared. They draw them into community where there is strength in numbers. They see human possibilities where others see no hope. Thus, power is born when caring others value another and believe in human potential. Experiencing "concern and unconditional regard, the patient's self-love and self-regard gradually increase. Self-regard begets a belief that one has the right to wish and act."[15(p. 339)]

ACKNOWLEDGMENT

The Florida Atlantic University Research Initiative Award funded research. Special thanks to Judy Chanin Robinson, RN, PhD candidate, for her review and suggestions.

REFERENCES

1. Mayeroff, M. (1971). *On caring.* New York, NY: Harper & Row.
2. Boykin, A., & Schoenhoffer, S. (1990). Caring in nursing: Analysis of extant theory. *Nursing Science Quarterly, 4,* 149–155.
3. Boykin, A., & Schoenhoffer, S. (1993). *Nursing as caring: A model for transforming practice.* New York, NY: National League for Nursing.
4. Mitchell, G. J. (1993). The view of freedom within the human becoming theory. In R. R. Parse (Ed.), *Illuminations: The human becoming theory in practice and research* (pp. 26–43). New York, NY: National League for Nursing.
5. Rafael, A. R. F. (1996). Power and caring: A dialectic in nursing. *Advances in Nursing Science, 19*(1), 3–17.
6. Rafael, A. R. F. (1998). Nurses who run with the wolves: The power and caring dialectic revisited. *Advances in Nursing Science, 21*(l), 29–42.
7. Flaskerud, J. H., Halloran, E. J., Janken, J., Lund, M., & Jetterlund, J. (1999). A glance back in time. Avoidance and distancing: A descriptive view of nursing. *Nursing Forum, 34*(2), 29–35.
8. Smith, M. (1999). Caring and the science of unitary human beings. *Advances in Nursing Science, 21*(4), 14–28.
9. Zerwekh, J. (1991). A family caregiving model for public health nursing. *Nursing Outlook, 39,* 213–217.
10. Swanson, K. (1993). Nursing as informed caring for the wellbeing of others. *Image, 25*(4), 352–357.
11. Ray, M. (1991). Caring inquiry: The esthetic process in the way of compassion. In D. Gaut, & M. Leininger (Eds.), *Caring: The compassionate healer* (pp. 181–189). New York, NY: National League for Nursing.
12. Hilfiker, D. (1994). *Not all of us are saints: A Doctor's journey with the poor.* New York, NY: Ballantine Books.
13. Cody, W. K. (1998). Critical theory and nursing science: Freedom in theory and practice. *Nursing Science Quarterly, 11*(2), 44–46.
14. Johnston, D. C. (1999). Gap between rich and poor found substantially wider. *New York Times,* Sept. 5, A14.
15. Yalom, I. D. (1980). *Existential psychotherapy.* New York, NY: Basic Books.

QUESTIONS FOR REFLECTION

Baccalaureate

1. Identify Swanson's five caring processes that Zerwekh discussed in terms of her research findings.
2. How does Zerwekh describe the concept of disenfranchised?
3. What research method guided Zerwekh's research? How many registered nurses were interviewed?

Master's

1. Are the themes identified in Zerwekh's research applicable to the disenfranchised living in your community? Why or why not?
2. How do you think registered nurses practicing within the community setting could use findings from this research to change their practice?
3. Is the metaphor of the Wall applicable to the disenfranchised living within your community? Why or why not?

Doctoral

1. What are the similarities and differences between the philosophical foundation of Zerwekh and Falk Rafael?
2. How would you replicate Zerwekh's research within your community?
3. Are the themes, metathemes, and subsequent Theory of Caring on the Ragged Edge developed by Zerwekh supported by the direct quotes of the participants? Please support your response in terms of the phenomenological research method.

VIII

Caring Leadership and Administration

Marian C. Turkel

Previous sections in this textbook have included an overview of the discourse of caring; conceptual, philosophical, and theoretical tenets of caring theory and caring science; seminal research, research designs, caring-based practice models, and caring within the community. As caring theory is integrated into nursing curriculum within the university setting, professional practice settings, and research to advance the discipline, the role of nursing leadership is integral. Nursing leaders need to role model and value caring science in terms of decision making and organizational mission, vision, and philosophy for innovations and outcomes to occur within organizations. The nurse leader can facilitate original caring science research or use research findings from studies conducted by caring scholars as a framework for clinical or administrative decision making. Caring science leaders are moving beyond the traditional, industrialized approaches, looking for authentic, collaborative relationships grounded in trust and shared values.

The sentinel articles reviewed in this section were written by caring scholars who were in nursing leadership roles in the practice setting or recognized as caring scholars. They were interested in how caring was lived and expressed within nursing leadership and how tenets from caring theory guided leadership philosophy and practice.

Nyberg's (1990) sentinel article was one of the first published research articles to examine the concepts of human care and economics within the hospital nursing environment. Nyberg (1990) referenced the sentinel work of Ray (1987, 1989), who was the first caring theorist to examine the moral conflict between the concepts of caring and economics with complex health care organizations. Literature related to human care and economics was reviewed and synthesized by Nyberg (1990). Her definition of human care was informed by Mayeroff (1971), Noddings (1984), and Watson (1985), and her thinking related to economics was focused on the traditional economic concepts of capitalism and socialism. Nyberg (1990) viewed health care in America as having elements of both. The element of capitalism includes independent buyers and sellers, free choice, and price; socialism influences of Medicare and Medicaid with the focus on equal distribution of services.

Nyberg (1990) cited the changes that have occurred within health care economics since the 1960s and reviewed the reimbursement measures in place to contain health care costs. At the time this article was published, health care systems were struggling to control costs. Administrators focused on cost control, while human care was valued by nursing. Nyberg's (1990) subsequent research focused on the ethical dilemma of nurses advocating for human caring in a cost-cutting economic environment.

The research study conducted by Nyberg (1990) included over 2700 registered nurses from seven hospitals in a western state completing a questionnaire designed by the researcher. The Nyberg Caring Assessment Scale (1990) identified caring attributes and was developed from various studies and supporting literature (Gaut, 1983; Larson, 1984; Mayeroff, 1971; Noddings, 1984; Nyberg, 1989; Watson, 1979). Nyberg (1990) added four open-ended questions to the questionnaire; two questions focused on economics and two focused on human care. In addition to registered nurses completing the Nyberg Caring Assessment Scale, the nurse executives of each hospital were interviewed and asked to define the characteristics of their hospital and their views related to human care and economics.

Quantitative findings indicated that registered nurses view caring as "very important" with a mean score of 4.1 out of 5, that they practice the attributes often with a mean score of 3.9 out of 5, and that they practiced the attributes about the same as 5 years ago with a mean score of 3 out of 5. The correlation between caring scores and the economic indicators of nursing hours per patient day and total nursing hours per patient day adjusted by Medicare case-mix index was calculated (Nyberg, 1990). Hospitals with higher numbers of nurses per patient had higher caring scores.

In terms of qualitative analysis to the open-ended questions registered, nurses responded negatively to the economic questions. They felt that economic pressure made it harder to provide human care and that the acuity levels of patients had increased, and they expressed deep concern and frustration over not having time to meet patients' basic needs. One comment included, "the emphasis on money is foreign and disgusting" (p. 16).

The responses to the questions regarding human care were very different. Nyberg's (1990) research acknowledged that nurses understand and value human care. Responses included providing care that honors the dignity of the patient, reaching out human to human, and dealing with the whole person. In terms of maintaining human care, nurses referred to trusting relationships, involving the family, and being open and knowing your limits. According to one nurse, . . ."it is caring that makes nursing unique and essential" (p. 16).

Nyberg (1990) made specific recommendations related to the interconnection of caring and economics based on findings from the research. One included the replication of this study on a national level. She urged hospital administrators to support and reward the practice of human care. Nyberg reminded nurse administrators to focus on quality care and to serve as advocates for needed resources. She also recognized the need to change the image of nursing administration from the "role of boss" to one of colleague and facilitator. Of interest, given the time of publication, was her recommendation of shared governance to allow nurses to be part of the decision-making process. Today (2012), shared governance has become the norm for professional nursing practice within many organizations; however, in 1990, this reflected visionary and innovative thinking related to the practice of nursing.

Turkel (2001) used a grounded theory approach to study the nurse–patient relationship within the context of economics and the changing health care environment. Turkel's study and thinking related to caring and economics was influenced by the writings of Buerhaus (1986), Miller (1987, 1995), Nyberg (1990, 1991, 1998), Ray (1987, 1989), Valentine (1989a, 1991, 1997), and Watson (1979, 1985). Turkel (2001) was concerned about sustaining the role of nursing as caring in the prevailing health care system and questioned if caring could be viewed as having economic value. She provided an overview of the current economic and political climate of health care reimbursement and the payment systems that do not value human caring or the nurse–patient relationship when allocating resource dollars. Turkel acknowledged that, despite the focus on cost and quality, there was limited research looking at the nurse–patient relationship within an economic context.

Literature related to nursing economics, caring, and economics was critiqued, reviewed, and synthesized with salient points highlighted. Turkel (2001) noted that before Medicare and Medicaid nursing students subsidized hospital nursing, the delivery of health care was not profitable, and nursing care was not considered an expense or revenue for hospitals (Lynaugh & Fagin, 1988). Turkel pointed out that as reimbursement changed from retrospective payment to prospective payment, the challenge to hospital administrators was to reduce costs, increase efficiency, and maintain quality. By the time nursing researchers (Bargagliotti & Smith, 1985; Curtin, 1983; McCormick, 1986; Walker, 1983) demonstrated the value of registered nurse staffing on patient outcomes, the move toward managed care had begun and hospital reimbursement constrained further.

Turkel (2001) recognized the work of nurse scholars who had previously studied the paradox between caring and economics. Buerhaus's (1986) question, "Can you tell me how much the nurse listening to you is worth?" served as the basis for questions asked by Turkel during her research to provide economic or dollar value data. Turkel (2001) cited Foa (1971), an exchange theorist who identified the interpersonal resources of love, status, and information. Turkel and Ray (2000) further expanded on Foa's concepts and referred to love as caring, status as the professional registered nurse, and information as teaching.

Turkel used a grounded theory approach and interviewed nurses, patients, and administrators from a 250-bed hospital. Interview questions focused on the nurse–patient relationship (where caring occurs) within a framework of cost-benefit parameters to examine the nurse–patient relationship as an economic resource. During the interview processes, Turkel (2001) asked more specific questions including describing specific caring nurse–patient interactions and the cost and benefits associated with these interactions. Data analysis involved the identification of categories from each participant group and the similarities and differences among the groups. The specific categories related to caring and economics served as the basis for the substantive theory.

According to Turkel's analysis (2001), nurses described practicing caring as being, knowing, and doing all at once, caring in the moment, caring beyond, and investing in patient education. Patients were interpreting the caring, and this was defined as distinguishing between caring and noncaring, caring making a difference, and valuing the educational process. The view of the administrators was slightly different. From a distance, they were judging caring and noncaring. This was further explained as defining caring, defining noncaring, wondering how they do it, and knowing the nurses are on call to everyone.

The category related to economics from the perspective of the nurse was entering a new reality, which included managing in the presence of costs, contending with costs, valuing the humanistic interaction, and fearing for patient's well-being. Patients felt threatened by the new reality, and this was further defined as surviving in the presence of chaos, deserving to be cared for despite the costs, and fearing for themselves. The administrators' were profiting in the new reality and this was described as accounting for the costs, accounting for the caring, valuing registered nurses, and positioning for future survival.

Turkel (2001) identified the substantive theory as struggling to find a balance, which referred to "sustaining the caring ideal in a new reality controlled by costs"

(p. 79). Nurses struggled to maintain humanistic caring in a cost-efficient managed care environment, patients desired caring, and quality care but did not want to pay for health care out of their own pockets, and hospital administrators were walking the fine line between making a profit and providing quality care.

This classic article represents one of the few published studies interviewing nurses, patients, and administrators on the topics of caring and economics. Of particular interest is the similarity of the nurses' responses to the concepts of caring and economics as noted in Nyberg's (1990) study conducted 10 years earlier. Turkel (2001) provided a view of caring in terms of an economic framework, contributed to the scholarly discourse related to the paradox between caring and economics, and discussed the relevance of the substantive theory to professional nursing practice. When this research was conducted, nurses, patients, and administrators were responding to economic changes mandated by managed care. Readers are asked to consider if the responses from nurses, patients, and administrators would be the same in 2012 as the government and insurance companies are reducing reimbursement to hospitals.

Valentine (1997) advanced the scholarship between the concepts of caring and economics by examining the relationship of professional nurse caring to costs. As a nursing leader, she was interested in the economics of caring and has developed a research trajectory in this area (1989a, 1989b, 1991a, 1991b, 1995). Valentine acknowledged the difficulty of studying the relationship between caring and costs as the terms are complex and ambiguous. She added to the scholarly discourse and reaffirmed that patients value humanistic interactions, while payers are consumed about the costs of health care.

The author identified caring and patient satisfaction as two outcomes of effective nursing practices. Valentine's (1997) definition of caring "as a multidimensional construct consisting of nurse attributes of professional knowledge and competence, vigilance, and therapeutic interactions with patients and families" (p. 72) was informed by the scholarship of Ray (1984, 1987) and Stiles (1990). Valentine proposed that in order for the profession of nursing to have resources allocated for caring, the definition of costs must be expanded to include patient outcomes.

She provided a systematic review of the nursing literature on institutional approaches for cost effectiveness related to the role of the registered nurse. Valentine (1997) questioned the practice of replacing registered nurses with unlicensed patient care technicians and advocated for the value of professional vigilance. According to Valentine (1989, 1991), professional vigilance has been identified as a crucial dimension of nurse caring, patients expect the registered nurse to have accountability and authority for the direct and delegated care provided to the patients.

Valentine (1997) expanded the discussion related to the traditional definitions of cost. From the author's perspective, costs need to include costs experienced by providers, patients, hospitals, and insurer as they are different. She challenged us to consider, "how do those costs differ for the patient, nurses, insurer, patient's family, and hospital?" (p. 74). According to Valentine materials, time, money, and human factors are all currencies used in the payment of health care costs. She also acknowledged the difficulty of calculating nursing costs from both research and practical perspectives.

Next, Valentine (1997) synthesized the nursing literature related to the definition and measurement of caring and acknowledged the contributions of Dr. Leininger to the scholarship of caring science. Leininger (1984) viewed caring as integral to healing process and believed that there could be caring without curing, but there could not be curing without caring. In Valentine's (1989) conceptual model of caring, the core elements of caring consisted of affective or cognitive psychologic elements put into action in an interaction and influenced by structural elements in the environment. These core elements have more of an effect in patient encounters than the philosophical or structural dimensions of caring (Valentine, 1989, 1995).

Based on the model and multidimensional definition of caring, Valentine (1989) developed the Patient Caring Questionnaire (PCQ) and the Nurse Caring Questionnaire (NCQ). Research findings from two different studies were presented and discussed (1989, 1992). Caring was measured by the NCQ and PCQ and costs were measured in relation to patient outcomes of length of stay, cost of nursing care, patient knowledge of medication, patient satisfaction with nursing care, and postoperative complications. Patient responses on the PCQ were correlated to their overall satisfaction with the hospital, supporting the value of nurse caring interactions in choices of where to go for health care. In addition, positive caring interactions had a healing effect on patients' recovery and positively impacted outcomes. Caring practices related to the knowledge of medications prepare patients for discharge and readiness to leave the hospital. Nurse caring positively correlated to patient satisfaction, postoperative clinical conditions, and length of stay.

Based on systematic research findings, the author made recommendations for practice. She reminded us of the need to continue with research related to cost and caring and to understand that although both are complex they are central components of the health care delivery system. Valentine (1997) acknowledged that caring is holistic, multidimensional, and integral to nursing care delivery systems. According to Valentine (1997), the issue of costs is central within health care organizations and will not go away; nurses must be prepared to ask questions, work with finance to better understand nursing care, and integrate costs and caring into clinical decision making. As Nyberg (1990) recommended, Valentine (1997) encouraged registered nurses to use the practice governance structure as way to focus on the relevant issues related to caring and costs.

Watson (2000) explored an inner path of transformational leadership guided by caring and healing, allowing nursing administrators and leaders to find purpose and voice through compassionate administrative services. This article is classic in terms of Watson's (2000) integration of Fox's (1991) work to illustrate how the fourfold path informs the personal and professional life journey through the four sacred directions. The philosophical, spiritual perspective grounded in the ontology and epistemology of caring science allows for the creation of authentic leadership practices. This is in stark contrast to the traditional organizational approaches of the time grounded in the industrial or management paradigm. Watson (2000) strongly believed that nursing administrators need to return to caring–healing modalities to inform practice in order for systems to sustain caring and healing.

Watson (2000) described how following the fourfold path (Fox, 1991) transforms the practice of nurse leaders. She recognized that the *Via Negativa* or dark side of our work has depleted the human spirit and invited nurse leaders to emerge from the darkness by rethinking about nursing's values, place, and purpose. The caring–healing visions cast light into the institutional darkness and healing occurs. Watson (2000) cited Arrien (1993) who suggested that the *Via Negativa* represents the path of the spiritual warrior. This *Via* honors the dark shadow, wounded aspect of self and systems, which must be named for intentional healing to occur.

Leaders choosing to follow the *Via Negativa* are led to the next path, the *Via Positiva* (Watson, 2000).

In the path of *Via Positiva*, nurse leaders are reminded of the need to pause and reflect on the privileged space they hold within systems. Nurse leaders bring forth loving, caring energy into the work place, which allows for the creation of caring–healing spaces and human-to-human connections, which in turn allows for caring–healing practices to unfold and flourish. Watson referred to the work of Arrien (1993) and acknowledged that this path represents the Way of the Healer as the nurse leader pays attention to what has heart and meaning. Watson (1988) encouraged nurse leaders to reflect on what has heart and reminded all of us that "Caring is a Passage to the Heart" (p. 3).

According to Watson (2000), as leaders continue the journey, they enter into the path of the *Via Creativa*, where they find their voice, role, and responsibility for caring and healing for self and system. On this path, leaders recognize the unique gifts and talents they offer while in compassionate service to others. Referring to the work of Arrien (1993), this *Via* represents the Way of the Visionary, and Watson reminds nurse leaders to name that which obstructs caring–healing practices and reflect on ways to connect and unite the whole system to sustain caring beyond the walls of the hospital.

The final part of the journey is the *Via Transformativa*. Leaders come full circle and emerge as energetic new beings open to new possibilities (Watson, 2000). Transformational leaders lead from the inside out, hold sacred space for caring–healing at all levels, remain open to unexpected outcomes, and are able to transform self and system (Arrien, 1993; Watson, 2000). Watson (2000) reminds the reader of the value to self and system when the transformed leader leads from caring.

Watson (2000) reflected on specific practices that illuminate leadership grounded in the fourfold path of caring and healing and called upon nurse leaders to move forward on the fourfold path to change the outdated, industrialized, medicalized systems. She reminded us that leading by giving voice and action to caring and healing was needed for nursing's survival in the 21st century.

Watson's (2003) philosophical reflection on love and caring within the practice of nursing is sentinel and reflects the author's innovative, creative integration of esthetic knowing as illustrated with the article beginning with a poem by Rumi. This is the first article related to the practice of nursing that draws on the philosophical views of Levinas (1991) and Logstrup (1997), integrates Watson's Transpersonal Caring Theory, and invites nurses to return to the heart and soul of humanity. This ontological and epistemological perspective of nursing practice is informed by metaphors, metaphysics, and meanings associated with the work of Levinas (1991) and Logstrup (1997), including "ethics of face" and "holding another's life in our hands." The reader is reminded of the need to reconnect with our own humanity while providing compassionate service to others grounded in love.

Watson's (2003) writing and thinking was informed by a profound personal loss and trauma, which she viewed as the gift of Spirit, experiencing life and spirit while in the midst of deep suffering. She invited us as nurses to bring love and caring back to our practice in order for professional survival to be sustained. According to Watson (2003), "it is our humanity that both wounds us and heals us, and those we serve; and in the end, it is only love that matters" (p. 199). Watson (2003) provided no specific answers but encouraged readers to reflect on the ethics of being and becoming through the lens of writings of Levinas (1991) and Logstrup (1997). For example, What does it mean to hold another person's life in ones' hand? How do we face our own humanity?

Watson (2003) continued the philosophical discussion related to the writings of Rumi (1999, 2000), Levinas (1991), and Logstrup (1997) in terms of the human soul, sustaining humanity, and connections among caring, loving, and humanity. She used the example of the caring moment where the nurse makes an energetic connection with a patient and how human presence affects another. She described her view of the metaphors of love, face, and hands as a metaphysics approach and related these views to transpersonal caring. Watson reminded us that our consciousness, intentionality, and presence make a difference, for better or for worse (p. 210). Practices related to the new space of love, caring, hands, and heart are presented for nurses to consider, and an eloquent quote on love serves as the profound ending to this reflective mastery of ethics, love, caring, infinity, hands, face, being, and becoming.

ONGOING REFLECTIONS

For caring to remain central to the practice of nursing, it is essential for nursing leaders to practice from the heart, envision new approaches to sustain humanity within the systems, and remain open to new ways of being and becoming within the role of leader. These classic articles can serve as a starting point for self-reflection and dialogue. The issues of economics, clinical decisions, medical paradigms, regulations, costs, land loss of values, and humanity were of concern to the authors as early as the 1980s, as they questioned if caring could be sustained within health care systems and health care in general. In 2012, the concerns remain; solutions from the past have not allowed for caring science to ground decision making in systems. However, a paradigm shift is occurring as

nursing leaders within the practice setting are using philosophical foundations of caring theory to create caring–healing environments, resulting in self and system self-actualization. I leave you, the reader, with these questions for reflection. What practice changes will emerge as caring science transforms systems? And in the year 2020, will human caring values inform all decisions within health care systems and health care in general?

REFERENCES

Arrien, A. (1993). *The four-fold way.* San Francisco, CA: Harper SanFrancisco.

Bargagliotti, A., & Smith, H. (1985). Patterns of nursing costs with capitated reimbursement. *Nursing Economics, 3*(5), 270–275.

Buerhaus, P. (1986). The economics of caring, challenges, and new opportunities for nursing. *Topics in Clinical Nursing, 8*(2), 13–21.

Curtin. L. (1983). Determining costs of nursing service per DRG. *Nursing Management, 14*(4), 16–20.

Foa, U. (1971). Interpersonal and economic resources. *Science, 171,* 345–351.

Fox, M. (1991). *Creation spirituality.* San Francisco, CA: Harper.

Gaut, D. A. (1983). A theoretic description of caring as action. In M. Leininger (Ed.), *Care: The essence of nursing and health.* Detroit, MI: Wayne State University.

Larson, P. (1984). Important nurse caring behaviors perceived by patients with cancer. *Oncology Nursing Forum, 11* (6), 46–50.

Leininger, M. (1984). The essence of nursing and health. In M. Leininger (Ed.), *Care: The essence of nursing.* Thorofare, NJ: Slack.

Levinas, E. (1991). *Totality and infinity.* Pittsburgh, PA: Duquesne University.

Logstrup, K. (1997). *The ethical demand.* Notre Dame, IN: University of Notre Dame Press.

Lynaugh, J. & Fagin, C. (1988). Nursing comes of age. *Image: Journal of Nursing Scholarship, 20*(4), 184–190.

Mayeroff, M. (1971). *On caring.* New York, NY: Barnes & Noble Books.

McCormick, B. (1986). What is the cost of nursing care? *Hospitals, 60,* 48–52.

Miller, K. (1987). The human care perspective in nursing administration. *Journal of Nursing Administration, 17*(2), 10–12.

Miller, K. (1995). Keeping the care in nursing care. *Journal of Nursing Administration, 25*(11), 29–32.

Noddings, N. (1984). *Caring.* Berkley, CA: University of California Press.

Nyberg, J. (1989). The element of caring in nursing administration. *Nursing Administration Quarterly, 13*(3), 9–16.

Nyberg, J. (1990). The effects of care and economics on nursing practice. *Journal of Nursing Administration, 20*(5), 13–18.

Nyberg, J. (1991). Theoretical explorations of human care and economics: Foundations of nursing administration practice. *Advances in Nursing Science, 1*(13), 74–84.

Nyberg, J. (1998). *A caring approach in nursing administration.* Niwot, CO: University Press of Colorado.

Ray, M. A. (1987). Health care economics and human caring in nursing: Why the moral conflict must be resolved. *Family Community Health, 10*, 35–43.

Ray, M. (1989). The theory of bureaucratic caring for nursing practice in the organizational culture. *Nursing Administration Quarterly, 13*(2), 31–42.

Ray, M. (1997). Existential authenticity: An ethical theory of nursing administrative caring art. *Canadian Journal of Nursing Research, 29*, 111–126.

Stiles, M. K. (1990). The shining stranger: Nurse–family spiritual relationship. *Cancer Nursing, 13*, 235–245.

Turkel, M. C. (2000). Relational complexity: A theory of the nurse–patient relationship within an economic context. *Nursing Science Quarterly, 4*(13), 106–113.

Turkel, M. C. (2001). Struggling to find a balance: The paradox between caring and economics. *Nursing Administration Quarterly, 26*(1), 67–82.

Valentine, K. L. (1989a). Caring is more than kindness: Modeling its complexities. *Journal of Nursing Administration, 19*, 28–35.

Valentine, K. L. (1989b). Contributions to the theory of care. *Evaluation of Program Planning, 12*, 17–24.

Valentine, K. L. (1989c). *The value of caring nurses: Implications for patient satisfaction, quality of care, and cost.* Ithaca, NY: Cornell University. Thesis.

Valentine, K. L. (1991). Comprehensive assessment of caring and its relationship to outcome measures. *Journal of Nursing Quality Assurance, 5*(2), 59–68.

Valentine, K. L. (1997). Exploration of the relationship between caring and cost. *Holistic Nursing Practice, 11*(4), 71–81.

Walker, D. (1983). The cost of nursing care in hospitals. *Journal of Nursing Administration, 13*(3), 13–18.

Watson, J. (1979). *The philosophy and science of caring.* Boulder, CO: Colorado Associated University Press.

Watson, J. (1985). *Human science and human care.* Norwalk, CT: Appleton-Century-Crofts.

Watson, J. (1988). *Brochure Information,* University of Colorado School of Nursing, Center for Human Caring.

Watson, J. (2000). Leading via caring–healing: The fourfold way toward transformative leadership. *Nursing Administration Quarterly, 25*(1), 1–6.

Watson, J. (2003). Love and caring. Ethics of face and hand—An invitation to return to the heart and soul of nursing and our deep humanity. *Nursing Administration Quarterly, 27*, 197–202.

33

The Effects of Care and Economics on Nursing Practice

Jan Nyberg

The moral conflict of care and economics was discussed by Ray, who placed value on human care through the use of a social exchange model.[1] In a more recent article, she showed that one's understanding of caring is strongly influenced by one's role and position within the organization.[2] For example, in administration, caring was defined in relation to the competition for human and material resources. In the clinical nursing units, caring was described as intimate and technical, as a team effort, and as patient advocacy. Ray's "theory of bureaucratic caring" included seven different dimensions.[2] She wrote:

> Understanding the full meaning and interpretation of caring in the organization as bureaucratic caring can give clearer direction to the formulation of more purposeful caring goals within health care organizations.

Others have discussed this problem as a cost–quality or efficacy–efficiency debate[3-6] and suggest various ways of achieving both quality and efficiency.

HUMAN CARE

Human care is the essence of nursing, and it is what clients want the most from the nursing profession.[7] Mayeroff said "to care for another person, in the most significant sense, is to help him grow and actualize himself."[7] In caring for someone, we must experience them as having potential and believe in our own ability to help the other grow.

Noddings wrote that to practice the "caring ethic," one must maintain a preparedness to care, which focuses on the welfare, protection, or enhancement of the one cared for.[8] Watson wrote about caring in nursing as a human science, which is a moral commitment to protect human dignity and preserve humanity.[9] Nurses care for patients in the sense that they help them attain optimal health, and they also care for them as unique human beings with their own personal strengths and weaknesses.

ECONOMICS

Economics "studies human behavior in response to the necessity of allocating scarce resources among alternative possible uses."[10] It assumes that people have unlimited desires, but limited resources for producing goods and services.

Two basic economic systems are capitalism and socialism. A capitalist system is based upon ownership of property, freedom of enterprise, self-interest, market competition, and limited government

From Nyberg, J. (1990). The effects of care and economics on nursing practice. *Journal of Nursing Administration*, 20(5), 13–18. Permission to reprint granted by Wolters Kluwer.

control. Conversely, in a socialist system, attempts are made to provide all members an equal amount of the wealth through strong central control and ownership.

Health care in America has shown elements of both capitalism and socialism. Fee-for-service medical care is capitalist (buyers and sellers are independent and free to choose, price is an important determining factor). The socialist influence can be seen in the federal programs, such as Medicare and Medicaid, whose goals are equal distribution of health services.

ECONOMICS AND HEALTH CARE

Health care economics have changed a great deal since the inception of Medicare and Medicaid in the 1960s. Those programs addressed the socialist issue of providing medical care for all Americans. The success of that approach also leads to the new problem of skyrocketing health care costs. While access to health care remains an American ideal, the emphasis in the past decade has been on cost-containment.

To address the problem of health care costs, a new method of payment was created based on the concept of prospective payment, or "pricing services," instead of automatically paying all costs retrospectively. Since the initiation of diagnosis-related groups (DRGs), economics has become more visible in the health care market. In particular, hospitals have felt the crunch of the government's insistence that health care costs be contained. In the past 5 years, nurses at all levels have learned a great deal about hospital economics. Hospital administrators recognized that nurses can control hospital costs more than any profession except medicine. By enlisting nurses' support of cost-containment methods, administrators introduced nursing to the arena of economics.

This study addresses nurses' responses to the intensified pressures for cost control during the past 5 years. While human care remains the most important concern of nursing, the new economic pressure calls for nurses to work more efficiently. The dilemma is this: How do nurses continue to advocate human caring in a cost-cutting economic environment?

THE RESEARCH STUDY

Our study explored nurses' reactions to the economic changes of the recent past. The study included 2,793 nurses from 7 hospitals in a western state. A total of 350 questionnaires (50 for each hospital) were sent to randomly selected nurses on staff at the various hospitals. There were 135 questionnaires returned (38.57%).

Interviews were conducted with the nurse executives of each hospital. The executives were asked to define the characteristics of their hospital and describe their impressions about human care and economics. Their organizations varied from profit to nonprofit, private to public, urban to suburban, teaching to nonteaching, and 125-bed to 400-bed. When asked about human care and economics, the nurse executives agreed that it is important for the two concepts to be viewed as interdependent; human care is the goal of nursing, but economics cannot be ignored. The nurse administrators also identified the nursing shortage as a serious problem for the delivery of patient care. One nurse administrator proposed a model, which placed caring as the mission of the hospital with economics, research, management, and education as supporting facets.

A questionnaire was developed (Figure 33.1), which identified caring attributes from a variety of previous studies.[7,8,11–13] The attributes included "deep respect for the needs of others," "expresses positive and negative feelings," "believes that others have potential which can be achieved," and "remains committed to a continuing relationship." A series of questions regarding Nyberg's attributes of

DIRECTIONS: Circle and fill in below the number that indicates the degree of your agreement with each of the following:
Are these caring attributes important to you?
Are they present in the most caring people you know?
Do they:

Extremely important 5
Very important 4
Somewhat important 3
Slightly important 2
Not important 1

1. Have deep respect for the needs of others.
2. Not give up hope for others.
3. Remain sensitive to the needs of others.
4. Communicate a helping, trusting attitude toward others.
5. Express positive and negative feelings.
6. Solve problems creatively.
7. Understand that spiritual forces contribute to human care.
8. Consider relationships before rules.
9. Base decisions on what is best for the people involved.
10. Understand thoroughly what situations mean to people.
11. Go beyond the superficial to know people well.
12. Implement skills and techniques well.
13. Choose tactics that will accomplish goals.
14. Give full consideration to situational factors.
15. Focus on helping others to grow.
16. Take time for personal needs and growth.
17. Allow time for caring opportunities.
18. Remain committed to a continuing relationship.
19. Listen carefully and be open to feedback.
20. Belive that others have a potential that can be achieved.

FIGURE 33.1

Nyberg Caring Assessment Scale.

caring[14] were asked: How important are the attributes (ideal scale)? How often do you use these attributes in your practice (actual scale)? How often does your supervisor use the caring attributes (supervisor scale)? How have the attributes changed in the past 5 years (5-year scale)?

> Hospital administrators recognized that nurses can control hospital costs more than those in any other profession except medicine.

In addition to the Nyberg caring attributes, Patricia Larson's CARE-Q tool was used.[14] That tool focuses on caring behaviors such as "checks on patient frequently," "suggests questions for the patient to ask his or her doctor," "sits down with the patient," and "knows how to give shots, IVs, and so on."

A pilot study of the questionnaire was conducted using graduate nursing students at the State University. Reliability for the subscales of the questionnaire (ideal, actual, 5-year, supervisor, CARE-Q) ranged from 0.87 to 0.98 using Cronbach's alpha coefficient. The reliability of the questionnaire for the study population ranged from 0.85 to 0.97, indicating excellent reliability for the whole questionnaire.

Mean scores and standard deviations were calculated to determine how the respondents rated the subscales of the questionnaires. Results indicated that nurses view caring as "very important" (score of 4.1 out of 5), that they use the attributes "often" (score of 3.9), that they practice the attributes "about the same" as 5 years ago (score of 3), and that supervisors scored lower than the nurses themselves (score of 3.4). The standard deviation for the supervisor scale was highest, indicating extreme scores; some supervisors were rated very high and others scored very low. The CARE-Q caring behaviors were also practiced "often" (score of 4.0).

A two-factor analysis of variance was conducted to determine whether there were significant differences between the subscales of the questionnaire and whether these differences were consistent across hospitals. It was found that there were significant differences between ideal, actual, 5-year, and CARE-Q scales, There were significant differences between hospitals only in the 5-year scale and the supervisor scale.

Finally, the correlation between caring scores and economic indicators was calculated. Two types of economic indicators were used: total nursing hours per patient day and total nursing hours per patient day adjusted by case-mix index. The case-mix index is a Medicare designation reflecting how acutely ill patients are in each hospital. Adjusting nursing hours by case-mix attempts to control the extraneous variable of patient acuity. The correlation coefficient for total nursing hours with caring scores was 0.59 ($P = 0.07$). The correlation coefficient for adjusted nursing hours and caring scores was 0.73 ($P = 0.04$). This indicated that hospitals that used higher numbers of nurses per patient exhibited higher actual caring scores.

At the end of the questionnaire, four open-ended questions were asked. The first two questions concerned economics and the last two questions concerned human care.

The economic questions were answered very negatively, and it was apparent that the vast majority of the study participants believed that current economic pressures are making it much harder to provide adequate human care. There were dozens of comments about how sick patients have become and how frustrating it is for nurses to not have time to meet patients' needs. The participants cited short-staffing as a major issue and said that administrators (including nursing administrators) are more interested in money than in what happens to patients. One nurse said that the emphasis on money is "foreign and disgusting," and several nurses expressed concern that patients who do not have money cannot obtain adequate health care services. Nurses' wages were cited many times as a problem, and nurses expressed feeling desperately rushed, having time to do "only the essentials," and feeling "more distant from patients."

The last two questions addressed human care and elicited very different answers. Nurses understand and value human care as follows:

- Providing care, which pays tribute to the dignity of the patient
- Being able to laugh and cry with patients
- Reaching out human-to-human
- Unconditional positive regard
- Dealing with the whole person
- Being concerned with the betterment of another

When asked how to maintain human care, nurses' answers were again warm and personal:

- Developing trusting relationships
- Involving the family

- Facilitating opportunities for growth
- Being an example to other professionals
- Being honest and knowing your limits

Most nurses seem to accept caring responsibilities with a great deal of pride and understanding. One nurse said that "nursing practice must have as its foundation the caring aspect of art/science. It is caring that makes nursing unique and essential."

RECOMMENDATIONS

An important overall conclusion from the study is that economics and human care are interrelated forces in today's hospital environment. Nurses' ability to provide care is dependent on economic resources. However, the study also showed that the hospital's ability to provide high levels of human care, thus ensuring economic viability, is dependent on nurses.

Further research is recommended to enhance the reliability of the tool and to validate the correlation between human care and economics. Limitations of the study relate to the geographic distribution and the moderate response rate of the questionnaires. A replicate study on a national basis with better follow-up to enhance the response rate would be needed to generalize the findings. Organizational assessments should be done to attempt to identify other barriers to human care and more efficient means of providing that care.

> The hospital's ability to provide high levels of human care, thus ensuring economic viability, is dependent on nurses.

Human care is the hope for nursing. Although the current economic environment is severe, this study showed that nurses continue to see caring as important and that they still use caring attributes and behaviors in their work. It was interesting to note that, although the economic resources (nursing hours per patient day) varied by over 200% in the study, the ideal and actual measurements of caring did not vary significantly across hospitals. This suggests that human caring is universally seen by nurses as their purpose and their achievement. Nurses' efforts to emphasize human care in their practice should be supported and rewarded.

This study also highlights the Lockian paradox of individual freedom versus the necessity of organization. In 1690, John Locke wrote that the enjoyment of total freedom is uncertain, and therefore, people choose to join societies that restrict individual freedom in exchange for security. Morgan wrote about restrictions imposed by organizations on their employees.[15] Nurses must practice under a certain amount of restrained individual freedom as long as they work in organizations and cultures. This does not mean that human care should be neglected because of economics. It does mean, however, that nurses should recognize that not all of the factors surrounding patient care are under the control of nursing. Nurses must accept the constraints while working optimally within them. As one nurse said, "the greater the economic pressure becomes, the more vigilant we must be to preserve human caring on a high level and the more creative we must be to allow it to continue in the face of greater and greater limitations of time and resources."

The next administrative recommendation is that nursing administrators maintain an awareness of the quality imperative. Donabedian[16] reminds us that, in the final analysis, there is no substitute for professional commitment and accountability. Quality of care remains our highest mission. One nurse in the study wrote that, in her hospital, she had been told to provide safe care rather than quality care. This is alarming because maintaining a quality approach in any business is necessary.[17] The problem currently seems to be that nurses are frustrated because they feel obligated to meet more and more patient needs with fewer and fewer resources. Identifying more efficient ways of providing care is a must, but sometimes the economics of an organization outstrip efficiency maneuvers. In such a case, nursing services should be defined by nurses in the organization in such a way that dollar cuts will translate into service cuts. If economic resources make it difficult to allow optimal patient care goals, the nurse administrator has a responsibility to obtain more resources from the organization or else work with nurses to redefine what expectations are realistic within given constraints, In this way, nurses' work is defined in such a manner that they can feel pride in the quality of the care that they do provide.

The last recommendation concerns nursing's place in the organization. Nurses in this study indicated that they felt controlled by "the system" and unable to affect decisions in the organization. Two ways in which nursing's participation in the organization can be enhanced are changing the image of the nursing administrators and changing the organization design.

Porter-O'Grady[18] wrote that it is time for the relationship between nurses and nurse administrators to change and that the nurse administrators of the future need to view themselves as facilitators rather than bosses. For nurses to feel they have input in organizational decisions, they need to view their nurse administrators as colleagues in the effort to provide optimal nursing care.

Changes in the formal organizational structure can also enhance nurses' perceptions of their effectiveness within the health care organization. Such systems as shared governance and participative management give nurses opportunities to become a part of the decision-making process. It is no longer appropriate for one nurse—the chief nurse executive—to be the only nurses' voice in the organization.[18] Rather, a philosophy of participation can be implemented, which allows many nurses to speak for patient care and nursing's interests.

CONCLUSION

Economics and human care must be viewed as interrelated forces within today's hospital environment. Economics was seen by nurses in this study as a constraining force in health care, while human care was recognized as nursing's responsibility and goal. Ray's theory of bureaucratic caring suggests that caring exists in the hospital in a variety of forms.[2] Tending to economics is a form of caring, in that it secures the organization's ability to support human care as it is expressed by nurses to patients. While it is clear that economic adjustments are necessary to maintain the viability of hospital organizations, the product of human care must be protected and encouraged for the welfare of patients, nurses, and hospital. Wisdom for the nurse administrator is in recognizing the realities of both human care and economics and integrating them into a system where the goals of patient care and organizational survival are mutually supportive.

REFERENCES

1. Ray, M. A. (1987). Health care economics and human care in nursing: Why the moral conflict must be resolved. *Family and Community Health, 10*(l), 34–43.
2. Ray, M. A. (1989). The theory of bureaucratic caring for nursing practice in the organizational culture. *Nursing Administration Quarterly, 13*(2), 31–42.

3. Fry, S. T. (1983). Rationing health care: The ethics of cost containment. *Nursing Economics,* 165–169.

4. Clifford, L. A., & Plomann, M. P. (1985). Cost and quality, two sides of the coin in cost containment. *Health Care and Financial Management,* 30–32.

5. Sisk, F., & May, J. J. (1986). Moving forward toward value: A new era in health care. *Health Care Financial Management,* 56–60.

6. Wyszewlanski, L., Thomas, J. W., & Friedman, B. A. (1987). Case-based payment and the control of quality and efficiency in hospitals. *Inquiry, 24,* 17–25.

7. Mayeroff, M. (1971). *On caring.* New York, NY: Barnes & Noble Books.

8. Noddings, N. (1984). *Caring.* Berkeley, CA: University of California Press.

9. Watson, J. (1985). *Human science and human care.* Norwalk, CT: Appleton-Century-Crofts.

10. Thaker, H. H. (1983). *Wage setting and evaluation: Economic principles for registered nurses.* Kansas City, MO: American Nurses Association.

11. Watson, J. (1979). *Nursing: The philosophy and science of caring.* Boulder, CO: Colorado Associated University Press.

12. Gaut, D. (1983). A theoretic description of caring as action. In M. Leininger (Ed.), *Care: The essence of nursing and health.* Detroit, MI: Wayne State University Press.

13. Nyberg, J. (1989). *Assessing attitudes of caring.* Unpublished.

14. Larson, P. (1984). Important nurse caring behaviors perceived by patients with cancer. *Oncology Nursing Forum, 11* (6), 46–50.

15. Morgan, G. (1986). *Images of organizations.* Beverly Hills, CA: Sage Publishers.

16. Donabedian, A. (1984). Quality, cost, and cost containment. *Nursing Outlook, 32*(3), 142–145.

17. Iacocca, L. (1988). *Talking straight.* Toronto, ON: Bantam Books.

18. Porter-O'Grady, T. (1986). *Creative nursing administration: Participative management for the 21st century.* Rockville, MD: Aspen Publication.

QUESTIONS FOR REFLECTION

Baccalaureate

1. Provide an example where caring and economics is an area of concern within your organization.
2. What do you think is the major economic issue influencing the delivery of health care at the national and international level?
3. Provide an example where caring practices have had a positive impact on patient/family/system outcomes.

Master's

1. Think of an example where caring and economics is an area of concern within your organization and identify practice changes you can initiate to demonstrate the economic value of caring.
2. What do you see as the future for nursing practice in the next 5 years, given the current economic issues at the national and international level?
3. What evidence-based practice changes can you make within your organization to demonstrate the economic value of caring within your system?

Doctoral

1. How have the economics of health care changed since this article was published in 1990? How have they remained the same?
2. Identify a quantitative research question looking at the economic value of caring.
3. Identify a qualitative research question looking at the economic value of caring.

34

Struggling to Find a Balance: The Paradox Between Caring and Economics

MARIAN C. TURKEL

As the United States is in the midst of radical health care delivery changes, the entire debate seems to focus on the concepts of managed care and health care economics. From an economic perspective, hospitals are a business enterprise first. The competition for survival among hospitals is becoming more intense as reimbursement decreases and cost controls become tighter. However, the element of human caring is missing from the economic discussion. In the economic debate, the sense of caring for the patients as the goal of hospitals has been lost. When patients are hospitalized, it is the caring attentiveness and compassion of the nurse that the patients perceive as quality care.[1] The concerns of patients are not about costs or health care finance. Patients are looking to develop a caring relationship with their nurses, built upon trust, mutual respect, and confidence.

However, in a climate increasingly focused on economics, nurses have been unable to document the economic importance of this caring relationship. Newer payment systems, such as managed care, do not look at human caring or the nurse–patient relationship when allocating resource dollars for reimbursement. The current payment systems, including health maintenance organizations (HMOs), managed care, Medicare, Medicaid, and private insurers, reimburse hospitals at a flat capitated rate. Subsequently, it is hospital administrators who must determine how these resource dollars will be allocated within their respective organizations.

The purpose of this research study was to use a qualitative grounded theory approach to study the nurse–patient relationship within the context of economics and the changing health care environment in a for-profit health care organization. Despite the significance of merging quality and cost in the current health care reform dialogue, there is limited research looking at the nurse–patient relationship within an economic context.

NURSING ECONOMICS

Nursing had its origins in poorly paid domestic work and charitable religious organizations. Before Medicare and Medicaid in 1965, health care delivery was not profitable for hospitals. Nursing students subsidized hospitals, and hospital-based nursing care was not considered an expense or source of revenue.[2]

From Turkel, M. C. (2001). Struggling to find balance: The paradox between caring and economics. *Nursing Administration Quarterly, 26*(1), 67–82. Permission to reprint granted by Wolters Kluwer.

Nursing students provided the labor, and hospital administrators made no attempt to identify the real cost of nursing care. As nursing education moved away from the hospital setting to colleges and universities in the late 1950s and the role of student nurse was reformed, hospital administrators began to account for the actual cost and revenue of hospital nursing care.[2] However, the introduction of Medicare and Medicaid in 1965 allowed for hospital profitability, and the issue of nursing care costs was not a major focus for administrators.

During the era of retrospective reimbursement from 1965 to 1983, the actual cost of nursing care was difficult to research because it was embedded in the daily hospital room charge. However, acute care hospitals were soon under scrutiny because of the rapidly escalating costs of health care. As a result of the change to the prospective payment system and the use of diagnosis-related groups (DRGs) in 1983, hospital administrators were pressured to increase efficiency, reduce costs, and maintain quality. Consequently, nursing administrators needed to develop systems to gather information relative to nursing costs and productivity. Research was conducted to examine the costs associated with nursing.[3-6] Common to all these studies was the use of a patient classification system that was time based and a predictor of the level of care needed for each class of patient. Data derived from these studies were used to calculate nursing costs per DRG, predict expenditures, and determine nursing productivity.

By the time nursing researchers had demonstrated the difficulty of costing out caring activities with patient classification systems and the effectiveness of registered nurse staffing on patient outcomes, patient satisfaction, and mortality, the move toward managed care had already begun. The economic environment was changing faster than nurse researchers could document the impact of these changes on professional practice. In a managed care environment, reimbursement to hospitals had been further constrained. As a response to shrinking operating budgets, many hospital administrators instituted registered nurse staff reductions or used unlicensed nursing assistants to replace registered nurses.

CARING AND ECONOMICS

The paradox between the concepts of human caring and economics has been studied by nurse scholars.[7-17] It is a challenge for nurses to combine the science and the art of caring within the economic context of the health care environment. However, human care is what patients want from the nursing profession.[11] Ray stated that the "transformation of American and other western health care systems to corporate enterprises emphasizing competitive management and economic gain seriously challenges nursing's humanistic philosophies and theories and nursing's administrative and clinical policies."[13(p. 31)]

Buerhaus challenged nurse researchers to conduct interviews that would yield economic or dollar value data when studying humanistic nursing behaviors. An example of this was to identify specific humanistic caring behaviors, such as a nurse sitting and talking about patients' fears and then to ask "Can you tell me how much the nurse listening to you is worth?"[18(p. 19)] The need to examine caring from the perspective of economic value was important because of the increasing pressure to reduce health care costs.

Numerous research studies have focused on caring in relation to patient outcomes and patient satisfaction.[19-22] The above studies explicitly linked nurse caring, patient satisfaction, and positive patient outcomes. The costs associated with human caring and the nurse–patient relationship were not as clearly articulated. This was in part because researchers used tangible economic indicators in an attempt to measure the intangible.

Foa, an exchange theorist, designed a theory that could bridge the gap between economic and noneconomic resources.[23] In the theory, love, status, and information were viewed as interpersonal resources and were correlated with the economic resources of money, goods, and services. According to Ray, "[t]he full inclusion of these resources is necessary and will require a major effort on the part of nurses and patients to see that they become an integral part of the health care economic analysis."[3(p. 40)]

This review of the literature on caring and economics has revealed the need to continue linking the concepts of economics and caring in nursing research. Most of the current studies have focused on patient satisfaction as an outcome of the caring between the nurse and the patient. However, as the nursing practice environment continues to change, research is needed to explore how nurses can continue to provide humanistic care with limited economic resources.

Interpersonal resources, such as love or caring, status or prestige, and information or teaching, are important in the nurse–patient relationship and to health care economic reform. To successfully merge the science of economics and the human art and science of caring in nursing, it was necessary to examine the dynamic patterns of the nurse–patient relationship as an economic health care resource.

A research study that focused on the nurse–patient relationship within a framework of benefit–cost parameters from the perspective of nurses, patients, and administrators responsible for health care system operations was conducted by the researcher. This type of research was seen as needed by the researcher so that caring would not be lost in the economics of the current health care environment.

METHOD

In this study, grounded theory techniques were used to guide data collection and analysis.[24,25] Considering the complexity of the nurse–patient relationship, grounded theory methodology allowed for discovery of patterns of the dynamic social process.

SETTING AND PARTICIPANTS

The 250-bed hospital selected for this study was part of a for-profit hospital network located in the southeastern United States. This specific setting was chosen because of the many changes that have occurred in the for-profit corporate health care system. Twenty-eight participants from the hospital were included in the study: ten registered nurses, ten patients, and eight top-level administrators.

The researcher approached the participants and requested their participation in the study. They were told participation involved a tape-recorded interview that discussed their experiences with the nurse–patient relationship. They were given the formal consent to read and asked if they had any questions before their agreement to participate in the study. Participants who agreed to be interviewed were then asked to select a convenient time for the interview within the next 24 hours.

DATA COLLECTION

Interviewing participants was the primary source of data collection. Participants' descriptions of their experiences provided the researchers with rich data for simultaneous data analysis. One interview,

30 to 60 minutes in length, was conducted with each participant. The interviews were semistructured, with the researcher allowing the participant to speak openly. The initial interviews began with a general open-ended question. Nurses, for example, were asked, "Tell me about a typical day on your unit. Start with 'I come to work. . . .'" Patients were asked, "Tell me about a day in the hospital." Administrators were asked, "How would you describe a typical day for a nurse from your understanding of the experience?"

As the interview process proceeded, more specific questions were asked, including describing specific caring nurse–patient interactions and the costs and benefits associated with these interactions. Use of the word *costs* was consistent with the challenge to nurse researchers by Buerhaus to conduct interviews that provide economic or dollar value data.[18] In relation to constant comparative analytic techniques, each interview involved exploration of topics arising from the preceding interviews. After each interview in this study was completed, the tapes were transcribed verbatim. The researcher read these transcripts and generated questions for the subsequent interviews.

DATA ANALYSIS

In the grounded theory method, data collection and analysis occur simultaneously. Through constant comparative analysis, data from each interview were used to enhance selection of questions in the next interview, leading toward identification of the social process and substantive theory.[25] Data were analyzed using the constant comparative method where each line, phrase, sentence, and paragraph from the transcribed interviews were reviewed. Each category was compared to other categories. Comparisons were made for similarities, differences, and patterns.

The first basic step of data analysis was open or substantive coding, which broke the data down into small segments. Data were analyzed line by line and significant words or sentences were highlighted. As the researcher proceeded with coding, categories or patterns of codes were identified. Level-two coding included the identification of categories and their properties. During this level of coding, the large number of substantive codes were subsumed into categories or patterns and moved to a higher level of abstraction. Theoretical coding, or level-three coding, was used to show how the categories related to one another. These theoretical codes conceptualize the relationship between the levels of coding.[25]

The researcher examined the data for relationships among categories for each group of participants: nurses, patients, and administrators. Subsequent relationships were also discovered by looking at similarities and differences among these three groups. This process of constant comparative analysis allowed the researcher to identify patterns within the data, leading to the identification of a basic social process and the substantive theory.

RESULTS: NURSE PARTICIPANTS

Findings revealed that the process of being part of the nurse–patient relationship followed a consistent pattern. The three categories that emerged from the data analysis included entering into the relationship, practicing caring, and entering into a new reality (Table 34.1). These categories overlapped and represented a continual ongoing process rather than being isolated and linear in nature. Each category was further divided into subcategories.

Entering Into the Relationship

The relationship was initiated when the nurse and patient met for the first time. This category involved establishing trust, creating the nurse–patient relationship,

TABLE 34.1 Results: Nurse Participants

Category	Subcategory
Entering into the relationship	Establishing trust
	Creating the nurse–patient relationship
	Maintaining the nurse–patient relationship
Practicing caring	Being, knowing, doing all at once
	Caring in the moment
	Caring beyond
	Investing in patient education
Entering a new reality	Managing in the presence of chaos
	Contending with costs
	Valuing the humanistic interaction
	Fearing for patient's well-being

and maintaining the nurse–patient relationship. Ways of establishing trust, as defined from the nurses' perspective, included "listening," "showing respect," "making eye contact," "instilling confidence," "using body language," "giving information," "sitting, talking, and meeting patients' needs." Establishing trust was characterized by attending to patients and providing for patients.

Once nurses began establishing trust with the patients, they actually pursued creating a relationship. Creating the relationship was characterized by personalizing the care and establishing that the patients prefer the registered nurse. Personalizing the care was described by nurses as "introducing one's self to the patient," "sharing personal knowledge," and "making them feel important." Nurses talked about patients wanting to know who the registered nurse was and wanting to be cared for by a registered nurse. Several nurses explained that "knowing they have an educated person" caring for them allowed the patients to feel more confident in their nurse. Other nurses acknowledged patients being "more relaxed and comfortable" knowing a registered nurse was taking care of them.

As the nurses finished creating a relationship, it became necessary to work on maintaining the nurse–patient relationship. Maintaining the relationship was operationally defined as establishing further rapport and letting the patients know they were not forgotten. During the course of the day, the nurses tried to get in the rooms as much as possible. Visiting with patients, spending some extra time, and anticipating individual patient's needs provided the nurses with an opportunity for establishing further rapport. Given the hectic schedule on the floor, increased acuity level of patients, and higher patient-to-RN ratios, the nurses were left with little time. However, the nurses still found ways of letting the patients know they were not forgotten.

Practicing Caring

Practicing caring was characterized by being, knowing, and doing all at once; caring in the moment; caring beyond; and investing in patient education. Caring reflected the art and science of nursing, which at times became lost within the chaos of practice, as more emphasis was placed on economics and the bottom line and just completing the necessary tasks.

Being, knowing, and doing all at once described professional caring. Being was the caring presence. Knowing referred to being competent, caring as knowing, and knowing the patient as a person. Doing all at once involved using a holistic approach to practice and seeing the whole person while meeting physical needs. As one nurse said, "Patients want to know that I know what to do if they have a heart attack while I'm with them" Caring requires knowledge when being used in the practice setting. Nurses valued and integrated knowledgeable caring into their practice. Using a holistic approach to practice was referred to by the nurses as "being aware of psychosocial needs" "looking at spiritual needs," "seeing the whole person," and "knowing my patient as a person."

Caring in the moment described nursing in the current practice environment. Faced with less time to spend with patients and shorter lengths of stay, nurses were constantly challenged to do it all and do it all now. No longer were nurses afforded the luxury of having lots of time to be with patients. Caring took place in that special moment when the nurse and patient were together and, often, the nurse only had a moment.

Caring beyond was manifested by sharing memories and feeling rewarded. Nurses reflected on the times they were able to transcend the usual limits of the caring experience. It was caring beyond what was often possible in the environment of practice, but doing it anyway. Nurses shared special memories they had with patients that involved caring beyond the moment and illustrated committed ongoing caring.

As nurses spoke about caring, all referred to teaching as part of the caring process. Often, there was little opportunity for teaching, and nurses were challenged to try and find the time to teach. However, because of the high value placed on teaching by the nurses and knowing that it has positive clinical and economic outcomes, teaching became a top priority for nurses. With limited resources available, the role of teaching has evolved

into investing in patient education. An important economic outcome of investing in patient education was preventing readmission to the hospital.

Entering a New Reality

As nurses were entering into the relationship and practicing caring, they were simultaneously entering into a new reality for practice that was controlled by costs. Entering a new reality was characterized by managing in the presence of chaos, contending with costs, valuing the humanistic interaction, and fearing for patients' well-being.

The pace on the floor was chaotic with "admissions and discharges coming and going," "getting six patients to the OR before 9:00 A.M.," and "trying to help a doctor during a procedure while the charts are piling up at the desk with orders." Often, the unit was so busy that nurses had "to squeeze it in to even go to lunch." Nurses described experiences of "going home and wondering if I did everything," "calling back to the floor because I forgot to chart something," "being unable to give medications on time," and "having a patient in a wet bed for hours till I had time to turn him." Nurses described this chaos as disturbing and distressing.

Contending with costs included costing as a foreign and distasteful idea, doing more with less, attempting to link cost and quality, and being afraid of the future. Although costs were synonymous with health care reform and the hospital focus was on reducing costs, the nurse participants had difficulty discussing costs as related to care provided at the bedside.

When asked to discuss the costs associated when interacting with patients, the nurses were perplexed. Their initial responses included "costs, I don't even know what that means," "I should know, but I don't," "I don't understand the question," or "costs are what the suits [administrators or managers] worry about." After a few minutes, the concept of costs was described as "time with one patient instead of another," "charging for teaching," "being exhausted" (personal cost), and "getting paid whether I do a good job or not." As the cost discussion continued, probes and cues from the researcher failed to yield a dollar amount related to specific interaction.

Although nurses were confronted with doing more for less, there was still an overwhelming value to retain humanistic caring and compassion while interacting with patients. This art of nursing was in danger of becoming lost in the economics of health care reform; however, the nurses valued caring. One nurse explained that she was actually leaving her current work place because of the high value she placed on having the time to be caring.

Facing the current challenges and looking ahead into the future has generated a sense of fear. Nurses described "seeing patient care suffer" as the hospital continued "making a profit at any cost." Nurses discussed diminishing human resources and ongoing hospital profitability as the way of the future. They described scenarios of deteriorating staffing and its negative consequences on patient care. The following quote reflected the concern for patient well-being:

It's gotten outrageous. The hospitals are wanting to make as much profit as in the past. I think the first that will go is nursing. You've got to cut back somewhere to get that profit, so we'll be the ones to go. Ultimately, the patient will pay for it. We may be a little more tired, a little more frustrated when we go home at night, but it's the patients that are going to go home without care.

RESULTS: PATIENT PARTICIPANTS

Regardless of the age of the patient or diagnosis, the process of being a part of the nurse–patient relationship followed a consistent overall pattern. The three categories included being in the relationship, interpreting the caring, and entering a new reality (Table 34.2). These categories converged and represented a continual ongoing process rather than being isolated events.

Being in the Relationship

In this category, the nurse and patient were getting to know each other and developing a mutual relationship. Being in the relationship encompassed developing trust in the nurse, recognizing the nurse–patient relationship, and having the nurse there for me. One patient explained, "If you don't feel safe with someone, you don't ever trust them," At times, patient

TABLE 34.2 Results: Patient Participants

Category	Subcategory
Being in the relationship	Developing trust in the nurse
	Recognizing the nurse–patient relationship
	Having the nurse there for me
Interpreting the caring	Distinguishing between caring and noncaring
	Caring making a difference
	Valuing the educational process
Feeling threatened by the new reality	Surviving in the presence of chaos
	Deserving to be cared for despite the costs
	Fearing for themselves

participants felt "you need to trust them that they know what they are doing" and then once "they got [sic] your confidence, it gets better." As the process of developing trust unfolded, it was important for patients to feel the nurse was keeping a commitment. Patient participants recalled "nurses coming back when they promised," "calling my family like they said," and "remembering to check on my lab results."

As patients developed trust and continued interacting with the nurse, they began to recognize the relationship that was forming. Patient participants described the start of the relationship when they began knowing the nurse was a person. Having this knowledge made it easier for patients to talk with the nurse and share personal feelings and experiences. As the personal exchange between nurse and patient evolved, so did the caring relationship.

Once the patient's physical needs were met, the humanistic, compassionate responses of the nurse were what mattered to the patient. The patient participants recognized the nurse being there for them as comforting, relaxing, giving hope, and providing support. As one patient participant stated, "Being there with you when you need her to be there, well it's just comforting." Another participant recalled, "Just her being there and holding my hand was like a guiding light."

Interpreting the Caring

Interpreting the caring encompassed the essence of the nurse–patient relationship. This category was illuminated by patients as distinguishing between caring and noncaring, caring as making a difference, and valuing the educational process. Caring was described by patients as "being there," "treating me with compassion," "helping me," "staying with me," "teaching me," "being empathetic," and "knowing just what

to say and do." Noncaring was talked about by patients as "being cold," "acting like it was a burden to answer my light," "being insensitive," "coming in to do something, but not speaking to me," "being rude," "just doing a job," "not answering my light," and "not meeting my needs in a timely manner." Patients felt angry and alone when the nurse was noncaring.

Patients discussed caring as making a difference. From their perspective, making a difference consisted of four outcomes: speeding the healing process, increasing my well-being, enhancing my learning, and reflecting quality. Patient participants believed they came out of the hospital experience better and faster when they had a caring relationship with their nurse. A second outcome of caring was the feeling of increased emotional well-being. Patient participants talked about feeling better mentally and being able to relax when they felt they had a caring nurse taking care of them. The third outcome of caring was enhancement of learning when the teaching was done by a caring nurse. Patient participants talked about being able to ask questions and wanting to learn when they had a caring nurse. They believed they could "remember better" with a caring nurse.

Quality care, as perceived by the patient participants, was the final outcome of caring. Patient participants referred to the caring as "why I came to this hospital" or "choosing to come back here because of the nurses." As patient participants continued to talk about caring, they discussed "being very satisfied with the nursing care" and "seeing this as quality care." One patient participant was recently diagnosed with leukemia. This diagnosis resulted in the patient having frequent admissions to the hospital. When, because of her age, her doctor wanted to admit her to another hospital closer to home, she refused.

Feeling Threatened by the New Reality

Patients felt threatened by the new reality of health care that was controlled by costs. From the patient perspective, conditions of this new reality included surviving in the presence of chaos, deserving to be cared for despite the costs, and fearing for themselves.

Patients recalled nurses running down the hall to answer a light or hearing call bells ringing and realizing no one was available to answer them. One patient remembered a time when he went out to the station looking for a nurse because he heard other patients calling for help. Although patients sensed the nurses scrambling around, they did not blame the nurses. Rather, they attributed the working conditions to "needing more help," "nurses having to do too much paperwork," and "system disorganization."

Patients became very vocal when the word *cost* was mentioned. When talking about costs and changes in health care and Medicare, patients became angry. There was an overwhelming consensus of deserving to be cared for despite the costs. Patients unanimously echoed that "costs shouldn't matter" when asked by the researchers to discuss the costs associated with interpersonal caring and humanistic interactions. Health care and health "caring" was a right and money should not matter.

As patients continued talking about costs, they began refocusing on the costs associated with caring interactions. They were attempting to assign a dollar value to the experience while simultaneously recognizing their inability to do so. The intangible nature of caring made it difficult to quantify in monetary terms. Patients described caring and humanistic interactions in terms of cost as:

> Sometimes a million dollars. Right? There's just nothing you can say. You can't put a monetary value on that, really. It's beyond that. You either have it or you don't.

No, probably not. Because it's just as important to the guy that only could pay $5.00 as it is to the chap who could pay $100 for it. So, you can't really put a dollar value on it.

Patients talked about the future of health care and expressed fear that hospitals would "dump the RNs" or "get rid of the nurses to save money." They questioned who would teach them about their medications or be there for them in an emergency, "It makes you feel like you should stay out if you're not going to get the care," one patient participant explained. Another patient participant echoed, "It's a scary thought, but you hate to come here anymore."

RESULTS: ADMINISTRATOR PARTICIPANTS

After data analysis of the nurse's and patient's interviews was completed, the researcher began analysis of the administrative interviews. This pattern consisted of four categories that overlapped and represented a continual ongoing process rather than being isolated and linear in nature. The four categories included viewing the nurse–patient relationship, judging caring and noncaring, recognizing the chaos, and profiting in the new reality (Table 34.3).

Viewing the Nurse–Patient Relationship

Administrators were not directly involved in the nurse–patient relationship; rather, they were observing this relationship from a distance. This category involved seeing the nurse entering into the relationship and having a vested interest in the nurse–patient relationship.

In order for the nurse to initiate the relationship, it was essential that they have strategies for establishing trust with the patients. According to the administrator, these strategies included introducing self, instilling confidence, reassuring patient and family, and anticipating patient needs.

TABLE 34.3 Results: Administrator Participants

Category	Subcategory
Viewing the nurse–patient relationship	Entering into the relationship
	Having a vested interest in the nurse-patient relationship
Judging caring and noncaring	Defining caring
	Defining noncaring
Recognizing the chaos	Wondering how they do it
	Knowing the nurses are on call to everyone
	Giving the nurses credit
Profiting in the new reality	Accounting for the costs
	Accounting for the caring
	Valuing registered nurses
	Positioning for future survival

Administrators explained the value and importance of the nurse–patient relationship. They discussed receiving letters from patients, scoring high on surveys, and getting positive verbal feedback for patients as indicators of positive nurse–patient interactions. This type of feedback validated the economic value of the nurse–patient relationship in terms of customer satisfaction. As administrators continued talking about the nurse–patient relationship, they linked this relationship to quality. From their point of view, quality care was defined by the patient's appraisal of the nurse–patient relationship and the quality of nursing care. All administrator participants saw the humanistic components of the nurse–patient relationship as key indicators when defining quality. Administrator participants looked at return business and viewed the nurse–patient relationship as central to patient referrals.

Judging Caring and Noncaring

Administrators easily differentiated between caring and noncaring nurses. These perceptions were based on personal observations made during rounds, letters from patients, and their own belief system concerning professional nursing practice.

Caring was defined as "teaching," "going one step further," and "using a holistic approach." Administrators recognized that caring was more than kindness or a friendly smile. These humanistic components were viewed as being essential to the nurse–patient relationship for patients to feel like they were being treated as an individual. One administrator participant stated, "We don't want our patients to be treated like a widget going through a process line, but more as a person."

Administrators also talked about behaviors and interactions they perceived to be uncaring. From the administrator point of view, "our business and return business is determined by how well we care for patients." Uncaring behaviors transmitted to patients have a negative impact on how patients judge the care they receive in the hospital. According to one administrator, "patients look at nursing for the caring over all the rest." Administrators acknowledged that there were often interruptions, distractions, and hindrances on the unit that made it difficult for nurses to be caring. However, as one administrator said, "I don't care how frustrated the nurse is, she can't transmit this to the patient."

Recognizing the Chaos

Administrator participants recognized the chaos on the nursing units. When administrator participants described a typical day for a nurse, they talked about the hectic work environment and all that was expected of the nurse. This category was operationally defined as wondering how they do it, knowing they are on call to everyone, and giving them credit.

Administrator participants were very complimentary of the wonderful job the nurses did of forming relationships with patients, given the current work environment. They acknowledged that in times of change and conflict, the most difficult role was the nurse on "the front line." There was a feeling that nurses are often given mixed messages from administrators, such as "give the best care, but keep the costs in line."

Administrators admitted that "nurses separate quality institutions from so-so institutions" and that nurses "are truly responsible for the patient." There was a sense that they have done a poor job letting the nurses know how they feel. "We get so mixed up in the business end of it," stated one administrator. And "by doing so, we forget who makes it all possible."

Profiting in the New Reality

Administrators viewed the nurse–patient relationship from a distance. However, as the discussions focused on costs and the future of health care, the administrators became directly involved in the process. They discussed cost, quality, and the need to provide the best care at the lowest cost. The great dilemma here was to increase the profits and provide high-quality care when reimbursement dollars have been greatly reduced.

Administrators were very vocal and articulate as they discussed the costs associated with health care and nurse–patient interactions. They detailed the associated costs and justified the reason for placing an emphasis on costs and the bottom line. When discussing the costs associated with nurse–patient interactions, administrators first identified reimbursement constraints. In their world, the issue of costs was synonymous with reimbursement. "Costs are irrelevant to me," stated one administrator. "I could charge whatever, but I'm only reimbursed at a certain level," explained another participant. In today's health care environment, administrators are faced with economic constraints. These constraints included "dealing with managed care," "receiving less Medicare dollars," and "treating all patients regardless of ability to pay." As one administrator stated, "The situation is changing much too fast and we have limited resource dollars available." Another stated, "We've become profit oriented, and we must be careful not to lose the humanistic approach in the process."

As administrator participants were accounting for costs, there was a concomitant accounting for the caring, which was part of the humanistic interactions between the nurse and the patient. When they discussed cost and quality, administrator participants were accounting for the caring.

One administrator viewed caring as a value-added interaction. From this point of view, "the benefits of the interaction outweigh the expense of the registered nurse." Another administrator felt "that given the educational preparation of RNs, they are going to be more attuned to creating a caring, empathetic tone." Administrators viewed caring as an "opportunity cost," "the cost of doing it right," and "the cost of providing quality," "If we want to be a quality institution, we need to realize the importance patients place on having a caring nurse," stated one administrator participant.

Administrators were actively involved and have responded to the changing health care environment. They viewed the future as a time of transition.

Continuing to do more with less was no longer a viable option, instead they were focused on finding ways to do it differently. From their perspective, hope for the future involved innovation and creativity. Profit-making strategies used by administrators as they were positioning for future survival included working with the community, streamlining the system, establishing new practice models, and marketing the hospital.

SUBSTANTIVE THEORY

Diminishing health care resources was the basic social problem encountered by nurses, patients, and administrators. The basic social process of the nurse–patient relationship in the current health care environment was "struggling to find a balance," which referred to sustaining the caring ideal in a new reality controlled by costs.

Nurses struggled to maintain humanistic caring and preserve the nurse–patient relationship in a cost-efficient managed care environment controlled by others. Caring as a relational concept was generally appraised as intangible, with little or no economic value in relation to cost. Nurses were practicing caring and continuing to value the nurse–patient relationship in an economic environment driven by the questions of "who will pay" and "how much will be paid."

Patients wondered what kind of health care would be available in the future. They desired quality care and caring when in the hospital but did not want to pay for health care out of their own pockets. There was a feeling of being entitled to care and caring despite the costs. Although many patients were fearful of being in the hospital in the future, there was a simultaneous recognition they could not afford to pay for private care either in the hospital or home. From their perspective, reducing reimbursement to hospitals translated into decreasing care.

Hospital administrators were walking the fine line between making a profit and providing quality care. They valued the caring relationship between nurse and patient while facing the challenge of shrinking reimbursement dollars. It was their responsibility to maintain profitability without sacrificing patient care.

IMPLICATIONS FOR NURSING PRACTICE

The substantive theory of "struggling to find a balance" has relevance to professional nursing practice. Nurses are practicing caring in an environment where the economics and costs of health care permeate discussions and impact decisions. The focus on costs is not a transient response to shrinking reimbursements; instead, it has become the catalyst for change within health care organizations. Nurses are entering into a new reality for practice that is controlled by costs.

Nurses are continuing to struggle with economic changes. It is a paradox in practice that nurses have fewer resource dollars and less time to provide patient education, while at the same time, the need is greater because of higher patient acuity levels. This means patients receive limited information on preventative care. As less information is available for patients to make future health care decisions, patients may be readmitted within 30 days after discharge with the same diagnosis. Recidivism is costly to patients and hospitals—costly to patients in terms of increased time required for recovery and costly to hospitals that may not be reimbursed for treatment. With a system goal of decreased length of stay and increased staffing ratios, nurses need to establish trust and initiate a caring relationship during their first encounter with a patient. As this relationship is being established, nurses need to focus on being, knowing, and doing all at once and being there from the patient perspective. For the nurse, this means completing a task while simultaneously engaging with a patient. This holistic approach to practice means knowing the patient as a person in all his or her complexity and then identifying the needs for professional nursing as they arise.

The foundation for professional caring is the blending of the humanistic and empirical aspects of care. In today's environment, the nurse needs to integrate caring, knowledge, and skills all at once. Given time constraints and reduced staffing, the art of caring cannot occur in isolation from meeting the physical needs of patients. When caring is defined solely as science, or as art, it is not adequate to reflect the reality of current practices. In this study, patients wanted a knowledgeable, competent, and confident registered nurse caring for them.

Nurses in this study valued caring and having a relationship with patients as important components of their practice. Economics and time constraints have made caring more difficult. Nurses are seeing the environment in which they practice reconfigured or redesigned in an effort to maintain the bottom line. However, their inability to understand and articulate the economics of practice has placed them in a situation where the only result is to contend with the cost constraints as they continue to deliver care at the bedside. Nurses felt frustrated and fearful in the current economic environment as they were struggling to provide for all the needs of their patients. Nurses are expected to care despite the obstacles; however, the nurses continue to care by trying to overcome obstacles and frustration. The resulting tension and struggle lets them go on.

While these nurses were frustrated, they still used caring in their practice. For example, caring in the moment suggested that even when there was only time to do the basics, nurses were communicating within a caring relationship while interacting with the patient. It was important for the nurses to find the time to be caring. The art of nursing, thus, is valued by nurses in practice.

IMPLICATIONS FOR NURSING ADMINISTRATION

The results of this study have implications for hospitals and nursing administration. Administrators state that they value caring and high-quality care. Their actions must then reflect these values to ensure that the caring philosophy of the hospital remains in the forefront of organizational profit making.

The issue of time constraints and inadequate staffing has been identified throughout this study. Nurses and patients viewed lack of time as a hindrance to forming a caring nurse–patient relationship. This points out the need for administrators to restructure the practice environment so that the maximum of nursing time is focused on caring nurse–patient interactions. Non-nursing tasks such as transcribing orders, making beds, and passing out water need to be redirected to ancillary personnel. If hospital administrators desire high levels of quality care, staffing ratios must be adequate in order to allow time for nurses to be with their patients.

Hospital administrators need to provide clear, concise information to the nurses on the topics of cost and quality. Presently, there are conflicting messages in which the top-level administrators say they value caring and high-quality care, but the meaning that is filtered down to the nurses is that the emphasis is on costs and making a profit.

CONCLUSION

Nursing practice occurs in the context of an environment that has been changing rapidly. Initially, the Clinton health care reform proposal identified nursing as a key resource for maintaining quality while decreasing costs.[26] Although major components of that proposal did not evolve as expected, the health care environment has changed drastically over the past eight years. Cost reduction pressure in terms of managed care and corporatization of health care has had an impact on nursing and hospitals.

Perhaps because the nursing profession did not clearly articulate various nursing roles and outcomes to others, cost-cutting efforts have been directed at registered nurses. Research in the areas of cost, caring, quality, and the nurse–patient relationship is necessary to shape health care policy and ensure the survival of professional nursing. This study represented a paradigm shift by examining the nurse–patient relationship within an economic context. The premise underpinning this study was to understand the experience of nurses who are practicing from a caring perspective in a changing environment focused on cost and quality.

Caring reflects quality and occurs in the interrelationship between nurse and patient. Although caring and economics may seem paradoxical, contemporary health care concerns emphasize the importance of understanding caring and quality in terms of cost. Findings from this study will help fill the gap among caring, quality, and cost in the current health care delivery system. Continued research in this area will provide essential information to the nursing profession for improving professional practice, advancing curriculum development, redesigning health care, and impacting health care policy.

ACKNOWLEDGMENTS

This research was part of a larger study sponsored by the Tri-Service Nursing Research Program (TSNRP#N95–017, MDA#905–95–Z–0038) and supported by a grant of $148,633 awarded to M. Ray, RN, PhD, Col. USAFR. The information or content and conclusions are those of the author and should not be construed as the official position or policy of, nor should any official endorsement be inferred by the Uniformed Services University of the Health Sciences, the Department of Defense, or the U.S. government.

REFERENCES

1. Hoggard-Green, J. (1995). *A phenomenological study of a consumer's definition of quality health care* (Ph.D. diss., University of Utah).
2. Lynaugh, J., & Fagin, C. (1988). Nursing comes of age. *Image: Journal of Nursing Scholarship, 20*(4), 184–190.
3. Bargagliotti, A., & Smith, H. (1985). Patterns of nursing costs with capitated reimbursement. *Nursing Economics, 3*(5), 270–275.
4. Curtin, L. (1983). Determining costs of nursing service per DRG. *Nursing Management, 14*(4), 16–20.
5. McCormick, B. (1986). What's the cost of nursing care? *Hospitals, 60*, 48–52.
6. Walker, D. (1983). The cost of nursing care in hospitals. *Journal of Nursing Administration, 13*(3), 13–18.
7. Miller, K. (1987). The human care perspective in nursing administration. *Journal of Nursing Administration, 17*(2), 10–12.
8. Miller, K. (1995). Keeping the care in nursing care. *Journal of Nursing Administration, 25*(11), 29–32.
9. Nyberg, J. (1990). Theoretical explorations of human care and economics: Foundations of nursing administration practice. *Advances in Nursing Science, 13*(1), 74–84.
10. Nyberg, J. (1991). The effects of care and economics on nursing practice. *Journal of Nursing Administration, 20*(5), 13–18.
11. Nyberg, J. (1998). *A caring approach in nursing administration.* Niwot, CO: University Press of Colorado.
12. Ray, M. (1987). Health care economics and human caring in nursing: Why the moral conflict must be resolved. *Family Community Health, 10*(1), 35–43.
13. Ray, M. (1989). The theory of bureaucratic caring for nursing practice in the organizational culture. *Nursing Administration Quarterly, 13*(2), 31–42.
14. Ray, M. (1997). Existential authenticity: An ethical theory of nursing administrative caring art. *Canadian Journal of Nursing Research, 29*(1), 111–126.
15. Turkel, M., & Ray, M. (2000). Relational complexity: A theory of the nurse–patient

relationship within an economic context. *Nursing Science Quarterly, 13*(4), 106–113.

16. Valentine, K. (1989). Caring is more than kindness: Modeling its complexities. *Journal of Nursing Administration, 19*(11), 28–34.

17. Valentine, K. (1991). Comprehensive assessment of caring and its relationship to outcome measures. *Journal of Nursing Quality Assurance, 5*(2), 59–68.

18. Buerhaus, P. (1986). The economics of caring, challenges, and new opportunities for nursing. *Topics in Clinical Nursing, 8*(2), 13–21.

19. Duffy, J. (1992). The impact of nurse caring on patient outcomes. In D. Grant (Ed.), *The presence of caring in nursing.* New York, NY: National League of Nursing.

20. Issel, L., & Kahn, D. (1998). The economic value of caring. *Health Care Management Review, 23*(4), 43–53.

21. Larson, P., & Ferketich, S. (1999). Patients' satisfaction with nurses' caring during hospitalization. *Western Journal of Nursing Research, 15*(6), 690–707.

22. Valentine, K. (1997). Exploration of the relationship between caring and costs. *Holistic Nursing Practice, 11*(4), 71–81.

23. Foa, U. (1971). Interpersonal and economic resources. *Science, 171*(29), 345–351.

24. Glaser, B., & Strauss, A. (1967). *The discovery of grounded theory: Strategies for qualitative research.* Hawthorne, NY: Aldine De Gruyther.

25. Glaser, B. (1978). *Theoretical sensitivity.* MillValley, CA: Sociology Press.

26. Marshall, W., & Schram, W. (1993). *Mandate for change.* New York, NY: Berkley Books.

QUESTIONS FOR REFLECTION

Baccalaureate

1. What substantive theory emerged from Turkel's research?
2. What research method was used by Turkel? Who were the participants?
3. What are the three interpersonal resources described by Foa and cited by Turkel?

Master's

1. Is the substantive theory still relevant to contemporary nursing practice? Why or why not?
2. How are the economics issues discussed by Turkel the same or different than those identified by Nyberg in 1990?
3. How was the concept of caring described by the registered nurses in Turkel's study? How was this similar or different to caring described by patients and administrators?

Doctoral

1. Buerhaus challenged nurse researchers to conduct interviews that would yield economic or dollar value when studying humanistic nursing behaviors. What questions would you ask of patients?
2. In response to the above question, what type of study design would you use? How would you do data analysis?
3. Review the administrators' responses to caring and economics. Are these still applicable to practice? Is cost still the major concern of administrators? Use cited references in response to the last question.

35

Exploration of the Relationship Between Caring and Cost

Kathleen L. Valentine

*I*ssues of cost are rarely considered part of holistic nursing practice. Yet in the United States, the economic forces of health care are integral to the effectiveness of nursing care delivery. Economic forces determine who can access health care, what their health services will be, which provider will deliver those services, and who will pay the service costs. Therefore, both cost and quality need to be addressed because they relate to patient outcomes through the examination of the costs and outcomes of nursing interventions performed.[1]

This chapter examines professional nurse caring as a holistic nursing process and explores its relationship to cost. This poses a challenge because *caring* and *cost* are complex and ambiguous terms that are often assumed to be simple and well understood. Such assumptions can lead to errors in decision making as they relate to both caring and cost and ultimately can affect the quality of patient care. The assumptions embedded in caring and cost need to be examined systematically and valid instruments for their measurement must be applied.

THE IMPERATIVE FOR COST EFFECTIVENESS IN NURSING CARE DELIVERY

As more emphasis is placed on cost containment and promotion of quality care in a cost-effective manner, the emphasis on cost and caring will also increase. This is true because payers are concerned about costs and consumers demand humanistic interventions. Patients wish to be treated as partners in, not passive recipients of, their care; to have information with which they can make informed choices; to have caregivers devote sufficient time to them so that their needs are met; to have their problems considered from a broad rather than a narrow perspective so that their total needs are assessed; to have caregivers show sensitivity to their unique ways of interpreting problems; and to have caregivers show sensitivity to their feelings.[2,3] Patients are more concerned with how humanely they are treated than with cost, convenience, or waiting time.[4]

Nurses can engage in the process of determining which services are most cost-effective through systematic measurement of nursing's contribution to the effectiveness of patient care.[5–7] The multivariate nature of clinical care and patient outcomes attributable to nursing practice must be examined.[8,9] Two outcomes relevant to the effectiveness of nursing practice are caring and patient satisfaction. Caring is a multidimensional construct that consists of attributes of the nurse such as professional knowledge and competence, vigilance, and therapeutic interactions with patients and families.[10–13] Inclusion of the consumer's perspective in the treatment

From Valentine, K. L. (1997). Exploration of the relationship between caring and cost. *Holistic Nursing Practice, 11*(4), 71–81. Permission to reprint granted by Wolters Kluwer.

process is essential "to study patients as people and not simply as organs, diseases, conditions, or disabilities."[14(p. 60)] Although quantitative exploration and measurement of caring are fraught with difficulty, "further development of caring outcomes is one way that nursing can balance the reductionistic focus of the current health care system."[6(p. 31)] In addition, nurses influence on health care policy changes will be enhanced through determination of the cost of nursing care.[15,16]

The real challenge, however, "is to develop measures of cost-effectiveness rather than of cost alone."[17(p. 70)] The monetary measures of cost must be expanded to include a broader definition of costs related to patient outcomes. Standardized definitions of cost and systems for patient classification are not currently applied regionally, nationally, or internationally through the use of a single nursing minimum data set. Thus, nursing's argument for resources to support caring lacks the necessary power and precision to convince health care policymakers and financiers to reallocate resources based on changing health care needs.

INSTITUTIONAL STRATEGIES FOR COST-EFFECTIVENESS

In response to economic pressures, many institutions are implementing cost containment nursing care delivery systems, in which registered nurses are being replaced with unlicensed patient care technicians.[18] These assistive personnel are not educated in the same manner as registered nurses to provide professional vigilance. The registered nurse is educationally prepared to detect subtle changes in patient condition that can lead to complications. Aiken[16] gives the example of a patient's request for a blanket. The registered nurse will assess the meaning of the patient's request in this situation by asking: Is this patient cold because of postoperative shock? Assistive personnel, on the other hand, may comply with what appears to be a simple request without further question.

This example is supported by research on differences in mortality rates. Higher mortality rates in some hospitals have been traced to a "failure to rescue."[16] That is, subtle changes in the patient's clinical condition are not recognized early enough, which leads to deterioration in the patient's condition. As acuity increases in hospitalized patients, there is less margin for error between observation and action. Clinical assessment and professional judgment cannot be delegated. Comprehensive caring requires professional vigilance, a crucial dimension of caring.[13,19]

Patient assessment becomes even more crucial as patients are admitted at higher levels of acuity and are discharged sooner. Determination of the proper mix of nursing personnel is an area of current research activity. Aiken's[16] national analysis of staffing trends found that the health care industry currently employs more registered nurses than ever before. It is surprising that the number of nursing assistive personnel employed in hospitals has actually declined, contributing to less total nursing care delivered. Furthermore, at a time when hospitalized patients are admitted with higher acuity and shorter lengths of stay, the ratio of registered nurses to hospitalized patients has remained steady. Therefore, determination of the optimal mix of registered nurses and assistive personnel to provide needed surveillance is crucial to patient safety, patient outcomes, and cost.[16]

Accountability and authority for both direct and delegated care are essential in the registered nurse's role for the coordination of all-care provided to the patient. Patients expect and acknowledge this role as a central component of caring.[20,21] This requires nurses to have professional autonomy, control over their practice, good communication with physicians, and organizational support for the primacy of patient care. Therefore, organization and management of the professional practice environment are essential for quality patient care.[16,21] Intentional creation of a care-focused practice environment staffed by the optimal mix of personnel can advance caring as a central, visible value in nursing practice.

PROBLEMS INHERENT IN THE DEFINITION OF COST

When costs associated with caring are examined, the following question needs to be asked: What costs and to whom? Costs are experienced by providers, patients, hospital/health care agencies, and insurers in different ways. What is the cost of a medication error to the nurse? To the patient? What is the cost of patients' dissatisfaction with a particular hospital or agency? How does the cost of this dissatisfaction differ for the insurer, health maintenance organization, and hospital? When practice is sub-optimal, what is the cost to the nurse in lost satisfaction with one's own performance in comparison with professional practice standards? How do those costs differ for the patient, nurse, insurer, patient's family, and hospital? How are different people in the system affected when the length of stay is different than anticipated? Who pays for health care costs and in what currency? Materials, time, money, and human factors are all currencies, used by individuals, families, organizations, and society in the payment of health care costs.

A recent dramatic example is the cost-shifting related to length of maternity stay in hospitals. Managed care organizations cut their costs through limiting maternity care to 24 hours or less. This shifted certain costs to mothers, families, and public health agencies. Nurses and others in society raised a collective outcry, which caused congressional and presidential review of the practice and federal intervention to stop such cost shifting. This is just one example of a broad definition of cost that extends beyond the dollars expended by a specific type of payer. Such cost-shifting is an attribute of all economic systems and happens regularly in our dynamic health care system. Principles of caring nursing practice call for nurses to be alert to other such examples and to examine the overall effect of such cost-shifting on the quality of patient care delivery systems.

MONETARY COSTS

Even if the definition of cost is narrowed solely to the financial costs incurred by a given institution, the lack of uniform definitions for direct, indirect, productive, and nonproductive nursing time makes it difficult to calculate costs even within a single institution. Comparisons across institutions become even more difficult and of questionable validity (i.e., are we really measuring what we think we are?). We need to be certain that we clarify how costs are derived and on what assumptions costs are based.

The goal appears simple enough: Identify what it is that nurses do for their patients, determine what it costs, and set a price to recover those costs. On review of the literature, however, it quickly becomes apparent that historically nursing charges have been buried in room and board charges. As a result, little research was done on this topic until prospective payment changed the way in which costs and revenue are examined within the health care industry. Disagreement about definitions and methods makes comparisons questionable. Nursing service, as a major component of hospitalization, must be able to identify its product, determine its cost, and price it competitively for the marketplace.

RELATED MARKET RESEARCH

Market research does broaden some definitions of costs to include patient satisfaction and patient choice of health care service setting. Market research examines the needs and wants of consumers as well as factors that motivate their purchasing behaviors. Nursing services have been found to be an important aspect of health care services marketing.[22] For example, a study of 156,000 patient admissions over 2 years and eight hospitals revealed that nurses' attitudes and nursing services accounted for 25% of the total satisfaction of patients. The next highest single category contributing to satisfaction was physician attitudes, at 2%. Therefore, based on this study, nursing services and nurse attitudes have a great deal to do with patient satisfaction.

Patient satisfaction is also considered important for marketing.[2] Satisfaction is achieved in part through provision of personalized care services, which has been shown to lower patient anxiety and increase patient satisfaction with care. This in turn has the effect of decreasing "shopping around" for health care, which increases continuity of care, patient compliance, and patient quality of life. With the expansion of managed care systems, consumers have a choice among plans. Enrollee satisfaction with services is a factor in the decision to continue with a particular plan or switch to an alternative.

Patient satisfaction, caring, and marketing are integrally related, although not identical constructs. In another study, a high perceived presence of caring correlated with high patient satisfaction with nursing care but had no relationship with other dimensions of patient satisfaction.[23]

RELATIONSHIP OF MARKET RESEARCH TO COST

Although patient satisfaction may be an important outcome indicator of nurse caring, patient satisfaction alone is not sufficient. Other factors, such as actual change in clinical condition and length of stay, are also important. If patients are satisfied but are not having a good recovery or if patients are satisfied but are overstaying the average length of stay, then the cost for obtaining that satisfaction is too high. If, however, patients can be satisfied, have good recovery, and do not exceed the length of stay, then the optimal conditions have been reached for health, marketing, and economics. It has been found that satisfaction with health services correlates with clients' perceived gain from treatment as well as with their realistic gain from treatment.[19,24]

Thus, the creation of caring treatment environments that address affect, cognition, actions, and interactions is good for patient outcomes and system outcomes. This supports the contention that nurses cannot simply attend to task but also must attend to both processes and patient perceptions of their effectiveness.

DEFINITION AND MEASUREMENT OF CARING

Professional nurse caring can be viewed as "those cognitive and culturally learned action behaviors, techniques, processes, and patterns that enable (or help) an individual, family, or community to improve or maintain a favorably healthy condition or life way."[25(p. 7)] Patterns include demonstration of professional knowledge and skill, surveillance, and reassuring presence; recognition of individual qualities and needs, promotion of autonomy, and time spent; and action taken to satisfy patient need. Satisfaction of the identified patient need is undertaken in a manner that conveys to the patient recognition and appreciation of the patient's worth and autonomy.[26]

Although there can be caring without curing, there cannot be curing without caring.[27] Caring is integral to the healing process. As mentioned earlier, caring can also be defined as a multidimensional construct that consists of attributes of the nurse such as professional knowledge and competence, vigilance, and therapeutic interactions with patients and families.[10,11,28,29]

In Valentine's[13] conceptual model of caring, the core of caring consists of psychologic elements (which are affective or cognitive in nature) put into action in an interaction that is either social or physical in nature. These core psychologic elements of caring are strongly influenced by philosophical beliefs, such as ethics, socialization processes, and cultural norms. Psychologic elements of caring are also influenced by structural elements in the environment, such as the available technology and resources, as well as by social organizational processes in the work environment. Thus, caring is understood to encompass affect, cognition, and action. These dimensions are then demonstrated in interactions with patients that are focused on communication processes, teaching and learning, or the provision of comfort care. The core elements of caring (affect, cognition, action, and interaction) have more of an effect in a particular caring encounter than philosophical and structural dimensions of caring.[13,21]

Multiple dimensions of nurse caring are well supported by other investigators.[10,11,25,30–33] Nurses' professional view of caring differs from patients' "folk" view of caring; this has been demonstrated empirically.[27,34] Patients view caring as a gestalt, whereas nurses view it as having distinct facets.[21,28] Less prominent in nurses' view of caring are cognitive and technical aspects of nurse–patient interactions, whereas these cognitive and technical aspects of caring are centrally integrated into patients' view of caring. This last point supports Weiss'[33] work, which suggests that, to be viewed as caring, nurses' must be competent. The reasons for these differences in patient and nurse perceptions of caring may be related to how nurses are educated about dimensions of caring. If they have learned that caring is something separate from competence, then they will separate the two ideas. Patients experience the caring encounter as a whole, inclusive of caring and competence.

MEASUREMENT OF CARING

Based on a multidimensional definition of caring, two 61-item, Likert type, paired surveys were developed: the Patient Caring Questionnaire (PCQ) and the Nurse Caring Questionnaire (NCQ).[23] The PCQ and NCQ are grounded in the combined experiences of both nurses and patients and examine the interaction between nurses and patients in specific encounters. This measurement approach represents the interactive phenomenon reflective of a shared experience between nurses and patients. This grounded experience of nurse–patient caring was derived from explorations of the contextual meaning of caring using various stakeholder groups (nurses, patients, nurse managers, nurse theorists, and health care administrators). The PCQ and NCQ both have three subscales. The Affective, Cognitive, Ethical (ACE) subscale measures those attributes of the nurse that tend to be interpersonal qualities rather than action behaviors. The Professional Vigilance (PV) subscale contains knowledge-based behaviors and processes that the nurse performs to help the patient be safe. The Interaction (INT) subscale includes communication processes, teaching/learning activities, and physical comfort measures.[19]

SPECIFIC RESEARCH LINKS BETWEEN CARING AND COST

In two different studies, specific measures of caring episodes in nurse–patient pairs were assessed in relation to outcome indicators of patient satisfaction, length of stay, and postoperative clinical condition. One study was conducted with 91 hysterectomy patients and the nurses who cared for them; the second study involved 350 male and female medical–surgical patients. The NCQ and PCQ paired surveys ($\alpha = 0.92$) were administered to patients and the nurses who cared for those patients after an 8-hour shift. The instruments measured each respondent's perceptions about the degree to which affective, cognitive, and interactional dimensions of caring were present during nursing encounters. Caring was measured by the NCQ and PCQ, and costs were measured by the following:

- *Patient length of stay*: The number of days in the hospital as determined by chart audit.
- *Cost of nursing care*: An isolation of the cost of nursing care per patient acuity point calculated for the individual patient's cost of nursing care. Patient acuity was based on the intensity of nursing services required. The higher the acuity, the greater the nursing services required. A second measure was based on trend data at the unit level and was based on nursing salaries per hour of patient care extracted from monthly cost accounting reports.
- *Patient knowledge of medication*: This was assessed before discharge by the nurse data collectors, who identified patients' discharge medications by chart review and by interview of the patient and nurse using the Nurse Continuous Improvement Indicators instrument.
- *Patient satisfaction with nursing care and the hospital*: Within 24 hours of anticipated discharge, patients answered questions related to satisfaction through interviews conducted by nurse data collectors.[35]
- *Postoperative complications*: This index was derived from chart audit after discharge. The index recorded whether

the patient had a return to surgery, postoperative fever greater than 101°F that required antibiotics, or other unanticipated results.[23]

RESULTS

Costs and benefits associated with caring are not only those directly associated with interactions between the registered nurse and the patient but also those associated with how that caring relationship affects the patient's perceptions of the hospital and his or her choice of where to seek future health care services. In two different studies that used the NCQ and PCQ to examine cost–caring relationships, patients' responses on the PCQ were substantially related to their overall satisfaction with the hospital. This supports the idea that positive experiences with caring in nurse–patient encounters affect consumers' choices of where to go for health services.[23,36]

Positive caring interactions can exert a healing effect on patients' recovery, which is consistent with a holistic view of health care, and can positively affect health outcomes. In one study, patients' perceptions of caring on the PCQ were predictive of their knowledge of medications at the time of discharge; nurses' perceptions of caring on the NCQ were also predictive of the patients' knowledge of medications at the time of discharge.[36] Thus, effective caring contributes to patients' readiness to leave the hospital. Patients and nurses agree that caring practices help patients know about their medications. This includes the ability to identify the medication, the reason to take it, and the time for administration as well as special instructions.

In the same study, patients' perceptions of caring correlated strongly with their perceptions of their satisfaction with nurses but weakly with their satisfaction with physicians or facilities.[36] This pattern suggests that patients' perceptions of caring, as measured by the PCQ, are specific to nurses and not a global measure of all caregivers' services or personal attributes (such items often appear on patient satisfaction questionnaires).

In another study, multiple regression analyses for responses to the NCQ and PCQ caring questionnaires were predictive of patient satisfaction, postoperative clinical condition, and length of stay.[32] In a repeat study with a larger sample, this pattern was not demonstrated at a statistically significant level, but patients' perceptions of caring correlated strongly with their overall rating of the hospital.[36] The greater the perceived presence of caring by patients, the higher their overall rating of the hospital. Interestingly, nurse and patient responses showed that these groups have different ways of predicting different outcomes. Specifically, patients' caring scores were consistently related to satisfaction but not as consistently related to length of stay or clinical outcome variables. Nurses caring scores, when compared against any outcome variables, were related to clinical outcomes and length of stay. This pattern of responses is interesting in that each group's perceptions of caring were related most strongly to the outcome variable with which the particular group was most familiar. Patients know about the nature of their own satisfaction. Nurses, by virtue of their role and expertise, are more aware of clinical outcomes.[36]

These different patterns of relationships with outcome variables provide further evidence of the differences between nurses and patients in the context of caring, which may be due to their role differences. Patients caring scores correlated primarily with patient satisfaction outcome variables. Their scores on the ACE subscale were consistently related to their satisfaction with the hospital overall. Their scores on the PV and INT subscales were related to satisfaction with

nursing care. This pattern of relationships is interesting because both these subscales have to do with what the nurse does rather than who the nurse is. What the nurse does contributes more to the patients' specific satisfaction with nursing care than a global judgment about the overall hospital. Hospital preference was most strongly related to the patients' and the nurses' scores on the INT subscale (teaching, learning, and interventions), which again represents nursing actions versus nurses' attributes. Other patterns identified included the following: Patients' scores were differentially related to satisfaction outcome variables, indicating a multidimensional rather than a unit-dimensional nature of caring; and patient caring items were strongly related to measures of satisfaction with nursing and not to satisfaction with physician care, housekeeping, or parking.[23]

IMPLICATIONS AND RECOMMENDATIONS

The measurement of caring and other subjective-judgmental phenomena, which often are key to quality patient care, goes beyond the tally of tasks completed and requires greater discrimination and the formulation of special techniques. "Measuring productivity by totaling the number of tasks is like measuring an author's work by counting the number of words."[37(p. 7)] Trying to assess the value and contribution of nursing in such a way ignores the essence of nursing's professional activity, which is caring. To answer questions about the relationship between caring and cost, individual institutions will need to implement studies that ensure that there are clear definitions of terms, variables, and the assumptions embedded within them. Full exploration of the meaning of cost and caring is necessary to avoid errors in data collection, analyses, and interpretation of results.

Thus, comprehensive studies that use a broad range of patient and system outcomes can provide better data for decision making about where to allocate resources for quality patient care delivery.

Both caring and cost are complex phenomena that are central to understanding health care service delivery systems. Because of their importance, issues of cost and caring require greater clarity and precision in measurement. The studies discussed in this chapter were focused on inpatient services; these concepts need to be explored further in other service sites.

For the practicing nurse, the following recommendations can be made:

- Realize the holistic and multidimensional nature of caring and what is known about its effect on nurse–patient encounters. Use this understanding when exploring nursing care delivery systems so that care-focused practice environments can be designed and delivered.
- Stay alert to issues of cost-shifting that go beyond short-term monetary considerations within your particular practice setting. Ask questions about how cost is being defined and calculated. Cost savings in one area may lead to cost over-runs in another. Short-term savings gained through the substitution of assistive personnel for registered nurses may lead to long-term costs in the form of less professional vigilance and its consequences for patient outcomes. Alternatively, overuse of registered nurses for nonnursing tasks may drive up the cost of services, ultimately denying fiscal support for other health care needs. Determining the right mix of personnel for the right functions is one of the most challenging issues that the health care system faces. Nurses need to be active in the discourse on these issues.
- Participate in the governance structures within your organization that deal with practice issues and include cost and caring issues as part of your focus. Participate in nursing organizations outside your agency to keep this concern part of nursing's agenda for action.
- If the cost of nursing care is being monitored in your agency, work within your governance structure to collaborate with finance to determine how nursing workload is defined and measured. Work with finance personnel to develop a definition of direct nursing costs that stays close to costs that are directly traceable to the delivery of patient care services. Also, determine definitions for indirect nursing costs and nonnursing costs.
- Work with the finance department to integrate clinical and financial information into a database that is useful for decision making.
- Classify patients using a reliable and valid patient classification system that reflects the essence of nursing and include nursing process elements as well as specific nursing tasks. The classification of patients must be related to the nursing care provided, not simply to what has been predicted as required, and it should be documented in the patient chart.
- Consider incorporating measures of caring (such as the NCQ and PCQ) into continuous quality improvement activities so that caring's importance is evident in core practice issues. As changes are made within care delivery systems, their impact on dimensions of caring can then be tracked and incorporated into improvements in practice.
- Accept costs as an inherent part of holistic nursing practice that requires attention. Nurses' detachment from issues of cost of care delivery leaves them without a voice to realize their vision of nursing care and contributes to errors in resource allocation decisions, which ultimately affect the quality of patient care.

REFERENCES

1. Wilson, A. (1993). The cost and quality of patient outcomes: A look at managed competition. *Nursing Administration Quarterly, 17,* 11–16.
2. MacStravic, R. S. (1986). Therapeutic pampering. *Hospital & Health Services Administration, 31,* 59–69.
3. Heffring, M. P., Neilsen, E. J., Szklarz, M. J., & Dobson, G. S. (1986). High tech, high touch: Common denominators in patient satisfaction. *Hospital & Health Services Administration, 31,* 81–93.
4. Anderson, R. M., Fleming, G. V., & Aday, L. A. (1981). The public's view as input for medical manpower training. In Center for Health Policy Research (Ed.). *Socioeconomic issues of health.* Chicago, IL: American Medical Association.
5. Hegyvary, S. T. (1992). Issues in outcomes research. *Journal of Nursing Quality Assurance, 5,* 1–6.
6. Lang, N. M., & Marek, K. D. (1991). Outcomes that reflect clinicai practice. In National Center for Nursing Research (Ed.), *Practice outcomes research: Examining the effectiveness of nursing practice.* Rockville, MD: National Center for Nursing Research.
7. Aiken, L. H., & Fagin, C. M. (1992). *Charting nursing's future: Agenda for the 1990s.* Philadelphia, PA: Lippincott.
8. Hinshaw, A. S. (1991). Welcome: Patient outcomes research conference. In National Center for Nursing Research (Ed.), *Practice outcomes research: Examining the effectiveness of nursing practice.* Rockville. MD: National Center for Nursing Research.
9. Murdaugh, C.(1991). Quality of life, functional status, and patient satisfaction. In National Center for Nursing Research (Ed.), *Practice outcomes research: Examining the effectiveness of nursing practice.* Rockville. MD: National Center for Nursing Research.
10. Ray, M. A. (1984). The development of a classification system of institutional caring. In M. Leininger (Ed.), *Care: The essence of nursing and health.* Thorofare, NJ: Slack.
11. Ray, M. A. (1987). Health care economics and human caring in nursing: Why the moral conflict must be resolved. *Family & Community Health, 10,* 35–43.
12. Stiles, M. K. (1990). The shining stranger: Nurse–family spiritual relationship. *Cancer Nursing, 13,* 235–245.
13. Valentine, K. L. (1989). Caring is more than kindness: Modeling its complexities. *The Journal of Nursing Administration, 19,* 28–35.

14. Crane, S. C. (1991). A research agenda for outcomes research. In National Center for Nursing Research (Ed.). *Practice outcomes research: Examining the effectiveness of nursing practice.* Rockville, MD: National Center for Nursing Research.
15. Huckabay, L. M. D. (1988). Allocation of resources and identification of issues in determining the cost of nursing sciences. *Nursing Administration Quarterly, 13,* 72–82.
16. Aiken, L. (1996). Restructuring hospitals: Considering patient outcomes. *Keynote address at the Midwest Alliance in Nursing 17th Annual Conference* September 12–14. Indianapolis, IN.
17. Johnson, M. (Ed.). (1989). *Series on nursing administration* (Vol. 2). Menlo Park, CA: Addison-Wesley.
18. Frusti, D. K. (1995). *Comparison of costs between two experimental nursing care delivery systems using new assistive roles and the current system.* Winona. MN: Winona State University, Thesis.
19. Valentine, K. L. (1991). Comprehensive assessment of caring and its relationship to outcome measures. *Journal of Nursing Quality Assurance, 5,* 59–68.
20. Valentine, K. L. (1989). Contributions to the theory of care. *Eval Program Plan, 12,* 17–24.
21. Valentine, K. L., Stiles, M. K., & Mangan, D. B. (1995). *Values, vision, and action: creating a care focused nursing practice environment.* New York, NY: National League for Nursing.
22. Casarreal, K. M., Mills, J. I., & Plant, M. A. (1986). Improving service through patient surveys in a multihospital organization. *Hospital & Health Services Administration, 31,* 41–52.
23. Valentine, K. L. (1989). *The value of caring nurses: Implications for patient satisfaction, quality of care, and cost.* Ithaca, New York, NY: Cornell University; Thesis.
24. Nguyen, T. D., Attkisson, C. C., & Stegner, B. L. (1983). Assessment for patient satisfaction: Development and refinement of a service evaluation questionnaire. *Eval Program Plan, 6,* 299–314.
25. Leininger, M. (1981). Some philosophical, historical, and taxonomic aspects of nursing and caring in the American culture. In M. Leininger (Ed.), *Care: An essential human need.* Thorofare, NJ: Slack.
26. Brown, L. (1986). The experience of care: Patient perspective. *Topics in Clinical Nursing, 8,* 56–62.
27. Leininger, M. (1984). Care: The essence of nursing and health. In M. Leininger (Ed.), *Care: The essence of nursing and health.* Thorofare, NJ: Slack.

28. Valentine, K. L. (1991). Nurse/patient caring: Challenging our conventional wisdom. In D. Gaut & M. Leininger (Eds.), *Caring: The compassionate healer.* New York, NY: National League for Nursing.

29. Stiles, M. K. (1988). *The shining stranger: A phenomenological investigation of nurse–family spiritual relationship.* Denver, CO: University of Colorado Health Sciences Center School of Nursing; Thesis.

30. Gaut, D. A. (1984). A theoretic description of caring as action. In M. Leininger (Ed.), *Care: The essence of nursing and health.* Thorofare, NJ: Slack.

31. Riemen, D. J. (1986). Noncaring and caring in the clinical setting: Patients' descriptions. *Topics in Clinical Nursing, 8,* 30–36.

32. Watson, J. (1985). *Nursing: Human science and human care.* Norwalk, CT: Appleton-Century-Crofts.

33. Weiss, C. J. (1986). Perceptions of nursing caring. *Dissertation Abstracts International, 47* (05), 1932. University Microfilms AdG86-18912.

34. Leininger, M. (1995). *Transcultural nursing: Concepts, theories, research and practices* (2nd ed.). New York, NY: McGraw-Hill.

35. Stiles, M. K., & Valentine, K. L. (1992). *A systems evaluation of the effects of two new nursing care delivery systems on the quality, effectiveness, and cost of patient care and on patient outcomes.* Proposal submitted to the Nursing Research Committee, Mayo Medical Center, Rochester, MN.

36. Valentine, K. L., & Stiles, M. K. (1993). *Nurses' effectiveness measured by caring questionnaires.* Proposal submitted to Studies of Clinical Outcomes and Nursing Practice, National Institute on Nursing Research, Rockville, MD.

37. Curtin, L. (1986). Nursing in the year 2000: Learning of the future. *Nurse Manage, 17,* 7–8.

QUESTIONS FOR REFLECTION

Baccalaureate

1. What type of patient satisfaction data is being collected in the organization where you are currently working or doing a practice rotation?
2. How does Valentine define caring? How does Valentine define cost?
3. Valentine discusses the concept of professional vigilance. Provide an example of how this concept is applied in the organization where you are currently working or doing a practice rotation.

Master's

1. What are the various definitions of caring (by scholars other than Valentine) that are discussed within this chapter?
2. Given the contemporary patterns of health care reimbursement, is patient length of stay still a valid measure of costs? Why or why not?
3. Valentine described positive caring interactions having a healing effect on patient's recovery. Provide an example of this within the organization where you are currently working or doing a practice rotation. If no example is available, what data would you review given the patient population being served?

Doctoral

1. Review the original Patient Caring Questionnaire and Nurse Caring Questionnaire. Are they still applicable to contemporary nursing practice? Support your response with cited references.
2. If you were going to add or delete any questions from the original Patient Caring Questionnaire and Nurse Caring Questionnaire, what would they be? Support your response with cited references.
3. What research question would you ask to replicate Valentine's original studies using the Patient Caring Questionnaire and Nurse Caring Questionnaire?

36

Leading Via Caring–Healing: The Fourfold Way Toward Transformative Leadership

JEAN WATSON

*I*n this waning hour of an outmoded era of nursing administration and health delivery that seeks sick and well care reform—an outdated era that applies economic indicators of care that view control, management, and health maintenance as cost containment; that acknowledges uncertainty, chaos, and complexity as a threatening norm; that is confused, if not hostile, to models of alternative-complementary medicine; that has distorted authentic caring practices—how is it that nursing administrators can survive? Especially, how can nursing administrators and leaders survive with their own vocational voice and form of authentic leadership that sustain systems of caring and healing? How can they remain intact with their own values? How can they sustain coherence and integrity for self, system, and society in a postmodern world that is turning upside down and inside out, seeking a new order in human health?

One way, one path, one road is the road less taken. The road I am referring to actually has four directions, four paths toward caring and healing, for self and system; this so-called fourfold way is inherent in any true transformative, visionary leadership.

Matthew Fox describes this fourfold path as the four *Via*.[1] It is a personal–professional journey through the four sacred directions of life itself, but ultimately leading to a new horizon, a new clearing, and a new vision of hope. This fourfold way—the path, the *Via*—can inform nursing administrators as they seek another way through the chaos and confusion during this critical transition and provide a turning point in health and human history.

VIA NEGATIVA

The *Via Negativa* is the path of acknowledging the shadow side of our lives and work. It requires going into the dark, shadowy side of our issues, realizing that we have been in an institutional desert during this modem era and have depleted ourselves and our systems of the human spirit that sustains and heals. From "daring the dark," as Fox says, we can put new light on our obstacles and difficulties. This path of entering and daring the dark, dealing with and naming the *negativa*, also allows us to enter and dwell in the space in which germination and patience reside, the space from which new life comes from the dark time of dormancy.

Nursing's dormant, value-based vision of caring and healing and wholeness

---

From Watson, J. (2000). Leading via caring–healing: The fourfold way toward transformative leadership. *Nursing Administration Quarterly, 25*(1), 1–6. Permission to reprint granted by Wolters Kluwer.

is emerging from the dark side of history to help to reestablish light and balance in systems and society that are out of balance. As nursing leaders rethink nursing's place and purpose, it is about to emerge from the dark and reenter the health care arena at this turning point in history. As it does, we see that new life, new germination, and new light is being brought into those spaces and places where there has been institutional darkness. Nursing's value-guided vision of care—caring for the human condition, for the embodied spirit seeking wholeness and healing—must gain voice as part of nursing leaders' true vocation.

From this *Via Negativa*, nursing leaders can acknowledge that nursing, and its phenomena of caring and the human health–illness healing experience, embraces the dark and light as the paradox of existence for both self and system. By the *Via Negativa*, nursing and nursing leaders draw upon the ancient voices from the past, from our ancestors, the mythological ancient ones who are the guardians of Mother Earth. From this rich heritage, nursing leaders call upon and bring forth healing energy from the four sacred directions—North, South, East, and West. These symbolize the primary elements of the universe: earth, air, fire, and water, which are essential for the survival of humanity and planet Earth alike.

Angeles Arrien suggests that this *Via Negativa* is the way of the (spiritual) warrior.[2] Through this path, this *Via*, we are called "to show up and choose to be present" to our purpose, authentically available and mindful of that which calls us toward compassionate service. This *Via* honors the shadow aspects, the wounded aspect of our self and our systems. This *Via* gives new voice and meaning to nursing's call to care in systems and settings in which care is perverted into slogans and platitudes and transmuted into economic jargon.

Underneath, there is a deep institutional and human wound needing to be named, in order for deep healing to occur at this time of crisis of noncaring in schools, systems, and society alike. By following the *Via Negativa*, we are led to the next path, the *Via Positiva*.

VIA POSITIVA

By following this path, nursing leaders can pause with gratitude for the special blessings, the privileged space and place we hold in the lives of humans and systems alike. It is by this path of bringing forth the light of positive, loving, caring energy into our work and world, wherever we may be, that we are replenished, and in turn we are more able to replenish others. As Fox said, by *Via Positiva* we can remind ourselves to "fall in love at least three times a day." This can occur whether it is falling in love with the new spring leaf on the budding tree; the snow flake on the eyelash; the miracle of the breath of life itself; or the look in the face of a friend, colleague, or patient that conveys the love and depth of human spirit, revealed whole to us in a given moment.

Once we open to the *Via Positiva*, we can find caring moments of joy and beauty, grace and gratitude, throughout all our day, every day. *Via Positiva* is an awakened consciousness that opens our hearts to carry the joy–sad heart paradoxically side by side, honoring the grace of both dark–light as the yin–yang of the human condition.

Through nursing leaders' ability to dwell in the grace and gratitude of the gifts of caring ·and healing, they offer human contact, human-to-human connection, creating healing environments, becoming ontological artists and architects,[3] creating spaces and a professional culture whereby caring–healing practices flourish. Through this path of *Via Positiva*, nursing leaders and administrators are nourished by the reciprocal processes of caring–healing. Thus, new energy, new light, new positive creations, and original solutions are more able to emerge from walking this *Via*.

Arrien's fourfold path corresponds to *Via Positiva* through what she acknowledges as the Way of the Healer—one who pays attention to what has heart and meaning. One takes this path from the inside out, finding one's own inner voice and unique gifts. That path in turn translates this inner voice into informed, compassionate action that serves both self and system. This *Via* reminds us that "Caring is a Passage to the Heart," and on this *Via Positiva*, nursing leaders give mindful attention to what has heart.[4]

VIA CREATIVA

Once we have honored the heartfelt journey of the *Via Negativa*, crossed into and learned to dwell in grace and gratitude with the *Via Positiva* of our existence and purpose; once we have begun to more clearly, more consciously assume our voice, our role and responsibility for caring and healing for self and system, then we are liberated into new horizons of fresh thinking. On this path of *Via Creativa*, we plumb new, deeper dimensions of self and our unique gifts and talents that we can offer as compassionate service on behalf of others. From this *Via Creativa*, creative energy and timeless, lasting solutions to our problems become more available, more accessible, more possible for self and others. From this direction we can creatively return to, articulate, and recreate a larger vision of nursing and health care. From this path the timeless values of caring and the compassionate healing health services manifest more openly, more publicly, as part of our leadership and responsibility for survival of the profession, as well as the survival of humane systems of health care.

This *Via* is the Way of the Visionary.[2] When nursing leaders reach this path, they are informed and fortified by nursing ancestors and voices across time that strengthen their vision and purpose, their mindful awareness, attention, and action that flows from the heart of nursing. When on this path, the nursing leader is more able to name that which obstructs and detours basic and human caring—healing practices for ourselves, our systems, and our public. From this *Via of Leader as Visionary*, nurse administrators are empowered from within, more able to tell the truth without blame or judgment.[2] On this *Via of Vision of the Visionary Leader*, one is allowed to care enough to make explicit the purpose and deeper meaning that connects and unites the whole value system, reminding self and others why nursing exists, why hospitals exist, why health care systems exist, why caring must be sustained beyond conventional institutional mindsets, and why we seek to move toward a healthful, caring society to better humankind.

VIA TRANSFORMATIVA

Finally, in taking this journey of the fourfold path, we enter *Via Transformativa*. On this mature path, we have come the full circle of the four sacred directions:

> North—*Via Negativa* (the dark—the spiritual warrior)
>
> East—*Via Positiva* (the light—the healer)
>
> West—*Via Creativa* (the water, flow—the visionary)
>
> South—*Via Transformativa* (the fire—the empowered teacher–leader).

Like an alchemy process, the leader emerges—reflective, cleansed, mindful, light-filled, and thus capable of birthing new beings, new possibilities. On the *Via Transformativa*, we have co-mingling of leaders and followers, each leading by following his or her own inner call and transformation. Here, having come through the test of fire, often literally as well as figuratively, we are repatterned with new energy to emerge through the alchemy of fire, to become the transformative leader, the spirit-filled teacher. From this *Via Transformativa*, visionaries, teachers, and healers for systems emerge, leading from the inside out. This form of leadership passes the test of time and position; this transformative leader is able to stand in place, to hold sacred space for caring–healing at all levels, while letting go of outcomes,[2] open to outcomes that may never be predicted nor controlled from conventional views of leadership.

Thus, through the fourfold path toward caring and healing, nurse administrators lead, follow, and co-create new forms, orders, and patterns of leadership. By the fourfold path, new levels of consciousness and awareness are more fully actualized, resulting in transformation of self and system.

Taking the fourfold path of leadership allows the growth and integration of the personal and professional journey. From this leading from the inner voice, nursing leaders emerge as spiritual warriors, leaders who are grounded in their own sense of being and becoming; their own *power*-with others; connected with and guided by that which is greater than self or system. In this form of deep leadership, the true leader is in balance with the deeper dimensions of life itself. This is the kind of leader who has been on the spiritual journey toward caring and healing in his or her own life.

It is this kind of leader and leadership path by which true transformation occurs. This transformed leader is a visionary, a value-guided navigator toward wholeness and hope. A transformed leader is one who leads from caring, yet follows one's own journey on the fourfold path,

honoring the four sacred directions of the universe and the lessons that each direction brings.

SO, HOW DOES ONE LEAD VIA THE FOURFOLD PATH OF CARING AND HEALING?

To lead *via the fourfold path of caring and healing* is to hear the inner call as to how to translate one's own unique talents and gifts into compassionate service.

To lead *via the fourfold path of caring and healing* is to paradoxically manifest one's full self, while simultaneously transcending ego self; to open to connections, visions of the whole, that are greater than any one person, but unite all.

To lead *via the fourfold path of caring and healing* is to lead from spirit-filled mindfulness and awareness; to lead by listening to others; to listen to the spirit of what is not said, as much as to what is said; to listen to the sound between the drum beats, detecting the emerging order arising from the comers of the chaos.

To lead *via the fourfold path of caring and healing* is to continuously learn—to learn about the sacred circle of life's journey, to awaken to deeper self and human nature, to learn to tap into and affirm the higher, deeper aspects of self and others that embrace and celebrate the diversity of human talents and experiences.

To lead *via the fourfold path of caring and healing* is to learn to pause, to center, to be still, to be authentically present in the midst of hectic paces and demands; to learn to experience a "caring moment" that transcends time and space and allows one to touch and connect spirit to spirit, releasing new energy, new possibilities of what might be, into a given moment.[3]

To lead *via the fourfold path of caring and healing* is to enable self and others, to experiment, to celebrate failures as well as successes, realizing that our failures are our lessons and blessings that transform into new successes; such a consciousness allows the wounds that hurt us to be the wounds that heal us, strengthen us.

To lead *via the fourfold path of caring and healing* is to learn to wait—to dwell in the void, the abyss, and await and coparticipate in the order that is emerging out of the chaos; that means attending and being alert to that which wants to emerge as a new path for self and system and society alike. It is often only in waiting that *Via Transformativa* can occur as we pause, on the fourfold journey, on the precipice, in the middle of our sentences, in the middle of our steps, on the sacred walk on the labyrinth of life.

Finally, transformed, nursing leaders reclaim their true vocation, in the full sense of the meaning of the word *vocation*; that is, rooted in the Latin for "voice."[5] Transformed nursing leaders at this crossroads in history are giving voice to their mission and vision of caring and healing. Transformed nursing leaders who walk the *fourfold Via* represent hope and order, the other way, for "leadership and the new science,"[6] in the midst of medicalized, industrialized, economized, clinical, and robotic models that are outdated as approaches to human health.

Perhaps it is from the *fourfold Via of caring and healing*, grounded in the spiritual journey of life itself, that leaders are both awaiting and shaping a new world of hope, a new path for new leaders and followers, for new systems, for a renewed health, for all.

In conclusion, as we move forward into this new century of nursing leadership and celebrate the 25th anniversary of *Nursing Administration Quarterly*, perhaps the *fourfold Via* can serve as a useful path to navigate our way through this turn of history in systems of decline—systems in dire need of transformation that can only come from transformed leaders. This fourfold path of leading, which gives voice and informed vocational action to the inner calling of caring and healing, may be the primary source of nursing's survival in this 21st century.

REFERENCES

1. Fox, M. (1991). *Creation spirituality*. San Francisco, CA: Harper SanFrancisco.
2. Arrien, A. (1993). *The four-fold way*. San Francisco, CA: Harper SanFrancisco.
3. Watson, J. (1999). *Postmodern nursing and beyond*. Edinburgh, Scotland, and New York, NY: Churchill-Livingstone/Harcourt-Brace.
4. Watson, J. (1988). *Brochure information*, University of Colorado School of Nursing, Center for Human Caring.
5. Palmer, P. (2000). *Let your life speak*. San Francisco, CA: Jossey-Bass.
6. Wheatley, M. (1999). *Leadership and the new science* (2nd ed.). San Francisco, CA: Berrett-Koehler.

QUESTIONS FOR REFLECTION

Baccalaureate

1. What are the four *Via* known as the fourfold path as described by Dr. Watson?
2. Provide an example of how each are being practiced within the organization where you are working or doing your practice rotation. If no example is available, what would this look like in practice?
3. From reading the nursing literature or professional experience, identify a transformational nursing leader. Why did you choose this leader?

Master's

1. Which of the four *Via* best describe your current leadership style?
2. Dr. Watson discussed authentic nursing leadership in order to sustain systems of caring and healing. What would this look like to you in the practice setting?
3. Describe a caring moment that you have experienced in your role as a nursing leader. This can be with a colleague, patient, or family.

Doctoral

1. How does the work of Matthew Fox inform Watson's reflections about nursing leadership and Watson's Theory of Human Caring?
2. Watson refers to a transformed leader as honoring the four sacred directions of the universe and the lesions that each direction brings. How do you honor each direction? What lessons have you learned from each direction over the course of your professional nursing journey?
3. Watson (2000) referred to systems of caring and healing. Based on contemporary nursing practice and cited literature, identify two systems that manifest caring and healing. Provide specific exemplars to support this decision.

37

Love and Caring: Ethics of Face and Hand—An Invitation to Return to the Heart and Soul of Nursing and Our Deep Humanity

Jean Watson

Let us fall in love again
And scatter gold dust all over the world.
Let us become a new Spring
And feel the breezes drift in the heaven's scent.
Let us dress the earth in green.
And like the sap of a young tree
Let the grace from within sustain us.
Let us carve gems out of our stony hearts
And let them light our path of Love.
The glance of love is crystal clear
And we are blessed by its light.

—Rumi[1(p. 117)]

We as nurses are invited, if not, required to unite at this cross roads in nursing history, at this new century of time and confusion and questioning of nursing's survival to reconsider what brings us together for a common purpose. Thus, this chapter and message are not to gather up new knowledge, although they may do that, but rather they are intended to gather nursing together for a more basic common purpose: perhaps to seek what Wittgenstein called "reminders"—reminders of what we already know at some deep human, experiential level, but continually pass over in our day-to-day living.

As Eliot[2] asked in the *Waste Land and Other Poems:* "Where is the life we have lost in living? Where is the wisdom we have lost in knowledge? Where is the knowledge we have lost in information?"

It seems the task of nursing and health and healing is related to the very nature of our shared humanity. In viewing nursing at this deeper level, we realize that our jobs have been too small for the nature of our work and the needs of those whom we serve, as well as too small for the evolution of our individual and collective humanity.

When working with others during times of despair, vulnerability, and unknowns, we are challenged to learn again, to reexamine our own meaning of life and death. As we do so, we engage in a more authentic process to cultivate and sustain caring healing practices for self and others. Such care and practices elicit and call upon profound wisdom and understanding, beyond knowledge, that touch and draw upon the human heart and soul.

In this reminder of basic values that transcend all circumstances and time and

From Watson, J. (2003). Love and caring. Ethics of face and hand—An invitation to return to the heart and soul of nursing and our deep humanity. *Nursing Administration Quarterly, 27*(3), 197–203. Permission to reprint granted by Wolters Kluwer.

place, we invoke the fullest and highest spiritual, spirit-filled dimensions into our work, allowing us to engage once again in compassionate service, motivated by love, both human and cosmic. From this place we offer to ourselves, and those whom we meet on our path, our compassionate response for fulfilling our chosen life's work and calling.

Just as it is in our personal lives that during crises of illness, tragedy, loss, or impending death that we ponder spiritual questions that go beyond the physical material world, it is here in our professional life, in its conventional, dispirited physical, technical, life form, deathbed of sorts, that we are given new freedom, new space to reconsider a deeper level of nursing. This may be the moment to reconsider what has always been the foundation of caring and healing, but must now be reconsidered again, for new/old reasons. Could the professional deathbed of sorts that we face in the conventional, medical, and nursing world be an opportunity for us as professionals to consider how we may live our lives if we had "only a year to live." What and how would we approach our last year to heal and be heated with so much unfinished business accumulated during this past century? How could we offer up our heart when we may be disheartened or in fear?

As Kierkegaard[3] might say, how do we encounter our *sickness unto death*, in this in-between existence—where spirit and matter have been torn off, split asunder, from our identity, our existence, our very being? Revisiting such foundational issues of infinity of humanity in relation to our caring may be the difference between life and death of a profession.

Having during the past few years come through a period of personal trauma and loss that was and remains deeply profound, I find that 1 was ironically given the gift of Spirit—the opportunity to fully experience life and spirit in raw form, in the midst of deep suffering.[4,5]

But the universal lesson from Buddha is that it does not matter how long you (we) have forgotten, only how soon you (we) remember. It is as if we have to be stopped to allow our souls/our soulful purpose to catch up with us. This insight may offer a moment of enlightenment for nursing as this crossroads of its survival, which may be the gift from this passage.

Perhaps, it is only when we acknowledge how much pain and suffering there is in our broken hearts and broken spirits, our broken world—within and without—that we can return to that which is timeless that can comfort, sustain, and inspire/inspirit us. It is here in this broken, wounded place that we can quiet the outer pace, bow down, and surrender to the loving presence of the universe and all its infinity.

So within this framework of caring and love, we now have a new call to bring us back to that which resides deep within us and intersects with the focus of this time and place to uncover the latent love in our caring work as well as connect us with contemporary philosophies that invite love and caring through our ethics of being-becoming. For example, the philosophy of Emmanuel Levinas[6] and his notion of the "Ethics of Face" help us connect with this ancient and contemporary truth. Likewise, I acknowledge the work of Knud Logstrup,[7] a Danish philosopher, who mirrors views similar to Levinas, but from the metaphor of "Hand," in that he reminds us that:

> holding another person's life in one's hand, endows this metaphor with a certain emotional power . . . that we have the power to determine the direction of something in another person's life . . . we're to a large extent inescapably dependent upon one another . . . we are mutually and in a most immediate sense in one another's power.[7(p. 28)]

Perhaps it is *love* that underpins and connects us through our metaphors of facing and holding another in our hands, reminding us of another dimension as to how to sustain our humanity at a deeper level at this point in human history.

Josephine Hart of the *London Times* wrote a compelling article on September 19, 2001, about the events of 9/11. Her article frames these issues more profoundly:

> We learnt a new moral alphabet this week.
>
> The letters which form the word love seemed empowered with more resonance, as though for all our lives we had not been spelling it correctly.
>
> We learnt that the dying understood that they would not be forgotten and that the manner of their leaving would determine their family's ability to survive their death. We learnt that, with death crashing towards them and with no means of escape, men and women absolved their families of the edge of grief that leads to madness. They did not scream in range "Why me?" nor babble in terror at what awaited them. They spoke a last "I love you," then turned towards their ghastly fate with unbelievable grace. They taught us another way to live and to die.[8(p. 9)]

With the crisis of meaning in our lives and work during this era in human history, we may paraphrase W.H. Auden to remember that in the end, love is all that really matters: The Native American Indians remind us that everyday we should do an act of power and an act of beauty. By reconsidering the role and power of love, light, and beauty in our life, we bring back reminders of what is truly valuable, serving ourselves with timeless reminders that in returning to our own inner light, and inner love, we offer an act of power and beauty to our self and those whom we serve.

Perhaps, the purpose of this manuscript and my writing of it is more specifically to remind myself and others of one other basic thing: *that it is our humanity that both wounds us and heals us, and those whom we serve; and in the end, it is only love that matters.* It is in entering into and participating with the great mysteries of the sacred circle of life and death that we engage in healing.

By attending to, honoring, entering into, connecting with our deep humanity, we find the ethic and artistry of being, loving, and caring. We are not machines as we have been taught, but spirit made whole.

From Rumi in the 13th century to Levinas (1906–1995)[6] and Logstrup (1905–1981)[7] in the twentieth century, we find the ancient truths of our work. We share the wisdom of these mystic poet-philosophers who captured the "Infinity and mystery of the Human soul, mirrored through the ethics of face" (Levinas's view); the fact that "we hold another's life in our hands" (Logstrup's view) and that "the glance," the mystical experience when eyes meet is ancient Rumi's reminder of how we mirror the human soul, through the eyes, the look, the glance.

In Rumi's words: "I see my beauty in you. I become a mirror that cannot close its eyes to your longing. . . . These thousands of worlds that arise from nowhere, how does your face contain them?" And ". . . out of eternity I turn my face to you, and into eternity. . . . "[9(p. 12)]

How can we dare to be so bold as to bring caring and loving and infinity of souls into our lives and work and world again? Because, without returning to this ancient place of cosmic power, energy, and beauty, we are inclined toward what Levinas referred to as a "totalizing of self and other"[6]—that is, a congealing of our humanity, separating us from any connection with spirit, with infinity, with the great divine—with no hope for healing and wholeness. A totalizing occurs when there is no relational engagement, no soul connection, thus no cosmic human field to engage our shared humanity. This totalizing of self and other, this turning away from the mystery of our shared humanity and divine connection, can be an act of cruelty to self and others; an inhumane act toward human civilization itself, perpetuating more inhumane acts, violence, and destruction of human spirit in our work and world.

So rather than asking *how can we dare* to bring love and caring together into our lives and work? We can ask: *How can we hear not to?*

Levinas reminds us the Infinity of the human soul mirrors the mystery of humanity back upon itself to us, through our shared human connections, through "the face," "the glance," the facing our own and others' shared souls as routes to this infinity and mysterious circularity of life.

To engage, to dwell in this new space of caring, living our mystery of being and dying, reveals the very situation in which we exist. This new space becomes our basic foundation for being and sustaining our humanity. This cosmic perspective, which invites spirit, mystery, and soul back into our lives and work, raises our courage to ethically engage in life and all its depths of being. Somehow, knowing that we can endure the pain with the joy; the hurts and humiliations with the forgiveness and praise; the suffering with endurance, dignity, grace, and poise, is tied to our infinite capacity to love and be loved, to become *love*.

To paraphrase Emily Dickinson: The mind is wider than the sky, cause it can hold it and Thee beside can be transposed to: The heart is as wide as the sky, because it can hold pain and joy side by side.

Though we can find this deep ethic of being, in Rumi, Levinas, and Logstrup and other poets and sages through the ages, we are invited now to be present to our own and others' deeply human soul conditions and connections that embrace all the vicissitudes of living and dying. As Rumi again reminds us: To die before we die—to find that delicate balance between self-discipline (dying of ego) and cosmic surrender.

CARING MOMENT AS RADIATING FIELD OF COSMIC LOVE

I recently heard it said that when a nurse enters into a patient's room, a magnetic field of expectation is created. In this deeper, more expanded way of thinking about the power, beauty, and energy of love, a *caring moment*[10,11] becomes an energetic vibrational field of cosmic love that radiates reciprocity and mutuality, which transcends time, space, and physicality confirming and sustaining our humanity and our connection with the Levinas' *Infinity* of the entire universe.[4,12]

The connections between caring, loving, and infinity become the process of facing our humanity as mystery, thus mirroring humanity of self and other back on itself. Such a human to-human act of caring within a given moment becomes a basic foundation for facing our humanity, uniting us and the cosmic energy of love, as one. In Rumi's words: "I am here, this moment, inside the beauty, the gift God has given . . . this gold and circular sign. . . ."[9(p. 10)]

Logstrup frames these issues and ethics of our artistry of being human, not only through the "look," the "face," the gesture, the glance, the voice, but also the Hands. He puts it this way:

> By our value/attitude to the other person we help to determine the scope and hue of his/her world; we make it larger or smaller, bright or drab, rich or dull, threatening or secure. We help to shape his world not by theories and views but by our very being and attitude toward him. Herein lies the unarticulated and one might say anonymous demand that we take care of life which trust has placed in our hands.[7(p. 19)]

These views remind us that one's human presence never leaves one unaffected. Expressed compassion and caring is not only the word that is spoken or the eye that sees, leading to action. The gaze itself is an expression; the word is also a gesture framed in a voice, an intonation. In the intuitive expression, what is said can be welcoming, receiving, affirming, but it also can be a careless phase, a looking away—nonfacing of an other's humanity and human condition . . . a "*totalizing* of another," setting and limiting, objectifying other . . . rather than an honoring of the "Infinity and mystery of the human condition and humanity" . . . a *facing* and connecting with the human soul and the infinity of the mystery therein. The opposite of this, a turning away from facing our humanity, can actually be an act of cruelty. So, in these deep ethical philosophical views of Levinas and Logstrup, which unite with caring theory, we acknowledge that through our very being, through our human presence toward facing self and other, we *bold others in our bands*, for better or for worse, either opening horizons to infinity or totalizing our own and others' humanity.

In this view of ethics and the metaphysics and metaphors of *love*, *face*, and *hands*, Levinas posited ethics as being beyond ontology: he placed ethics as the first principle of philosophy. It is acknowledging the ethical responsibility for the other, understood as vulnerability and proximity. In this view, love is originary. Love watches over other demands, such as justice.[13] The subject as *other* is an incomprehensible, infinite otherness. The human face is not a concept, it is not a figure in which message can be captured by knowledge. It is the face in its exposedness, its nudity, as an opening toward the infinite that makes the one responsible for the *other*.

This view is beyond philosophy; it is not an ontology, it is not a normative theory, it is a metaphysics: it explains how *being-for-the-other* precedes *being-with-the-other*. This approach critiques Heideggerian ontology by positioning ethics as preceding ontology. Within this metaphysics, we dwell in originary love, cosmic, and divine.[13]

Finally, what is traced in Levinas' *Ethic of Face*, in Rumi, *mystic-ecstatic love* and mystery, and in Logstrup's holding another in one's *band* is central to all professions involved in human care; it comes before and informs clinical judgments and can serve as an epistemological foundation for any clinical care.[13]

To frame these profound truths as foundational to our humanity, we can relate for new reasons to some theoretical notions of transpersonal caring:[11,14]

- Each thought and each choice we make carries spirit energy into our lives and those of others
- Our consciousness, our intentionality, our presence, makes a difference, for better or for worse
- Calmness and mindfulness in a caring moment beget calmness and mindfulness
- Caring and love beget caring and love
- Caring and compassionate acts of love beget healing for self and others
- Transpersonal caring becomes transformative, liberating us to live and practice love and caring in our ordinary lives in nonordinary ways.

To enter into this new space of love, caring, hands, and heart that sustain infinity of our humanity, we can consider the following practices:

- Suspending of role and status: honoring each person, their talents, gifts, and contributions as essential to the whole
- Speaking and listening without judgment, working from heart-centered space; working toward shared meaning, common values
- Listening with compassion and an open heart, without interrupting; listening to another's story is a healing gift of self
- Leaning to be still, to center self while welcoming silence for reflection, contemplation, and clarity

- Recognizing that a transpersonal caring–loving practice transcends ego self and connects us human-to-human, spirit-to-spirit, where our life and work are divided no more
- Honoring the reality that we are part of each other's journey: we are all on our own journey toward healing as part of the infinity of the human condition: when we work to heal ourselves, we contribute to healing of the whole.

In conclusion, the crisis in modern medicine and health in this new millennium seems to lie in the lack of a meaningful perspective on the very nature of our humanity. It seems that somewhere along the way modern medicine has forgotten that it is grounded and sustained by and through the very nature of our being and becoming more human.

We have forgotten that we are nurtured and sustained by love, by grace, by the beauty, and by depth of life. We are reminded that through our wounded humanity, including our vulnerability, suffering, and joy, the light and shadows of our teeming humanity, we enter into and contribute to connecting with the infinity of the human soul, life itself, and all the vicissitudes that encompass and surround our humanity.

Addressing the role of our being and becoming more human, through the phenomenon, the metaphysics, and ethic of love and caring allows us to more fully "face our humanity." These considerations are critical to engage in healing practices for ourselves and for those whom we serve.

This process of connecting with Logstrup's and Levinas's ethic of first principle[6] of belonging-being and sustaining our humanity is the same as sustaining our dignity, our divinity—reminding us of the sacred world of the infinity of existence; thus, humanity is ultimately floating in, trusting in the spirit, energy, and grace of cosmic love.

This ethic of love and caring become first principles for facing and sustaining the infinity of our profession. If we follow this ethical demand, nursing has a critical role in moving humanity toward the omega point, ever closer to God and the mysterious sacred circle of living, trusting, loving, being, and dying,

I conclude with a Teilhard de Chardin quote:

> Love in all its subtleties is nothing more, and nothing less, than the more or less direct trace marked on the heart. . . . This is the ray of light which will help us to see more clearly. . . . [15(p. 265)]

NOTE

Parts of this chapter are based upon a presentation at the International Reflective Practice Conference, Amsterdam, The Netherlands, June 2002

REFERENCES

1. Rumi. (2001). *Hidden music* (pp. 117). (M. Mafi&A. M. Kolin, Trans.) Hong Kong: HarperCollins.
2. Eliot, T. S. (1934). Two choruses from "The Rock." In *The waste land and other poems* (pp. 81). New York, NY: Harcourt, Brace & World.
3. Kierkegaard, S. (1941). *Fear and trembling and the sickness unto death*. Princeton, NJ: Princeton University Press.
4. Watson, J. (1999). *Postmodern nursing and beyond*. New York, NY: Churchill/Harcourt Brace.
5. Watson, J. (2002). Illuminating the spiritual journey, Jean Watson tells her story. In P. Burkhardt & M. G.Nagai-Jacobson (Eds.), *Spirituality: Living our Connectedness* (pp. 181–186). New York, NY: Delmar.
6. Levinas, E. (1991). *Totality and infinity*. Pittsburgh, PA: Duquesne University.
7. Logstrup, K. (1997). *The ethical demand*. Notre Dame, IN: University of Notre Dame Press.
8. Hart, J. (2001). Editorial. *The Times*. September 19,9.
9. Rumi. (1999). "I see my beauty in you." In C. Barks (Trans.) *The glance songs of*

soul-meeting (p. 12). New York, NY: Penguin Group.

10. Watson, J. (1999). *Nursing human science and human care. A theory of nursing.* Sudbury, MA: Jones & Bartlett.

11. Watson, J. (2002). Intentionality and caring-healing consciousness: A practice of transpersonal nursing. *Holistic Nursing Practice, 16*(4), 1–8.

12. Quinn, J. (1992). Holding sacred space: The nurse as healing environment. *Holistic Nursing Practice, 6*(4), 26–35.

13. Norvedt, P. (2001). Clinical sensitivity: The inseparability of ethical perceptiveness and clinical knowledge. *Scholarly Inquiry for Nursing Practice, 15*(3), 1–19.

14. Watson, J., & Smith, M. C. (2002). Caring science and the science of unitary human beings: A trans-theoretical discourse for nursing knowledge development. *Journal of Advanced Nursing, 37*(5), 152–461.

15. de Chardin, T. (1964). *The future of man* (p. 265). New York, NY: Harper & Row.

QUESTIONS FOR REFLECTION

Baccalaureate

1. Perform an online literature search on Rumi. Find a poem that is meaningful to you. Why did you select this poem?

2. Logstrup as cited in Watson wrote "we hold another's life in our hand." What does this mean to you?

3. Watson wrote about listening with compassion and an open heart, without interrupting. Provide an example where you did this with a patient or family member.

Master's

1. Watson wrote "that it is our humanity that both wounds us and heals us, and those whom we serve; and in the end only, it is only love that matters." What does this mean to you? Are you comfortable with the word love in terms of those you serve? Why or why not?

2. Levinas as cited in Watson wrote about the ethics of face. What does this mean to you? Provide a practice example where this helped you understand the mystery of the human soul.

3. Watson wrote about learning to be to still, to center self while welcoming silence for reflection, contemplation, and clarity. How do you center self? How can you learn to be still? Identify a ritual that allows for this and see if this makes a difference in your personal life and professional practice of nursing.

Doctoral

1. Discuss the similarities and differences among the writings and thinking of Rumi, Levinas, and Logstrup. How does each inform Watson's Theory of Human Caring.

2. Watson refers to practices for us to consider as we enter this new space of love, caring, hands, and heart. Identify a qualitative research question around three of the practices.

3. Watson explains that being-for-the-other precedes being-with-the-other. What does this mean to you? How is this supported in other literature written by Watson?

IX

Synthesis and Epilogue

MARLAINE C. SMITH, MARIAN C. TURKEL, AND ZANE ROBINSON WOLF

The original idea for this book arose from a dialogue among a group of caring scholars and members of the International Association for Human Caring (IAHC), while attending the 23rd IAHC conference, *Creating Communities of Caring-Global Initiatives* (2001), in Stirling, Scotland. We were part of the energetic dialogue focused on honoring the early works of caring scholars, preserving the legacy of caring, and making the work easily accessible at the international level. The dialogue continued at the 25th IAHC conference, *Calling the Caring Circle* (2003) in Boulder, Colorado. During this conference, we reflected on the importance of the 25th anniversary of the IAHC, and intently discussed the need to move from energy and ideas to formal publication. We identified the need for the first book to be *Caring Classics*, representing the sentinel works of caring scholars. We also talked about a series of books on caring focused on specific content such as education, administration, research methods, history, and expressions of caring within the everyday practice of nursing. The dialogue continued, and at the 26th IAHC conference, *Caring, For a Renewed Care* (2004) in Montreal, we had an in-depth discussion, and Dr. Zane Wolf came prepared with a list of manuscripts for inclusion in *Caring Classics*.

In 2008, Dr. Marilyn Parker and Dr. Marlaine Smith started an e-mail communication restating the need for this work

for doctoral education in caring science. At the same time, Dr. Turkel was becoming involved with the Watson Caring Science Institute (WCSI), and registered nurses were increasingly implementing Watson's Theory of Human Caring in the practice environment. The nurses wanted to learn about caring science, the history of caring in nursing, and how caring scholarship could be used to guide practice. Dr. Watson supported the idea of *Caring Classics* and encouraged Dr. Turkel to contact Alan Graubard, Acquisitions Editor at Springer Publishing. To be fair and inclusive to the process, the original participants in the book discussions were contacted via e-mail, and three of us agreed to be the editors and honor the legacy of caring science. During dialogues with Alan Graubard, the need to have a faculty resource book originated, and Dr. Wolf and Dr. Turkel agreed to coauthor this book, so our colleagues in academia and staff development could use our material. So 11 years later, we have come full circle; the vision from 2001 is reality, and we want to honor the ideas and inspiration of many of our colleagues who started the initial journey.

Selecting the caring classics in this book provided the editors with the unique opportunity to examine the original and important work on nurse caring, perhaps more closely than previously. We went through a sorting process over several months and kept to the task.

We reviewed and ranked published works and organized them thematically. After our initial review by the publisher, we reduced the number of contributions due to the practicality of page counts for textbooks. We hoped that we would carry out the preservation of some of the original material on nurse caring, so that others would have easy access.

We understood that nurse caring had multiplicative antecedents, beginning with unrecorded situations where one individual was vulnerable and another took on the responsibility of helping. It is easy to say that the starting place of caring goes back to centuries and that respect for human dignity was the value on which it centered. Nursing scholars recognized the importance of bringing what might have been considered hidden work forward and making it visible. Lone nursing scholars began putting their ideas into print. Nurse–patient relationship was central in many publications.

Moreover, there was growing attention to the scholarly works on caring. A significant amount of interest resulted as the worth of such writing gradually permeated the consciousness of professional nursing in the mid to later part of the 20th century. Care and caring scholarship took root and flourished. Scholars from other disciplines joined nurses, and many nurses enjoyed reflecting on the work of Milton Mayeroff, Martin Buber, Henri Nouwen, Willard Gaylin, and Emmanuel Levinas, and orienting their writing in such conceptualizations. Nurses created and tested caring theories and models.

Perhaps the pioneers who addressed nurse caring reacted to some of the efficiency studies of the mid 20th century. For them, nursing practice was more than procedural and technical. The intrusion of technology into nursing practice made the studies on nurse caring even more important, because some feared that it interfered dramatically with the quality of the nurse–patient relationship. They started with the assertion that caring was the essence of nursing and the unifying focus of the discipline and profession. This assertion has continued, repeated many times over the last decades.

Although caring conferences appealed to few scholars initially, attendance grew and those who came were attracted to the prospect of listening to the ideas, research, and theories on caring that were shared. Nurses continued to create and disseminate caring scholarship, wrestling with assumptions, propositions, concepts, emerging theories, and qualitative research on caring. The national conferences soon became an international scholarly forum for nurses interested in the advancement of knowledge and caring within nursing. What followed is evidenced by the numerous works that have been published.

THE FUTURE OF CARING SCIENCE

The year 2013 marks 35 years from when Dr. Madeline Leininger and Dr. Jean Watson and a group of doctoral students gathered for the first conference to present research and philosophical reflections related to caring and nursing. This group continued to meet every year to reflect, dialogue, and share research and philosophical assumptions about caring. In 1988, the group formalized and became known as the IAHC. From this group, numerous contributions to the scholarship of caring science have emerged; the scholarly discourse continues and is disseminated via our annual nursing conferences and the *International Journal for Human Caring*. New ideas, theoretical assumptions, and research continue to unfold, and nurses in practice are looking to caring theory as a return to the values of the profession. Caritas coaches are working intentionally to create caring–healing relationships with self, colleagues, patients, and families. Health care systems are changing from the industrial, medical, technical focus to a caring, healing, person-centered focus. In the future, we question the following: Whether these changes will be sustained? Will they differ across regions and countries? How will economics influence human caring? How will caring and technology be complementary? How will the early work of caring scholars inform practice? How will caring interventions merge across disciplines and affect outcomes of caring, such as being healed, being comforted, having quality of life, being satisfied with care, and having more healthy physiological changes?

We invite our readers to reflect on caring from your personal frame of reference whether it be scholarship, practice, education, research, or philosophical assumptions. Consider the following:

> Is caring the essence of nursing and the unifying focus of the discipline?

> Is caring theory serving as a framework for your practice of nursing?

> Are the thoughts from 1980s relevant to contemporary nursing practice?

> Are we moving from the medical paradigm with a focus on curing to a caring science humanistic paradigm with a focus on caring and healing?

> What will the practice of nursing grounded in caring look like in 2020?

> What outcomes of caring are important?

> Do we need to change the way caring informs nursing education?

> Are the current research methods adequate to capture the lived expressions of caring?

> Will caring become part of the metaparadigm of nursing?

> If a second edition of *Caring Classics* was republished in 2020, what would it look like?

> Will concepts such as authentic presence, love, caritas processes, sacred space, rituals, and reflection become part of the language of caring in everyday practice or remain only in scholarly discourse?

Index

ACE subscale, *See* Affective, Cognitive, Ethical subscale

ACN, *See* Attending Caring Nurse

activities, concept of nurses', 386

administration, nursing, 403, 466
  implications for, 493

administrators
  caring categories of, 315
  hospital, *See* hospital administrators
  non-nurse, 313
  nurse, *See* nurse administrators
  perception of nurse caring, 90

aesthetic knowing patterns, 229–230

Affective, Cognitive, Ethical (ACE) subscale, 501, 503

AHNA, *See* American Holistic Nurses Association

ambiguity about caring, 46, 133

American Holistic Nurses Association (AHNA), 426, 447

American Nurses Association, 397

American Nurses Credentialing Center (ANCC), 423

analysis of caring, 265, 271

ANA *Social Policy Statement*, 285

ANCC, *See* American Nurses Credentialing Center

anthropocentrism, 448

anthropological approach, to study care and caring, 132

anthropological perspectives, of caring, 11

anthropological questions, 35–36

antineoplastic drugs, 446

appreciating pattern, 50–51

artistic nurses, 12

arts, caring, 1, 251–253

art work of Hildegard of Bingen, 188, 189

attachment, caring as, 273–274

Attending Caring Nurse (ACN), 389, 419–420

Attending Nurse Caring Model (ANCM), 388, 389, 419, 420
  pilot project, 421
  proposed theory-guided evidence program, 420–421

attention, care as giving, 273

attitudes, nurse, 294–295

attributes of caring, 36–37, 117, 166
  process, 15–16, 106
  professional caring, 22
  reflections on, 165

awareness, caring condition, 276–278

behaviors
  noncaring, 294–295, 297
  nurturant, caring as, 311
  physical action–oriented helping, 299
  scientific caring, 306

behaviors, nurse caring, 10, 78–80, 267, 348, 374
  for cancer patients, 283–290, 300, 302–305
  defined, 266, 285
  evaluation of, 305–306
  perceptions of, 299–306

Being-Caring, human caring skills of, 255

being-in-caring-healing-relationships, 255

being modes, *See* mode of being

"believing in a good death," 325–326, 329

Benner's helping role of nurse, 219

bioactive mode, 94, 123, 202, 206

biocidic mode, 94, 123, 201–203

biogenic mode, 94, 202, 206

biopassive mode, 94, 123, 201, 202, 205

biostatic mode, 94, 123, 201–202, 204

blended model, 397–401

bracketing, 212

Buber, Martin, 159, 160

bureaucracy
  criticisms of, 311
  mediating with, 459–460
  organizations as, 310–311

bureaucratic caring, 268, 269, 312
   formal theory of, 314, 316
   for nursing practice, 309–318
   structure, 317

Calling the Caring Circle (2003), 521
cancer patients
   CARE-Q instrument using for, 286–289,
      300–302, 305
   nurse caring behavior for, 283–290
   oncology nurses vs., 299–306
capacity for caring, 14, 61, 62–64
capitalism, 465, 473
Carative Factors (CFs), 117, 119–120, 238–239,
     244, 255–257, 396
   cultivation of sensitivity, 151–153
   humanistic-altruistic value system, 148–149
   instillation of faith-hope, 149–151
   in nursing, 146
   overview of, 147–148
   transpersonal teaching–learning, 425, 435,
     438, 439
   in Watson's theory, 433
carative processes, 436
care diversities, 25
caregivers, 25, 337, 373–374
   guideline used by, 24
   standard of care for caring, 380
care provider, 334
CARE-Q, *See* Caring Assessment Report
     Evaluation Q-Sort instrument
care receiver, 25
care themes, 348
caring actions, 61, 78
   future directions for Level IV inquiry, 85, 89
   inductively derived, 86–89
   qualitative inquiry, 85
   quantitative inquiry, 78–85
*Caring: A Feminine Approach to Ethics and Moral
     Education* (Noddings), 216
Caring Assessment Instrument, 348
Caring Assessment Report Evaluation Q-Sort
     (CARE-Q) instrument, 78, 266–268, 284,
     286, 348, 349
   format and sorting directions, 287
   patients' rating of items, 288
   subscale rankings, 81, 84
   tool, 475
   using for cancer patients, 286–289,
     300–302, 305
Caring Assessment Tool (CAT), 90
caring-based nursing practice models
   ANCM, 388, 389, 419, 420
   moving forward, 389–391
   ongoing reflection, 391–392
   Quality-Caring Model©, 386, 404
   relevance to practice, 411–412

caring-based professional practice, 385, 387
Caring Behavior Inventory (CBI), 78, 81, 335,
     336, 347, 349, 350, 391
   dimensions of, 353
   factor analysis of, 351–353
caring behaviors, 26–27, 138
   measuring, 78
   of nurses, 118
Caring Behaviors Assessment (CBA), 78, 81
caring consciousness, *See* consequences of
     caring
caring dimension, 202
caring–healing, 347, 354, 374, 469–471
   consciousness, 122
   leading *Via*, 507–511
   modalities, related to pain management, 389
   practices, 389, 390
     environment, 416
caring ingredients, 226
caring inquiry, esthetic process in, 334, 340–344
caring interactions, 409
caring literacy, 253–254
   dimensions of, 254–255
   examples of, 254
   framework of, 255
   ontological competendes in, 255
caring literature, 357
   analyses of, 46
   review, 373–375
caring model, 299, 357, 364
caring nursing leaders, 409, 412
caring nursing practice, evidence for, 403
caring on ragged edge, 457
   method, 452
   pervasive fear, 454–455
caring organizations, 408–409
caring person, 35, 36
   capacities of, 63–64
caring practices, 363, 407, 469, 507
caring process, 118, 123, 134, 424, 434–436, 462
   attributes of, 15–16, 106, 107–108
   being with in, 216
   clinical, *See* clinical caring processes
   conceptual cross-validation of, 219
   definitions of, 214
   dynamics of human, 246
   expert nursing practice, 107
   knowing in, 215–216
   subdimensions of, 215
caring relationships, 122, 196, 387, 399
   characterizing nurse–patient
     relationships, 94
   cultural variations in, 108
   devotion for, 5
   with nurses, 397
   outcomes from, 397
   social benefits of participating in, 93

caring rituals, 138
Caring Satisfaction Scale (CARE/
    SAT), 81
caring scholars, 388, 408, 465
Caring Science, 233, 249–251
    as academic discipline, 198
    arts and humanities, 251–253
    assumptions, 119, 147, 250
    balancing with humanism, 144
    development of, 194–196
    essential characteristics of, 145
    formulation of new questions, 193–194
    hermeneutic dimension in, 194
    humanistic development thinking
        in, 193
    leaders, 465
    nursing as, 143–144
    practitioners of, 197
    premises for, 146–147, 250–251
    research, 465
    theory, 197, 198
    upward causation model of, 187
    vs. humanities, 144–145
    working definition of, 251
Caring Science as Sacred Science (Watson), 247
caring scientists, 198
Caring Theory, 24–25, 389, 391, 420, 427, 451,
    465, 471
Caritas consciousness
    love, basics for, 262
    practice of loving kindness and equanimity,
        262–263
Caritas Nursing, emergence of, 259–260
Caritas Processes (CPs), 126, 255, 256
    core principles/practices, 258–259
    fluid aspects of, 257
    moving from carative to, 258
    nursing and nurse, emergence of, 259–260
Caritas, value assumptions of, 261–262
case-mix index, 466, 476
CBI, *See* Caring Behavior Inventory
CFs, *See* Carative Factors
challenges in nursing, 456
characteristics of nursing staff, 350
clarification concept of caring
    critique of, 48
    process for, 48–49
Clean Air Act, 446
clinical caring processes, 387, 396, 399,
    400, 404
Clinical Nursing Models Project, 215–216
    caring and, 213–214
clinical practice, implications for, 296–297
clinical setting, noncaring and caring in,
    293–297
clinical units, caring categories on, 315–316
coding strategy, of caring, 105, 106

cognitive knowledge, for health consultative
    acts, 365
collaborative relationships, 399
commitments, 37, 39, 61, 66–67, 121, 168–169,
    176–178, 205, 225, 364
    of caring, 14
    cultural origins of, 65
    future directions for Level II inquiry, 68
communicating caring, 27
communication, Six Cs of nurse, 417
community assessment tool, 439
community caring, 425, 438
community connection, 427, 458–460, 462
community health nurses, 425, 426, 431, 439
community health nursing practice, 424, 425,
    426, 428, 431
    conceptual framework for, 436–440
community health nursing praxis, 428
Community Nursing Practice Model, 428
community spirit, 437
compassion, 36, 38, 121, 167, 170–172
    and caring, 469, 481, 509, 516, 517
    esthetic process in way of, 339–344
competence, 36, 37, 39, 117, 167–168, 172–173
competent clinical skills, 365
complementary–alternative–integrative
    medicine, 252
components of caring, 12, 24, 111,
    274–275, 299
comportment, 121, 169, 178–179
composite description, 366
    of responses, 359
concept analyses of caring, 104–106
conception of reality, 193–194
concept of caring, 4, 127, 129, 130, 271, 274
conceptual context, caring as, 311
conceptualization of caring, 28, 212
conceptual models
    of caring, 469, 501
    nursing, 385
    for transcultural nursing care, 137–140
concerns, 61, 66–67, 364
    of caring, 14
    cultural origins of, 65
    future directions for Level II inquiry, 68
conditions, 61, 68
    of caring, 274–275
    future directions for Level III inquiry, 75
    nurse-related, 71–75
    organization-related, 75, 76–77
    patient-related, 69–70
conducive environment, 109–110
confidence, 37, 121, 168, 173–174
conscience, 37, 121, 168, 174–176
consciousness
    caring–healing, 181
    theory, 424, 432

consequences of caring, 3, 27–29, 61, 89–90, 92–93
  for clients and nurses, 91–92
  future directions for Level V inquiry, 93
  positive and negative, 14
  quantitative investigation of, 90
constant comparative method, 484
constitutive meanings of caring, 49
  appreciating pattern, 50–51
  attuning to dynamic flow, 51–52
  infinite experiencing, 52
  inviting creative emergence, 52–53
  manifesting intentions, 50
contemporary nursing, 181–183
  practices, 238, 387
  theoretical systems, 185
content analysis of caring, 338, 375–376, 379
context of caring, 337, 366
co-researchers, 203, 204
  conceptions of, 207
cosmic love, caring moment as radiating field of, 516–518
cost–caring relationships
  implications and recommendations, 503–504
  results, 502–503
cost effectiveness
  institutional strategies for, 498–499
  in nursing care delivery, 497–498
costs, 489, 491
  caring and, 501–502
  concept of, 487
  definitions of, 468, 499
  of nursing care, 502, 504
cost-shifting, 499
  issues of, 504
covenantal relationship, for nursing ethics, 228
CPs, *See* caritas processes
Creating Communities of Caring-Global Initiatives (2001), 521
criticism of physicians, 328
cultural care, 36, 38
cultural variations, 119
  in caring relationships, 108
culture, organizational
  bureaucratic caring, 309–318
  differential caring, 315–316
  strategies for recreating, 410–411
cultures, organizations as, 310
Cumulative Index of Nursing and Allied Health Literature (CINAHL), 104
curative factors, 119

data analysis, 105–106, 467
  in grounded theory method, 484
data collection, 333, 337
  in grounded theory method, 484
  instrumentation and procedures for, 375–377

definition of caring, 135–136, 218–220, 468, 500–501
Delphi technique
  results, 377–380
  standard of care for caring, 337, 371–382
Denver Nursing Project in Human Caring, 241
devotion, 5, 177
diagnosis-related groups (DRGs), 474, 482
dialogues, 390
differential caring, 269, 312, 314
  in organizational culture, 315–316
dignity living, 457
dimensions of care, task and affective, 365
dimensions of nurse caring, 90, 335–336, 373
  method, 349–351
  results, 351–353
disciplinary dialogue on caring
  analysis of, 46–47
  historical background, 43–45
disciplinary matrix of caring, 249
discipline of nursing, 2, 227–230, 249, 253, 398
  caring as central to, 3–4
  foundation for, 258
disenfranchised patients, 426
distinctive qualitative method, 334
"doing for" in caring process, 85, 88, 216–217, 462
domain for nursing, 131–132
"do-not-resuscitate-order," 328
DRGs, *See* diagnosis-related groups
dynamics of human caring process, 246

economics, 473–474
  and health care, 474
  human caring and, 482–483
    administrator participants, 489–492
    data analysis, 484
    data collection, 483–484
    method, 483
    nurse participants, 484–487
    patient participants, 487–489
    nursing, 481–482
    recommendations, 477–478
    research study, 474–477
education, caring, 165–166, 306
effective caring, 147, 250, 502
elements of caring, 362–363
emerging model, nurse hospitalist as, 417–418
emerging science of caring, 1
empirical knowing pattern, 12, 37, 38–39
empowered caring, 451
enabling in caring process, 89, 217, 462
energy dimensions, of transpersonal caring, 184

environment
  caring–healing practices, 416
  concept of, 428
  definition of, 426, 446
  healing, 411
  health care, 410
  high-speed ICU, 327
  nursing and, 446
environmentalism, 445
epistemological questions, 37–40
epistemological standpoints, 196–197
epistemology of caring, personal knowing
    patterns, 37, 229
Eriksson's theory, assumptions of, 122,
    194–196
essential patterns of caring, 336, 359, 363–364
esthetic act, 340
  of compassion, 334, 339
  phenomenology of, 341, 343–344
esthetic knowing pattern, 12, 39–40
  in caring research, 340
esthetic phenomenological hermeneutic
    inquiry, 335
esthetic process, in caring inquiry, 334,
    339–344
ethical knowing pattern, 12, 37, 39
ethics preceding ontology, 197
ethnoscientific approach, to caring, 132
evidence-based practice model, 386, 408,
    418, 421
expert nursing practice, in caring process, 107
exploratory factor analysis, 351, 379
"expressing moral awareness," 328–329, 330
extant theory analysis
  anthropological questions, 35–36
  epistemological questions, 37–40
  ontical questions, 36–37
  ontological questions, 33–35
  pedagogical questions, 40–41

face-to-face human encounter, 6, 7
factor-naming theory, 212
faith-hope instillation
  astrological and biorhythmical charts, 150
  humanistic-altruistic value system, 151
  therapeutic effects of, 149
  Yalom's factor, 149
family legacy, nurses, 456
family members
  caring, 108
  patients and, 108
feelings
  caring for well-being, 285
  of distress, 326–327, 330
  sensitivity to, 151–153
feminine, caring in nursing practice, 47
Feng Shui, 411

fondness, caring as, 273–274
formal theory, 269, 312
  of bureaucratic caring, 314, 316
  in caring, 14
  concept of caring in, 14
fourfold path, 469, 470
  toward transformative leadership, 507–511
framing caring, 105

Gaut's philosophical analysis, 218
general nursing theory, 229
grounded theory approach, 105, 466, 467,
    481, 483
  data analysis, 484
  data collection, 483–484
  results
    administrator participants, 489–492
    nurse participants, 484–487
    patient participants, 487–489
growing in caring, 124, 223–224, 231, 233–234

HCI, *See* Holistic Caring Inventory
healing
  arts, diverse categories of, 253
  environment, 407
  gardens, 388, 411
  interaction pattern, 364
  modality, 388
  patterns, 366
  process, 468
  room for nurses, 388, 411
  spiritual dimensions of, 252
health
  definition of, 424, 437, 438
  education, 425, 439
  promotion, 438
health care
  economics, 474
    changes in, 465
  environments, 410
  and nursing, 401
  organizations, 388, 397, 407, 410
  outcomes, 395
  technological aspects of, 299
health care practices, 371
health care providers, 372–373, 381
health care systems, 122, 522–523
  corporate culture of, 309
helping clients, with human needs, 365
helping role of nurse, dimensions of, 219–220
helping–trusting relationship, 434
hermeneutic dimension, in caring
    sciences, 194
high-speed ICU environment, 327
Hildegard of Bingen, art work of, 188, 189
holistic approach, 429, 437
  to practice, 486, 493, 497, 504

Holistic Caring Inventory (HCI), 90, 373
holistic nursing perspectives, 446–447
holistic theory, 424
holographic theory, 185
honesty, ingredients of caring, 5
hospital administrators, 493
hospital care delivery models, reorientations
    for, 416–417
hospitalist nurse model, 417–418
hospital treatment delivery model, 416
human being, 122, 452
    mission of, 196
human caring, 447–448, 473, 474
    beliefs about, 136–137
    core aspects theory of, 255–258
    dimensions of transcendence in, 184–185
    and economics, 482–483
    framework, 182
    future of, 492
    philosophy of, 385, 447
    process of, 25, 182, 420
    quality health care and, 397–401
    quality of care and, 401–402
    recommendations, 477–478
    research study, 474–477
    skills of being-caring, 255
    value, 476
Human Caring Model, 398
Human Connection, 427, 458, 462
human dignity, 122, 196
    protection of, 39
human dimensions of caring, 188–189
human encounter, face-to-face in, 6, 7
human health, caring and, 119
human interaction, 396
humanistic-altruistic value system, 148–149
humanistic caring, 134
    behavior, 482
    with limited economic resources, 483
    nurses struggled to maintain, 468, 492
humanistic nursing, 120
    authentic commitment, 158
    choice and intersubjectivity, 158–160
    foundations of, 155
    framework of, 160–162
    process of, 158–160
    theory of, 120, 160
humanistic value system, 146
humanity, 35, 251–253, 470
    experience of, 456
    honoring, 458
    knowing, 458
    nursing and, 513–518
    preservation of, 39
    shared, 458
human mode of being, caring as, 165–179

human potential, 156
human science of nursing, 229, 473
human situation, in humanistic nursing,
    160–162
human trait of caring, 10, 21–22
humility, essence of, 38
hypotheses about caring, 137

IAHC, *See* International Association for
    Human Caring
ICC, *See* International Caritas Consortium
ICUs, *See* intensive care units
importance of caring, 129
    to nursing profession, 131
independent relationships, 387, 399
individual freedom, 477
ingredients of caring, 5
inquiry, caring, 340–341
instantiation of caring concept, 49, 53–55
instrumental caring activities, 306
instrumental perspective on caring, 46
instrument development design, 335
intellectualization, 448
intensive care nursing, 269
    methodological and ethical considerations,
        323–324
    moral obligations and work responsibilities
        in, 321–331
    participants
        responses, 324
        selection of, 322–323
        study background, 322
        typical features of examples, 324
    themes for, 324–329
    theoretical perspective, 321–322
intensive care units (ICUs), 269
    natural death in, aspects of, 329–330
    nurses and physicians in, 321
intentional caring, 275
intentional response pattern, 365
intention of nurses, 266, 285
interactions
    human, 396
    noncaring, 267, 294, 296
    pattern, 337
Interaction (INT) subscale, 501, 503
intermediate outcomes, 401
International Association for Human Caring
    (IAHC), 1, 333, 336, 338, 372, 521
    caring conferences and investigations, 265
    goal of, 426, 448
    members of, 375, 381
International Caritas Consortium (ICC), 254
interpersonal sensitivity, in caring process,
    107–108
interpersonal theory of nursing, 125

interpretive investigations, 60
intersubjective transaction, 156–157, 159
intimate relationships, in caring, 108
INT subscale, *See* Interaction subscale
intuiting, phenomenology, 212–213
investigators, research designs for, 333, 336
inviting creative emergence, 52–53

knowing patterns, 229
  empirical, 38–39
  esthetic, 39–40
  ethical, 39
  personal, 37–38
"knowing the course of events," 269
knowledge
  caring conditions, 277–278, 299
  of human behavior, 337, 365, 366

labyrinth walk, 411
learning activities, 40–41
legal restrictions, 68
Leininger's Theory of Transcultural Care
      Diversity and Universality, 10
level of inquiry
  capacity for caring, 63
  caring actions, 85–89
  commitments and concerns, 68
  conditions, 75
  consequences of caring, 93
levels of caring knowledge, 61
Levinas, Emmanuael, 6, 7
liberal arts education, 143–144
life-destroying mode, *See* biocidic mode
life-giving mode, *See* biogenic mode
life-neutral mode, *See* biopassive mode
life-restraining mode, *See* biostatic mode
life-sustaining mode, *See* bioactive mode
Likert-like scale, 333, 337
  4-point, 349, 350, 354
  6-point, 354
limiting, issues of caring, 46
listening, caring behavior, 284, 300
literacy, caring, *See* caring literacy
literature on caring, 4, 13
living caring, 124–125, 223–225, 232, 234
love
  caring and, 260–261
  Caritas consciousness, 262

Magnet hospitals, 385
Magnet Recognition Program®, 423
maintaining belief in caring process, 85,
    86, 218
Making Self-care Possible, 427, 457, 460–461
manifesting intentions, 49–50
man–living–health theory, 122

Maslow's theory, 433
Mayeroff, Milton, 5, 6
measurement of caring, 500–501, 501
Medicaid, 459, 465, 467, 474, 482
Medicare, 465, 467, 474, 482
medication, patient knowledge of, 502
mental well-being of nurses, 110
metaparadigm, 426
  of nursing, 423
meta-synthesis
  design, 336
  qualitative analyses of caring, 357–368
  studies, 337
metasynthesis of caring in nursing
  attributes
    expert nursing, 107
    interpersonal sensitivity, 107–108
    intimate relationships, 108
    process, 107
  conceptualization of caring, 110–111
  conducive environment, 109–110
  consequences, 110
  data analysis, 105–106
  four-factor structure, 111
  methodology, 103–104
  moral foundations, 109
  needs and openness, 108–109
  overview, 106–107
  process of caring, 106
  professional maturity, 109
  purposive sampling, 104–105
meta-themes, 427, 457, 458
middle range theory of caring, 14, 61, 85, 117,
    118, 123, 211–212, 391
  caring and miscarriage, 213
  clinical nursing models project, 213–214
  method, 212–213
  in newborn intensive care unit, 213
mind–body–spirit, 252, 424, 432, 433, 434
miscarriage, caring and, 213, 214
model of caring, *See* caring model
mode of being, 33, 34, 123, 157, 165–179, 201,
    202, 204–206
modern medicine, crisis in, 518
monetary costs, 499
moral foundations, caring, 109
"moral ideal of nursing," 34
moral imperative/ideal, caring as, 22
morality of care, 269
more–being, health–illness quality of, 155–156
mortality rates, in hospitals, 498
mutuality of caring, 362, 368

National Caring Conferences, 127–140
natural caring, 26
natural death in ICU, aspects of, 329–330

NCQ, *See* Nurse Caring Questionnaire
Neuman's theory, 431
newborn intensive care unit (NICU), 213–216
New Dimensions of Human Caring Theory, 238
Nightingale, Florence, 134, 135
noncaring
  behaviors, 294–295, 297
  in clinical setting, 293–297
  consequences of, 91–92, 93
  interactions, 267, 294, 296
  patients' perceptions of
    behaviors and attitudes, 294–295
    nurses, 295
nongeneralizable caring, 47
non-nurse administrators, 313
nurse administrators, 313, 408
  caring, effects of, 90
  nurses and, 409, 478
nurse caring behaviors, 10, 78, 267, 348, 374
  for cancer patients, 283–290, 300, 302–305
  defined, 266, 285
  evaluation of, 305–306
  perceptions of, 299–306
Nurse Caring Questionnaire (NCQ), 469, 501,
    502–503
nurse communication, Six Cs of, 417
Nurse Continuous Improvement Indicators
    instrument, 502
nurse educators, 143, 403
nurse hospitalist
  as emerging model, 417–418
  model, 389
nurse investigators, 63, 68, 93, 211, 372
nurse leaders, 407, 410, 411
nurse–patient relationship
  being in relationship, 487–488
  entering into relationship, 484–485
  entering new reality, 486–487
  feeling threatened by new reality, 489
  grounded theory approach, 466, 467,
    483–492
  interpersonal, 10, 23, 483
  interpreting caring, 488
  judging caring and noncaring, 490
  practicing caring, 485–486
  profiting in new reality, 491–492
  recognizing chaos, 491
  viewing, 489–490
nurse-related conditions, affect caring, 71–75
nurses' activities, concept of, 386
nurses' knowledge pattern, 337, 365, 366
nurses' personal attributes, 365
nurse subscale rankings, Larson's CARE-Q, 84
nursing act, 155, 157
nursing administration, 403, 466
  implications for, 493

nursing as caring
  assumptions, 223
  nursing situation, 232–235
  perspective of persons as caring, 223–227
  relationship grounded in, 232
  theory of, 231, 235
nursing care
  definitions of, 135–136
  delivery systems, 469, 498, 504
    cost effectiveness in, 497–498
  quality, 373, 391
nursing, challenges in, 456
nursing conceptual models, 385
Nursing: Human Science and Human Care
    (Watson), 237
*Nursing: Human Science and Human Care:
    A Theory of Nursing* (Watson), 125, 244
nursing leaders, 387, 388, 452, 465, 468, 470, 508
nursing literature, caring in, 3
  perspectives on, 46
nursing metaparadigm, 2
  critique of, 45
  requirements for, 45
nursing model development, 234
Nursing Quality Management and Research
    Council, 373
*Nursing's Agenda for the Future: A Call to the
    Nation*, 404
nursing situation, caring, 120–121, 124,
    232–235
nursing studies of caring, 284–285
nursing theory, 24–25, 385, 423, 424, 447
  foundations from, 451–452
  levels of, 229
Nursing: The Philosophy and Science of Caring
    (1979) (Watson), 125, 126, 243, 244
nursing work, technical and medical aspects
    of, 396–397
nurturant behavior, caring as, 311
Nyberg caring assessment scale, 466, 474

observantia respect, 277
On Caring (Mayeroff), 224
oncology nurses, 453
  vs. cancer patients, 299–306
ongoing reflections, caring, 429
ontical questions, caring, 11–12, 36–37
ontological competencies, caring, 125, 253–254
ontological questions, caring, 11, 33–35, 195
ontology of caring, 165, 225, 428
Orem's Self-Care Deficit Theory of Nursing, 10
organizational culture
  bureaucratic caring for nursing practice in,
    309–318
  differential caring in, 315–316
  strategies for recreating, 410–411

organization-related conditions, affect caring, 75–77
organizations
　as bureaucracies, 310–311
　as cultures, 310
Ottawa Charter
　for health promotion, 438
　principles in, 439

pain management, 387
　caring–healing modalities related to, 389
pain theory, 420
patient care facilitator (PCF), 390–391
Patient Caring Questionnaire (PCQ), 469, 501, 502–503
patient/family–nurse independent relationship, 399–400
patient knowledge of medication, 502
patient-related conditions, affect caring, 69–70
patients' perceptions of noncaring
　behaviors and attitudes, 294–295
　nurses, 295
patient subscale rankings, Larson's CARE-Q, 84
patterns of caring, 363–364
patterns of knowing, *See* knowing patterns
PCF, *See* patient care facilitator
PCQ, *See* Patient Caring Questionnaire
pedagogical questions, caring, 40–41
personal awareness, 364
personhood, 225
persons as caring, perspective of, 223–227
persons live caring, 124
person-to-person
　caring, 11
　relationships, 226
perspectival caring, 46–47
perspective of nursing, 2
phenomenological–hermeneutical theory, 341, 343
phenomenological hermeneutics, 334, 340
　inquiry, 334, 335, 340–341
phenomenologic investigations, 78
　in nursing practice, 62
phenomenology
　basic steps in, 212–213
　of esthetic
　　act, 335, 341, 343–344
　　research, 340–341
phenomenon of caring, 130, 136–137
phenomenon of nursing, 155, 156, 160
philosophical foundations of caring, 5–7
philosophy and science of caring, 243
　balancing with humanism, 144
　nursing, 249–250
　vs. humanities, 144–145

physical action–oriented helping behaviors, 299
physician hospitalist model, 417
positive caring interactions, 502
positive change condition, 278–279
Postmodern Nursing (Watson), 125
Postmodern Nursing and Beyond (1999) (Watson), 246
potential of caring, 131–132
practice, nursing
　bureaucratic caring for, 309–318
　caring behaviors, 306
　implications for, 318, 492–493
　models, 385–392
practicing caring, 93, 467, 485–486
process of caring, 25–26, 106, 366
　conceptual cross-validation of, 219
　subdimensions of, 214, 215
process of nursing, 158–160
profession of nursing, 227–230
professional attachment development, caring, 206
professional caring, 135, 176, 177, 179, 207
professional encounters, caring, 400
professional maturity in caring, 25–26, 109
professional nursing care, defined, 135
professional nursing practice models, 385, 386
professional nursing services, 396
　aspect of, 397
professional vigilance (PV), 468, 498
　subscale, 501, 503
professionally practicing caring, 93
psychiatric nurse, 458, 460
psychologic elements of caring, 501
public health nursing practice, 425, 431, 436, 440
PV, *See* professional vigilance

Q-methodology, 266, 286, 305
Q sorts, 266, 286, 300, 301
qualitative inquiry, caring, 61, 85
qualitative investigations, caring, 62, 65, 90
qualitative reports of caring, 105
qualitative studies
　of caring, 15, 104–105
　caring from patient's perspective, 360–362
　on nurse caring, 333, 337
Quality-Caring Model©, 386, 403
　accuracy of, 402–403
　assumptions of, 401
　components of, 386–387, 397–401
　nursing's work, 396–397
　outcomes, 387, 401
　process, 387, 399
　proposition of, 401
　purpose of, 387
　structure, 386, 398

quality nursing care, 373, 391
quality of care, 306, 401–402, 488, 490
quantifying caring, 27
quantitative inquiry, caring, 61, 78–85
questionnaire
    healthcare economics, 474
    NCQ and PCQ, 469, 501, 502–503

rationale for studying caring, 133–135
rational-legal principles, 310
recidivism, 492
refinement of caring conditions
    awareness, 276
    caring as respect for persons, 276–277
    knowledge, 278
    positive change condition, 278–279
    respect, 277–278
    welfare-of-x-criterion, 279
regard, caring as, 273–274
relationship-centered professional
        encounters, 387
repertory grid techniques, 68
research
    approach, 311
    to caring, 265–270
    designs on caring, 333
    implications for, 305–306
    qualitative, purpose of, 309
respect for persons, caring as, 276–277
responses, nurse and cancer patient, 302–304
responsible, caring as, 273

saints, 208
Science of Unitary Human Beings (SUHB), 43,
        48, 54
    Rogers' framework of, 12
    theoretical niches of, 13
scientific caring behaviors, 306
self-actualization, concept of, 432–433
self as caring person, 226
self-care, 24, 388, 408
    theory, 24
Self-care Deficit Theory of Nursing, 24
self-renewal, value of, 409–410
self sensitivity, 151–153
semantic analysis, caring, 265, 271
semantic expressions of caring
    appreciating pattern, 50–51
    attuning to dynamic flow, 51–52
    infinite experiencing, 52
    inviting creative emergence, 52–53
    manifesting intentions, 50
senses of caring, 271
sensitive caring, 373
sensitivity cultivation to self and others,
        151–153
shared humanity, 458

Six Cs, caring, 121, 166
social conception of nursing, 227–230
socialism, 465, 473–474
social support, definition of, 212, 218
sociocultural environment of patient, 435
speculations, caring, 448–449
standard of care for caring, 371–382
statistics of nursing staff and patients, 350
structural caring categories, 313–314
structure–process–outcomes health model, 395
"struggling to find a balance," 492
students of nursing, 40–41
substantive analysis of caring, 13
substantive theory, 268–269, 312–313, 467, 492
SUHB, *See* Science of Unitary Human Beings
supportive nurse caring, 90
Supportive Nursing Behaviors Checklist
        (SNBC), 78, 81

task-orientated nursing care, 324
teaching in caring, 12, 40–41, 365
themes for caring, 324–325
    "believing in a good death," 325–326, 329
    "expressing moral awareness," 328–329, 330
    "feelings of distress," 326–327, 330
    "knowing the course of events," 326
    "reasoning about physicians' doings,"
        327–328
theoretically adequate description of caring,
        271–279
theoretical niches, identifying, 48–49
theory
    bureaucratic caring, 309, 409, 473, 478
    caring, *See* caring theory
    development in caring, 118
    human care, 24–25, 121, 237–240, 397,
        424, 425
    nursing, *See* nursing theory
    nursing as caring, 390
    transcultural care diversity and
        universality, 25
Theory of Human Caring, 117, 122, 125, 126,
        182, 367–368, 385, 424, 448
theory-generating model, 139
therapeutic intervention, caring as, 23–24
therapeutic model, 337
    developing, 366–367
think-tank theory, 128
transcultural nursing care theories, conceptual
        model for, 137–140
transcultural nursing theory, 119
transformative leadership, 469, 470
    fourfold path toward, 507–511
        Via Creativa, 470, 509
        Via Negativa, 469, 507–508
        Via Positiva, 470, 508–509
        Via Transformativa, 470, 509–510

transpersonal caring, 11, 35
   healing, 185–187
   relationship, 433, 434
transpersonal caring theory, 347–348, 354
   energy dimensions of, 184
   extended science-upward causation
      perspective, 187–188
   holographic-extended science metaphor,
      185–187
   transcendence in human caring, 184–185
transpersonal teaching-learning, carative
     factor, 425, 435, 438, 439

ubiquitous caring, 46, 47
uncaring dimension, 202
uncaring nurse, 204
uniform state, caring as, 26–27
unitary pattern appreciation, 50
universe, caring, 165–166
upward causation model of science, 187
uses of caring, 271–272, 273

Watson Caring Science Institute (WCSI), 117,
     391, 521
Watson's caring theory, 239–240, 374–375

Watson's *Caritas* literacy dimensions,
     254–255
Watson's conceptualization of health, 432,
     437, 438
Watson's theory, 424
   of human caring, 10, 386, 388, 432–436,
      439, 521
      for community health nursing,
        436–440
Watson's Transpersonal Caring Theory,
     336, 470
WCSI, *See* Watson Caring Science Institute
welfare-of-x-criterion, caring condition, 279
well-being
   elaboration of caring for, 461–462
   health–illness quality of, 155–156
WHO, *See* World Health Organization
Wingspread Caring Conference,
     13, 60
World Health Organization (WHO),
     437, 438
worldview approach, to study care and
     caring, 132

Yalom's curative factor, 149